Essentials of Uroradiology

Essentials of Uroradiology

E. Stephen Amis, Jr., M.D.

*Associate Professor of Radiology,
Columbia University College of Physicians and
Surgeons; Chief, Section of Uroradiology,
Columbia-Presbyterian Medical Center,
New York City*

Jeffrey H. Newhouse, M.D.

*Professor of Radiology,
Columbia University College of Physicians and
Surgeons; Director, Abdominal Imaging Division,
Columbia-Presbyterian Medical Center,
New York City*

Little, Brown and Company
Boston/Toronto/London

First Edition

Library of Congress Catalog Card No.
90-61841

ISBN 0-316-03735-4

Printed in the United States of America

HAL

For Richard C. Pfister, M.D., who taught us

Contents

Preface

Both of us teach uroradiology at the viewbox and in the fluoroscopic suite on an almost daily basis. Our residents at Columbia-Presbyterian Medical Center are constantly seeking recommendations for reading in the subspecialty of uroradiology. We found ourselves recommending sections in the general textbooks of diagnostic radiology and occasionally referring them to the several multivolume treatises on uroradiology for reading on specific topics. But we noted that an up-to-date, concise textbook of uroradiology did not exist. Further, in our interactions with the urology residents we found that they, too, were seeking a concise source of imaging information in their specialty. Therefore, we accepted the challenge of writing such a textbook. Having worked together for several years, we elected to write the text ourselves to ensure consistency of style and to prevent overlap.

Although we originally planned a shorter book highlighting only those areas seen in the daily practice of uroradiology, we found that anything less than coverage of the large majority of disease processes encountered in the genitourinary system would result in a book with very little real value. Based on our cumulative experience of about 40 years in the field of uroradiology, we have included the salient clinical and imaging facets of these disease processes as we teach them at the viewbox and in our lecture series.

Just as the text cannot be exhaustive in a book of this size, neither can the illustrations. Even the large multivolume texts, with their thousands of illustrations, cannot depict all the possible variables that can be encountered in clinical practice. Unfortunately, we could not illustrate all of the disease processes mentioned. However, the more common lesions are illustrated with what we think are classic examples of these entities, in the hope that the reader will be guided to the correct diagnosis for a clinical case based on these typical findings. In some instances, we have elected to use drawings to elucidate pathologic or physiologic processes and even to represent radiographic findings.

Every effort was made to keep our bibliographies as concise and current as possible, though where appropriate, classic articles are referenced. It is our intention that the references at the end of each chapter also be used as a guide for further reading.

Uroradiology is defined as the subspecialty area that covers the imaging spectrum encountered by urologists in their practice. Therefore, we have covered the imaging of the urinary system in both males and females and the genital system in the male. Generally the book is organized according to the organs found in the urinary system and the male genital system. Certain disease processes, because of their clinical significance and complexity, are dealt with in separate chapters. We have concentrated on the diagnostic aspects of uroradiology. Interventional therapeutic techniques are mentioned where appropriate, but no attempt has been made to describe these in detail.

As we completed this book, we found it to be less than a comprehensive survey of the field but certainly far more than a cursory look for the neophyte. It is designed to be easily read and reread during rotations on uroradiology. We hope it will also prove to be a useful vehicle for review for the board examinations in both diagnostic radiology and urology.

E.S.A.
J.H.N.

Acknowledgments

The time and efforts of many individuals helped make this book possible. Susan Pioli, our editor at Little, Brown and Company, provided encouragement, guidance, and a great deal of leeway regarding style and content. Many members of our department were constantly willing over many months to search their teaching files and current cases to provide illustrative material for the book. Deserving of special mention in this regard are Linda Sanders, M.D., Chris Ng, M.D., Walter Berdon, M.D., Ronda Bixon, M.D., Karen Laffey, M.D., Joel Rosen, M.D., David Seldin, M.D., David Grant, M.D., and Jacqueline Brunetti, M.D. Several members of our specialty organization, the Society of Uroradiology, also provided case material: John J. Cronan, M.D., Alan J. Davidson, M.D., Isabel Yoder, M.D., and Matthew Rifkin, M.D.

Our secretaries, Ruth Harvey, Anna Calderin, and Madeline Cannella, deserve special thanks for their transcription of our original dictations followed by multiple revisions. Of special note, Ruth Harvey is responsible for completion of approximately 75 percent of the manuscript.

Our medical illustrator, Kevin Somerville, was most responsive to our requests for revisions of his original drawings, and we think he has produced a set of clear and easily understood illustrations.

Our wives, Anne and Nancy, deserve special mention for their forbearance during the evenings and weekends we spent working to meet our deadline.

Richard C. Pfister, M.D., to whom this book is dedicated, was our mentor during the time we spent at Massachusetts General Hospital. Probably no other individual has influenced our careers more than he, and for this reason he deserves our deepest appreciation.

Finally, we wish to thank the residents at Columbia-Presbyterian Medical Center, whose questioning minds brought us to our decision to write this text. We hope they will find it useful.

Essentials of Uroradiology

Notice

History of Uroradiology

The announcement of the discovery of x-rays on December 28, 1895, resulted in hundreds of investigations within a period of months. As early as 1898, case reports of plain-film findings of renal and ureteral calculi could be found in various American journals. In 1901, two American physicians reported the use of a radiopaque wire that could be cystoscopically inserted into the ureter; this served not only to outline the ureter but also partially to separate ureteral stones from other incidental calcifications within the abdomen [2]. For the next few years, oxygen and other gases were injected into the urinary tract in retrograde fashion as a means of visualizing the collecting systems, ureters, and bladder. However, this technique never gained wide acceptance as there was considerable confusion with preexisting abdominal gas shadows.

The true beginning of uroradiology occurred in 1905, when German urologists discovered the technique of retrograde injection of a silver colloid suspension, collargol, into the ureters and renal pelves, resulting in the first real retrograde pyelogram [2]. At the Mayo Clinic, Dr. William Braasch, over the next several years, gained significant clinical experience, and in 1915 he wrote a book describing virtually all of the urinary structural lesions recognized today [1].

In the early 1920s the concept of intravenous or oral administration of a sodium iodide solution for opacification of the urinary tract was studied. Unfortunately, the upper urinary tract was only faintly visualized or not at all, though the bladder was almost always adequately opacified. While unsuccessful, these attempts led the way to the development of our current iodinated contrast agents

About 1928, Drs. Binz and Rath, biochemists at the Chemical Institute in Berlin, developed a compound called Selectan-Neutral for the treatment of coccus infections. At about the same time, Dr. Emanuel Leibman of the Mount Sinai Hospital in New York awarded a fellowship for foreign study to one of his medical interns, Dr. Moses Swick. After arriving in Germany, Dr. Swick heard of these new drugs, and it occurred to him that since they contained 54 percent iodine they might be of use in visualizing the urinary tract. Swick then conducted various studies on Selectan-Neutral and found that in rabbits and humans the kidney parenchyma and bladder could be visualized after intravenous administration of the drug. For the most part however, the renal pelvis and ureter were poorly seen. Furthermore, patients receiving this compound complained of diplopia, nausea, vomiting, and headache. Swick's investigations were then transferred to the St. Hedwigskrankenhaus in Berlin, a 200-bed urologic hospital under the direction of Professor Alexander von Lichtenberg. There, Swick was able to work closely with Dr. Binz and made suggestions for diminishing the toxicity, increasing the solubility, and increasing the iodine content of Selectan-Neutral. These efforts resulted in a new preparation, Uroselectan, the earliest precursor of our modern contrast agents [5]. After several successful intravenous pyelograms were performed on patients at the hospital, Swick informed von Lichtenberg, who was lecturing at urologic meetings in the United States at the time, of the momentous news. von Lichtenberg apparently spoke with enthusiasm of this development during the remainder of his travels in the United States. Upon his return, a presentation was planned at the 1929 meeting of the German Urologic Society in Munich. Since the final work had been done in his institution, von Lichtenberg evidently felt he should be the principal author. Unfortunately, Swick was to be relegated to a minor role in the presentation. However, because of the intervention of Professor Lichtwitz, at whose clinic Swick's early work was begun, the first presentation at that historical meeting was done by Swick alone. Swick's presentation concerned the developmental work done on animals and human beings. A second presentation was on clinical applications and was given by both von Lichtenberg and Swick. There is apparently no historical argument that Binz and Rath actually prepared the compounds. How important Swick's suggestions were in creating Uroselectan is unprovable, but his role in redirecting the biochemist's goals and in conducting animal and human experimentation on the end product was undoubtedly important. von Lichtenberg's role in providing Swick with facilities to conduct his clinical studies was also important, though secondary [3].

On his return to the United States, Swick, in 1933, was successful in attaching useful quantities of iodine to a natural metabolite, hippuric acid, resulting in the compound Hippuran. The descendants of Hippuran are our current ionic contrast agents. Until the past decade, opacification of the hollow viscera of the genitourinary system by these agents was the mainstay of urologic diagnosis. However, in recent years newer imaging modalities have had a profound impact on uroradiology. As a result, most radiology departments in the United States have experienced a significant reduction in the volume of urography performed [4]. Coincident with this decrease in the number of urograms has been an increase in the use of sonography and computerized tomography (CT).

Also coincident with the development of the newer imaging and interventional techniques has been a change in the way urology is practiced. As recently as two decades ago, all renal masses discovered by intravenous urography or retrograde studies were subjected to surgical exploration. With the advent and subsequent wide acceptance of percutaneous cyst aspiration, simple cysts could be diagnosed without surgical intervention. Then came renal sonography, which for a time was used to guide the cyst punctures. As ultrasound became more sophisticated, however, it became obvious that it alone was needed to establish the diagnosis of a simple cyst; this remains a standard of practice to this date.

As another example, about 15 years ago percutaneous techniques for chemical dissolution of certain renal stones (struvite, uric acid, cystine) began replacing the need for their surgical removal. This technique was rapidly supplanted by percutaneous fragmentation and extraction of most stones found in the collecting system. To a large degree even this technique is being supplanted by the relatively recent development and current wide use of extracorporeal shock wave lithotripsy for noninvasive fragmentation of renal stones into particles small enough for spontaneous passage down the ureter.

While the list of changes resulting from the evolution of the newer imaging and percutaneous interventional techniques is long, it is clear that the subspecialty area of uroradiology is rapidly changing and continually modifying and facilitating the practice of urology.

REFERENCES

1. Braasch, W.F. *Pyelography.* Philadelphia: Saunders, 1915.
2. Cunningham, J.J., and Friedland, G.W. Early American uroradiology 1896-1933. *Urol. Surv.* 32:226, 1972.
3. Marshall, V.F. The Controversial History of Excretory Urography. In D.M. Witten, G.H. Myers, Jr., and D.C. Utz (eds.), *Emmet's Clinical Urography* (4th ed.). Philadelphia: Saunders, 1977. Pp. 2–5.
4. Pollack, H.M., and Banner, M.P. Current status of excretory urography: A premature epitaph? *Urol. Clin. North Am.* 12:585, 1985.
5. Swick, M. The discovery of intravenous urography: Historical and developmental aspects of the urographic media and their role in other diagnostic and therapeutic areas. *Bull. N.Y. Acad. Med.* 42:128, 1966.

2

Embryology, Anatomy, and Physiology

This chapter will address the embryology, anatomy, and physiology of the urinary system in both males and females, and the genital system in the male. The adrenal gland, though not a part of these systems, will also be described since it is usually considered within the purview of uroradiology. Discussions will be brief and will emphasize points necessary for better understanding of uroradiology. The reader is encouraged to pursue further information in any of the many excellent textbooks that cover these subjects.

EMBRYOLOGY

The adrenal gland is composed of two separate functional units, the cortex deriving from mesodermal tissue and the medulla from ectoderm. Though these originate separately, during their development they fuse into a single organ and become encased in a common capsule.

The kidney originates from the nephrogenic mesoderm, which is part of the intermediate mesoderm extending caudally from the level of the seventh somite. Glomeruli and tubules form in the nephrogenic mesoderm beginning cephalad and progressing caudally. The pronephros, or most superior and earliest "kidney," appears in the fourth week of embryonic life and only rarely has been shown to contain glomeruli in humans. The pronephros is succeeded by the mesonephros, which is fully developed by the second month and totally resorbed by the fourth month. At 13 weeks, the ureter appears as a dorsal bud (metanephric duct) arising from the wolffian (mesonephric) duct, which is an extension of the duct from the pronephros. This bud grows and meets undifferentiated mesenchyme, the metanephric blastema, lying caudal to the mesonephros (Fig. 2-1A). By 21 weeks the ureteric bud branches to form several secondary buds, which eventually become the renal pelvis and calices. The collecting ducts are eventually formed from the sixth through eleventh generations of branchings of the original ureteral bud. The metanephric vesicle, or primitive renal tubule, originates in the metanephric blastema and eventually differentiates into the nephron, which connects with the collecting ducts arising from the ureteral bud.

Once the embryonic human kidney has been formed at the second or third sacral vertebral level, ascent begins. The kidney reaches the level of the second or third lumbar vertebra by the end of the third month and by term comes into contact with the adrenal gland at the level of the first lumbar vertebra. During this ascent, the renal pelves originally face anteriorly and then rotate 90 degrees to terminate in their medial location. The fetal kidney usually contains about 10 to 14 lobes, or renunculi, which are functional parenchymal units of the kidney developing in concert with the minor calices. This lobation is usually lost with maturation, and the characteristic adult shape of the kidney results.

At about the fifth week, cloacal division begins. This division into the urogenital sinus anteriorly and rectum posteriorly is complete by the seventh week. The perineal body appears at this point, and subsequent anterior and posterior perforations result in the urogenital and anal orifices, respectively. As development proceeds, the urogenital sinus differentiates superiorly into the vesicourethral canal, from which the bladder and upper urethra are formed, and inferiorly into the definitive urogenital sinus, the progenitor of the main part of the urethra (Fig. 2-1B). By the fourth month, the vesicourethral canal has enlarged and assumed the shape of the urinary bladder. The allantois eventually becomes the urachus, which loses its lumen in the late stages of gestation because of the proliferation of fibrous tissue.

In the male, the posterior urethra proximal to the verumontanum develops from the distal part of the vesicourethral canal, as does the entire

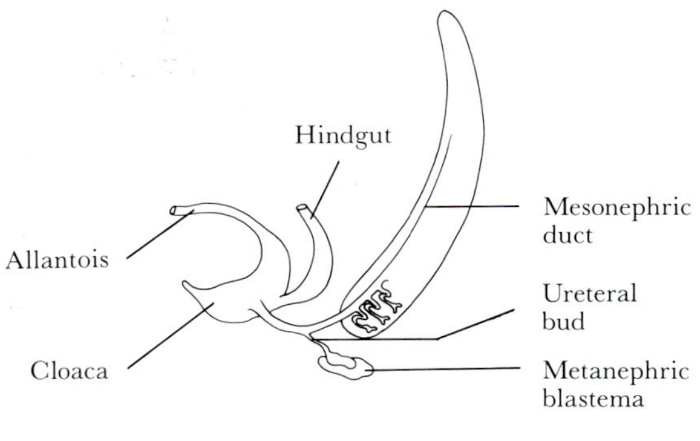

A

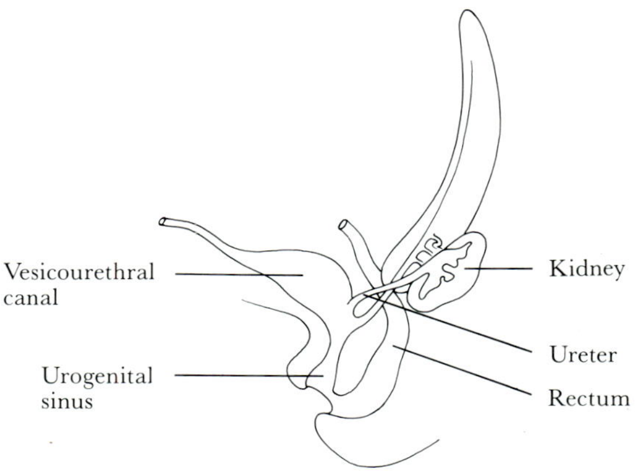

B

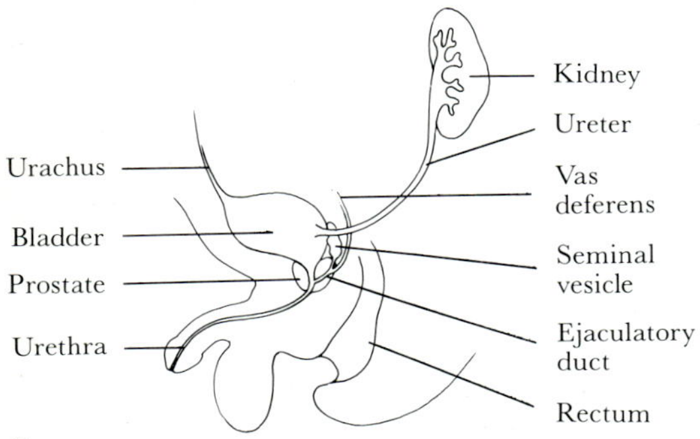

C

Figure 2-1. Embryologic development of the urinary tract. A. Cloacal stage. B. Differentiation into vesicourethral canal and definitive urogenital sinus. C. Embryologically complete.

female urethra. The remainder of the male urethra arises from specific parts of the definitive urogenital sinus; the distal prostatic and membranous urethra form from the pars pelviana and the penile urethra from the pars phallica. The prostate then arises by budding from the posterior urethra.

The wolffian duct joins the cloaca laterally before giving rise to the ureteral bud. As the wolffian duct migrates caudally, the ureteral bud is absorbed into the growing bladder, giving rise to the ureteral orifice. The wolffian duct then continues its caudal migration to the level of the posterior urethra, where it differentiates into the ejaculatory duct, the vas deferens, and the epididymis (Fig. 2-1C); the last joins the testis in the retroperitoneum. The seminal vesical arises from a diverticulum of the convoluted portion of the vas deferens.

The müllerian ducts, arising shortly after the appearance of the wolffian ducts and lying lateral to them, atrophy in the male. However, traces of the müllerian ducts can persist, the superior end forming the appendix testis and the caudal ends fusing to form the utricle. In the female, the müllerian ducts form the uterus, vagina, and fallopian tubes.

The testes and ovaries undergo similar development in both sexes, arising from the genital ridge, which is a thickened epithelial layer high in the retroperitoneum. After formation of the testis, the gubernaculum testis, a cord of tissue extending from the skin in the inguinal region that will become the scrotum, attaches at its superior end to the lower body and epididymis of the testis. The gubernaculum does not lengthen as the body grows and in fact may shorten, resulting in a steady downward migration of the testis into the scrotum. In the female, a gubernaculum is also responsible for descent of the ovary, but only to the level of the uterine fundus.

Table 2-1 lists the embryonic derivations of the genitourinary organs.

ANATOMY

RETROPERITONEUM

The adrenals, kidneys, and ureters lie in the retroperitoneum. The bladder is found in the pelvis, below the inferior peritoneal reflection. The retroperitoneal space is defined anteriorly by the posterior parietal peritoneum and posteriorly by the transversalis fascia. It is bounded superiorly by the diaphragm and extends inferiorly to the pelvis. Three compartments of the retroperitoneum are recognized: the anterior pararenal space, the perirenal space, and the posterior pararenal space [8] (Fig. 2-2). These spaces are created by two coronally oriented, dense connective-tissue sheets within the retroperitoneal space, one anterior and one posterior to the kidney, which are fused superiorly, join laterally to form the lateroconal fascia, communicate medially with corresponding sheets on the contralateral side, and remain widely separated inferiorly as they disappear into the pelvic fat. The net result is the formation of an inverted cone, Gerota's fascia, which contains the adrenal, kidney, and proximal ureter. The space inside the cone surrounding the kidney and otherwise filled with fat comprises the perirenal space. This fat is more abundant posteriorly and inferiorly, and provides an excellent radiolucent frame for visualization of the kidney during urography. The adrenal, in the most cephalad portion of the cone, may or may not be separated from the kidney by a thin connective-tissue septum. Other thin septae randomly traverse the perirenal fat. Gerota's fascia is normally about 1 mm in thickness. Greater thickness may indicate renal or other abdominal conditions such as infection or neoplasm, though on occasion the finding is nonspecific [1]. The communication of Gerota's fascia across the midline, at least in some patients, results in a potential space around the great vessels through which fluid or infection can spread [7].

The anterior pararenal space, bounded anteriorly by the posterior parietal peritoneum and posteriorly by the anterior leaf of Gerota's fascia, extends across the midline, and contains the pancreas, most of the duodenum, and the ascending and descending colon. The duodenal sweep lies in close relation to the right renal hilus. The posterior pararenal space has as its anterior boundary the posterior leaf of Gerota's fascia and is bounded posteriorly by the transversalis fascia. It contains fat but no viscera.

ADRENAL GLANDS

The adrenal glands are located close to the anteromedial surface of the upper poles of the kidneys within the most superior region of Gerota's capsule. Their shape is highly variable, though the maximum thickness of any portion of the gland should not exceed 1 cm. The arterial supply of the adrenals, while also variable, is

Figure 2-2. Retroperitoneal anatomy. Note the potential for communication between the right and left perirenal spaces across the midline. (IVC = inferior vena cava.)

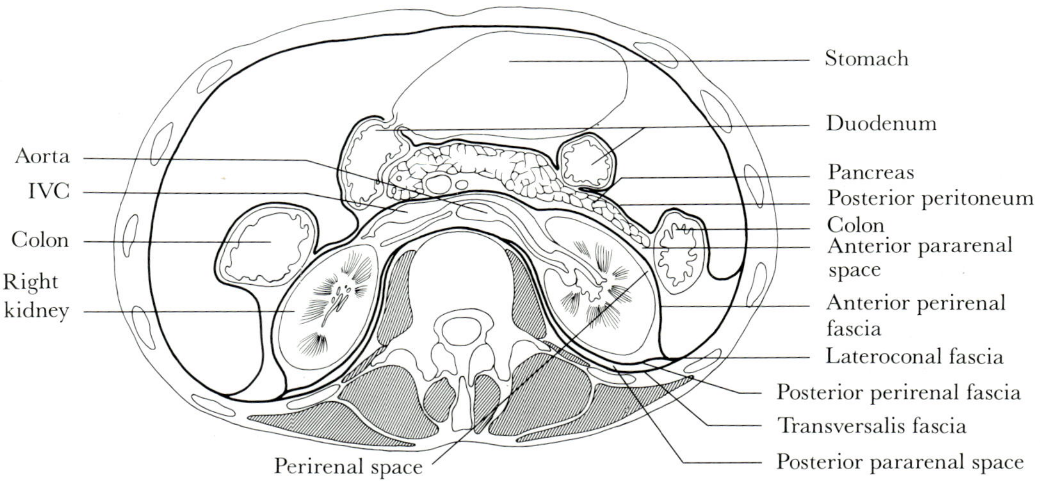

Table 2-1. Embryonic sources of genitourinary organs

Organ	*Embryonic source*
Adrenal	Mesoderm and ectoderm
Kidney	Metanephric blastema
Collecting ducts Calices Infundibula Renal pelvis/ureter	Ureteral bud from Mesonephric duct
Bladder	Vesicourethral canal
Proximal posterior urethra	Vesicourethral canal
Distal posterior urethra	Urogenital sinus
Membranous urethra	Urogenital sinus
Anterior urethra	Urogenital sinus
Prostate	Buds from urethra
Seminal vesicle	Bud from mesonephric duct
Ejaculatory duct	Mesonephric duct
Vas deferens	Mesonephric duct
Epididymis	Mesonephric duct
Testis	Genital ridge
Ovary	Genital ridge
Fallopian tubes	Müllerian duct
Uterus	Müllerian duct
Vagina	Müllerian duct

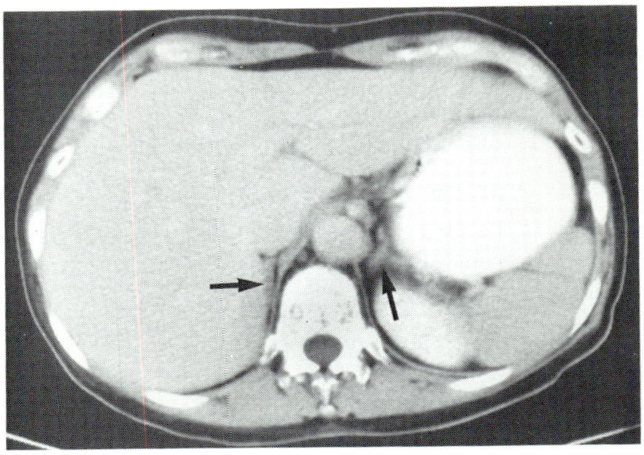

Figure 2-3. Normal CT of the adrenals. The right adrenal is seen as a vertical soft-tissue streak (arrow) behind the inferior vena cava and sandwiched between the medial surface of the liver and the diaphragmatic crus. The left adrenal is shown as a Y-shaped soft-tissue structure (arrow) anteromedial to the upper pole of the kidney.

usually via three paths: the superior adrenal artery arising from the inferior phrenic artery, the middle from the aorta, and the inferior from the renal artery. Venous drainage, also variable, is usually a single trunk emptying into the inferior vena cava on the right and into the renal vein on the left after joining the inferior phrenic vein. Of clinical note, the adrenals in the fetus and neonate are relatively large in relation to the kidneys and have a more rounded shape. Significant shrinkage is noted within a few weeks after birth.

On nephrotomography the right adrenal can occasionally be seen as a single streak or a V- or Y-shaped structure above the right kidney. On the left, the adrenal is less frequently seen. Coronal ultrasonographic views may demonstrate the adrenals as hypoechoic structures surrounded by echogenic fat. CT identifies the adrenals in almost every study (Fig. 2-3), especially if thin sections are obtained. The right adrenal is found behind the inferior vena cava in sections below its intrahepatic segment. It may be seen as a thin vertical soft-tissue streak sandwiched between the medial surface of the liver and the diaphragmatic crus; occasionally two parallel limbs are seen, or a transverse limb can be seen on other sections. The left adrenal is typically found anteromedial to the upper pole of the kidney and has a V- or Y-shaped appearance. MR imaging of the adrenal is similar to that described for CT. On T1 weighted images, the adrenals exhibit medium signal intensity surrounded by bright fat.

KIDNEYS

After their ascent from the pelvis, the kidneys finally come to rest at the level of the upper lumbar vertebrae, their hila usually being found at the level of L-1–L-2. The renal artery, which divides into anterior and posterior branches, passes through the renal hilum, as do the renal vein, nerves, and lymphatics. It is not uncommon to find multiple renal arteries originating from the aorta at various levels. The renal lymphatics function as an alternate route for drainage of the kidney during obstruction of the ureter [5]. The renal sinus, a potential space surrounding and containing the collecting system within the kidney, is otherwise occupied by fatty tissue, vessels, lymphatics, and nerves, and communicates with the perinephric space via a medial notch—the renal hilum. Sinus fat can also extend to the midlateral margin of the kidney between incompletely fused lobes as a normal variant; this is called the junctional parenchymal defect and is occasionally recognized on sonography as an echodense focus on the lateral margin of the kidney [4].

The functional unit of the kidney is the nephron, with each kidney containing approximately 1 million of them. This U-shaped structure begins at the glomerulus, then becomes the proximal tubule, the loop of Henle, and finally the distal tubule, which joins one of many collecting ducts emptying into the calices via openings on the renal papilla. The renal cortex, peripherally located and also extending in columns between the medullary pyramids, contains the glomeruli and proximal and distal tubules. The medulla is composed of pyramidal structures that contain the loops of Henle and whose medially pointed apices become the renal papillae, which communicate with the calices of the collecting system. Each pyramid with its adjacent cortex constitutes a lobe of the kidney.

The long axis of the kidney normally parallels the psoas margin, though in individuals with large amounts of retroperitoneal fat, the kidneys have a tendency to "float," resulting in displacement away from the psoas and changes in their axes. About 90 percent of the time, the left kidney is located 1 to 2 cm higher than the right. Both upper poles lie more posteriorly than the lower poles, a fact that influences nephrotomographic imaging. This will be discussed in more detail in the chapter on imaging techniques. The kidneys move freely with respiration, the maximal excursion often reaching 3 or 4 cm.

Renal size is of importance in evaluating patients with medical renal disease and suspected renovascular hypertension. During urography the average length of the right kidney is 12.7 cm in males and 12.4 cm in females, while the left kidney averages 13.2 cm and 12.8 cm, respectively [11]. Though the left kidney is usually about 5 mm longer than the right, this size differential is reversed in approximately 5 percent of cases. In fact, the left kidney can be up to 2.0 cm longer than the right and the right up to 1.5 cm longer than the left and still be considered within the range of normal. One caveat refers to the kidney with partial or complete duplication of its collecting system, whose length may be significantly greater than its nonduplicated mate and still be considered normal. Renal lengths on urography are larger than in true life because of a magnification factor and swelling secondary to the osmotic diuresis induced by contrast medium. Conversely, sonographic renal lengths are usually slightly less than the true lengths, even presuming the kidney is measured in its longest imaged dimension, a factor dependent on the operator [2]. Table 2-2 compares urographic and sonographic renal lengths with actual lengths determined at autopsy. More significantly, it must be realized that true normal renal size, regardless of imaging technique, is dependent on several factors, including body habitus, fluid balance, sex, and age. For example, the length of the kidney can decrease with aging by 10 percent or more from its maximum length. A more useful frame of reference for determining the normalcy of renal size is comparison of the renal length urographically with the upper four lumbar vertebral bodies. Approximately 95 percent of normal kidneys will be between three and four vertebral bodies in length.

The majority of normal kidneys have 10 to 14 minor calices. The term calix means cup. The papilla of the medullary pyramid protrudes into the larger, open portion of the cup, and the rim of the cup is known as the fornix of the calix. The fornix normally forms an acute angle; blunting of this angle is one of the earliest signs of mild obstruction, and it is at the fornix that extravasation occurs with more severe obstruction (see Fig. 15-11). In roughly three-fourths of the population, calices in one or both poles are compound in nature, with several papillae protruding into a minor calix without benefit of individual infundibula. Minor calices drain via minor infundibula into a major infundibulum.

The renal pelvis may be located primarily within the renal sinus (intrarenal pelvis) or have

Table 2-2. Comparison of average renal sizes as determined by urography, sonography, and autopsy studies

	Right (cm)	*Left (cm)*
Sonography	10.7	11.1
Autopsy	11.2	11.8
Urography	12.6	13.8

a large extrarenal component. The radiographic appearance of the pelvis is thus highly variable, and a capacious extrarenal pelvis associated with normally cupped calices and good drainage should not be mistaken for obstruction.

Vascular structures can indent the major infundibula (usually in the upper pole) or renal pelvis, occasionally mimicking filling defects. Distention of the collecting system by compressing the ureters during urography can prove the extrinsic nature of such defects. The collecting system from the calices to the proximal urethra is lined with transitional epithelium.

During urography, the calices are seen to be delicately cupped and located equidistant from the renal margins (Fig. 2-4). The interpapillary line, connecting the tips of the papillae, is about 1.5 to 2.0 cm from the renal margin at the midpoint of the kidney, and up to 3 cm from the margin at the poles (Fig. 2-5). A focal decrease in this distance usually indicates parenchymal scarring. Fetal lobation, or smooth indentations of the renal margin between calices, is not pathologic and should be recognized and reported as a normal variant (Fig. 2-6).

Other normal variants may mimic renal masses on occasion. These include the dromedary hump, prominent column of Bertin, and suprahilar or infrahilar "bumps" [13] (see Fig. 2-6). The dromedary hump is a masslike prominence of the midlateral portion of the left kidney that is formed because of molding of the

Figure 2-4. Normal urographic anatomy of the kidney. A. Nephrogram 30 seconds after bolus injection of contrast shows cortical opacification. Cortical columns can be seen extending between the lucent pyramids. B. Film after 5 minutes shows contrast-filled collecting system. The nephrogram is now homogeneous. (From J.H. Newhouse and R.C. Pfister. The nephrogram. *Radiol. Clin. North Am.* 17:213, 1979.)

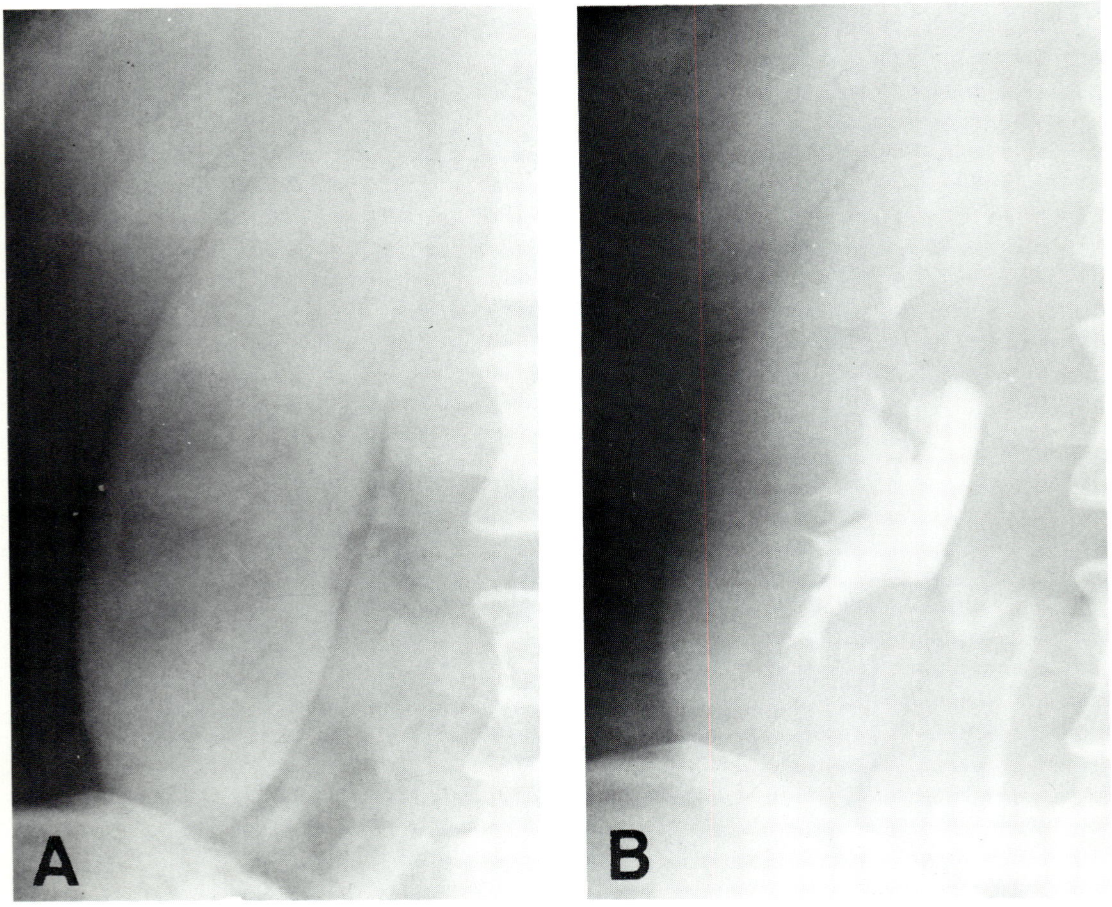

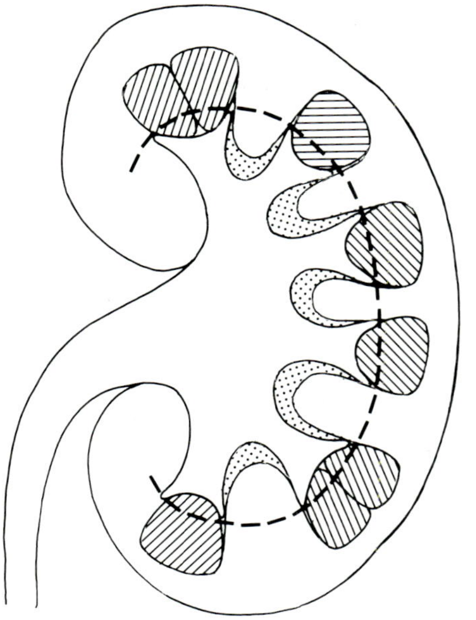

Figure 2-5. Interpapillary line. A line connecting the calices is usually equidistant from the lateral renal margin, though this distance is slightly greater at the poles. Striped areas represent medullary pyramids.

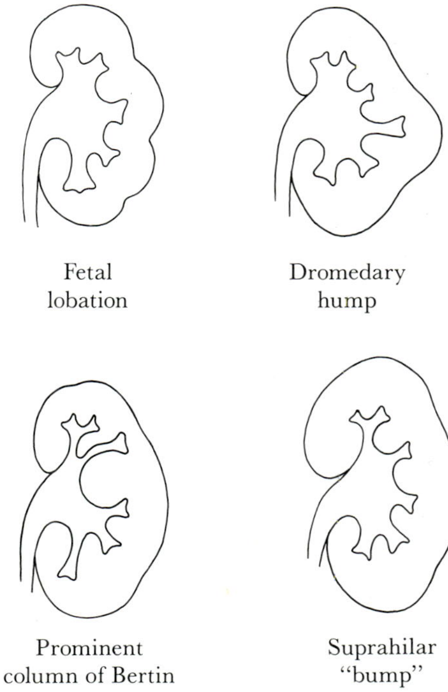

Figure 2-6. Renal pseudotumors. Prominence of either lip of the kidney can occur, resulting in suprahilar or infrahilar "bumps."

kidney by the superiorly and laterally located spleen. The calix serving this area usually extends outward, maintaining the normal parenchymal thickness beyond the interpapillary line, unlike the medial caliceal displacement which would be found with a true renal mass in this area. Cortical columns of Bertin extending into the medulla may be prominent and simulate a mass. These are usually found at the junction of the upper third with the lower two-thirds of either kidney. Prominent renal parenchyma above or below the renal hilum may also resemble masses but are often symmetrical bilaterally and do not displace calices. All pseudotumors opacify similar to adjacent parenchyma during the nephrographic phase of urography. Renal scintigraphy using a radiopharmaceutical that labels the kidney parenchyma is a helpful examination in determining the true nature of a pseudotumor; a pseudotumor will show radioactivity like the adjacent parenchyma while a true renal mass (cyst or tumor) will demonstrate a "cold" area.

When imaged by sonography, the normal renal cortex is homogeneously echogenic, the echoes being slightly less dense than those of liver parenchyma (Fig. 2-7). Cortical columns of Bertin can be seen extending into the medulla between the hypoechoic pyramids. The corticomedullary junction can be recognized in some patients by the discrete, high-level echoes of the arcuate arteries. The renal sinus, which contains

Figure 2-7. Normal sonographic anatomy of the right kidney. The renal parenchyma is less echogenic than the adjacent liver while the pyramids (arrows) are almost sonolucent. Echogenic foci adjacent to the lateral margins of the pyramids represent the arcuate arteries.

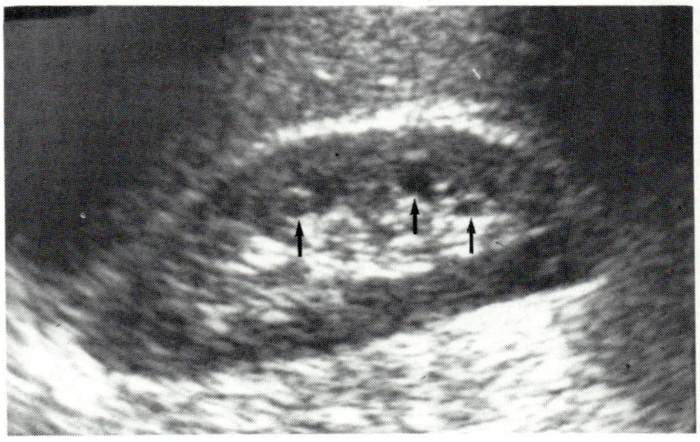

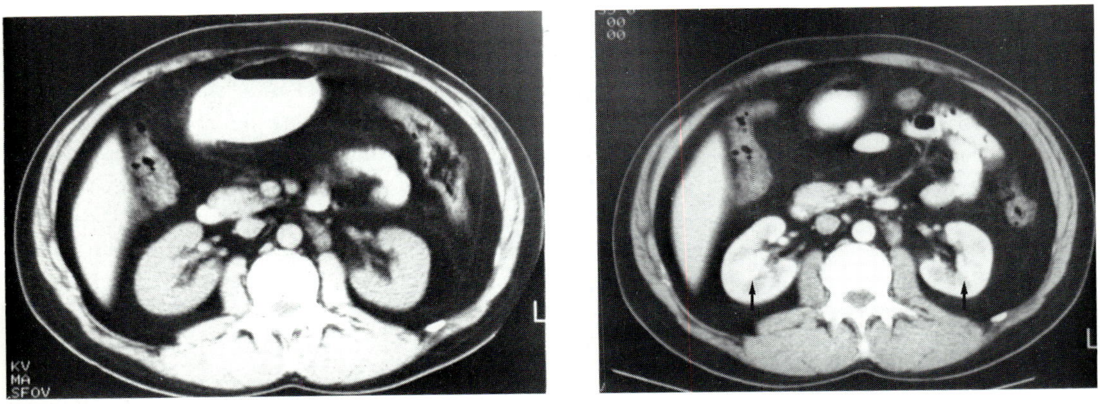

A B

Figure 2-8. Normal CT anatomy of the kidneys (transverse plane). A. Precontrast scan shows the kidneys to be of homogeneous soft-tissue density. B. Dynamic scanning after bolus of intravenous contrast shows corticomedullary differentiation. Note the cortical columns of Bertin extending between the medullary pyramids (arrows).

fat, is seen in longitudinal images as an oval, hyperechoic area centrally located in the kidney; on transverse views, this central echo complex has a round configuration.

Transverse CT sections through the kidney demonstrate its anterior and posterior margins well because of the inherent contrast provided by perinephric fat (Fig. 2-3). Fat surrounding the collecting system in the renal sinus has a negative attenuation value similar to that of perinephric fat. The renal parenchyma is of uniform density and usually measures 30 to 50 Hounsfield units. The collecting system, with the exception of any extrarenal portions of the renal pelvis, is not well defined until it is opacified by intravenous contrast. After a rapid bolus injection of contrast material, parenchymal attenuation can reach 80 to 120 Hounsfield units; corticomedullary differentiation can be seen during the first minute or so after the injection. The renal artery and vein can almost always be seen if contiguous sections are obtained.

The appearance of the normal kidney on MRI is dependent on technique and the hydration status of the patient. Generally speaking, on T-1 weighted images the cortex has a moderately high signal intensity while the medulla is of moderately low intensity; the cortical columns extending into the medulla can be easily seen (Fig. 2-9). Corticomedullary definition is di-

Figure 2-9. Normal MRI anatomy of the kidneys. A. T-1 weighted image shows good corticomedullary differentiation. B. T-2 weighted image show kidneys to have homogeneous moderately high intensity.

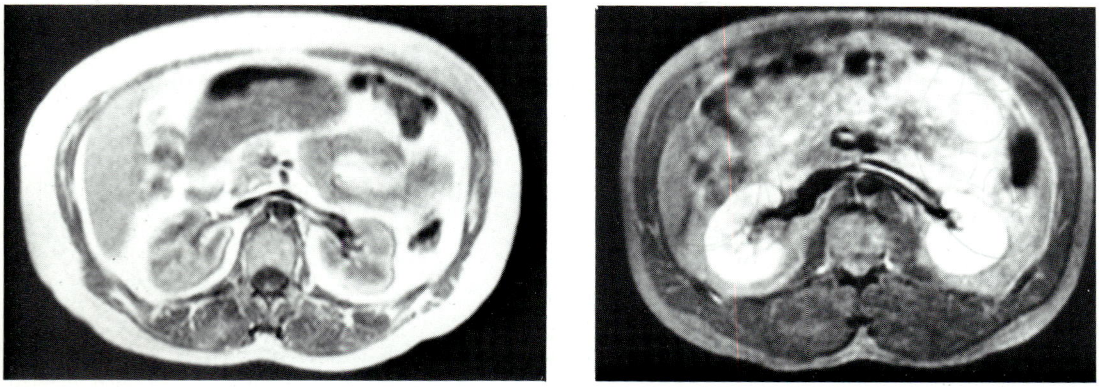

A B

rectly related to the degree of hydration of the patient. With T-2 weighting, corticomedullary distinction diminshes to the point where the entire kidney appears of uniformly high intensity. These imaging findings are the same whether the kidney is imaged in the transverse, coronal, or sagittal planes.

When opacified during renal arteriography (Fig. 2-10), the main renal artery is seen to bifurcate near the renal hilum into anterior and posterior branches. These in turn further branch into segmental arteries, which give rise to interlobar arteries that run in the columns of Bertin to the corticomedullary junction; there they arch over the pyramids as the arcuate arteries. Tiny intralobular arteries originate from the arcuates and extend into the renal cortex. Throughout this branching, there is a progressive decrease in size of the arteries. The venous anatomy of the kidney has a similar branching pattern (Fig. 2-11).

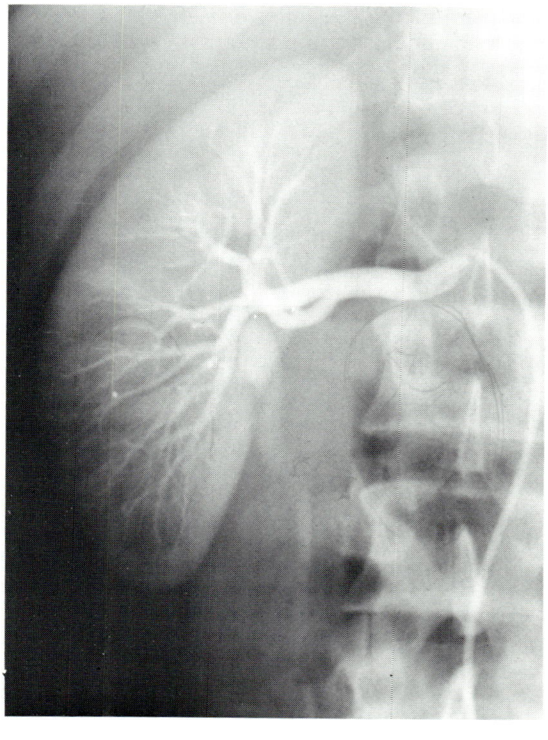

Figure 2-10. Normal renal arteriogram. Selective injection of the renal artery results in excellent opacification of the branching arterial tree. The arcuate and interlobular arteries are not defined.

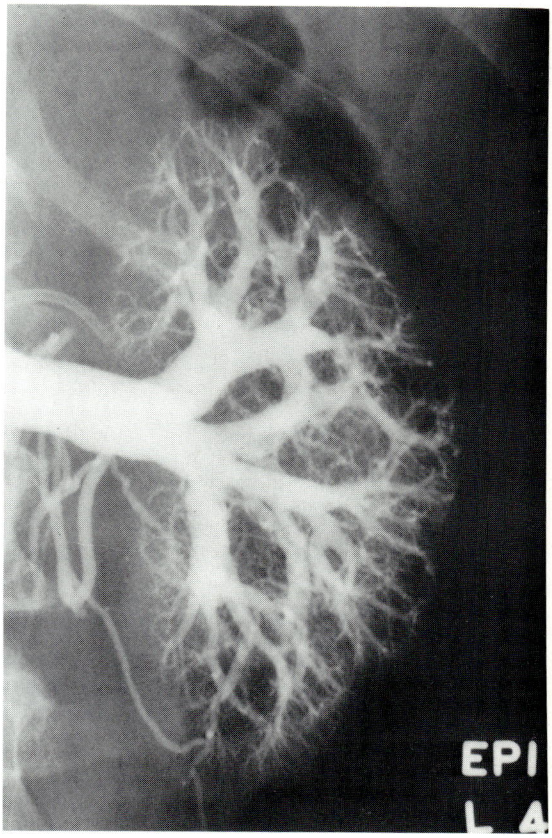

Figure 2-11. Normal renal venogram. Selective injection of the renal vein shows the branching venous system of the kidney. This study was enhanced by the prior injection of epinephrine into the renal artery to diminish arterial flow and allow more complete filling of the venous system.

URETERS

The ureters extend from the ureteropelvic junctions (UPJs) to the bladder. Proximally, they may parallel the psoas margin for a short distance before deviating medially to course toward the bladder on a path that will carry them near or over the tips of the lumbar transverse processes. More commonly, the ureters course anterior to the psoas from the level of the UPJs. They are straightest during full expiration, when the kidney is at its highest position. During inspiration, they may exhibit a series of nonobstructing kinks or twists. On reaching the pelvic inlet, they exhibit a smooth lateral curve, following the contours of the bony pelvis, and enter the bladder base at the lateral margins of the trigone (ureterovesical junctions) (Fig. 2-12). The ureteral diameter varies considerably, the narrowest portions being at the UPJ, at the point of crossing the iliac vessels, and at their entry into the bladder. It is not unusual to see one or both of the midureters widen to about 1 cm in diameter before they cross the iliac vessels, forming what is called the ureteral spindle. When the opacified ureter is observed fluoroscopically, it is seen to be a dynamic organ with a constantly changing diameter due to peristalsis. While significant deviations of the course of the ureter may indicate retroperitoneal or pelvic pathology, there can often be pronounced medial deviations of the midureters in muscular individuals with prominent psoas muscles [3] (Fig. 2-13). Generally speaking, the normal course of the ureters can be quite variable, even when comparing the right and left

Figure 2-12. Normal ureteral course. Urography shows well-opacified ureters describing a normal course to the bladder bilaterally.

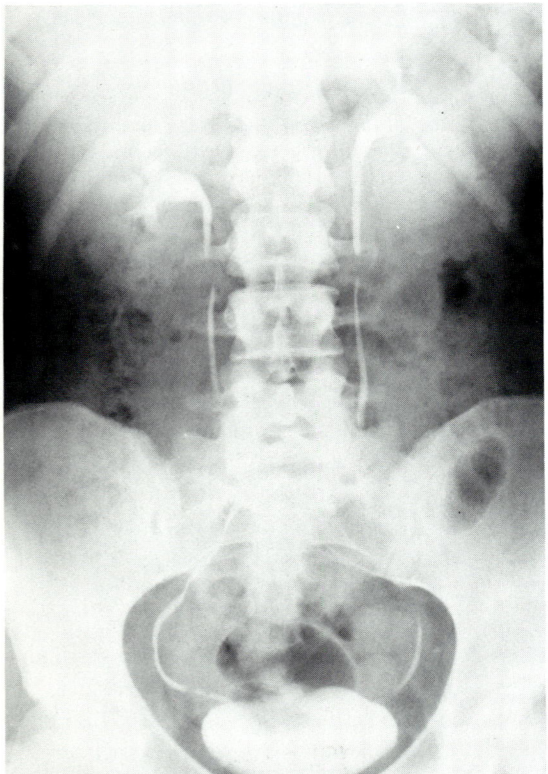

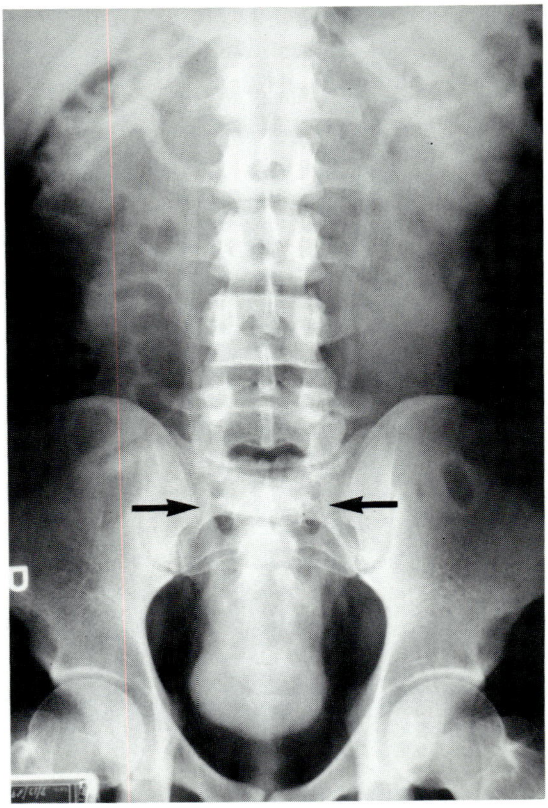

Figure 2-13. Medial deviation of the ureters and teardrop configuration of the bladder caused by prominent ileopsoas muscles (normal variant). Urography in muscular individual shows significant medial location of ureters over sacrum (arrows) and bilateral compression of the bladder.

sides in the same individual.

The ureters are aganglionic organs that receive their blood supply from a periureteral arterial plexus whose branches arise from the aorta and ipsilateral renal and iliac arteries.

BLADDER

The bladder, as the urinary reservoir, varies widely in size and contour, depending on the degree of filling. Its normal capacity may vary from 300 to 1,000 ml. When partially filled, the sides and dome of the bladder can be indented by adjacent organs, the most common being the uterine fundus, which causes a superior impression. Distended loops of the rectosigmoid colon can also result in extrinsic impression on the bladder laterally, superiorly, or posteriorly; these indentations usually disappear as the full state is reached. When full the bladder may be round, ovoid, or even exhibit a somewhat rectangular appearance. The wall of the distended bladder is 2 to 3 mm thick. Prominent ileopsoas muscles may impart a teardrop configuration to the bladder (see Fig. 2-13), though pathologic causes should also be considered when this configuration is seen [14]. The normal bladder base lies just above, and parallels, the superior margin of the pubic symphysis. Impressions on the bladder contour at the midbase usually indicate prostate pathology in the male, and may have multiple causes in the female. These will be discussed in subsequent chapters, as will other extrinsic lesions that can change the bladder contour.

During urography, a dense, rounded accumulation of contrast may be seen above the trigone (Fig. 2-14). While this is sometimes mistaken for a posteriorly located bladder diverticulum, in reality the finding is due to contrast, which is heavier than urine, layering out in the bas fond, or most dependent portion of the bladder in the supine patient. Contrast can also be trapped in lateral folds of the almost empty bladder in females, resulting in the erroneous diagnosis of small diverticula.

Figure 2-14. Bas fond. Coned view of urogram shows oval-shaped area of increased density in bladder (arrows) representing contrast pooling in the most dependent portion of the bladder, above the trigone, in this supine patient.

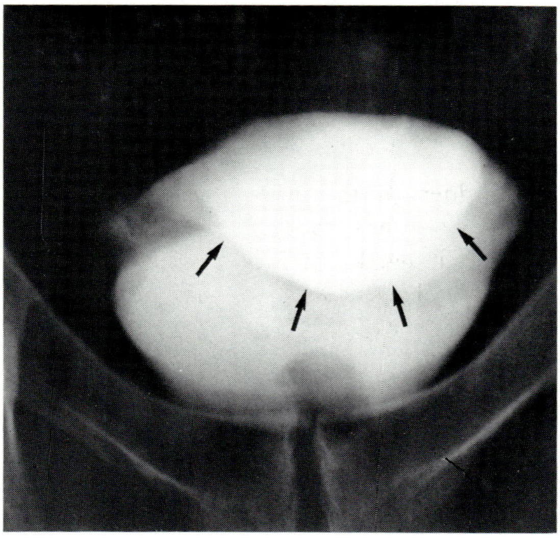

The nerve supply to the bladder is via a reflex arc derived from the second through fourth sacral cord segments. Blood supply is from the paired superior, middle, and inferior vesical arteries originating from the anterior trunks of the hypogastric arteries.

PROSTATE AND SEMINAL VESICLES

The prostate, an accessory sex organ, is a firm, elastic gland located at the base of the male bladder. It is approximately the size of a walnut in its healthy state and weighs 15 to 20 g. Its shape is that of an inverted pyramid, the bladder resting on its base superiorly, and its apex terminating at the urogenital diaphragm (Fig. 2-15). The prostatic urethra and paired ejaculatory ducts traverse the prostate, the latter emptying on the distal surface of the verumontanum, a small mound of tissue situated posteriorly in the distal prostatic urethra. A small indentation in the middle of the verumontanum, the utricle, is a müllerian remnant that is homologous to the female uterus. The prostatic glands drain into the floor of the prostatic urethra via 30 to 40 small openings surrounding the verumontanum.

Figure 2-15. Anatomic relationship of bladder and prostate. The prostate is shaped like an inverted pyramid with its base supporting the bladder and its apex abutting the urogenital diaphragm (B = bladder; P = prostate; SV = seminal vesicle; R = rectum.)

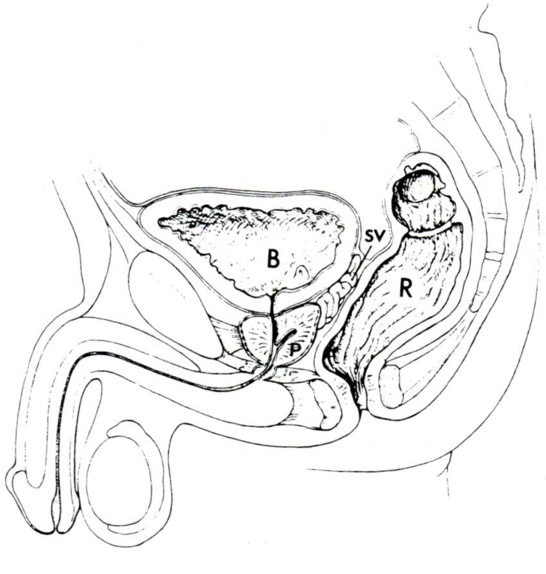

Classic descriptions of prostate anatomy enumerate five lobes that confluently form the gross gland. These include the two lateral lobes, the anterior lobe, the posterior lobe, and the median lobe. Further, vestigial prostatic tissue can be found behind the bladder neck and trigone, which, if hypertrophied, is classically referred to as the lobe of Albarrán. However, dissections of the prostate do not reveal clear demarcations of the gland along lobar divisions; more recent studies of the prostate indicate that the anatomy is zonal rather than lobar in nature [10] (Fig. 2-16). However, median lobe and lobe of Albarrán hypertrophy remain useful and descriptive terms for specific radiographic patterns that will be discussed in the chapter on prostatic diseases. Zonal anatomy applies when imaging the prostate by transrectal ultrasound or MRI. A small transitional zone, comprising only about 5 percent of prostate volume, surrounds the prostatic urethra. This zone appears to be the site of origin of benign prostatic hyperplasia. The remaining bulk of the glandular prostate is posterior to the urethra and is composed of central and peripheral zones. The peripheral zone occupies almost the entire posterolateral portion of the prostate and the prostatic apex, cupping the central prostate as a baseball glove would cup a baseball. Carcinoma of the prostate and prostatitis are generally felt to originate in the peripheral zone. The anterior zone is composed of fibrous tissue anterior to the urethra.

The arterial supply to the prostate is from branches of the inferior vesical arteries, which, as previously noted, originate from the anterior divisions of the hypogastric arteries. A periprostatic venous plexus (Santorini) drains into the hypogastric veins. There are also anastomoses between the prostatic veins and Batson's venous plexus, which invests the lumbar spine, sacrum, and iliac wings, explaining the high incidence of bony metastases from cancer of the prostate in these regions.

The seminal vesicles are paired, saccular organs extending superolaterally above the prostate between the bladder and rectum. The ducts from these glands join the vasa deferentia to form the ejaculatory ducts.

URETHRA AND PERIURETHRAL STRUCTURES

The female urethra is straight and about 3 to 4 cm in length. In men, the urethra is more complicated and is composed of three segments: the prostatic or posterior urethra, the membranous urethra, and the anterior urethra

Figure 2-16. Zonal anatomy of the prostate. (C = central zone; P = peripheral zone; T = transitional zone; U = urethra; V = verumontanum; A = anterior zone; SV = seminal vesicle.)

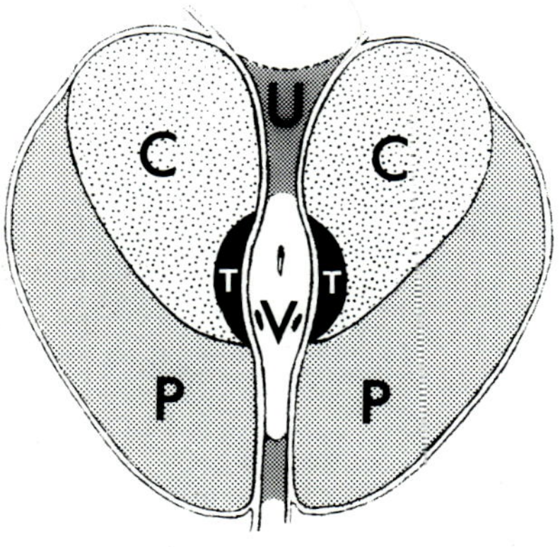

Coronal view

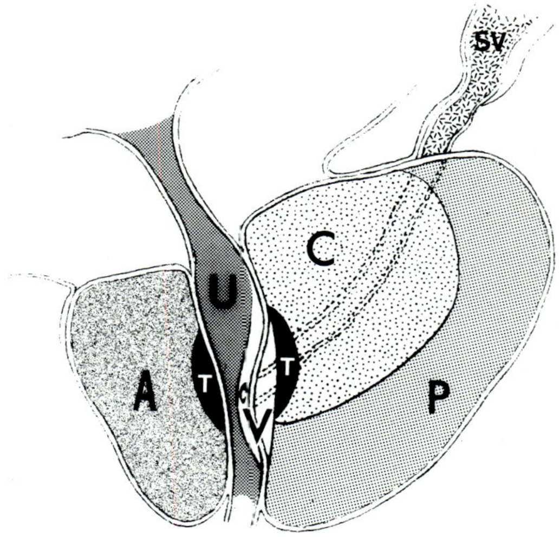

Sagittal view

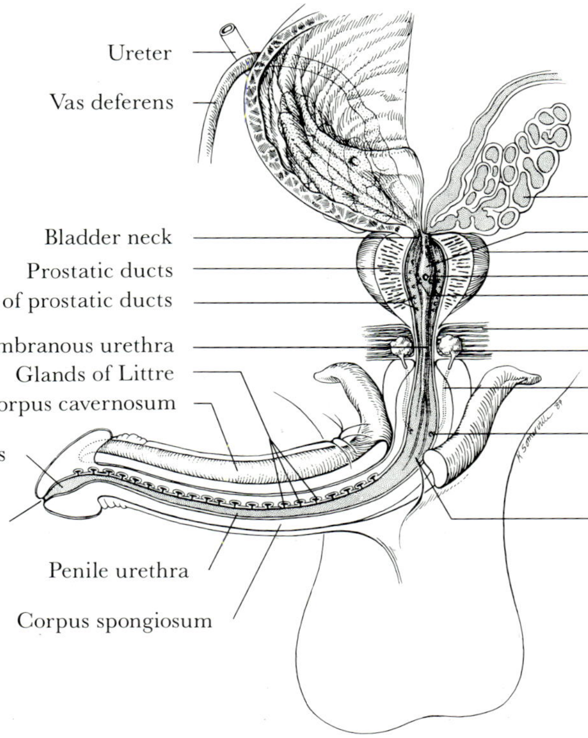

Figure 2-17. Make urethra and periurethral structures. (From E.S. Amis, Jr., J.H. Newhouse, and J.J. Cronan, Radiology of male periurethral structures. *A.J.R.* 151:321–324. © American Roentgen Ray Society, 1988.)

(Fig. 2-17). The prostatic urethra extends from the bladder neck to the apex of the prostate, where it meets the membranous urethra, whose length is about 1 cm as it traverses the urogenital diaphragm. Radiographically, the proximal landmark for the membranous urethra is the distal end of the verumontanum, while the distal landmark is the proximal bulbous urethra, which has the shape of a smoothly tapered cone. The anterior urethra is encased in the corpus spongiosum and is comprised of the bulbous urethra, which extends from the urogenital diaphragm to the penoscrotal junction, and the more distal penile or pendulous urethra. The distal 2 cm or so of the penile urethra, the fossa navicularis, is slightly widened. The paired corpora cavernosa lie dorsal to the anterior urethra. The posterior urethra is lined with transitional epithelium, while the anterior urethral lining is columnar in nature with the exception of the most distal segment, where squamous epithelium is found.

The paired accessory sex glands of Cowper are about the size of peas and lie between the leaves of the urogenital diaphragm on either side of the membranous urethra. Their ducts pierce the inferior leaf of the diaphragm and extend approximately 2 cm before separately entering the proximal bulbous urethra. The glands of Littre are multiple, small lubricating glands surrounding the anterior urethra. These are more numerous in the bulbar region.

There are three urethral sphincters in the male: the smooth muscle internal sphincter at the bladder neck, and the intrinsic (smooth muscle) and external (striated) sphincters surrounding the membranous urethra within the urogenital diaphragm [9] (Fig. 2-18).

MALE GENITALIA

The pertinent anatomy of the male genital system is discussed fully in the chapters on the scrotum, male infertility, and impotence.

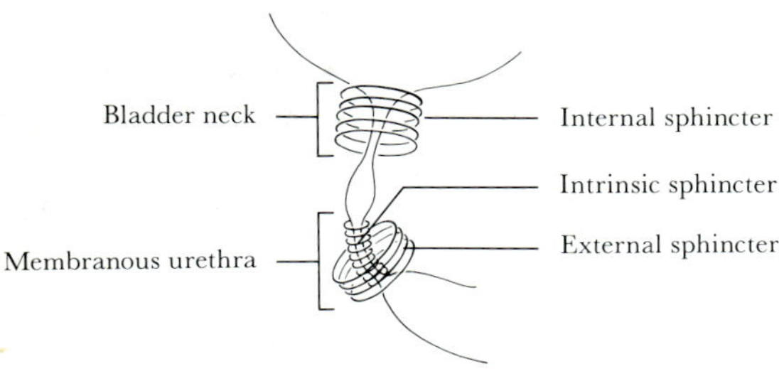

Figure 2-18. Urethral sphincters. (Modified from R.W. McCallum. The adult male urethra: Normal anatomy, pathology, and method of urethrography. *Radiol. Clin. North Am.* 17:227, 1979.)

PHYSIOLOGY

KIDNEY

Adrenal physiology is beyond the scope of this book, as is a detailed discussion of renal function. Simply speaking, the kidney forms concentrated urine as a mechanism for relieving the body of waste materials. This is accomplished by filtration of the blood at the glomerulus, resulting in a protein-free ultrafiltrate of plasma. The kidneys are perfused by about one-fourth of the cardiac output, resulting in a renal blood flow of 1,250 ml per minute. The glomerular filtrate averages 125 ml per minute, which must then be reduced to the normal urine output of about 1 ml per minute. This is in large part accomplished by the absorption of water from the proximal tubule. The countercurrent multiplier system of the loop of Henle then acts to create a high solute concentration in the medulla by active transport of sodium out of the ascending limb of the loop, resulting in a high osmotic gradient between the medulla and the collecting ducts descending through it. This gradient, in conjunction with antidiuretic hormone (ADH) secreted by the posterior lobe of the pituitary, allows water to diffuse from the collecting ducts into the medulla and results in a concentrated urine. Body acid–base balance is maintained by the ability of the kidney to secrete hydrogen by the formation of titratable acid and excretion of ammonium and its ability to reabsorb bicarbonate selectively in exchange for hydrogen. The kidney is also instrumental in erythropoiesis, being the chief site of either the activation or production of erythropoietin. Erythrocytosis is seen with some renal tumors, while renal insufficiency results in anemia. Radiographic contrast material is almost completely excreted by glomerular filtration and will be discussed further in the chapter on contrast agents.

COLLECTING SYSTEMS AND URETERS

After formation by the kidney, urine is delivered to the bladder by the collecting system and ureter. The calices function independently and asynchronously in transmitting urine to the renal pelvis. While the location of a pacemaker for coordinated peristalsis is not precisely known, it is felt that the first propagating wave begins in the pelviureteric region in response to urine distending the renal pelvis. This wave then passes down the ureter in a coordinated fashion via an electrical impulse that passes through nexi connecting smooth muscle cells in the ureteral wall [6]. As one segment of the ureter contracts to propel the urine bolus caudad, another immediately below relaxes to accept the bolus, this sequence repeating until the bolus reaches the bladder. Peristaltic waves occur at a rate of approximately three per minute but are inhibited as pressure in the bladder rises. For effective propulsion of a urine bolus, the ureteral walls must be able to coapt, or meet. Therefore, while peristaltic contractions can be seen fluoroscopically in a dilated ureter, they are often not able to move the bolus, and an uninterrupted column of urine from renal pelvis to bladder results.

BLADDER

A knowledge of the innervation of the bladder is necessary for understanding bladder function. The micturition reflex arc is parasympathetic and derived from the second through fourth sacral cord segments. The external sphincter has a somatic innervation. Receptors in the bladder wall initiate the micturition reflex via afferent fibers in the arc in response to bladder distention. This voiding reflex can then be inhibited or facilitated by activity originating in the cerebral cortex and extending down the spinal cord to the sacral level. During voiding, the bladder detrusor (musculature) contracts and actively funnels the bladder neck; the sphincters surrounding the membranous urethra then relax, allowing complete expulsion of the bladder contents. Between voidings, the intravesical pressure remains at a low and steady level because of control of the reflex arc by the inhibitory effect of the central nervous system as well as the elastic properties of bladder smooth muscle. In the normal patient, urinary continence is maintained by the internal and intrinsic sphincters combined, though the intrinsic sphincter at the level of the membranous urethra can maintain passive continence in patients who have loss of the internal sphincter after prostatectomy. Neurogenic dysfunction of the bladder will be discussed in Chap. 20.

SEXUAL FUNCTION

Normal sexual function in the male requires penetration of the vagina by the erect penis and deposition of semen therein. Penile erection may result from psychic or local stimulation and is physically due to engorgement of the corpora cavernosa and corpus spongiosum by inflow from the internal pudendal arteries. Erection is initiated by sympathetically controlled release of adrenergic neurotransmitters, which results in relaxation of smooth muscle in the walls of sinusoids filling the corpora. As these sinusoids fill with blood, small peripheral veins draining the corpora are compressed between the distended sinusoids and the dense tunica albuginea surrounding the corpora cavernosa, effectively halting venous outflow from the penis [12]. This mechanism is illustrated in Chap. 27.

During ejaculation, which is also mediated by the sympathetic system, secretions from the testes, seminal vesicles, and prostate are deposited in the posterior urethra. The sphincters around the membranous urethra then relax while the bladder neck remains closed, and semen is propelled through the urethral meatus by the perineal and bulbocavernosus muscles. In the average ejaculate volume of 3.5 ml, 2.0 to 2.5 ml are from the prostate and seminal vesicles, 0.5 ml from the glands of Cowper and Littre, and the reminder from the testes. The seminal vesicle secretions are rich in fructose, which provides an energy source for the spermatozoa. The primary function of the prostatic portion of semen appears to be liquification of the semen, which is initially a gelatinous clot. Lubrication of the urethra is provided by Cowper's glands and the glands of Littre.

REFERENCES

1. Barbaric, Z. Renal fascia in urinary tract disease. *Radiology* 119:561, 1976.
2. Brandt, T.D., et al. Ultrasound assessment of normal renal dimensions. *J. Ultrasound Med.* 1:49, 1982.
3. Bree, R.L., et al. Medial deviation of the ureters secondary to psoas muscle hypertrophy. *Radiology* 118:691, 1976.
4. Carter, A.R., et al. The junctional parenchymal defect: A sonographic variant of renal anatomy. *Radiology* 154:499, 1985.
5. Clark, R.L., and Cuttino, J.T. Microradiographic studies of renal lymphatics. *Radiology* 124:307, 1977.
6. Hanna, M.K., et al. Ureteral structure and ultrastructure. Part I. The normal human ureter. *J. Urol.* 116:718, 1976.
7. Kneeland, J.B., et al. Perirenal spaces: CT evidence for communication across the midline. *Radiology* 164:657, 1987.
8. Love, L., et al. Computed tomography of extraperitoneal spaces. *A.J.R.* 136:781, 1981.
9. McCallum, R.W. The adult male urethra: Normal anatomy, pathology, and method of urethrography. *Radiol. Clin. North Am.* 17:227, 1979.
10. McNeal, J.E. Normal and pathologic anatomy of prostate. *Urology (Suppl.)* 17:11, 1981.
11. Moell, H. Size of normal kidneys. *Acta Radiol.* 46:640, 1956.
12. Sidi, A.A., Koleilat, N., and Fraley, E.E. Evaluation and treatment of organic impotence. *Invest. Radiol.* 23:778, 1988.
13. Thornbury, J.R., McCormick, T.L., and Silver, T.M. Anatomic/radiologic classification of renal cortical nodules. *A.J.R.* 134:1, 1980.
14. Wechsler, R.J., and Brennan, R.E. Teardrop bladder: Additional considerations. *Radiology* 144:281, 1982.

Techniques and Modalities

There are several specific techniques useful in imaging the urinary tract. Furthermore, most imaging modalities have specific indications for evaluating various conditions in the genitourinary system. This chapter will discuss these techniques and modalities, particularly with regard to how they should be performed. As the various disease processes that can affect the urinary tract are discussed throughout the remainder of this book, the most efficacious use of the proper imaging study or modality for that specific disease process will be stressed.

EXCRETORY UROGRAPHY

Urography has now been refined to a point at which the renal margins and parenchyma, as well as the entire collecting system including the ureters and the bladder, can be diagnostically visualized. This requires "tailoring" of the urogram to answer the pertinent clinical questions for any given patient [2].

INDICATIONS

Most patients suspected of having urologic disease will be referred for excretory urography. However, this may vary from hospital to hospital because of the acceptance and availability of newer imaging modalities. Furthermore, there is variability in the preference and experience of referring clinicians. The more common indications for urography include urinary colic, hematuria (microscopic or gross), prostatism, trauma, suspected neoplasm, neurogenic bladder dysfunction, congenital anomalies, and evaluation of the postoperative patient. There are several indications for emergency urography. These include trauma involving the genitourinary system, massive gross hematuria, suspected vascular accident involving the kidneys, sepsis that may derive from a source in the urinary tract, and suspected ureteral calculus. Clinical experience indicates that many patients with other urologic diseases will also eventually undergo urography at some point during diagnosis or treatment. However, urography is not felt to be useful in the evaluation of acute pyelonephritis (unless obstruction is suspected), in cases of nephrologic disease, or in renal failure. There are currently differences of opinion regarding the use of urography for the investigation of benign prostatic hypertrophy and as a screening examination for renal vascular hypertension.

The hypertensive urogram involves obtaining views of the kidneys in a rapid sequence immediately after bolus injection of contrast. The minimum series includes films at 1, 2, and 3 minutes postinjection and a 30-minute film. Radiographic criteria for a renal vascular cause of hypertension include delayed contrast visualization in the collecting system of the affected side, decreased size of the involved kidney, and delayed washout of contrast medium from the affected kidney on the late film. Reports indicate that urography is a nondiscriminatory test for renal vascular hypertension. The true positive rate has been reported as only 60 percent, and the predictive value for favorable surgical outcome in hypertensive patients with positive hypertensive urograms was only 24 percent [35].

The urogram should not be considered a reliable test for quantitating functional impairment of the kidneys. Modern contrast agents result in such high plasma concentration of the agent that even kidneys with significantly decreased function may yield diagnostic studies. Though useful information can be gained with regard to the presence or absence of obstruction in some patients with renal failure, a better modality for evaluating such patients is renal ultrasound, which is an excellent screening examination for hydronephrosis.

CONTRAINDICATIONS

There are no absolute contraindications to urography. However, there are several conditions for which the potential risks of the examination must be weighed against the possible diagnostic benefits. These include pregnancy, history of previous reactions to contrast media, and renal failure associated with diabetes mellitus.

If it is essential to perform urography during pregnancy, a limited study composed of a preliminary film and single 30-minute postinjection film will minimize radiation exposure. Urography should be avoided in patients who are undergoing either diagnosis or treatment of thyroid disease, since the iodine-containing contrast agent may block the thyroid uptake of radioisotopes of iodine being administered for diagnostic or therapeutic reasons.

Statistics indicate that the use of urography has declined significantly over the past two decades. This is most likely a result of the advent of the newer cross-sectional imaging modalities and the increased concern about reactions to intravenous contrast media as well as about contrast-induced renal failure.

PATIENT PREPARATION

Patients scheduled for nonemergent urography are usually instructed to take nothing by mouth (NPO) after midnight on the day of the examination and to undergo a mild bowel preparation to reduce gas and feces that partially obscure the urinary tract.

It has been well established that no significant dehydration occurs with the degree of fluid restriction recommended. Rather, the NPO past midnight regimen is primarily to ensure that the patient will have an empty stomach; this minimizes the risk of aspiration in the uncommon cases in which contrast administration results in nausea and vomiting. With regard to bowel preparation, enemas are to be condemned as, in some cases, large amounts of gas are actually introduced into the colon during the enema. Many bowel preparation kits are commercially available. However, bisacodyl (Dulcolax) tablets, two to four 5-mg tablets at bedtime on the day before the study, usually provide adequate bowel preparation.

The need for informed consent prior to urography remains controversial, though the trend is toward requiring its use. Whether used or not, the patient should be queried regarding risk factors for the administration of contrast material, informed of the possibility of contrast reactions, and informed that he or she is likely to experience a warm flushed feeling, a metallic taste in the mouth, and perhaps a mild wave of nausea during and immediately after the injection.

EXPOSURE FACTORS (PHYSICS OF UROGRAPHY)

Both the preliminary film and the urogram should be exposed at 66 to 70 kVp. The mean energy of polychromatic radiation is about one-third to one-half of its peak energy. Therefore, the mean energy of the recommended x-ray beam will be about 30 kV, which is very close to the K-shell binding energy of iodine (33.2 keV). Since the binding energy of iodine and the mean energy of the x-ray beam are roughly the same, interactions at the K-shell level will be maximized. This allows the photoelectric effect to dominate and results in maximum attenuation of the x-ray beam by the contrast agent. If the radiation energy is increased, Compton scattering becomes more apparent and attenuation decreases.

Another advantage of the 66-to-70-kVp beam energy is the enhanced ability to image calcifications. As the energy of the x-ray beam is increased, differential attenuation between calcium and soft tissue decreases, resulting in reduction of image contrast. Small stones that are easily seen at 70 kVp may not be seen at 100 kVp.

All urograms should be obtained with a Bucky diaphragm. Generally speaking, a medium-speed screen–film combination is most desirable for urography. Higher-speed systems, while reducing motion artifact, may result in some loss of detail and increase in quantum mottle. Tomographic study of the kidneys should use linear motion along the long axis of the kidneys. Since there is an inverse relation between the magnitude of the arc and the thickness of the cut obtained, the greater the arc the thinner the section. A 40-degree arc provides a section of sufficient thinness to provide good detail. However, as the section thickness decreases, more tomographic cuts may be needed for complete evaluation of the renal parenchyma. With very thin cuts, contrast may be diminished, canceling the advantages of sharper detail. Tube sweep times of less than 1 second require generation of very high current. On the other hand a tube sweep time of more than 2 seconds invites patient motion and tube sway or unsmoothness.

PRELIMINARY FILM OF THE ABDOMEN

The preliminary film of the abdomen during urographic examination is also known as the KUB (kidneys, ureters, bladder), the scout film, or plain film of the abdomen. This is an indispensable adjunct to excretory urography, and no attempt to interpret the urogram should be made if a preliminary film is not available. The most common deficiency of the preliminary film is failure to demonstrate the upper or lower reaches of the urinary tract. It has been reported that the entire urinary tract is included on a single 14×17 in. film in only 17 percent of adult patients of average height. Therefore, in a significant percentage of patients, coned plain views of the kidneys or pubic area may be necessary to complete the preliminary evaluation. One report indicates that two preliminary films should be obtained in all but the smallest adults [19]. In this technique, a 14×17 in. film is exposed with the inferior margin of the pubic symphysis positioned about 6 cm above the lower margin of the cassette and the x-ray tube angled 10 degrees toward the patient's feet. An 11 × 14 in. upper film is centered 2 to 4 cm above the umbilicus with the x-ray tube angled 10 degrees cephalad.

When calcifications are seen overlying the renal shadows on the preliminary film, confirmation of their renal location can be obtained by appropriate oblique views. A right posterior oblique view is necessary for evaluation of calcifications possibly within the right kidney, and a left posterior oblique is useful to evaluate left-sided calcifications. If the calcifications remain in constant relation to the renal shadow on the oblique views, it can be reasonably assumed that they are renal in origin. Calcifications anterior to the kidney will be projected lateral to the renal shadow on ipsilateral posterior oblique views, and calcifications posterior to the kidney will be projected medial to the renal shadow. This will aid in making diagnostic comment as to their specific cause.

Figure 3-1 depicts the location and configuration of calcifications commonly seen in the abdominal area on plain films. Gallstones or pancreatic calcifications might aid in elucidating upper abdominal pain of unknown cause. Vascular calcifications in the aorta or in splenic, renal, or iliac arteries may be incidental findings; however, when both walls are calcified and widely separated, aneurysmal dilatation can be diagnosed. Arterial calcifications can occasionally extend throughout the intrarenal arterial tree (Fig. 3-2). Incidental calcifications include those in the costochondral cartilage, splenic and hepatic granulomas, calcified mesenteric nodes, and either old hemorrhage or granulomatous disease in otherwise normal-sized adrenal glands. Phleboliths are seen as small rounded calcifications in the pelvis, usually with lucent centers. These are thought to result from thrombosis in the deep pelvic veins, one cause for which is postulated to be straining at stool. While these are usually also incidental findings they can lie over the course of the distal ureters and be confused for distal ureteral calculi. Prostatic calcifications are seen as an aggregate of multiple small calcific densities usually protruding above the pubic symphysis. These may be idiopathic or secondary to infection. Calcification of the vasa deferentia is of clinical significance, since almost 90 percent of men with this diagnosis have diabetes mellitus (Fig. 3-3). While calcifications associated with the urinary tract are obviously of greatest importance in interpreting the preliminary film, mention of the calcifications described above or other significant abnormalities should be made in the dictated report.

NEPHROTOMOGRAPHY

Since nephrotomography should be a routine part of the urogram, a scout tomographic section should be obtained before contrast injection to ensure that the tomographic series will be adequate for evaluation of the renal outlines. The midpoint of the kidneys (distance from the table top) can be easily determined by multiplying the thickness of the abdomen in centimeters at the level of the lower costal margin by

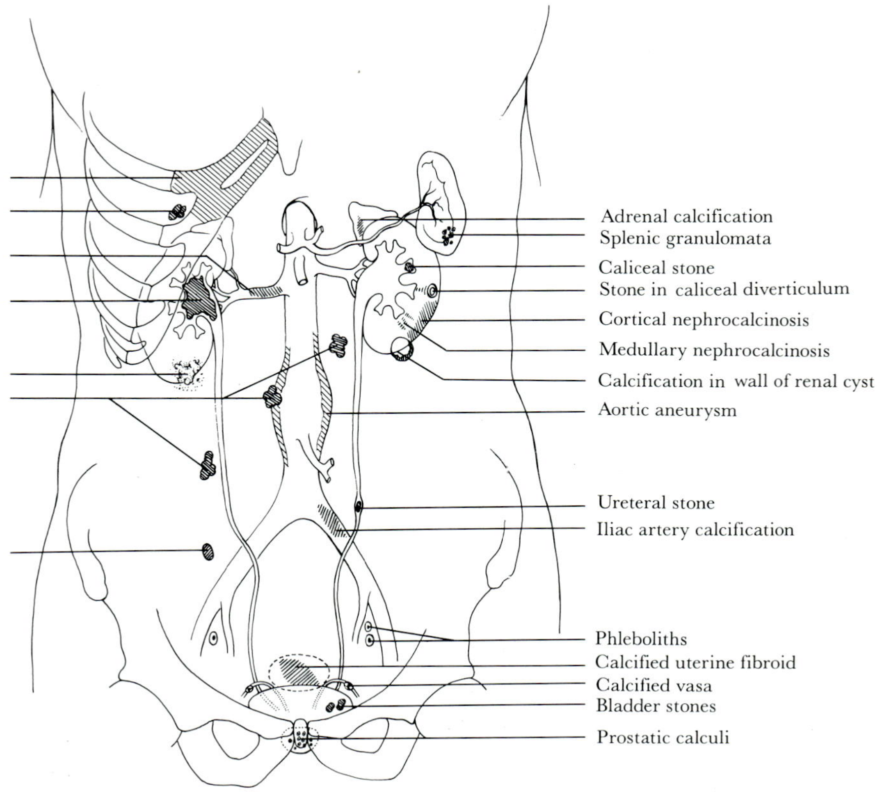

Figure 3-1. Diagram showing common origins of calcifications on abdominal plain films.

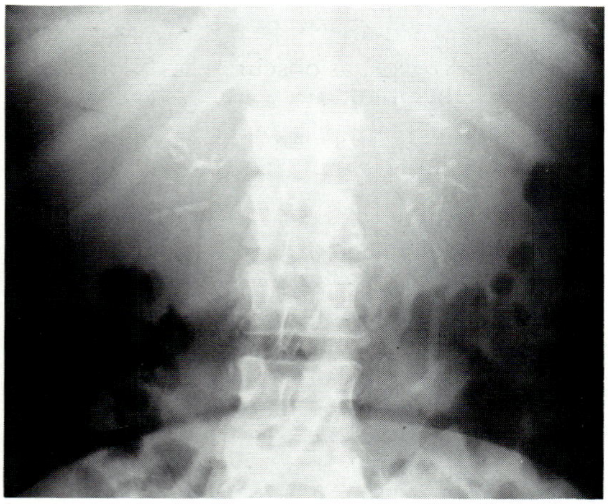

Figure 3-2. Intrarenal arterial calcifications. Plain film of upper abdomen shows branching, linear calcifications over both renal shadows.

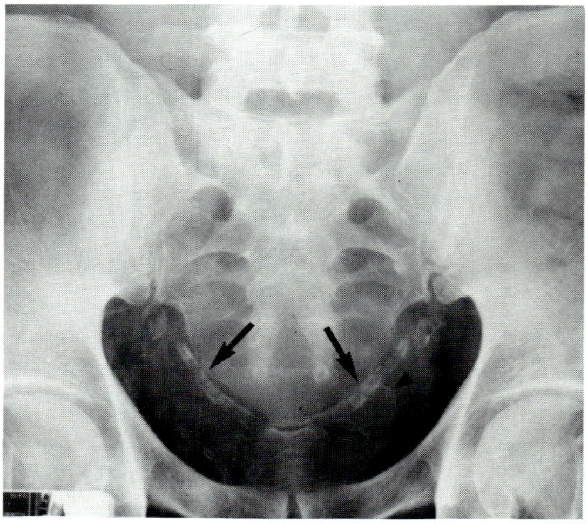

Figure 3-3. Calcification of vasa deferentia and seminal vesicles in diabetic man. Plain film of pelvis shows tubular calcification in vasa (arrows) and curvilinear calcification in left seminal vesicle (arrowhead).

0.4 [6]. The figure obtained is then rounded to the nearest whole number and becomes the middle of tomographic sections. The preliminary tomographic section should reveal a reasonably large portion of the renal outline as an indicator that the planned section levels will delineate the entire renal outline after contrast injection.

The long axis of the kidney is slightly oblique to the long axis of the body, with the upper pole of the kidney lying more posterior and the lower pole more anterior. Figure 3-4 demonstrates that three tomographic sections are usually adequate for visualization of the entire renal outline in the normally positioned kidney. However, in the low-lying kidney, the lower pole may be anteriorly displaced over the iliac crest with a resultant exaggeration of the angulation of the kidney in relation to the axis of the body. In this case, six or more tomographic sections may be necessary to visualize the renal outline completely. This is also true of transplanted kidneys in the iliac fossa and in congenital anomalies such as horseshoe or pelvic kidneys. The limitation of nephrotomography is that renal margins are only seen when they are situated tangential to the x-ray beam. Therefore, abnormalities of the renal contour or renal masses in other areas (specifically the anterior or posterior renal surfaces) may be missed.

Figure 3-4. Tomographic sections required to show complete renal outline in normal and low-lying kidneys. Note that six or more sections may be necessary if kidney is significantly tilted in relation to table top. (From E.S. Amis, Jr. Excretory Urography. In J.M. Taveras and J.T. Ferrucci (eds.), *Radiology: Diagnosing-Imaging-Intervention*, Philadelphia: Lippincott, 1988.)

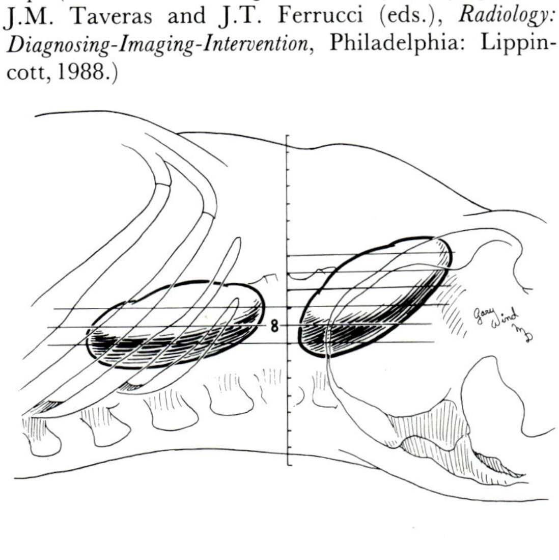

On occasion, the fluid-filled fundus of the stomach presents as a round, soft-tissue mass several centimeters in diameter above the left kidney on tomography (Fig. 3-5A). The true nature of this mass can be demonstrated by obtaining a prone film of the upper abdomen; in this position the fundus will fill with air (Fig. 3-5B).

CONTRAST ADMINISTRATION

There has been controversy in the past regarding the advantages of bolus injection versus infusion of contrast material. While there are advantages to both, the bolus technique is currently widely used, as it allows the maximum plasma concentration of iodine. The bolus should be administered rapidly through an 18- or 19-gauge needle into a large arm vein when possible. The needle should then be left indwelling during the remainder of the examination as a safety precaution, as it could be needed for treatment of a contrast reaction.

Table 3-1 lists recommended dosages of contrast material for children and adults. A routine dose is important, since there are no ideal ways of calculating an optimal dose for each patient. In children, however, the weight of the patient is a more prominent factor, and recommended doses are based on this parameter.

FILM SEQUENCES

After satisfactory preliminary filming, the urogram can proceed after injection of contrast. In the infant, if bowel gas obscures the kidneys to a significant degree, intake of a commercial soft drink that contains carbon dioxide will produce distention of the stomach and provide a window for visualization of the kidneys. Prone filming can also be helpful since it acts as a form of compression and displaces colon and stomach gas away from the renal areas. While bowel gas may be bothersome in the adult, the routine use of tomography usually allows adequate visualization of the kidneys.

All urographic exposures should be made with the patient in deep expiration. This results in straightening of the ureter and reduces the possibility of tortuosity or kinking. Furthermore, the patient should have been instructed to void

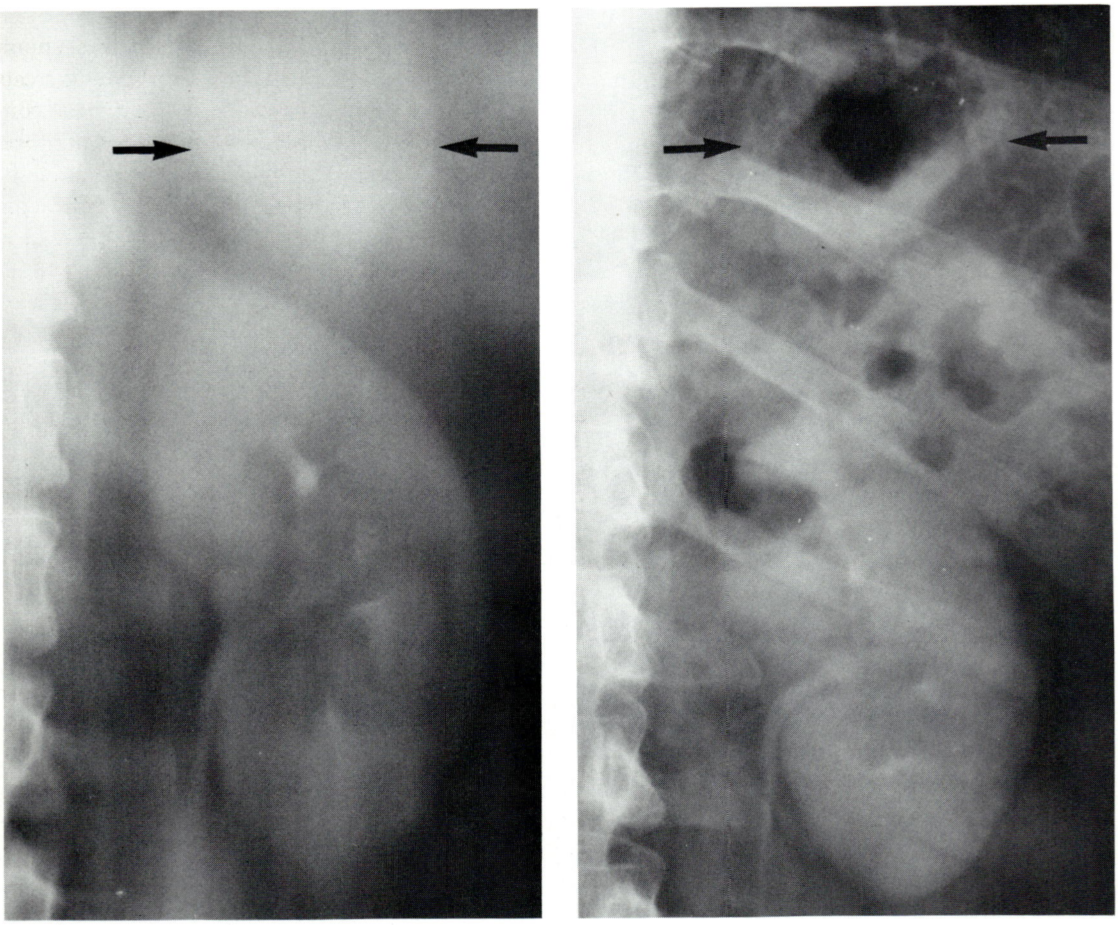

Figure 3-5. Fluid-filled fundus of stomach presenting as pseudotumor. A. Nephrotomography shows soft-tissue mass above left kidney (arrows). B. Prone plain film of upper abdomen shows air in stomach fundus (arrows) in region of previously noted "mass."

Table 3-1. Dosages of radiographic contrast medium

Children	
Less than 5 lb	2 ml/lb
Newborn (5–10 lb)	10 ml
10–50 lb	1 ml/lb
50–100 lb	50 ml
Over 100 lb	75 ml
Adults	
Over 100 lb	75–100 ml

prior to the study to allow for dense opacification of the bladder on later films.

There is no standard sequencing of films that must be followed. Indeed, it would be rare to find two institutions performing exactly the same sequence of films. Table 3-2 lists a recommended sequence of filming that can be used as a basic guide.

Tomographic sections of the kidneys should probably be obtained in all adults undergoing urography. Certainly, they are mandatory in patients with a history of trauma, hematuria, or a suspected renal mass. If it is elected not to use tomography in young patients without a specific indication, good visualization of the renal outlines and full thickness of a parenchyma can be obtained by exposing a single coned view of the kidneys at 1 to 2 minutes after bolus injection of contrast. When a full tomographic series is obtained, the first film in the series should be exposed within 1 minute after injection and the remainder obtained as rapidly as possible.

Table 3-2. Recommended urographic film sequence

Pediatric urography
Plain film of abdomen (appropriate size and collimation)
Postbolus injection
1-minute full view
10-minute full view
Adult urography
Plain film of abdomen
Full view
Coned view as necessary to include kidneys or prostate area
Oblique views as necessary for calcifications over kidneys
Scout tomogram
Postbolus injection
1-minute tomograms, 3–6 views as necessary
(Apply compression)
15-minute full view with compression in place
(Release compression)
Bilateral oblique full views
Full view postvoiding

Routine application of ureteral compression is recommended unless specifically contraindicated (Table 3-3). The most significant contraindication is aortic aneurysm. This requires careful scrutiny of the preliminary film for calcifications in the aortic walls that suggest aneurysmal dilatation.

Compression can be applied immediately after obtaining the tomographic series. One of the more effective compression devices consists of two inflatable rubber balloons that are held in place by a plastic block and flexible cloth band that is placed around the patient. The belt should be tightly applied while the patient is in deep expiration prior to inflating the balloons.

Table 3-3. Contraindications to compression

Suspected or known aortic aneurysm (check KUB for typical calcifications)
Evidence of obstruction on early urographic films
Recent abdominal surgery
Urinary diversion
Severe hypertension
Recent trauma
Renal transplant
Abdominal distention
Bladder distention
Bowel ostomies
Abdominal pain on application of compression device

When inflated, the balloons should nearly touch in the midline and their upper edges should parallel the superior margins of the iliac crests. Pain in the renal areas after application of compression usually indicates that there has been rupture of a caliceal fornix and subsequent extravasation of urine. This is usually of no clinical significance, but compression should be released immediately. On the other hand if the patient is known to have infected urine, appropriate antibiotic treatment is indicated. After compression has been applied for approximately 10 minutes, a full view of the abdomen is obtained. With adequate compression, there will be complete opacification of the intrarenal collecting system and upper ureters (Fig. 3-6). Mild distention of the collecting system due to the minimal degree of obstruction caused by compression may be seen. Return to a normal, nondistended state should be seen after release of compression. After this release, bilateral full-length oblique views are obtained rapidly. The distal ureters

Figure 3-6. Compression film. Full-view 15-minute film with compression band properly applied (arrows show tops of inflated balloon at level of iliac crests) results in excellent opacification of upper urinary tract.

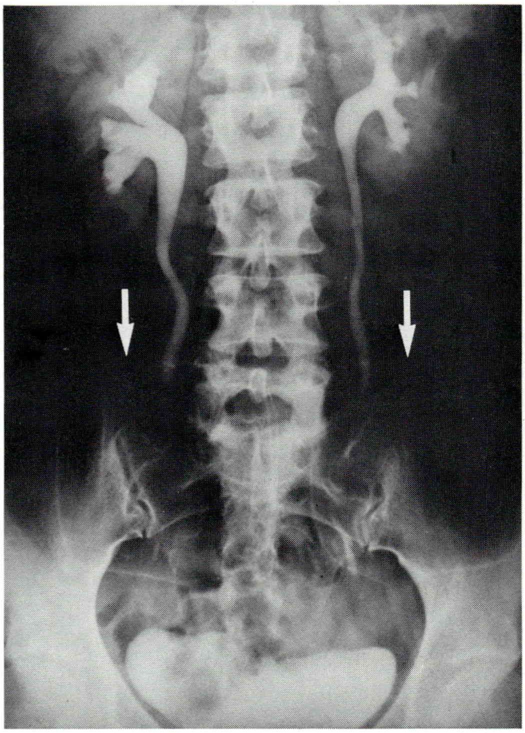

should be visualized on these films because of the rapid passage of contrast from the upper tracts.

After the patient voids in privacy, a full postvoiding view is obtained as soon as possible. The presence and amount of postvoid residual urine should be noted in the radiographic report. However, since the environment in most radiology departments is often not conducive to normal full voiding, any postvoid residual may or may not reflect the patient's inability to empty his/her bladder fully.

If the urogram is being tailored (monitored after each exposure), appropriate deviations from the standard sequence can be used to evaluate abnormalities. These may include oblique tomographic sections, coned oblique views of the kidneys, or a prone view, which may provide better filling of the distal ureters. Coned oblique views of the bladder are useful for imaging filling defects in the bladder as well as the ureterovesical junctions. The right posterior oblique coned view of the bladder will allow visualization of the left ureterovesical junction and vice versa. A coned postvoid view of the bladder is very helpful when evaluating questionable filling defects, as it often enhances a persistent defect.

The level or cause of a ureteral obstruction may not be clearly defined during a standard urogram. Delayed films are then essential. A recommended sequence for these delayed views is 30 minutes, 1 hour, 2 hours, 4 hours, 8 hours, and even 24 hours if necessary to allow complete opacification of an obstructed collecting system. The patient should always be instructed to void prior to obtaining a delayed film so that a calculus in the distal ureter will not be obscured by a full bladder. In most cases of obstruction, at some point during the sequence of delayed films contrast medium can be seen forming a column in the ureter to the point of obstruction. If this has not occurred by 24 hours, further films are not indicated. In such cases, antegrade or retrograde pyelography or CT may be necessary to define the anatomy of the obstructed system.

UROGRAPHIC INTERPRETATION

All parts of the urinary system must be examined thoroughly. These include the renal outlines and parenchyma as seen on tomographic sections, the opacified collecting system including each calix and its infundibulum, the ureters in their entirety, and the opacified bladder.

The peak nephrogram density lasts for up to 2 or 3 minutes after bolus injection. In very early tomograms, the peripheral cortex and vertical columns of Bertin dipping into the medulla are more intensely opacified than the medulla (see Fig. 2-3). This corticomedullary distinction is soon lost, resulting in a diffusely homogeneous nephrogram. Bilateral prolonged dense nephrograms may indicate a hypotensive response to contrast material, and the patient should be examined immediately. A unilateral prolonged nephrogram is most frequently caused by obstruction, but since acute ischemia may produce the same finding, delayed films should be obtained to see if the collecting system is dilated or not. Tomographic sections during this nephrogram phase allow evaluation of the renal outlines and parenchyma. Renal contour abnormalities or rounded areas of decreased nephrographic density indicate the probability of a renal mass.

In normally functioning kidneys, contrast is first seen in the calices 2 minutes after bolus injection. By 3 minutes there is usually complete opacification of the intrarenal collecting system. Maximum collecting system opacification occurs between 5 and 10 minutes.

The ureters begin to opacify about 3 minutes after contrast injection. Maximal opacification, as in the intrarenal collecting system, occurs between 5 and 10 minutes after injection. While complete filling of one or both ureters can be seen on individual films, persistent filling of the entire ureter is known as "columning" and may suggest some degree of distal obstruction.

It is important to visualize the entirety of both ureters, especially in patients with hematuria. This may require segmental reconstruction of the ureter by visualization of the various films in the sequence. Comment should be made in the written report regarding the portions not visualized. This is especially important since an abnormality may reside in a nonopacified ureteral segment without causing any abnormality in the visualized proximal ureter.

Within 5 minutes after bolus injection, a small

amount of contrast agent can usually be seen in the bladder; progressive filling is found on subsequent films. The bladder does not usually distend to maximal capacity during the time allowed for routine urography. When the bladder is incompletely distended, care must be taken in interpreting trabeculation of the bladder wall. Therefore, unless the wall is grossly thickened and irregular with cellules or diverticula, the diagnosis of bladder trabeculation is best left to the cystoscopist.

Densely opacified urine may obscure pathologic findings in the full bladder. Therefore, the postvoiding film should always be scrutinized for filling defects as well as for degree of emptying; also, mucosal detail is better evaluated in the postvoid view.

VOIDING CYSTOURETHROGRAPHY

Voiding cystourethrography (VCUG) is a technique for studying the lower urinary tract by filling the bladder with contrast material in a manner designed to simulate the normal physiologic filling of the bladder by urine. Voiding is then observed and recorded. This allows evaluation of the capacity, contour, and mucosal detail of the bladder; filling defects within the bladder; the presence or absence of vesicoureteral reflux; urethral anatomy; sphincter function; and postvoiding residual.

INDICATIONS

Indications for VCUG include upper urinary tract infections in children, recurrent lower urinary tract infections at any age, lower abdominal trauma (especially when pelvic fractures are involved), neurogenic dysfunction of the bladder, and suspected urethral pathology. VCUG is an especially important study in patients with urinary tract infection as it evaluates the ability of the bladder to empty completely and the competence of the ureterovesical junction in preventing reflux. When reflux does occur, it is especially important to note the presence or absence of intrarenal reflux, as this is thought to be a significant factor in subsequent renal scarring.

TECHNIQUE

No special preparation is necessary for VCUG, though the patient should void just before the examination. Sterile preparation of the glans penis in males or the periurethral area in females is then performed. While females require no local anesthesia for catheter insertion, in adult males and boys over the age of 3 to 5 years 0.5 percent lidocaine (Xylocaine) jelly can be instilled into the urethra and left in place for several minutes by application of a Zipser clamp to the distal penis. The Zipser clamp applies only very loose compression to the urethra and can also be used during the voiding study to allow greater distention of the urethra.

A self-retaining (Foley) catheter is not necessary for this study. Any small-caliber catheter that will allow a reasonably rapid flow of contrast for filling the bladder may be used. An 8 French pediatric feeding tube is ideal, as is an 8 to 12 French Robinson catheter. In catheterizing the male, resistance may be met in the region of the external sphincter. Exertion of gentle pressure at this point will eventually result in relaxation of the sphincter and easy passage of the catheter into the bladder. Any residual urine encountered in the bladder is emptied prior to progressing with the study.

The bladder is then filled with 30 percent contrast material using a gravity drip. The container of contrast medium should be positioned approximately 50 to 75 cm above the level of the bladder to allow filling without exceeding normal maximal intravesical pressure. In children, the contrast will usually stop dripping when the capacity of the bladder is reached. Another end point is the severe urge to urinate. In babies, voiding around the catheter occurs automatically when the normal capacity of the bladder is achieved. Fluoroscopic monitoring of the filling sequence should be intermittent. Filming, using a 105-mm camera or spot films, should be minimized. The bladder should be filmed when full in the anteroposterior (AP) position as well as in both oblique positions. If reflux does not occur, the renal areas are filmed to confirm this finding. If reflux does occur, the degree of this reflux should be documented, which may require a full film of the abdomen. Finally, the catheter is removed as the patient begins voiding, and the urethra is filmed during this voiding phase (AP view for females and oblique for males). The amount of residual urine in the bladder (and collecting system if reflux has occurred) on completion of voiding should also be filmed.

NORMAL FINDINGS

In males, pressure on the undersurface of the penis by the collecting vessel can result in compression of the urethra and be mistaken for a stricture. With radiopaque urinals, this artifact is easily recognized. However, a cardboard or plastic urinal may not be seen on the radiographs and may lead to misinterpretation of the study unless the radiologist is aware of this artifact. On the other hand, because of the bend in the urethra at the penoscrotal junction, the caliber of the penile urethra may normally be smaller than the caliber seen on retrograde urethrography. More proximally, during voiding the bladder neck opens 1 to 2 cm and there is moderate distention of the prostatic urethra. The membranous urethra will usually distend to approximately 7 mm in diameter in the adult, and there is loss of the normal proximal conic configuration of the bulbous urethra.

The female urethra has a variety of normal configurations but is usually seen to be ovoid or tubular during voiding. Mild funneling of the bladder base is usually noted. In the female, especially young girls, the presence and amount of vaginal reflux should be noted, as it may explain wetting after voiding.

RETROGRADE URETHROGRAPHY IN THE MALE

INDICATIONS

Indications for retrograde urethrography include trauma, obstructive symptoms not shown to be due to prostate enlargement, initial hematuria (hematuria clearing with voiding), and penile masses or fistulas.

TECHNIQUE

A small Foley catheter (10 French) is inserted into the distal urethra so that the balloon, when inflated, will be in the fossa navicularis, approximately 1 cm from the meatus. The balloon is inflated in the fossa navicularis with approximately 2 ml of saline. The patient should be in the oblique position, facing the radiologist, with the down leg flexed. The penis, with the indwelling catheter, is stretched over the flexed leg and the catheter is placed on mild traction by taping it to the thigh. This allows a tangential study of the urethra.

Using a 50-ml syringe, 30 percent contrast is injected under fluoroscopic control. Steady gentle pressure on the syringe will usually overcome external sphincter resistance and allow opacification of the posterior urethra. Two or three films are obtained during the injection procedure.

NORMAL FINDINGS

In the normal urethra, important landmarks are the symmetric conical shape of the proximal bulbous urethra, the verumontanum (visualized as an ovoid filling defect within the distal prostatic urethra), and the bladder neck. The membranous urethra can be consistently localized between the tip of the cone of the bulbous urethra and the most distal portion of the verumontanum [27]. During retrograde studies, the membranous and posterior segments of the urethra are poorly distended. Therefore, unless there is gross irregularity in the region of the membranous urethra, it is difficult to diagnose stricture in this area. Filling defects in the posterior urethra can usually be easily seen. The internal sphincter at the level of the bladder neck can be delineated by a jet of contrast medium flowing into the bladder. Generally speaking, however, retrograde urethrography best demonstrates the anterior urethra.

Several normal variations can be seen during urethrography. A slight annular constriction of the proximal bulbous urethra below the cone is due to contraction of the musculus compressor nuda. This is physiologic and should not be misconstrued as a stricture. On rare occasions, the bulbocavernosus muscle can flatten or actually indent the floor of the proximal and mid bulbous urethra. This indentation is smooth and extraluminal.

RETROGRADE FEMALE URETHROGRAPHY (DOUBLE-BALLOON URETHROGRAM)

INDICATIONS

This technique is usually performed for the demonstration of a suspected urethral diverticulum that has not been visualized by conventional techniques such as the postvoid film from a urogram or voiding cystourethrogram [18].

TECHNIQUE

The double-balloon catheter is basically a Foley catheter with a second proximal inflatable balloon. One such catheter has inflatable balloons that are fixed in position. Another catheter has a proximal inflatable balloon that is movable on the shaft of the catheter. The latter catheter is preferred since the movable balloon provides better isolation of the urethra.

The catheter is passed into the bladder and the distal balloon is inflated and seated gently at the bladder neck. The second balloon is inflated outside the patient and then moved along the shaft of the catheter until it is seated snugly against the external urethral meatus. Contrast medium injected under fluoroscopic control flows out of the catheter only through a side hole between the two balloons, thus opacifying the urethra (Fig. 3-7). This should be performed under fluoroscopic control, and spot films are obtained in various obliquities to document the appearance of the urethra.

Figure 3-7. Double-balloon female urethrogram. Contrast medium enters the urethra via the catheter opening between the balloons occluding the bladder neck and external urethral meatus. If present, a urethral diverticulum (arrow) is usually found communicating with the urethra posteriorly.

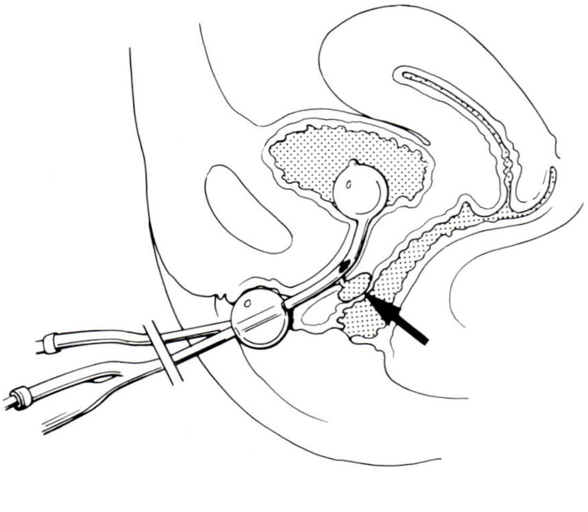

NORMAL AND ABNORMAL FINDINGS

The female urethra is seen as a poorly distensible, tubular or ovoid structure. Rounded collections of contrast adjacent to the urethra are consistent with a diverticulum. These are more commonly seen in the middle or distal portions of the urethra posteriorly but can also occur adjacent to the proximal urethra or even anterior to the urethra.

RETROGRADE PYELOGRAPHY AND URETEROPYELOGRAPHY

INDICATIONS

Indications for retrograde studies of the upper urinary tract usually include incomplete opacification of portions of the upper tracts during urography in patients with hematuria, or a need for visualization of the upper tracts in patients for whom urography is contraindicated. Another reason for performing a retrograde study is to delineate the point of ureteral obstruction that has not been well demonstrated on a urogram.

Retrograde studies are generally felt to be safe in patients who have previously demonstrated a reaction to intravenous contrast material. In the typical retrograde study, less than 10 ml of contrast medium is used, and it has been shown that less than 1 percent of this is absorbed via the urothelium [26]. While it is conceivable that a reaction to this amount of absorbed contrast medium might occur, in reality, contrast reactions following retrograde studies are exceedingly rare.

TECHNIQUE

These studies are performed by the urologist using a cystoscope. In retrograde pyelography, a small-caliber catheter is passed through the length of the ureter to the renal pelvis. Three to five milliliters of contrast material is then injected for opacification of the intrarenal collecting system. As the catheter is withdrawn, contrast medium can be continually injected, resulting in a "pullout" ureterogram. Retrograde ureteropyelography is accomplished by inserting a bulb-tipped catheter into the ureteral orifice, thus occluding it. Seven to ten milliliters of contrast medium is then injected for opacification of the ureter and intrarenal collecting system. After either procedure, a drainage film is obtained after 10 to 15 minutes. These studies are usually submitted to the radiologist for formal interpretation.

NORMAL AND ABNORMAL FINDINGS

Although attempts are made to flush the catheters with contrast before performing the study, it is not unusual to see air bubbles in the ureter or intrarenal collecting system in retrograde studies. These are rounded in configuration and usually change position on serial films.

Since these studies are frequently performed without fluoroscopic control, on rare occasions there will be overdistention of the intrarenal collecting system with extravasation ("backflow") of contrast into various structures (Fig. 3-8). The most common type of extravasation is pyelosinus. In this case, there is rupture of the fornix of one or more calices with tracking of contrast medium into the renal sinus and possibly through the renal hilum. Contrast material thus may be seen surrounding the proximal ureter. Pyelovenous backflow results in opacification of the renal vein, which is seen as a band of contrast angling obliquely upward toward the vena cava from the renal hilum. Pyelolymphatic backflow causes opacification of the renal hilar lymphatics, which are seen as thin irregular bands of contrast medium extending horizontally from the calices or renal hilum. Pyelotubular backflow implies opacification of the collecting ducts in the papilla. These are seen as thin streaks of contrast medium radiating fanlike from the tip of the papilla. Pyelointerstitial backflow is contrast material extravasated into the interstitium of the kidney. This has a more amorphous appearance than pyelotubular backflow, and contrast medium may track through the entire thickness of the renal parenchyma and collect in the subcapsular area. The final type of extravasation is pyelocancerous or pyelotumoral. This occurs when a necrotic process in the kidney, such as a hemorrhagic

Figure 3-8. Various types of "backflow" that can be seen during retrograde studies. Pyelotubular backflow can also be found in cases of severe vesicoureteral reflux, and pyelosinus backflow (extravasation) is not uncommon with ureteral obstruction.

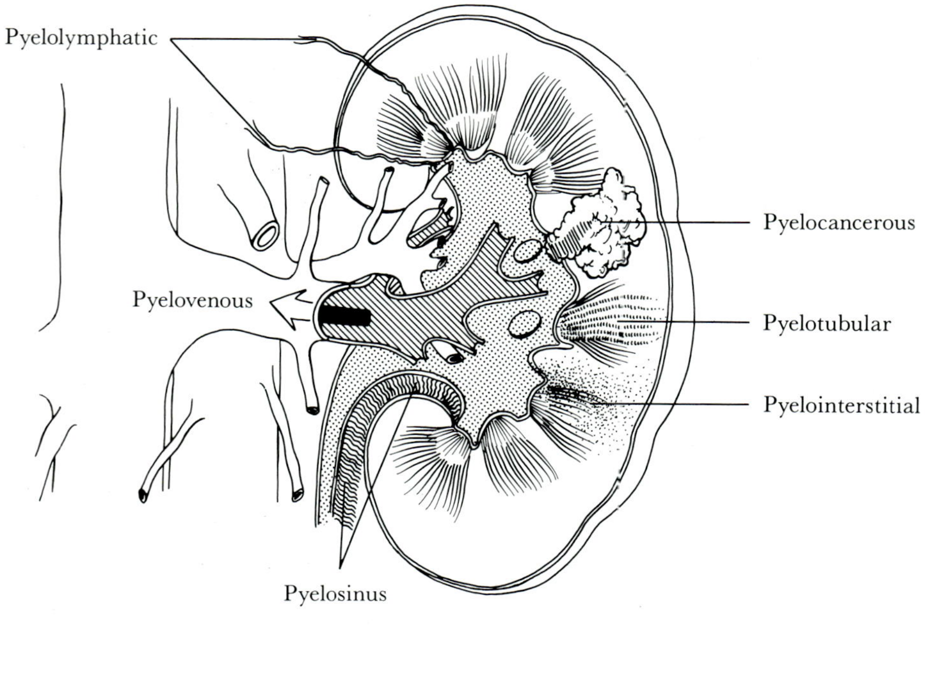

renal-cell carcinoma or tuberculous abscess, ruptures into the collecting system. On retrograde studies, contrast medium can be seen filling an irregular cavity adjacent to the collecting system. When this last pattern is seen, an obvious abnormality of the kidney should be reported. The other types of extravasation are usually not clinically significant.

LOOPOGRAPHY

INDICATIONS

Radiographic evaluation of the patient with a bowel conduit urinary diversion usually involves only excretory urography. This study establishes stability of the upper tracts. However, progressive dilatation, inflammatory scarring, or stone formation in the upper tracts are indications for loopography. Other indications include stomal stenosis, hematuria, and positive urine cytology.

Most bowel conduit urinary diversions are constructed using small-bowel segments. On occasion, large-bowel conduits may be seen. Small-bowel conduits are constructed to be freely refluxing, while large-bowel conduits have antirefluxing ureteroconduit anastomoses [36]. More recently, urinary diversion has been accomplished by continent pouches constructed from bowel segments.

TECHNIQUE

Loopography of small-bowel conduits is performed using a 14 French Foley catheter with a 5-ml balloon inflated in the conduit below the level of the fascia [3]. The catheter is placed on gentle traction to occlude outflow and is then filled with 30 percent contrast material by gravity drip under fluoroscopic control. In large-bowel conduits, a larger catheter with a 30-ml balloon is used. The study is then conducted in similar fashion to that described for small-bowel loops. The technique for studying continent pouches, while similar to the above, is described in detail in Chap. 26.

NORMAL AND ABNORMAL FINDINGS

Loopography defines the length, position, luminal size, and integrity of the conduit as well as the presence or absence of reflux (Fig. 3-9).

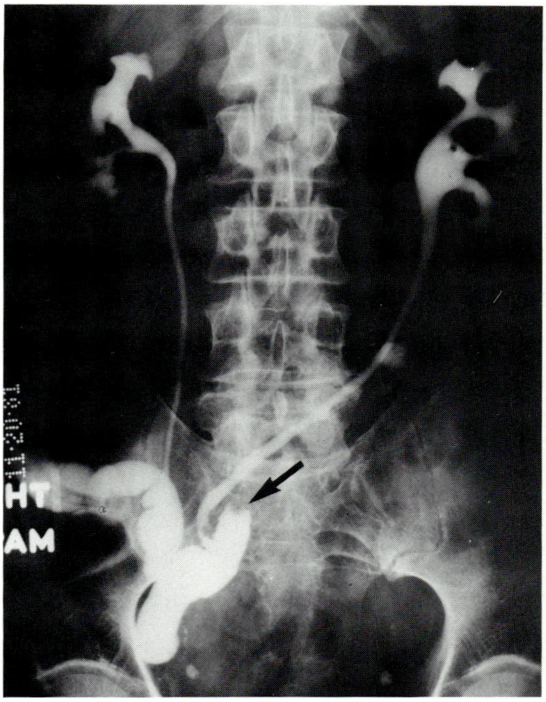

Figure 3-9. Normal loopogram. Contrast agent has filled the conduit via a Foley catheter. Bilateral reflux results in minimal fullness of the upper tracts. Small defect in proximal end of loop (arrow) is a construction artifact due to multiple-layer closure.

The ability of the conduit to empty can be assessed by drainage films or by fluoroscopy. Complete emptying requires active peristalsis, and this can be evaluated easily under fluoroscopy. Persistent narrowing or fixation of the conduit may represent fibrosis and should be reported, as should any persistent filling defects. In large-bowel conduits, reflux, if it occurs, will usually be seen at high conduit pressures. These pressures can be determined by incorporating a simple manometer in the drip line with its base at the level of the conduit. In a freely refluxing conduit, mild dilatation of the upper tracts is commonly seen [10].

When there is absence of reflux at loopography in a small-bowel conduit, obstruction is likely. Since urography may not have adequately visualized the obstructed upper tracts, percutaneous antegrade pyelography may be necessary for further delineation of the obstructed system.

STENTOGRAPHY

INDICATIONS

Ureteral stents are often placed in retrograde fashion for relief of an obstructive lesion of the ureter. Stents may also be placed at the time of surgical repair of ureteropelvic junction obstruction or any procedure requiring ureteral anastomosis. Stentography allows determination of the patency and adequate drainage of the upper urinary tract.

TECHNIQUE AND FINDINGS

If stents have been externalized through the urethra or skin, stentography can be performed by dripping 30 percent contrast medium through the distal end of the stent. This procedure allows visualization of the intrarenal collecting system. If drainage is adequate, no dilatation will be seen. After opacification of the intrarenal collecting system, the drip is continued and contrast material is visualized fluoroscopically as it opacifies the ureter around the stent. This allows visualization of any operative site for edema and obstruction or for extravasation. Flank pain or increasing distention of the intrarenal collecting system are indications that the procedure should be halted. Otherwise, the end point of the study is complete visualization of the upper urinary tract with passage of contrast around the stent into the bladder. Once the upper tract is maximally opacified, overhead films should be obtained to demonstrate the urinary tract in toto. This is most effective when obtained with the drip still running at a slow rate. A drainage film should be obtained 10 to 15 minutes after completion of the study to ensure that the stent is providing adequate drainage.

NEPHROSTOGRAPHY

INDICATIONS

Nephrostomy tubes may be placed percutaneously or at the time of surgical procedures that involve the collecting system. A nephrostogram is usually obtained prior to removing the tube to ensure that drainage is adequate and that there is no extravasation.

TECHNIQUE AND FINDINGS

This study should be performed with the drip technique previously described and monitored fluoroscopically. As with stentography, flank pain or increasing distention of the collecting system during the study should prompt cessation of the drip. Extravasation, when seen, should be documented in multiple oblique views if necessary to determine its exact point of origin. Without obstruction or extravasation, the intrarenal collecting system will opacify and contrast material will be seen passing down the ureter to the bladder. If this is the case, the nephrostomy tube should be clamped and a drainage film obtained in 10 to 15 minutes to ensure physiologic emptying of the upper tract.

ANTEGRADE PYELOGRAPHY

Direct opacification of the intrarenal collecting system and ureter may be accomplished by injecting contrast through a needle inserted percutaneously into the collecting system specifically for this purpose. Imaging guidance may be performed by fluoroscopy, CT, or ultrasound. Choice of the imaging modality depends on the procedure ultimately to be performed. If antegrade pyelography is the only procedure, fluoroscopy alone may be used. Alternatively, a portable ultrasound device may be used to localize the intrarenal collecting system.

Percutaneous needle puncture of the collecting system is usually performed with the patient in the prone or prone oblique position. In general, a track should be planned so that the needle traverses renal parenchyma and enters a calix rather than entering the wall of the renal pelvis directly after passing through the perinephric space; also, an approach directly into the renal pelvis risks puncturing the major renal blood vessels. A slight oblique rather than direct posterior approach is usually preferable, in order not to puncture the paraspinous muscles. The needle track should also be subcostal whenever possible; although occasionally a superiorly located kidney may require an intracostal approach, the latter carries a higher risk of pneumothorax. A 22-gauge needle of appropriate length is satisfactory for this study.

Providing the above rules are followed, the exact site of puncture of the intrarenal collecting system is not critical for antegrade pyelography. If, however, the needle track is subsequently to be used as a track for ureteral catheterization, the path of the needle becomes more important, and is critical if percutaneous nephrostomy, stone extraction, or ureteral stenting is planned.

After satisfactory needle placement, 30 percent contrast medium is injected and fluoroscopic monitoring is performed until the collecting system is sufficiently opacified to answer the clinical question necessitating the exam. The study should be stopped if contrast medium extravasation is seen or the patient complains of pain in association with distention of the collecting system.

All patients should give informed consent and should have appropriate blood coagulation studies performed. The puncture should be made using sterile technique and local lidocaine anesthesia; systemic sedation or analgesia is usually not necessary for simple antegrade pyelography, at least in adults.

THE WHITAKER TEST

The Whitaker test is designed to measure ureteral resistance to the flow of urine and thus to provide a measure of upper urinary tract obstruction. It measures resistance by recording the pressures of fluid in the renal pelvis and in the bladder as the fluid is flowing down the ureter at a constant rate and thus has the advantage of directly quantitating ureteral obstruction. It is, however, an invasive test and provides no estimation of renal function.

To perform the Whitaker test, there must be direct access to the lumen of the renal pelvis or a calix and to the lumen of the bladder (Fig. 3-10). The latter is usually provided by catheterizing the bladder through the urethra; the former can be accomplished either by needle puncture of the collecting system or by using an indwelling

Figure 3-10. Whitaker test. Dilute contrast material is pumped into the collecting system via a percutaneously placed needle. When a steady state is reached (collecting system completely opacified and configuration stable) for a given flow rate (usually 10 ml/min), pressures are measured via the percutaneous needle and bladder catheter. The difference in these pressures is the resistance to flow that urine encounters between the renal pelvis and the bladder.

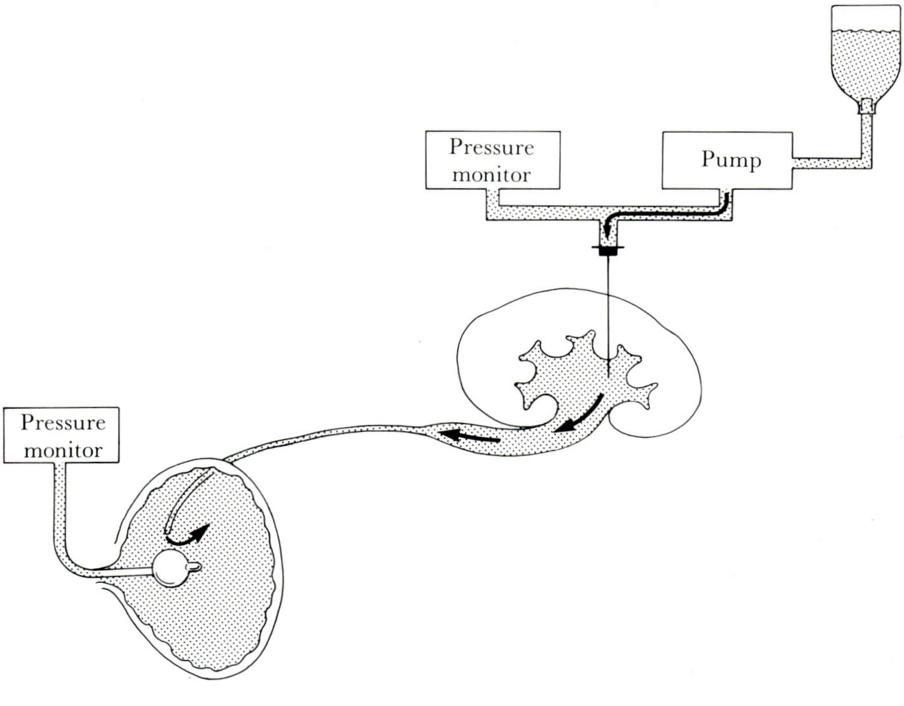

nephrostomy catheter in any patient who has had one inserted for other reasons.

The test is usually performed on a fluoroscopy table with the patient in the prone position. Fluid (either saline or dilute contrast medium) is infused into the renal collecting system; contrast medium permits fluoroscopy and radiography of the ureter as the test progresses. Fluid is commonly infused at the rate of 10 ml per minute, and the fluid flow is maintained long enough to reach a steady state—that is, long enough to reach a constant volume of the collecting system and constant flow rate down the ureter into the bladder. The bladder is usually drained. If the nephrostomy tube is a large-bore catheter, pressure in the collecting system can be measured simultaneously with the infusion of fluid; if the fluid is infused through a needle, the infusion must be halted for a few seconds in order for pressure to be measured through the needle. Pressure in the bladder should be measured simultaneously with measurements of pressure in the collecting system. Fluid infusion may be accomplished by any simple pump, or may even be performed using a large-capacity syringe that is steadily emptied at an appropriate rate, determined by watching a clock. Pressures may be measured by simple water manometers or by using calibrated electronic pressure transducers. The perfusion pressure is calculated by subtracting the bladder pressure from the renal pelvic pressure; at a flow rate of 10 ml per minute, this pressure should not exceed 13 cm H_2O in normal subjects. Pressures above this level indicate varying degrees of partial obstruction. The examination should not be attempted in patients with complete ureteral obstruction.

PERCUTANEOUS NEPHROSTOMY

Percutaneous access to the intrarenal collecting system [16, 30] has now become not only a common procedure for draining an obstructed upper urinary tract, but also a common way to provide access to the collecting system and ureter for a variety of therapeutic techniques.

Preprocedure preparation of the patient should be carried out as for antegrade pyelography. A route that avoids traversing the major paraspinal muscle groups should be planned. The route should be subcostal if possible (intracostal access routes are occasionally necessary, but run the risk of traversing the pleural space), should traverse renal parenchyma rather than puncturing the collecting system directly, and if possible should enter a calix rather than the renal pelvis. When it is intended to follow the procedure by attempts to stent the ureter or remove collecting system stones, a collecting system entry site and direction should be planned so that the catheter that enters the collecting system should be pointing toward the proximal ureter or toward the calix that it ultimately needs to reach.

A number of technical variations have been described for inserting catheters. The most common one involves placing a 0.038-in. guide wire into the collecting system. This may be performed in several ways. After the collecting system has been opacified (possibly through a 22-gauge needle puncture), an 18-gauge needle is inserted along the planned nephrostomy track and the guide wire is inserted through it. Conical dilators of increasing size are serially passed over the wire into the collecting system; finally, a nephrostomy tube—often an 8.3 French pigtail catheter—is passed over the guide wire, and the guide wire is subsequently removed. Alternatively, a 0.018-in. guide wire may be inserted into the collecting system through a 22-gauge needle; after the needle is removed, a special dilator whose end hole is the appropriate size for the 0.018-in. guide wire, but that also has a side hole through which a 0.038-in. guide wire can be advanced, is inserted over the smaller guide wire. The smaller guide wire is removed and the larger one is inserted through the side hole; once the dilator is removed, the larger guide wire is used in the same way as described above. Finally, a system is available in which a 22-gauge needle is first inserted along the planned nephrostomy track; over it a 18-gauge needle is placed coaxially, the 22-gauge needle is removed, and a 0.038-in. guide wire is inserted through the 18-gauge needle; the guide wire ultimately serves to permit dilation of the upper tract and insertion of the final nephrostomy tube.

For some procedures, a large nephrostomy

track is required; these procedures include stone extraction, percutaneous ultrasound stone disintegration, and nephroscopy. For these, either serial dilators or balloon dilators can be used, each guided by a 0.038-in. wire, so that ultimately a large-bore sheath may be inserted into the collecting system to provide a route for grasping devices, scopes, and ultrasound contact lithotriptors.

RENAL CYST PUNCTURE

Diagnostic puncture of renal space-occupying lesions that are thought probably to be benign cysts, but that may be tumors, is performed much less frequently than it was prior to the advent of high-quality ultrasound and CT. It is occasionally thought to be necessary, however, so the technique is worth a brief review.

As with any invasive procedure, informed consent, coagulation studies, sterile technique, and local lidocaine anesthesia should be used. The examination is almost always performed with the patient in the prone position; the needle track should be planned to avoid the renal hilar vessels, pleural space, liver, spleen, and gut. Ultrasound, CT, and fluoroscopy have all been used to guide the puncture. A 22-gauge needle of adequate length should be used.

When the needle enters the lesion, several milliliters of fluid should be aspirated. The color, consistency, and odor of the fluid should be recorded; mandatory laboratory examinations include cytologic examination and culture and sensitivity. If no fluid can be aspirated from the lesion, and imaging shows that the needle tip is without question in the lesion, biopsy should be performed by using a syringe to apply strong suction while twisting the needle and inserting and withdrawing it for short distances through the lesion.

If the lesion is cystic, radiographs of the interior should be performed by replacing aspirated fluid with an equal volume of soluble contrast. Fluoroscopy-guided radiographs should be obtained in all possible obliquities so that as many of the lesion margins as possible are demonstrated on the film. After radiography, as much of the fluid should be aspirated from the lesion as possible prior to removing the needle.

TECHNIQUES OF URINARY TRACT ULTRASOUND

Ultrasound examination of the urinary tract has developed to the point at which it is a mainstay of urinary tract imaging practice [4, 14, 33]. The choices of proper instrumentation and technique are critical; at this time, it has become a cliché to state that the examination is very operator-dependent; the real thrust of this comment is that it is not only important to use the correct equipment and proper technique [17] but also that in order to do successful urinary tract examination it is essential that the examiner be experienced in performing urinary tract ultrasound, be able to acquire the best possible images, and be sufficiently well versed in urinary tract diseases so that each examination is certain to include all of the appropriate anatomic parts.

INSTRUMENTATION

Real-time gray-scale devices are now the norm for all transabdominal imaging of the urinary tract. The well-known principle that higher-frequency transducers produce finer detail but less penetration must be kept in mind, so that the highest-frequency transducer capable of imaging the appropriate parts of the urinary tract should be chosen for each patient and for each segment of the examination. In adults, 2.25-MHz or 3.5-MHz transducers are usually appropriate for transabdominal scanning; transrectal imaging of the prostate and imaging of the scrotum require 7.0-MHz to 10.0-MHz transducers.

Doppler ultrasound can detect the flow of blood in vascular structures, and by virtue of frequency shifts and flow characteristics is useful in detecting arterial stenoses, venous thrombi, the vascular nature of various cystic-appearing lesions, and other vascular diseases.

POSITIONING

The right kidney is usually best imaged using the liver as an acoustic window. Imaging is usually begun with the patient supine. Coronal or anterior sagittal views, or angled views between the two, and transverse views of the kidney are recorded. Turning the patient toward the left lateral decubitus position may be helpful. The right adrenal may not be visualized in all cases when it is normal; the enlarged right adrenal is usually visible, however; an anterior view that demonstrates the adrenal immediately posterior to the inferior vena cava is usually best. In some patients, posterior views of the kidney obtained with the patient in a prone position may provide satisfactory images.

The left kidney is slightly more difficult to demonstrate, since gas in the stomach and splenic flexure often obscure the kidney. The spleen may be used as an acoustic window, so that a lateral approach is often necessary for transverse and longitudinal views of the kidney. The right lateral decubitus position may aid in demonstrating the kidney; occasionally, posterior views in prone patients may image the kidney as well. When it is normal the left adrenal is more difficult to visualize with certainty than the right; again, left lateral views in the supine or right lateral decubitus position are usually the best. Both kidneys are usually easiest to see in suspended inspiration.

The normal ureters cannot be visualized by ultrasound; dilated ureters may or may not be visible in their retroperitoneal course, depending on the body habitus and the amount of gas in the individual patient. The most proximal portion of a dilated ureter may be seen in examinations of the kidney; the distal centimeter or two of each ureter may be visualized through the bladder when it is distended with urine. The bladder itself is best demonstrated by the transabdominal route; although the bladder is best demonstrated when filled, scanning immediately after voiding may be useful if an estimate of postvoid residual is desired. Although some experimental work has been done with transurethral imaging of the bladder wall via transducers in the bladder lumen, this technique is not in common clinical use.

Transrectal imaging is the method of choice for displaying the prostate, although a gross estimate of prostate size may be achieved by transvesical imaging. Transrectal probes may be linear array, phased array, or mechanical sector scanners and may produce images that are either transverse or longitudinal. There is no real consensus regarding whether longitudinal or transverse scanning is better; when time and equipment permit, the best prostate examinations are probably performed with imaging in both planes. Imaging is performed with a 7.0-MHz transducer that is covered with a condom before being inserted into the rectum; the space between the transducer and the condom is filled with water and the patient is examined in the lithotomy or decubitus position. The seminal vesicles can also be easily imaged with transrectal transducers.

For ultrasound imaging or the scrotum, the patient is placed in a supine position. The scrotum should be suspended on a towel that has been stretched across the thighs; the penis may be placed in the anatomic position. A 7.5- or 10.0-MHz transducer should be used, and a water balloon or other stand-off device should be used both to improve visibility of the immediate subcutaneous structures and to make the examination more comfortable for the patient. The entirety of each hemiscrotum should be evaluated in transverse and longitudinal images.

As with CT scanning, the exact protocol to be followed with ultrasound imaging of the urinary tract depends on the clinical question to be answered and on the pathology encountered. The most important principle to follow is that when disease is encountered that may have manifestations in body parts other than that in which it is initially found, that body part should be examined as well. If a mass is encountered in the kidney or adrenal gland, masses should be carefully excluded in the other kidney or adrenal, in the liver, and in the upper retroperitoneum. If hydronephrosis is found, the upper retroperitoneum should be imaged, as should the bladder and distal ureters to search for the cause of any obstruction. When ultrasound evidence of primary tumors of the bladder or prostate are encountered, the retroperitoneum, kidneys, adrenals, and liver should be demonstrated to search for metastatic disease. Testicular abnormalities that may represent tumor should be followed with ultrasound examinations of the retroperitoneum in the region of the renal hila. Any male patient without two intrascrotal testes should have the inguinal regions and pelvis examined to search for undescended testes and any masses that may have arisen from such ectopic organs.

TECHNIQUES OF URINARY TRACT CT

Successful examination of the urinary tract by CT depends on appropriate control of tehnique [5, 23, 28]; specifically, oral and intravenous contrast agents, scan timing, slice thickness and spacing, and anatomic extent of the examination each need to be appropriate if the most accurate diagnoses are to be made.

ORAL CONTRAST

Despite the fact that many urinary tract lesions may be adequately evaluated by CT without oral contrast, most CT scans of the urinary tract should be performed with an opacified bowel. The reason for this is that unexpected masses in the peritoneal cavity may be present, and certain urinary tract lesions may protrude into anatomic regions in which they may be confused with unopacified bowel loops. On occasion oral contrast may be omitted, such as when a renal lesion discovered on a recent previous scan is being reevaluated with extra slices or with additional variations of intravenous contrast administration. But as a routine, an oral contrast agent should be administered in sufficient volume and in sufficient time prior to the scan that the entire gut can be opacified.

SLICE THICKNESS

For most scans, 1-cm slices provide sufficient anatomic resolution. Specific circumstances require thinner slices, however; when searching for small adrenal masses, when investigating a renal mass to see if it contains small amounts of fat, or when trying to eliminate partial volume averaging to determine whether a small renal lesion is enhanced after administration of intravenous contrast medium 5-mm slices may be necessary. For most applications, contigous slices should be used. For a survey of the urinary tract in which the likelihood of disease is low, slice gaps up to 1 cm may be employed.

INTRAVENOUS CONTRAST

For almost all applications in the urinary tract, intravenous contrast medium should be used. Large doses are usually not necessary; 50 ml of 50 to 60 percent contrast agent given as a bolus is usually sufficient to opacify the kidneys; excreted contrast medium from such a dose is more than adequate to opacify the ureters and bladder. Rarely, additional boluses may be necessary to distinguish between retroperitoneal nodes and vessels or to distinguish small adrenal masses from adrenal vein varices or tortuous splenic arteries. As mentioned above, scans before the administration of the contrast agent are usually not required in the urinary tract. There are specific circumstances in which these scans are necessary, however [12]. Scans without contrast are usually required to visualize faint parenchymal or renal mass calcifications; to diagnose urinary tract stones and to distinguish them from other lesions that produce filling defects in the collecting system, ureter, or bladder; and to distinguish hematomas from space-occupying lesions, which may become relatively dense after contrast administration. Renal masses should always be studied with scans both before and after administration of the contrast agent.

ANATOMIC EXTENT OF SCAN

Determination of the extent of a scan requires tailoring of the examination to meet the requirements of the specific clinical situation. When scanning the adrenals for metastatic disease, all other body parts at risk for metastases should be included. A scan protocol to search for pheochromocytoma should extend at least from the dome of the diaphragm to the base of the bladder. Scans to evaluate the adrenal glands for other benign diseases can probably be limited to the glands themselves. When scanning the kidneys, the scans may be limited to the organs or the extent of their contained pathology unless lesions are encountered that may have spread to other body parts; for example, renal cell carcinoma patients should have the entire upper abdomen scanned and probably should undergo scanning of the chest as well. Scans of structures contained in the pelvis should include the region from the iliac crest to the symphysis pubis; if the patient has lymphadenopathy from malignant pelvic disease, the scans should be extended superiorly in order to exclude other retroperitoneal lymphadenopathy. When searching for undescended testes, the scan should begin below the pubic symphysis and continue cephalad until the testis is identified or until the lower abdomen has been included. When evaluating patients with testicular tumor, the retroperitoneum at the level of the kidneys should be examined, as should the mediastinum and chest.

TECHNIQUES OF URINARY TRACT MRI

During the years in which urinary tract MRI has been developed, a variety of technique variations [11, 25], including differences in field strength, pulse sequences, slice thickness and gaps, data acquisition times, and coils, have been tried. The technique is still in a state of evolution, but many of the factors have now come into common use, so at the time of writing, most practitioners would be in general agreement with regard to technique.

MAGNETIC FIELD STRENGTH

Very-low-field magnets have not found general acceptance for urinary tract imaging. Medium-field (0.3 to 0.6 T) magnets appear to be satisfactory for imaging the upper urinary tract [8, 21, 22] and to be not unsatisfactory in imaging the bladder [15] and (provided surface coils are used) the scrotum. High-field (1.5 T) magnets are best when the particular imaging task requires T2 weighted images and relatively small fields of view and relatively thin slices and involves structures not subject to respiratory motion; the obvious application for which high-field magnets are best suited is prostate imaging. Obviously, very few practices or institutions have the luxury of magnets available at more than one field strength; if the available magnet is 1 to 1.5 T, virtually all urinary tract structures may be imaged in a satisfactory way; medium-strength magnets will be satisfactory for all imaging except high-quality prostate imaging or possibly imaging of small bladder abnormalities.

RADIOFREQUENCY COILS

Satisfactory upper urinary tract imaging can be performed using standard body coils. Although in thin or small patients the kidneys and adrenals may be sufficiently close to the skin that surface coils can be used, clear-cut clinical advantage has not been demonstrated for using these coils to image these structures. Most imaging of the pelvis and lower urinary tract has also been performed using standard body coils. At the time of writing, preliminary work has shown that intrarectal coils or sandwich-type pelvic surface coils show promise but are not in current widespread use. The scrotum, however, absolutely requires surface coils for high-quality imaging [31].

PULSE SEQUENCES

Most urinary tract imaging has been performed with standard spin–echo pulse sequences. Inversion recovery sequences have not found widespread use, and although gradient echo sequences that produce strong signals from blood moving in venous structures have been advocated for evaluating the renal veins and the inferior vena cava for thrombi, these sequences are also not universally used.

Most urinary tract MRI imaging requires T1 weighted images. For these images, the TE range should be as short as possible to maximize signal strength and remove as much T2 weighting as possible from the images. The TR is less critical; very few important abnormalities are visible on strongly T1 weighted images that are not also visible on images with only moderate T1 weighting. TRs as long as 600 or 700 msec have no significant disadvantages with regard to shorter TRs and can provide images with satisfactory signal levels [24]. The number of signal acquisitions, or measurements, chosen involve the usual compromise between signal to noise level and imaging time; four groups of measurements, or numbers of acquisitions, are commonly used for T1 weighted images.

T2 weighted images are essential in imaging the scrotum, prostate [7], and bladder wall; when imaging the kidney, T2 weighted images may be omitted if T1 weighted images are normal, and it is not certain that T2 weighted images are even always necessary for characterization of renal lesions detected on T1 weighted images. T2 weighted images should always be added to T1 weighted images in imaging adrenal masses. TR values ranging from 1,800 to 2,500 msec have been advocated for spin–echo

T-2 weighted imaging; despite the longer imaging time required for the longer values, longer TRs may be useful for high-field magnets in order to remove as much T-1 weighting as possible. TEs of approximately 100 msec are useful; with stronger magnets, the increased T-2 weighting associated with TEs as long as 130 msec may be advantageous. Constraints on imaging time usually limit the number of measurements or acquisitions to two when long TRs are used.

SLICE THICKNESS, SPACING, AND ORIENTATION

The increased anatomic resolution made possible by decreasing slice thickness is offset by a decrease in signal-to-noise ratio. Therefore, in structures in which areas of abnormalities may be relatively large, the slice thickness should usually not be reduced below 1 cm. But when the abnormalities to be imaged are small, such as small adrenal masses or small focal abnormalities in the prostate, slices as thin as 5 mm may be necessary. The gaps or spaces between slices also require compromise: although small gaps or contiguous slices reduce the possibility of missing small lesions, effects from adjacent slices may add unwanted T1 weighting to the images and cause overall image degradation. This problem may be avoided by retaining gaps between slices of at least several millimeters in thickness or by interleaving contiguous slices. When imaging the adrenal and kidney, transverse slices are almost always sufficient and have the advantage of producing images comparable in anatomic display to those produced by C.T. Occasionally, sagittal or coronal images may be useful in distinguishing adrenal from upper-pole renal masses, in demonstrating extensive caval thrombi, and in evaluating planes between tumors and adjacent viscera. In the bladder, transverse slices image the anterior, posterior, and lateral walls well, but coronal or sagittal images may be necessary to evaluate lesions involving the dome or base of the organ. When imaging the prostate, T2 weighted images may be required in the coronal and sagittal as well as the transverse plane. Surface coil imaging of the scrotum is most often best accomplished with coronal images.

TECHNIQUES OF URINARY TRACT ANGIOGRAPHY

The techniques of introducing catheters into the abdominal vasculature [13, 34] are beyond the scope of this book, as are intravascular therapeutic procedures and pharmacoangiography. Some information regarding the specifics of radiographic visualization of the renal vasculature are in order, however.

Aortography plays a part in searching for supernumerary renal arteries. This may be necessary prior to renal transplantation or partial nephrectomy and in evaluating patients for arterial stenosis located at the renal artery orifices. For this technique, 50 ml of 76 percent contrast agent injected at 25 ml/sec usually provides a satisfactory contrast dose; filming in slightly oblique projections may be necessary to visualize the renal artery orifices adequately. A filming sequence that is often satisfactory consists of three exposures per second for 2 seconds, followed by two exposures per second for 2 seconds and one exposure per second for 4 to 6 seconds.

Selective renal arteriograms may be performed using 10 ml of 76 percent contrast agent injected at 5 ml/sec or 14 ml of contrast agent given at 7 ml/sec. Several filming runs may be necessary. Anteroposterior and both posterior oblique views may be necessary. Exposures may be obtained at two exposures per second for 4 seconds followed by one exposure per second for 6 seconds. Contrast dose may be markedly reduced if digital subtraction angiography [20] is used; there is at least moderate loss of high-frequency spatial resolution when this technique is used, however. Digital subtraction aortography has been found useful by some radiologists, especially for screening for renal artery stenosis.

RENAL VENOGRAPHY

If direct opacification of the renal vein is necessary, this vessel may be catheterized and opacified; an injection and filming technique that usually suffices consists of injection of 15 to 30 ml of 76 percent contrast medium at 15 to 20 ml/sec; three films per second are obtained for 4 seconds. If the intrarenal branches of the renal vein need to be opacified, flow in them may be reduced by the administration into the renal artery of 12 μg of epinephrine [1] immediately prior to venous injection.

NUCLEAR MEDICINE TECHNIQUES

Nuclear medicine studies have multiple applications in evaluating the genitourinary system. However, they are usually performed by specialists in this area [9, 29, 32]. Their sophistication and computer-aided analysis further remove an in-depth discussion of these techniques beyond the scope of this book. Rather, the indications for specific radionuclide examinations and a review of the expected findings will be discussed in the chapters covering various disease processes that might be more clearly defined by the use of these studies.

REFERENCES

1. Abrams, H.L. The response of neoplastic renal vessels to epinephrine in man. *Radiology* 82:217, 1964.
2. Amis, E.S., Jr. Excretory Urography. In J.M. Taveras and J.T. Ferrucci (eds.), *Radiology: Diagnosis-Imaging-Intervention.* Philadelphia: Lippincott, 1989.
3. Amis, E.S., Jr., Cronan, J.J., and Pfister, R.C. Filling defects in small bowel urinary conduits. *A.J.R.* 137:787, 1981.
4. Amis, E.S., Jr., and Hartman, D.S. Renal ultrasonography 1984: A practical overview. *Radiol. Clin. North Am.* 22:315, 1984.
5. Aronberg, D.J. Techniques. In J.K.T. Lee S.S. Sagel, and R.J. Stanley (eds.), *Computed Body Tomography.* New York: Raven, 1983.
6. Cantwell, K.G., and Press, H.C., Jr. Evaluation of the renal outline by excretory urography. *Radiology* 137:223, 1980.
7. Carrol, C.L., et al. The abnormal prostate: MR imaging at 1.5 T with histopathologic correlation. *Radiology* 163:521, 1987.
8. Choyke, P.L., et al. Focal renal masses: Magnetic resonance imaging. *Radiology* 152:471, 1984.
9. Conway, J.J., et al. Detection of vesicoureteral reflux with radionuclide cystography. *A.J.R.* 115:720, 1972.
10. Cronan, J.J., et al. Renal obstruction in patients with ileal loops: US evaluation. *Radiology* 158:647, 1986.
11. Dikengil, A., and Newhouse, J.H. Urinary Tract Magnetic Resonance Imaging. In J.M. Taveras and J.T. Ferrucci (eds.), *Radiology: Diagnosis-Imaging-Intervention.* Philadelphia: Lippincott, 1989.
12. Englestad, B., McClennan, B.L., and Levitt, R.G. The role of precontrast images in CT of the kidney. *Radiology* 136:153, 1980.
13. Fankuchen, E., Techniques of Renal Angiography. In J.M. Taveras and J.T. Ferrucci (eds.), *Radiology: Diagnosis-Imaging-Intervention.* Philadelphia: Lippincott, 1989.
14. Feinberg, H.J. Renal ultrasound: Anatomy and technique. *Semin. Ultrasound* 2:7, 1981.
15. Fisher, M.R., et al. Urinary bladder MR imaging. II. Neoplasm. *Radiology* 157:471, 1984.
16. Goodwin, W.E., Casey, W.C., and Woolf, W. Percutaneous trocar (needle) nephrostomy in hydronephrosis. *J.A.M.A.* 157:891, 1955.
17. Grant, D. Ultrasound of the Genitourinary Tract. In J.M. Taveras and J.T. Ferrucci (eds.), *Radiology: Diagnosis-Imaging-Intervention.* Philadelphia: Lippincott, 1989.
18. Greenberg, M., et al. Female urethral diverticula: Double-balloon catheter study. *A.J.R.* 136:259, 1981.
19. Hattery, R.R., et al. Intravenous urographic technique. *Radiology* 167:593, 1988.
20. Hillman, B.J., et al. Digital video subtraction angiography of renal vascular abnormalities. *Radiology* 139:277, 1981.
21. Hricak, H., et al. Magnetic resonance imaging in the diagnosis and staging of renal and perirenal neoplasms. *Radiology* 154:709, 1985.
22. Hricak, H., et al. Nuclear magnetic resonance imaging of the kidney: Renal masses. *Radiology* 147:765, 1983.
23. Lee, J.K.T., and Balfe, D.M. Pelvis. In J.K.T. Lee, S.S. Sagel and R.J. Stanley (eds.), *Computed Body Tomography.* New York: Raven, 1983.
24. Lee, J.K.T., et al. Magnetic resonance imaging of abdominal and pelvic lymphadenopathy. *Radiology* 153:181, 1984.
25. LiPuma, J.P. Magnetic resonance imaging of the kidney. *Radiol. Clin. North Am.* 22:925, 1984.
26. Lytton, B., Brooks, M.B., and Spencer, R.P. Absorption of contrast material from the urinary tract during retrograde pylography. *J. Urol.* 100:779, 1968.
27. McCallum, R.W. The adult male urethra. *Radiol. Clin. North Am.* 17:227, 1979.
28. McClennan, B.L., and Lee, J.K.T. Kidney. In J.K.T. Lee, S.S. Sagel, and R.J. Stanley (eds.), *Computed Body Tomography.* New York: Raven, 1983.
29. O'Reilly, P.H., et al. Diuresis renography in equivocal urinary tract obstruction. *Br. J. Urol.* 50:76, 1978.
30. Pfister, R.C., and Newhouse, J.H. Interventional percutaneous pyeloureteral techniques. II. Percutaneous nephrostomy and other procedures. *Radiol. Clin. North Am.* 17:351, 1979.

31. Rholl, K.S., et al. MR imaging of the scrotum with a high-resolution surface coil. *Radiology* 163:99, 1987.
32. Rosen, J.M. Scintigraphic Examination of the Urinary Tract. In J.M. Taveras, and J.T. Ferrucci (eds.), *Radiology: Diagnosis-Imaging-Intervention.* Philadelphia: Lippincott, 1989.
33. Rosenfield, A.T., et al. Ultrasound of the renal sinus: New observations. *A.J.R.* 133:441, 1979.
34. Seldinger, S. Catheter replacement of the needle in percutaneous arteriography: A new technique. *Acta Radiol.* 139:368, 1953.
35. Thornbury, J.R., Stanley, J.C., and Fryback, D.G. Hypertensive urogram: A nondiscriminatory test for renovascular hypertension. *A.J.R.* 138:43, 1982.
36. Yoder, I.C., and Pfister, R.C. Radiology of colon loop diversion: Anatomical and urodynamic studies of the conduit and ureters in children and adults. *Radiology* 127:85, 1978.

Contrast Media

PHARMACOLOGY

The contrast agents currently in widespread use for urography, computed tomography (CT), and angiography are triiodinated derivatives of benzoic acid salt (Fig. 4-1). These salts dissociate nearly completely in aqueous solution. The anion, which contain the three iodine atoms, may be diatrizoate, iothalamate, metrizoate, or iodamide; the first two of these are the most widely used in the United States. Although any given preparation has only one kind of anion, the cation may be sodium, methylglucamine (meglumine), or a mixture of the two. These contrast agents are available in a number of concentrations for urography and CT; doses ranging from 20 to 60 gm of iodine are commonly used in adults.

The practical upper limit of concentration is established by the high viscosity of the more concentrated solutions. Both the cations and the anions are monovalent, so that complete dissociation produces two osmotically active particles per molecule; since there are three iodine atoms per molecule, a solution of contrast medium contains 1.5 iodine atoms per osmotically active particle. In the concentrations commonly employed, the osmolalities of solutions of contrast medium are much higher than that of plasma.

In order to reduce the osmolality, while keeping the amount of iodine per unit volume of contrast high enough to be radiographically visible, newer contrast molecules have been designed that have a higher number of iodine atoms per osmotically active particle (see Fig. 4-1). Some of these are ionic agents, in which the anion is a dimer of benzoic acid; an example of this type is ioxaglate. Others are nonionic compounds similar in structure to the anions of the ionic monomers. The first of these to be developed was metrizamide, which is not in current widespread use for intravascular administration since it must be stored as a lyophilized powder; more practical nonionic monomers are iopamidol and iohexol.

For a given amount of iodine per milliliter of contrast agent,the iodine dimers and nonionic monomers have approximately half the osmolality of the ionic monomers, although they are still hypertonic to plasma (Table 4-1). Unfortunately, in the United States they are much more expensive than the high-osmolality agents. It is clear that the low-osmolality contrast agents produce much less pain when given intraarterially and are frequently used for angiographic studies. Any increased safety they may enjoy over the standard contrast agents when used intravenously, however, has been much more difficult to demonstrate, so they are not the most commonly used agents for urography or CT. Practices vary with regard to the accepted indications for intravenous administration of lower-osmolality contrast agents, and the decisions are usually based on a number of factors, including local standards, legal precedent, perceived safety, cost, and government policies [44]. Currently, the number of patients being given low-osmolality agents appears to be rising rapidly.

CONTRAST AGENT DISTRIBUTION AND TISSUE OPACIFICATION

The patterns of opacification of renal parenchyma and other tissues are determined by the site, dose, and duration of administration and by the pharmacodynamics of the contrast medium itself. The salient features of contrast pharmacology consist of its high solubility in water, its extremely rapid exchange between blood plasma and extracellular fluid, its exclusion from the intracellular space, and its primary excretion through the kidneys via glomerular filtration.

When injected as an intravenous bolus, all of the standard and low-osmolality contrast agents

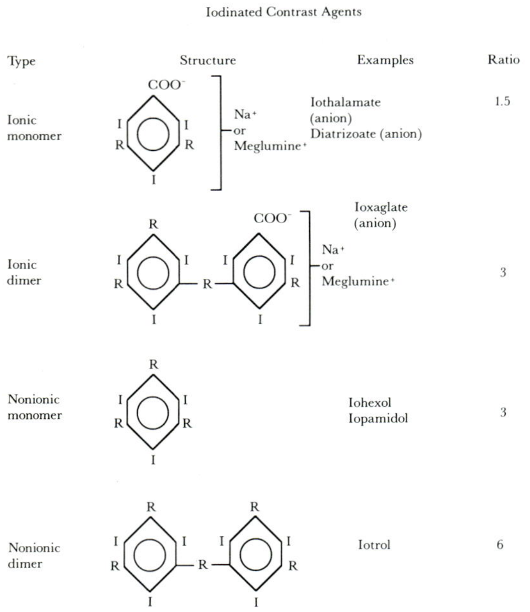

Figure 4-1. Generic formulae of contrast agents. Short side chains are denoted by the letter "R." The ratio is the number of iodine atoms per osmotically active particle.

are mixed rapidly throughout the entire blood volume, and, as soon as they are exposed to a capillary bed, diffuse very rapidly from the plasma to the extracellular space (with the exception of the brain, where the blood–brain barrier limits contrast primarily to the intravascular space).These processes cause the high concentration of contrast agent in the initial bolus to drop rapidly to a considerably lower concentration in the plasma and to reach an approximately equal concentration in the plasma in all parts of the circulation. There is also an approximate equality of concentration of contrast material between plasma and the extracellular fluid space, but since the extracellular fluid volume is much greater then the plasma volume, the total amount of contrast in the extracellular space is several times higher than that in blood. This situation is reached within a minute or two after the contrast agent is administered.

The dose and rate of administration of contrast medium affect the time course of these concentration changes considerably. In general, if different doses are given as short boluses, immediately after administration the levels of contrast medium in blood and extracellular fluid are roughly proportional to the doses. If the agent is administered as an infusion, the plasma and interstitial fluid levels begin to rise at the beginning of the infusion, at first rapidly and then more slowly; if the infusion lasts for many minutes, a steady state will be achieved with a relatively constant concentration throughout the latter part of the infusion. For a given dose, the longer the infusion, the lower will be the plasma and interstitial fluid concentrations ultimately achieved.

The opacification of tissue observed on CT examination is proportional to the total amount of contrast agent in the tissue at the instant of the scan, which consists both of the contrast material in the extravascular and intravascular spaces. Except for extremely rapid boluses and extremely rapid scanning, tissue opacification is produced to a much greater extent by extravascular than by intravascular contrast.

When contrast material reaches the kidney, it is excreted the same way that mannitol or creatinine is [55]. It is filtered at the glomerulus and neither secreted nor absorbed by the tubules. It is present in glomerular filtrate in the same concentration as in plasma. Seventy to eighty percent of filtered water is absorbed in the proximal tubule, and varying fractions of the remainder in the distal tubule. Concentration of contrast medium is many times higher in the tubular lumina and urine than in the plasma. Contrast material traverses the entire length of the nephron from glomerulus to calix within a minute or two. The kidney, therefore, is opacified by contrast in a unique combination of fluid compartments: the intravascular, extravascular, and intratubular compartments. The last of these contains by far the largest proportion of contrast agent that contributes to renal parenchymal opacification.

Opacification of the renal parenchyma is known as the nephrogram [26]. This effect is seen on almost all urograms, contrast-enhanced CT examinations, and arteriograms. If the contrast is administered intravenously, the density of the nephrogram is roughly proportional to the administered dose. The nephrogram produced by an infusion of contrast medium will never be

Table 4-1. Comparison of some commonly used standard and low-osmolality contrast agents

Product	*Manufacturer*	*Generic name*	*Iodine content (gm/100 ml)*	*Osmolality (mOsm/l)*
Standard contrast agents				
Conray	Mallinckrodt	MG iothalamate	28	1500
MD-60	Mallinckrodt	MG/Na diatrizoate	29	1539
Renografin 60	Squibb	MG/Na diatrizoate	29	1450
Hypaque Meglumine 60%	Winthrop	MG diatrizoate	28	1415
Low-osmolality contrast agents				
Hexabrix	Mallinckrodt	MG/Na ioxaglate (ionic dimer)	32	600
Optiray	Mallinckrodt	ioversol	32	702
Isovue 300	Squibb	iopamidol	30	616
Omnipaque 300	Winthrop	iohexol	30	676

MG-meglumine; Na-sodium

as dense as that produced by the same amount given as a bolus, but it will have a longer period of maximum density. Since the nephrogram is primarily produced by contrast material within intratubular fluid, and since this fluid requires a minute or two to move from glomerulus to calix, the density of the nephrogram at any instant is proportional to the average contrast concentration in plasma during the minute or two preceding the radiograph or CT image.

If rapid radiographic or CT exposures are taken after the administration of an intravenous bolus, the nephrogram will be seen first to be limited to the cortex as the fluid filtered at the glomerulus fills the proximal tubules. A minute or so later, the corticomedullary opacification difference will have disappeared, and the nephrogram will appear of approximately uniform intensity throughout the renal parenchyma. High-quality urogram films and CT images often reveal that the nephrogram subsequently becomes very slightly denser in the region of the papilla. This effect, due to final concentration of the tubular fluid in the collecting ducts, is called a "papillary blush" and is normal; it is not to be confused with the striated papillary nephrogram seen in patients with benign tubular ectasia or medullary sponge kidney.

Since the tubules concentrate contrast agent to many times the levels found in plasma because of resorbed water, but not contrast agent, from the tubular lumina, the density of the nephrogram is considerably higher than the density of tissue opacification produced in virtually any other solid tissue. This principle is worth remembering: When analyzing morphologically unusual renal lesions on CT examinations, it is a useful rule that no abnormal tissue opacifies as densely as the normal nephrogram.

The choice of contrast agent [62] has not been shown to have an effect on the nephrogram [63]. If the iodine dose, duration of administration, and site of injection are held constant, the choice of cation or anion for standard contrast agents or the use of nonionic or dimeric agents has not been shown to alter the nephrogram effect in any appreciable way [42].

Once contrast material has traversed the entire length of the tubules, it emerges through the collecting ducts into the calices. It has, by this time, become concentrated in the urine to many times the concentrations found in filtered plasma (except in the case of a selective renal arteriogram). The concentration of iodine in the urine depends on a number of factors, including the total dose, duration of administration, choice of contrast agent, state of hydration of the patient, and the time after administration that the urinary iodine level is measured.

For very low doses of contrast agent, the concentration of iodine in the urine rises as the dose rises. But at the doses currently in common use for urography and CT, the contrast material acts as an osmotic diuretic and thus lowers the amount of water that can be resorbed from the distal tubule; the increase in excreted water causes there to be little or no increase in iodine concentration as the administered doses continue to rise. However, the increased urine flow tends to cause the caliceal system to distend, so that even if an increased dose gains little in the way of urinary iodine concentration, the amount of urine in the path of an x-ray beam used to produce a urogram may continue to increase; thus the overall density of the calices and remainder of the collecting system and ureter may continue to increase as the dose rises.

Opacification of the collecting system [16, 20, 51, 71, 72] may vary depending on the choice of contrast agent. Ionic agents dissociate in solution, and though both sodium and methylglucamine are freely filtered at the glomerulus, much more sodium is resorbed than methylglucamine, so that the methylglucamine acts as an osmotic diuretic and may diminish the concentration of iodine in the resultant urine [5, 17, 23]. But the decreased concentration of urinary iodine when methylglucamine is used may be at least in part offset by the increased caliceal distention caused by the added diuresis; therefore, while some investigators have reported improved caliceal visibility using agents with sodium as a cation, others have not, and any real difference is probably slight [68]. Dimeric and nonionic agents are able to deliver a greater amount of iodine to the distal tubule for a given osmotic load, and therefore offer a slight, but real, improvement in caliceal opacification.

The contrast agents used for urography and CT examinations are excreted almost entirely via the kidneys because they are barely bound to plasma. Some degree of protein binding occurs, however, and the bound contrast material is susceptible to active uptake and excretion by hepatocytes; the small amount of contrast agent thus excreted by the liver may be seen in the delayed hepatic opacification effect seen by CT and in the opacification of the gallbladder sometimes seen when delayed films are obtained as a part of a urogram. The fraction of contrast material excreted by the liver increases as renal function decreases. This is called vicarious excretion of contrast [46].

SYSTEMIC REACTIONS TO CONTRAST AGENTS

The intravenous administration of iodinated radiographic contrast agents may produce a variety of side effects [60] that range from some very mild or subclinical effects to life-threatening ones and even death. In this section, the reactions themselves and their incidence, prophylaxis, and therapy will be discussed. The pathophysiology of most of them, about which there is continuing controversy, is beyond the scope of this book, as are the reactions caused by intraarterial contrast administration.

Minor reactions occur much more frequently than major ones [3]. A frequently quoted figure for the incidence of all reactions is about 5 percent. Estimates of the incidence of death caused by intravenous contrast medium range from 1 in 10,000 to 1 in 150,000 patients, with figures between 1 in 40,000 to 1 in 75,000 being frequently quoted [3, 31, 59, 60]. Statistical variations and differences in techniques of data acquisition probably account for the wide range of figures.

If all adverse reactions are considered together, roughly half occur between the beginning of the injection and 2 minutes after injection; almost all of the remainder have appeared within 10 minutes of the injection. Contrast reactions that appear many minutes to several hours after the injection are extremely unusual.

The minor reactions include nausea and vomiting, and integumentary reactions such as pruritus, hives, and angioneurotic edema; other symptoms include sneezing, transient dizziness, a sensation of heat throughout the entire body, a peculiar taste, and headache. Some of these tend to occur during or immediately after the injection, including nausea and vomiting, taste sensation, dizziness, and sensation of heat; these symptoms usually resolve within a minute or so after the injection ends. Others, including the development of hives, may take several minutes to appear, and the itching associated with them may persist for many minutes to several hours.

In addition to the symptoms described above, a number of subclinical physiologic alterations have been described that appear rather commonly but do not cause symptoms. These include bronchial constriction [41], electrocardiographic abnormalities [6, 35, 50, 63], and blood pressure changes. Mild asymptomatic bronchial constriction occurs in a majority of patients who receive contrast agents; bronchial constriction is slightly worse in patients who have a history of previous allergic phenomena. A variety of patterns of immediate blood pressure changes have been described after administration of contrast medium [24]. A biphasic response consisting of an initial transient rise in pressure followed by a mild and slightly more prolonged fall in base-line pressure is the most frequently described change; other patterns that have been found include biphasic changes in which a mild pressure drop is followed by a mild rise, uniphasic mild rises, or mild falls in pressure. The asymptomatic ECG changes that have been described include transient changes in heart rate (usually mild tachycardia), premature atrial and premature ventricular contractions, prolongation of the P–R interval, ST-segment depression, and short runs of ventricular tachycardia. Clearly, any of these subclinical changes may progress to symptomatic and even severe or life-threatening reactions, but they do so only infrequently

More severe reactions may be circulatory, respiratory, or neurologic. The incidence of severe reactions requiring treatment varies depending on the quoted series; a reasonable estimate for this group is approximately one in a thousand cases.

Occasionally, during attempts to inject contrast medium intravenously, it may extravasate into the subcutaneous tissues. Voluminous extravasation can be avoided virtually always if the person injecting the agent monitors the venipuncture site continuously and the contrast is injected by hand or gravity infusion. Massive extravasation may be caused if a poorly positioned needle or cannula is used with a power injector. Local pain, swelling and erythema are caused by relatively small amounts of extravasated contrast material; larger amounts may produce sloughing of skin and subcutaneous tissues.

Probably the most frequently encountered severe reaction requiring therapy is systemic hypotension. In the commonest form, hypotension is accompanied by sinus tachycardia; occasionally, severe bradycardia—presumably vagally mediated—may accompany the hypotension [65]. The hypotension may be profound, with unobtainable diastolic pressures and systolic pressures of 20 to 40 mmHg. At the extreme, there may be complete circulatory collapse with no detectable systolic pressure. A severe drop in blood pressure may be manifested by loss of consciousness; moderately severe pressure drops may be experienced by the patient as air hunger, disorientation, anxiety, or dizziness. Obviously, severe ventricular arrhythmias may also be accompanied by hypotension; vital sign monitoring and electrocardiography are needed for diagnosis. Severe hypotension may produce myocardial infarction.

Patients with severe hypotension may demonstrate a particular nephrogram effect [52]. If the hypotension appears immediately after injection of contrast, the nephrogram appears very slowly but ultimately becomes very dense and disappears slowly. If the hypotension is very severe, no nephrogram may appear at all. Alternatively, if the hypotension appears several minutes after the contrast agent is administered, the early nephrogram and pyelogram may appear normal but the nephrogram may then persist and become relatively dense (Fig. 4-2).

Respiratory reactions may involve the lower or upper airways. Bronchospasm or bronchial edema may present as wheezing, with or without shortness of breath. Laryngeal edema produces stridor and hoarseness or other voice

Figure 4-2. Severe hypotension caused by intravenous administration of contrast. This film was obtained 15 minutes after contrast was given; the patient had become very hypotensive. The nephrograms are dense and symmetrical, and there is negligible contrast in the collecting systems.

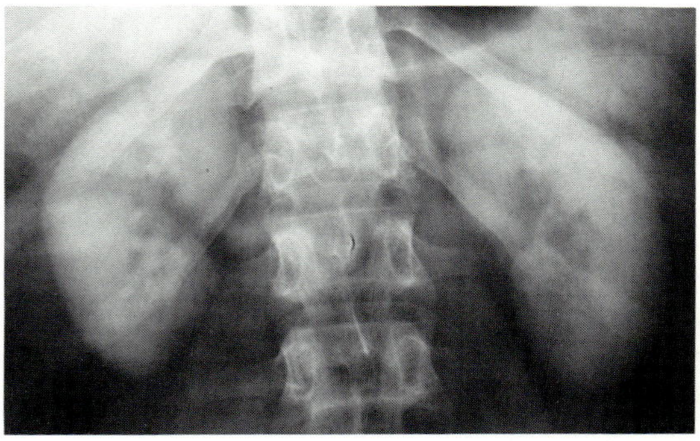

changes; very severe or sudden laryngeal edema may appear as apnea.

The most important, albeit infrequent, neurologic complication is seizure [57].

A number of factors have been proposed that, when present, place the patient in a higher-risk category. Dose and rate of administration [34] of contrast medium, at least for intravenous use and within the clinically useful ranges, do not seem to have a great effect on likelihood of severe reactions. Faster administration of a given dose does seem to increase the risk of ECG abnormalities, however [64]. Age is important; patients in the third and fourth decades seem to be at highest risk for most reactions, but elderly patients with coronary artery disease and preexisting arrhythmias are at particular risk for arrhythmias and myocardial ischemia induced by contrast agents. No sex predilection has been found. A history of asthma or allergic phenomena of any kind appears to increase the risk of reaction by approximately a factor of 2; some investigators feel that this relationship holds only for the minor reactions, however. It is thought that a history of a life-threatening previous reaction to contrast material constitutes a particular risk factor for subsequent contrast administrations; as might be expected, no large controlled series has been reported that permits estimation of the actual risk. It is important to keep in mind that no combination of factors has been shown to place a patient at high risk; since the risk of severe reactions appears to be so low for the general population of patients, the increased risk associated with histories of allergy (for example) still places an individual patient at risk of serious reaction that is much less than 1 percent. A practical approach is to assume that the risks for all patients are low, albeit variable, and that one should be prepared to treat a reaction in any patient, no matter what his history. Pretesting patients by administering small doses of contrast medium has been abandoned as a measure of risk.

Use of low-osmolality contrast agents has been proposed to decrease the risk of reaction [8, 32]. Certain minor reactions have been shown relatively conclusively to be less frequent with lower-osmolality agents; these include nausea, vomiting, and sensation of heat. The issue of whether low-osmolality contrast media carry a lower risk of life-threatening reactions or death is less easy to determine from the literature, since the incidence of these reactions is so low to begin with (and hence the statistical power of any but the largest series is marginal). In addition, the available series lack proper controls, compare figures gathered by different means, and have not standardized the doses of specific contrast agents. Nevertheless, there is a growing consensus that low-osmolality agents may really carry a lower risk of life-threatening reactions and death [36, 48, 56], but their considerably greater costs [25, 33] (at least in the United States) and the incompleteness of scientific data have prevented an immediate switch to these agents. Their use, however, is becoming unquestionably more common.

PROPHYLAXIS

Certain measures have been proposed to diminish the risk of reactions to contrast agents. Pretreatment of patients with steroids has been suggested [40]; a particularly well carried out study suggests that 32 mg of oral methylprednisolone administered 12 hours and 2 hours prior to administration of contrast medium significantly reduces the incidence of both major and minor reactions. In keeping with the theory that at least some of the observed contrast reactions are mediated by histamine release, pretreatment with cimetidine, 300 mg intravenously (IV), has been suggested, but the effectiveness of this regimen has been less well established. Pretreatment with diphenhydramine (Benadryl), although occasionally suggested to reduce the incidence of minor allergic reactions, has not been proven to be effective by any well-designed studies.

Since many preurogram or pre-CT regimens require fluid restriction, because some severe reactions involve hypotension, and since the hypotension may respond to fluid replacement, administration of intravenous fluid before administering contrast medium has also been suggested as a prophylactic measure. Straightforward as the reasoning may appear, no large series has been performed that shows this method reduces the incidence of contrast-agent–induced hypotension.

THERAPY

Many mild reactions require no specific therapy other than reassurance that the symptoms will be transient. These include nausea, vomiting, sensation of heat, and local discomfort from the injection. Certain skin reactions—particularly pruritus and hives—may be treated with diphenhydramine; 50 mg of the drug may be administered orally, intramuscularly, or intravenously. Since the hives may appear relatively rapidly, the oral and sometimes even the intramuscular routes may cause sufficiently delayed absorption so that the drug is not particularly effective. Intravenous administration of the drug is obviously the most rapidly effective; unfortunately, hypotension (as well as the more common drowsiness) may accompany the rapid administration of diphenhydramine, so the drug should not be administered indiscriminately, and patients who receive it parenterally should be monitored. Very severe integumental reactions, such as conjunctival edema or angioneurotic edema, can be treated with epinephrine (0.3 or 0.4 ml of a 1:1000 solution subcutaneously). Contrast material that extravasates in small amounts may require no more than transient elevation of the affected limb and compression of the puncture site. Large amounts of contrast material may cause necrosis and sloughing of the affected tissues no matter what first aid is applied; although many regimens involving infiltration of various drugs or enzymes into the affected regions have been described, none has been conclusively shown to be beneficial. Reconstructive plastic surgery is sometimes necessary.

Severe circulatory, respiratory, or neurologic reactions may be life threatening, but many of the therapeutic maneuvers available to treat them are not entirely without risk. Therefore, a cardinal rule of managing patients who may have severe reactions to contrast agents is to evaluate their clinical status quickly and to continue to monitor them until it is clear that the reactions and their sequelae have subsided [1]. At the very least, such assessment should include accurate vital signs monitoring, mental status checks, chest and airway auscultation, and electrocardiography. It is probably true that a significant amount of morbidity has been caused by erroneous or unnecessary treatment of patients who were thought to be having a life-threatening reaction but who in fact were not.

The main initial objective of therapy for severely hypotensive patients is to increase systemic venous cardiac return [1, 14]. The patients should immediately be placed in the Trendelenburg position, oxygen should be administered by mask, and a large-bore intravenous catheter should be inserted. (Many practitioners recommend leaving the needle used for administration of contrast medium in place for 5 or 10 minutes after the administration in order to begin intravenous therapy if necessary.) Intravenous fluids should be started immediately [69]; saline or lactated Ringer's solution are usually effective. The volume of fluid necessary to restore pressure varies; on occasion, as little as 500 ml may be effective [47], but at other times as much as 2 to 3 liters may be necessary.

Pressors should be used only if fluid therapy alone is not effective; although the first impulse of many practitioners is to administer epinephrine whenever a severe reaction is suspected, this drug may not be successful in restoring systemic pressure and, especially in elderly patients, may precipitate serious arrhythmias. If necessary, epinephrine may be given subcutaneously (an initial dose of 0.3 to 0.5 ml of 1:1000 solution may be augmented with one or two additional equal doses if absolutely necessary). In order to increase the speed of action and diminish the variability of absorption, epinephrine may also be given intravenously. The 1:1000 solution should be diluted to 1:10,000 and infused slowly; 3 to 5 ml of the dilute solution may be administered. Electrocardiographic monitoring is especially important when using epinephrine in order to detect any arrhythmias. Steroids (hydrocortisone, 300 to 900 mg) may be administered; acute administration of steroids is a relatively safe maneuver and may both reduce fluid loss into the interstitial space and increase vascular reactivity.

In patients in whom the hypotension is accompanied by severe bradycardia, atropine (0.4 to 0.5 mg IV) may be useful to restore normal rhythm and blood pressure; simultaneous fluid therapy may be needed as well. The dose may be repeated if necessary.

Ventricular arrhythmias may be treated with intravenous lidocaine (50 mg IV over a period of about a minute is a good initial dose and may be repeated if necessary). The drug needs to be used with care, however, since it may occasionally exacerbate hypotension.

Dyspnea alone may not require specific therapy. Obviously, any patients complaining of difficulty breathing should be evaluated quickly, and specific conditions should be treated. Air hunger may be associated with hypotension and should be treated as for dyspnea. Oxygen should be administered to any patient who begins to demonstrate respiratory insufficiency. Bronchospasm should be treated with epinephrine in the dose described above; diphenhydramine is ineffective in treating this condition. Aminophylline may also be administered; 250 to 500 mg (for adults) may be injected slowly or infused. For laryngeal edema, epinephrine (see above for dosage) is the pharmacologic agent of choice; diphenhydramine is not indicated.

If further respiratory assistance is required, intubation or emergency tracheotomy should be performed. Although it is sometimes suggested that insertion of a large-bore needle in the cricothyroid membrane is useful, this maneuver does not provide a sufficiently wide airway to sustain life.

As mentioned above, seizures, though rare, constitute the primary neurologic reaction requiring therapy. Most seizures induced by contrast agents are short lived, so that placement of an oral airway to prevent respiratory obstruction and prevention of trauma to the patient is sufficient therapy. If the seizure is prolonged, diazepam (Valium), 5 to 10 mg IV, may be administered slowly; the dose may be repeated at 10- to 15-minute intervals up to maximum of 30 mg.

CONTRAST NEPHROTOXICITY

The intravascular administration of iodinated contrast agents may be followed by a period of renal dysfunction [11, 43, 45]. The incidence, risk factors, pathogenetic mechanisms, natural history, and prophylaxis of these cases of contrast nephrotoxicity have been described in a voluminous literature [7, 9], but there is little agreement regarding them. The causes for the lack of agreement in experiments and reported clinical series include failure to standardize doses, routes of administration, the studied populations, coincident causes of transient renal failure, the degree of renal functional change that constitutes nephrotoxicity, and statistical analysis. Despite all this, it is incumbent on the radiologic practitioner to establish standards of practice that are in the best interests of his or her patients both to avoid undue risks and to avoid deferring examinations for putative "risks" that are really trivial. It is also incumbent on radiologists to be aware of the disputed issues since, in medicolegal practice, rigorous science and "expert" legal testimony may not coincide.

INCIDENCE

The reported frequency of nephrotoxicity in response to contrast medium varies tremendously [15, 38, 71]; estimates range from less than 1 percent in series in which the incidence was too low to measure [22] to as high as 76 percent in a selected population with moderate to severe existing chronic renal failure and longstanding diabetes mellitus [30]. It is probably true that, in the absence of preexisting risk factors, the administration of sufficient contrast agent to perform a standard urogram, CT, or angiogram rarely causes clinically significant renal failure. All other things being equal, the risk is probably a little higher for contrast agents administered directly into the renal arteries or into the abdominal aorta above the renal arteries than for contrast medium given intravenously.

RISK FACTORS

A sizable list of preexisting risk factors have been postulated to predispose to contrast nephrotoxicity [13, 66]; these include chronic [58] or acute renal failure present at the time of administration of contrast medium, diabetes mellitus [19, 54] (especially longstanding disease), multiple myeloma, dehydration, hypertension, generalized vascular disease, advanced age, and proteinuria [54]. Only a few of these have been supported as risk factors in multiple studies. The most important is preexisting chronic renal failure. The severity of the renal dysfunction appears to be particularly important: The higher the serum creatinine at the time of the administration of contrast medium, the more likely it is that contrast nephrotoxicity will occur, will be severe, and will not be short lived. The degree to which preexisting acute renal failure constitutes a risk factor is much harder to establish, primarily because in most cases of acute renal failure the daily alterations of renal function are so great that it is difficult to determine the degree to which the administration of contrast medium caused changes in renal function.

Diabetes mellitus is the other risk factor that has been supported by a considerable number of studies. It may or may not be a factor entirely distinct from chronic renal failure. Some investigators have found that diabetic patients without chronic renal failure do not have a measurable increase in the incidence of contrast nephrotoxicity, but there is a consensus that if chronic renal failure has been caused or is accompanied by diabetes mellitus [49], the likelihood, severity, and duration of contrast nephrotoxicity are all increased. Indeed, at one extreme, in a group of patients with severely elevated serum creatinine and diabetes mellitus that had been present since early in life, the incidence of renal dysfunction after contrast agent administration was 92 percent. But for the group of all patients with chronic renal failure and diabetes, the incidence of contrast nephrotoxicity is probably an order of magnitude less than this.

Early studies describing a group of patients with contrast nephrotoxicity who had preexisting multiple myeloma led to the assumption that this disease was an important risk factor. Subsequent examinations investigating larger numbers of patients, however, have failed to implicate multiple myeloma as a severe risk factor [57]. Proteinuria for reasons other than myeloma has also been mentioned as a possible risk factor but has also failed to be confirmed in well-controlled experiments.

Since the preparation for certain examinations requires withholding fluid and administration of laxatives, dehydration has been thought to be a risk factor for contrast nephrotoxicity. Yet no well-controlled study has clearly shown that patients in this condition are at greater risk than well-hydrated patients; indeed, severe dehydration is probably almost never brought about by preparation protocols for imaging studies.

Generalized vascular disease, systemic hypertension, and being more than 60 years of age have also been suggested as risk factors; these, too, have failed to be confirmed in well-controlled studies.

Some investigators have suggested that contrast nephrotoxicity increases in incidence as the dose of contrast agent rises [39]. Although it is hard to imagine that there is not some degree of dose-dependence for contrast nephrotoxicity, a clear-cut relationship between incidence or severity and dose has never been established. It has been suggested that repeated doses of contrast medium—given sufficiently rapidly so that the later doses were received at the time when any contrast nephrotoxicity from earlier doses would be expected to be reaching its peak severity—probably does compound the risk, but again, multiple, carefully controlled series have failed to show multiple doses to be a definite factor.

The use of low-osmolality contrast media—as opposed to conventional ionic agents—has not been shown to lower the incidence of contrast nephrotoxicity [67].

Given the tremendous variety of opinions regarding risk factors, it simply becomes impracticable—and probably not necessary—to withhold examination from all patients who exhibit any one of them. In patients who have chronic renal failure, especially if accompanied by diabetes mellitus, however, it is certainly advisable at least to review the necessity for the proposed examination even more carefully then usual and to discuss the potential benefit of information to be expected from the exam against the risk of contrast nephrotoxicity with the referring clinician. Prophylactic measures may be useful if clinical indications lead to administration of contrast medium despite the risks.

PATHOPHYSIOLOGY

The pathogenetic mechanisms of contrast nephrotoxicity are not known. It has been proposed that renal ischemia, tubular luminar obstruction by precipitates of one sort or another, or direct tubular toxicity [61] might be responsible; indeed, the proposed mechanisms are similar to those that have been proposed for other types of acute renal failure, and there is as little agreement on the causes of one group as on those of the other.

There are several reasons to suspect that renal ischemia, or hypoxia, might be responsible. Diminished renal blood pressure and flow [27] have been demonstrated in both animals and humans after administration of contrast medium [10]. The hyperosmolality of contrast media has been implicated, as have renin- and prostaglandin-mediated alterations in renal vascular tone. In certain circumstances, contrast medium has been shown to increase the propensity of circulating red cells to form rouleaux and to sludge, and even to shift the hemoglobin–oxygen dissociation curve [53] such that renal tissues may become hypoxic. To date, however, none of these mechanisms has been shown conclusively to be the major cause for contrast nephrotoxicity in humans.

Renal tubular obstruction has been postulated as well. Some work has implicated the precipitation of Tamm-Horsfall protein in tubular lumina [18]; other studies have suggested that contrast medium may produce precipitation of uric acid crystals in hyperuricemic states [37]. Precipitation of Bence-Jones or light-chain proteins in patients with multiple myeloma has also been implicated. Again, none of these mechanisms has been reliably shown to operate in clinical cases of contrast nephrotoxicity.

Finally, direct tubular toxicity [61], suggested by the demonstration of enzymuria [12, 28] and by the demonstration of histologic abnormalities in the tubules after contrast agent administration, has also been postulated, but as with the other mechanisms, this pathogenesis has not been clearly established as the most important cause or even a common one. Certain experiments have shown that contrast-agent–induced proteinuria and enzymuria are less marked when low-osmolality agents are used, but to date, these agents have not been shown to reduce the incidence of clinically important contrast-induced renal dysfunction.

DIAGNOSIS AND NATURAL HISTORY

The renal dysfunction associated with contrast nephrotoxicity is usually transient [2]. Serial measurements of serum creatinine and blood urea nitrogen will show that these levels rise after the administration of contrast agent, typically reaching a peak approximately 3 days after administration. The most common clinical course is for them then to fall to their base-line values over a period of time that varies but typically might last a week or more. During this period of dysfunction, glomerular filtration rate and effective renal plasma flow are diminished.

Less frequently, blood urea nitrogen (BUN), or creatinine levels, or both, will rise and then decline only partially to base-line values [70]; even less frequently, BUN and creatinine levels will rise and never decline [29]. Dialysis may be required. As might be expected, the worse the dysfunction, the greater the likelihood that renal function will not return to base-line.

Most cases of contrast nephrotoxicity are not accompanied by oliguria or anuria, although the most severe cases may be. Some cases may go entirely unnoticed, since outpatients may not have renal functional studies and usually do not have oliguria or anuria. And even in patients who have transient renal dysfunction after contrast agent administration, it may be difficult to establish with certainty that the contrast agent was responsible. There is no specific clinical or biochemical marker for contrast nephrotoxicity. A persistent nephrogram seen in abdomen radiographs or CT examinations after the administration of contrast medium may provide an indication that acute renal dysfunction exists, but the sensitivity of this sign is not known, and there is no reason to think that it can discriminate between contrast nephrotoxicity and acute renal dysfunction of any other cause.

PROPHYLAXIS

It is true that the best way to prevent contrast nephrotoxicity is not to administer contrast agents at all, but since good radiologic practice requires the performance of necessary examinations just as it requires the avoidance of needless ones, this maneuver is not always available. It has been suggested that intravenous hydration of patients prior to the administration of contrast medium may lower the incidence [21], but this technique is by no means a proven or commonly accepted one, and it may interfere with the quality of the urograms. There is some evidence that instituting therapy designed to induce a lengthy diuresis immediately after contrast agent administration may be helpful [4]. Mannitol, 20 percent in 250 ml of normal saline, possibly accompanied by furosemide, may be administered during the hour following contrast agent administration; thereafter, for a period of 24 hours, urinary fluid losses should be replaced with saline. Assuming there are no contraindications for this therapy, administration of fluid and diuretics is relatively safe and presumably worth trying in patients with clear-cut risk factors in whom examination using a contrast agent cannot be replaced by a less-risky procedure.

REFERENCES

1. American College of Radiology Commission on Public Health and Radiation Protection, Committee on Drugs. Prevention and management of adverse reactions to intravascular contrast media. Reston, VA: American College of Radiology, 1977.
2. Ansari, Z., and Baldwin, D.S. Acute renal failure due to radio-contrast agents. *Nephron* 17:28, 1976.
3. Ansell, G. Adverse reactions to contrast agents: Scope of problem. *Invest. Radiol.* 5:374, 1970.
4. Anto, H.R., et al. Infusion intravenous pyelography and renal function. *Arch. Intern. Med.* 141:1652, 1981.
5. Benness, G.T. Urographic contrast agents: A comparison of sodium and methyglucamine salts. *Clin. Radiol.* 21:150, 1970.
6. Berg, G.R., Hutter, A.M., Jr., and Pfister, R.C. Electrocardiographic abnormalities associated with intravenous urography. *N. Engl. J. Med.* 289:87, 1973.
7. Berkseth, R.O., and Kjellstrand, C.M. Radiologic contrast-induced nephropathy. *Med. Clin. North Am.* 68:351, 1984.
8. Bettmann, M.A. Angiographic contrast agents: Conventional and new media compared. *A.J.R.* 139:787, 1982.
9. Byrd, L., and Sherman, R.L. Radiocontrast-induced acute renal failure: A clinical and pathophysiologic review. *Medicine* 58:270, 1979.
10. Caldicott, W.J.H., Hollenberg, N.K., and Abrams, H.L. Characteristics of response of renal vascular bed to contrast media. *Invest Radiol.* 5:539, 1970.
11. Carvallo, A., et al. Acute renal failure following drip infusion pyelography. *Am. J. Med.* 65:38, 1978.
12. Cavaliere, G., et al. Tubular nephrotoxicity after intravenous urography with ionic high-osmolal and nonionic low-osmolal contrast media in patients with chronic renal insufficiency. *Nephron* 46:128, 1987.
13. Cochran, S.T., Wong, W.S., and Roe, D.J. Predicting angiography-induced acute renal function impairment: Clinical risk model. *A.J.R.* 141:1027, 1983.
14. Cohan, R.H., Dunnick, N.R., and Bashore, T.M. Treatment of reactions to radiographic contrast material. *A.J.R.* 151:263, 1988.
15. Cramer, B.C., et al. Renal function following infusion of radiologic contrast material. *Arch. Intern. Med.* 145:87, 1985.
16. Dacie, J.E., and Fry, I.K. A comparison of sodium and methylglucamine diatrizoate in clinical urography. *Br. J. Radiol.* 44:51, 1971.
17. Davidson, A.J., et al. An evaluation of the effect of high-dose urography on previously impaired renal and hepatic function in man. *Radiology* 97:249, 1970.
18. Dawnay, A.B. St. J., et al. Tamm-Horsfall glucoprotein excretion and aggregation during intravenous urography. *Invest. Radiol.* 20:53, 1985.
19. Diaz-Buxo, J.A., et al. Acute renal failure after excretory urography in diabetic patients. *Ann. Intern. Med.* 83:155, 1975.
20. Dure-Smith, P., et al. Physiology of the excretory urogram. III. A densitometric and subjective assessment of changes in contrast medium concentration. *Invest. Radiol.* 9:104,1974.
21. Eisenberg, R.L., Bank, W.O., and Hedgcock, M.W. Renal failure after major angiography can be avoided with hydration. *A.J.R.* 136:859, 1981.
22. Eisenberg, R.L., Bank, W.O., and Hedgcock, M.W. Renal failure after major angiography. *Am. J. Med.* 68:43, 1980.
23. Evill, C.A., and Benness, G.T. Solute excretion during intravenous urography: A comparison of sodium and methylglucamine iothalamates. *Invest. Radiol.* 10:148, 1975.
24. Fischer, H.W., et al. Systemic response to excretory urography. *Radiology* 151:31, 1984.
25. Fischer, H.W., Spataro, R.F., and Rosenberg, P.M. Medical and economic considerations in using a new contrast medium. *Arch. Intern. Med.* 146:1717, 1986.

26. Fry, I.K., and Cattell, W.R. The nephrographic pattern during excretion urography. *Br. Med. Bull.* 28:227, 1972.
27. Gates, G.F., and Green, G.S. Transient reduction in renal function following arteriography: A radionuclide study. *J.Urol.* 129:1107, 1983.
28. Goldstein, E.J., et al. Enzymatic evidence of renal tubular damage following renal angiography. *Radiology* 121:617, 1976.
29. Gomes, A.S., et al. Acute renal dysfunction after major angiography. *A.J.R.* 145:1249, 1985.
30. Harkonen, S., and Kjellstrand, C.M. Intravenous pyelography in nonuremic diabetic patients. *Nephron* 24:268, 1979.
31. Hartman, G.W., et al. Mortality during excretory urography: Mayo Clinic experience. *A.J.R.* 139:919, 1982.
32. Holtas, S. Iohexol in patients with previous adverse reactions to contrast media. *Invest. Radiol.* 19:563, 1984.
33. Jacobson, P.D., and Rosenquist, J. The introduction of low-osmolar contrast agents in radiology. *J.A.M.A.* 260:1586, 1988.
34. Jensen, N., and Dorph, S. Adverse reactions to urographic contrast medium: Rapid versus slow injection rate. *Br. J. Radiol.* 53:659, 1980.
35. Kappelman, N.B., et al. Electrocardiographic changes with intravenous pyelography in healthy individuals. *Urology* 9:88, 1977.
36. Katayama, H., et al. Adverse reactions to ionic and nonionic contrast media. A report from the Japanese committee on the safety of contrast media. *Radiology* 175:621, 1990.
37. Krumlovsky, F.A., et al. Acute renal failure. Association with administration of radiographic contrast material. *J.A.M.A.* 239:125, 1978.
38. Kumar, S., et al. Low incidence of renal failure after angiography. *Arch. Intern. Med.* 141:1268, 1981.
39. Lang, E.K., et al. The incidence of contrast medium induced acute tubular necrosis following arteriography. *Radiology* 138:203,1981.
40. Lasser, E.C., et al. Pretreatment with corticosteroids to alleviate reactions to intravenous contrast material. *N. Engl. J. Med.* 317:845, 1987.
41. Littner, M.R., et al. Evaluation of bronchospasm during excretory urography. *Radiology* 124:17, 1977.
42. Levorstad, K., Kolbenstvedt, A., and Loyning, E.W. Iohexol compared with metrizoate in urography. *Acta Radiol. Diagn.* 24:337, 1983.
43. Mason, R.A., Arbeit, L.A., and Giron, F. Renal dysfunction after arteriography. *J.A.M.A.* 253:1001, 1985.
44. McClennan, B.L. Low-osmolality contrast media: Premises and promises. *Radiology* 162:1, 1987.
45. Mudge, G.H. Nephrotoxicity of urographic radiocontrast drugs. *Kidney Int.* 18:540, 1980.
46. Nelson, C.M.K., Brown, R.C., and Culp, D.A. The extrarenal excretion of urographic contrast material. *J. Urol.* 110:109, 1973.
47. Obeid, A.I., et al. Fluid theraphy in severe systemic reaction to radiopaque dye. *Ann. Intern. Med.* 83:317, 1975.
48. Palmer, F.J. The RACR survey of intravenous contrast media reactions: Final report. *Australas. Radiol.* 32:426, 1988.
49. Parfrey, P.S., et al. Contrast material-induced renal failure in patients with diabetes mellitus, renal insufficiency, or both. *N. Engl. J. Med.* 320:143, 1989.
50. Pfister, R.C., et al. Contrast-medium-induced electrocardiographic abnormalities: Comparison of bolus and infusion of methylglucamine iodamide and methylgucamine/sodium diatrizoate. *A.J.R.* 140:149, 1983.
51. Rankin, R.N., and Eng, F.W.H.T. Iohexol vs. diatrizoate: A comparative study in intravenous urography. *Invest. Radiol.* 20(suppl.):S112, 1985.
52. Robbins, J.S., III, Mittemeyer, B.T., and Neiman, H.L. The persistent nephrogram: A sentinel sign of contrast reaction. *J. Urol.* 114:758, 1975.
53. Rosenthal, A., Litwin, S.B., and Laver, M.B. Effect of contrast media used in angiocardiography on hemoglobin-oxygen equilibrium. *Invest. Radiol.* 8:191,1973.
54. Pillay, V.K.G., et al. Acute renal failure following intravenous urography in patients with long-standing diabetes mellitus and azotemia. *Radiology* 95:633, 1970.
55. Saxton, H.M. Urography, *Br. J. Radiol.* 42:321, 1969.
56. Schrott, K.M., et al. Iohexol in excretory urography. *Fortschr. Med.* 104:153, 1986.
57. Scott, W.R. Seizures: A reaction to contrast media for computed tomography of the brain. *Radiology* 137:359, 1980.
58. Shafi, T., et al. Infusion intravenous pyelography and renal function: Effects in patients with chronic renal insufficiency. *Arch. Intern. Med.* 138:1218, 1978.
59. Shehadi, W.H. Adverse reactions to intravascularly administered contrast media. *A.J.R.* 124:145, 1975.
60. Siegle, R.L., and Lieberman, P. A review of untoward reactions to iodinated contrast material. *J. Urol.* 119:581, 1978.
61. Skaarup, P., and Thomsen, H.S. Urinary protein profiles following urography with iothalamate. *Acta Radiol.* 28:335, 1987.
62. Smith, H.-J., et al. High dose urography in patients with renal failure. *Acta Radiol. Diagn.* 26:213, 1985.
63. Spataro, R.F., et al. High-dose clinical urography with the low-osmolality contrast agent Hexabrix: Comparison with a conventional contrast agent. *Radiology* 162:9, 1987.

64. Stadalnik, R.C., et al. Electrocardiographic response to intravenous urography: Prospective evaluation of 275 patients. *A.J.R.* 129:825, 1977.
65. Stanley, R.J., and Pfister, R.C. Bradycardia and hypotension following use of intravenous contrast media. *Radiology* 121:5, 1976.
66. Swartz, R.D., et al. Renal failure following major angiography. *Am. J. Med.* 65:31, 1978.
67. Taliercio, C.P., and Burnett, J.C. Contrast nephropathy, cardiology and the newer radiocontrast agents. *Int. J. Cardiol.* 19:145, 1988.
68. Thompson, W.M., et al. Iopamidol: New, nonionic contrast agent for excretory urography. *A.J.R.* 142:329, 1984.
69. vanSonnenberg, E., Neff, C.C., and Pfister, R.C. Life-threatening hypotensive reactions to contrast media administration: Comparison of pharmacologic and fluid therapy. *Radiology* 162:15, 1987.
70. VanZee, B.E., et al. Renal injury associated with intravenous pyelography in nondiabetic and diabetic patients. *Ann. Intern. Med.* 89:51, 1978.
71. Webb, J.A.W., et al. Renal function after high dose urography in patients with renal failure. *Br. J. Radiol.* 54:479, 1981.
72. Winfield, A.C., et al. Iohexol for excretory urography: A comparative study. *A.J.R.* 141:571, 1983.

5

Congenital Anomalies

The incidence of all major malformations detected at birth has been estimated at slightly over 2 percent. For major urinary tract anomalies, the incidence has been reported as 0.14 percent. However, up to 10 percent of all live births are afflicted with some degree of anomalous formation of the urinary system. These range in severity from very minor anomalies to major malformations incompatible with postnatal life. As many as half of patients with renal malformations will have coexistent anomalies occurring in other portions of the urinary tract or in other organ systems [12]. These associations are typified by the "VATER" syndrome, which is an acronym for the multiple organ systems involved: *V*ertebral, *A*nal, *T*racheal, *E*sophageal, *R*adial bone, and *R*enal [16].

On occasion, physical characteristics of the infant may suggest the possibility of significant genitourinary anomalies. In the past supernumerary nipples have been suggested as one of these signs. However, one report found that only 1 of 49 infants with supernumerary nipples had a renal anomaly [10]. On the other hand, up to 25 percent of infants with hemihypertrophy, an uncommon condition characterized by a congenital enlargement of one side of the body, have congenital defects, especially genitourinary anomalies. This finding also has a high association with malignant neoplasms of the kidney, adrenal gland, and liver.

Hereditary polycystic diseases of the kidney and multicystic dysplastic kidney, though congenital, are both classically considered in the category of renal cystic diseases and will be discussed in Chap. 8. Furthermore, ureteropelvic junction obstruction and primary megaureter are also congenital diseases, though they will be covered in more detail in subsequent chapters. Vesicoureteral reflux and duplex collecting systems, because of their prevalence and clinical significance, are deserving of their own chapters.

KIDNEY

SUPERNUMERARY KIDNEY

A third, or supernumerary, kidney is probably the rarest of all renal malformations. It is defined as a mass of renal tissue that has no parenchymal connection with the definitive kidneys. It is usually found within the perinephric space lying below one of the normally situated kidneys. While it may be as large as a normal kidney, it is usually smaller and comprised of only one or two lobes. On urography, ureteral drainage is seen to be via a separate renal pelvis into the ipsilateral normal ureter.

AGENESIS OF THE KIDNEY

Renal agenesis, a far more common abnormality, can be unilateral or bilateral. It results from a failure of the ureteric bud arising from the mesonephric duct to meet and organize the metanephric blastema into a definitive kidney. Bilateral renal agenesis is more common in males by a ratio of 2:1. Most of these cases are characterized by maternal oligohydramnios, and the infants exhibit the so-called Potter facies, with a beaklike nose, receding chin, and rather large, low-set ears. Pulmonary hypoplasia is also a constant finding. This abnormality is incompatible with life.

The incidence of unilateral renal agenesis is approximately 1 in 1,000. It is more common in males and affects the left kidney more than the right. Coexistent genital anomalies are quite common in such cases, especially in females, in whom the incidence is approximately 50 percent. The most common associated genital abnormalities in the male are ipsilateral cryptorchidism and seminal vesicle cysts. In women, the genital anomalies include bicornuate or unicornuate uterus, uterine didelphys, or less commonly, vaginal abnormalities such as atresia or hypoplasia. The single developed kidney almost always exhibits compensatory hypertrophy, but it is usually otherwise normal. On cystoscopy, the ipsilateral trigone and ureteral orifice are often absent.

On urography there is no function on the side of the absent kidney. No renal outline is seen on plain film of the abdomen, but this is not always found even when there is a kidney present. If the contralateral kidney is large, if no ectopic location of the kidney is seen, and if the ipsilateral ureteral orifice is absent, agenesis can be presumed. Renal agenesis may result in abnormal orientation of other organ systems. The ipsilateral adrenal, which is usually not absent, is located in the paraspinal region and has a disk shape when studied by CT [9]. The tail of the pancreas can also be seen on CT to be displaced posteriorly and medially into the area of the left renal fossa with left renal agenesis. This can also be found with ectopic left kidney or prior left nephrectomy. Furthermore, with congenital absence of the left kidney or ectopic left kidney, the anatomic splenic flexure of the colon occupies the left renal fossa. Demonstration of a normal splenic flexure by barium enema in patients without a functioning left kidney precludes renal agenesis [15].

COMPENSATORY HYPERTROPHY OF THE KIDNEY

Compensatory hypertrophy of the kidney denotes enlargement of the nephrons rather than an increase in number. It can result from the loss of contralateral renal function from any cause. Certainly the degree of compensatory enlargement is greatest in younger patients; the degree of enlargement declines if contralateral renal function is lost after the age of 40. On urography the hypertrophied kidney may be up to five vertebral bodies in length.

RENAL HYPOPLASIA/DYSPLASIA

Renal hypoplasia presumes a congenitally small kidney (Fig. 5-1). This condition is rare; most smooth, small kidneys have an acquired cause, which may be vascular compromise, inflammatory disease, or atrophy on the basis of obstruction or reflux. In the absence of acquired disease, true hypoplasia is usually defined as a reduction in size by more than 50 percent in a kidney that contains a reduced number of calices (in comparison with the normal count of 10 to 14). Hypoplasia must be differentiated from dysplasia, which is an unrelated lesion. A dysplastic kidney usually results from ectopic insertion of its ureter. Radiographically, while the true hypoplastic kidney functions essentially normally and has characteristics as described above, the dysplastic kidney, while also small, is grossly distorted and functions poorly, if at all.

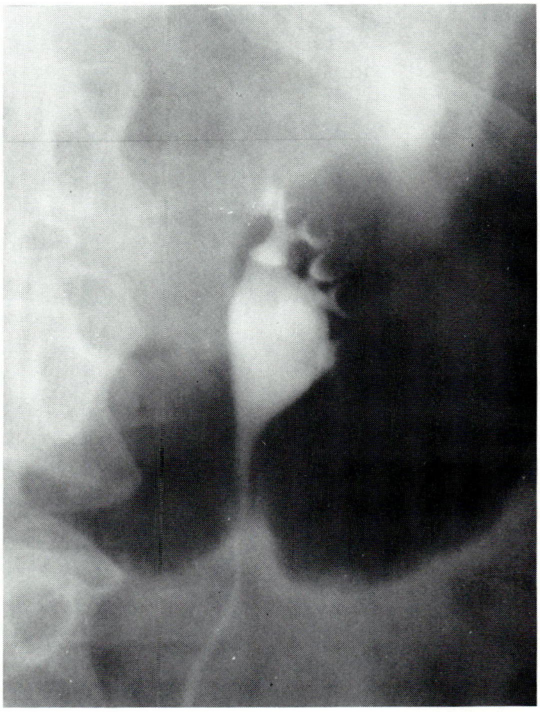

Figure 5-1. Hypoplastic kidney. Retrograde pyelography demonstrates the normal appearance of the tiny collecting system in this kidney, which functioned on urography and was only 4 cm in length. Note that there are fewer than the normal number of calices.

Historically, the Ask-Upmark kidney has been considered a variant of hypoplasia. This kidney is small and characteristically bears a deep transverse groove or grooves on its lateral cortical surface near the upper pole. In the past this has been considered a variant of true hypoplasia occurring in girls or young women and frequently associated with hypertension. However, most of these kidneys have been found in patients with urinary infection and vesicoureteral reflux. Therefore, current thinking is that this is a kidney scarred by chronic pyelonephritis and not a true congenital lesion [1].

ROTATIONAL ANOMALIES OF THE KIDNEY

Rotational anomalies of the kidney can result in bizarre urographic presentations. As the kidneys ascend from the pelvis during fetal life, they undergo a medial rotation of approximately 90 degrees about their longitudinal axes. If this rotation does not occur or is less than 90 degrees, the renal pelvis as seen on urography will remain anteriorly or anteromedially situated (Fig. 5-2). This is termed incomplete rotation. Tomography and oblique views usually allow evaluation of the parenchyma of these kidneys. On rare occasions the kidney may rotate beyond 90 degrees, resulting in the pelvis facing posteriorly or even laterally. This is termed excessive rotation. Rotational anomalies are quite common in both ectopic and fused kidneys, further contributing to the bizarre appearance of these anomalies.

ECTOPIC KIDNEYS

The kidney is normally found in the upper lumbar region. Though the kidney may be ectopically located in the thoracic cavity, this is usually acquired rather than congenital and results from passage of the kidney through a herniation in the diaphragm, which may be either congenital (foramen of Bochdalek) or acquired. In renal ptosis, another acquired condition, the lower pole may be well below the iliac crest. In such cases the ureter is of normal length and the renal artery arises from the aorta at the normal level.

Figure 5-2. Incomplete rotation of the kidney. Urography shows a bizarre appearance of the right collecting system whose pelvis and ureter face anteriorly because of failure to rotate 90 degrees medially.

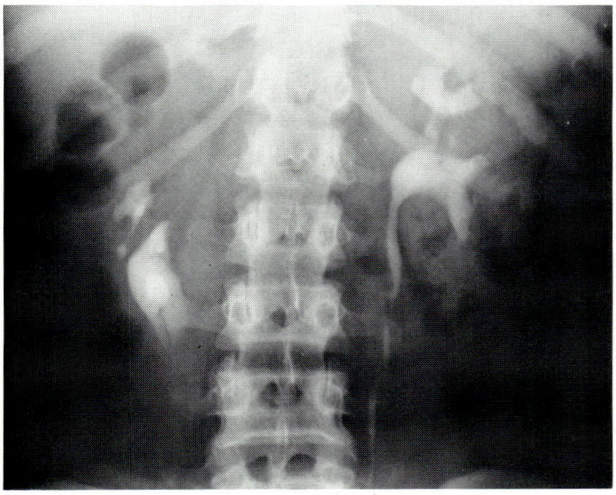

True ectopy of the kidney involves a permanent location of the kidney at the level of the lower lumbar spine, at the level of the iliac vessels, deep in the true pelvis behind the bladder, or across the midline below the normal contralateral kidney. Ipsilateral ectopy into the pelvis results from failure of normal ascent of the kidney during fetal life. The blood supply of such kidneys is usually from the lower aorta, from the iliac arteries, or from both. Pelvic kidneys have poor drainage of urine, which predisposes them to infection and stone formation. However, most pelvic kidneys remain asymptomatic throughout life. While normal pregnancy and vaginal delivery is the rule in women with pelvic kidneys, the ectopic kidney may obstruct delivery in up to one third of cases, thus necessitating cesarean section.

Urographically, the pelvic kidney may be difficult to visualize since it frequently overlies the bony pelvis (Fig. 5-3). A careful search in the pelvis for the opacified collecting system should be made whenever a single, normal-sized kidney is visualized. Oblique views may be helpful. Tailored nephrotomography may help in evaluation of the pelvic kidney, though retrograde pyelography may be necessary to define the collecting system. On occasion, CT or ultrasound will be required to image the pelvic kidney.

The crossed kidney almost invariably lies inferior to the normally located contralateral kidney and in the large majority of cases is fused with it. On urography, its ureter can be seen crossing the midline and draining in normal position into the bladder.

FUSIONS OF THE KIDNEY

Some degree of renal fusion is found at approximately 1 in 250 autopsies. The most common fusion is the horseshoe kidney, which is classically seen as attachment of the lower poles of

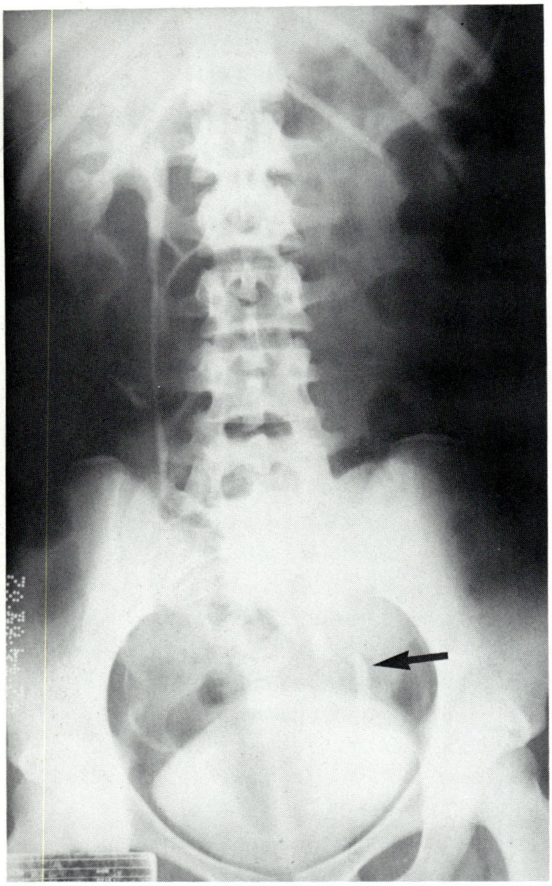

Figure 5-3. Pelvic kidney. Urography shows a normally located right kidney. The left kidney, lying in the pelvis, is difficult to see since it lies over the bony pelvis. However, its ureter (arrow) can be seen entering the bladder normally.

the kidneys by an isthmus of renal tissue crossing the midline anterior to the great vessels (Fig. 5-4). While this isthmus usually contains normally functioning renal tissue, it may be a simple fibrous band. In rare instances, a fusion may occur at the level of the upper pole or even in the midpolar regions of the kidney. Even rarer is fusion at both the upper and lower poles, resulting in a "ring" or "doughnut" kidney. The vascular supply of a horseshoe kidney, especially to the isthmus, is highly variable and usually consists of multiple renal arteries from various levels of the aorta.

Radiographically, the collecting systems in a horseshoe kidney exhibit some degree of incomplete rotation. Furthermore, there is a reversal of the normal longitudinal axis of the collecting systems, the lower calix usually being more medially situated than the upper on both sides. The ureters from the anteriorly located pelves cross the isthmus anteriorly. It is not unusual on urography to see mild dilatation of the collecting systems due to this anterior angulation of the ureters. The resultant urinary stasis predisposes the horseshoe kidney to infection and stone formation. On occasion the isthmus is difficult to see on urography; in such cases fusion of the lower poles can be suspected by the bilateral medial deviation of the lower poles. Renal tumors may occur in the isthmus and be difficult to see on urography, though more anterior tomographic sections should be obtained in an effort to demonstrate the isthmus. CT is recommended for imaging the horseshoe kidney when pathologic involvement is suspected.

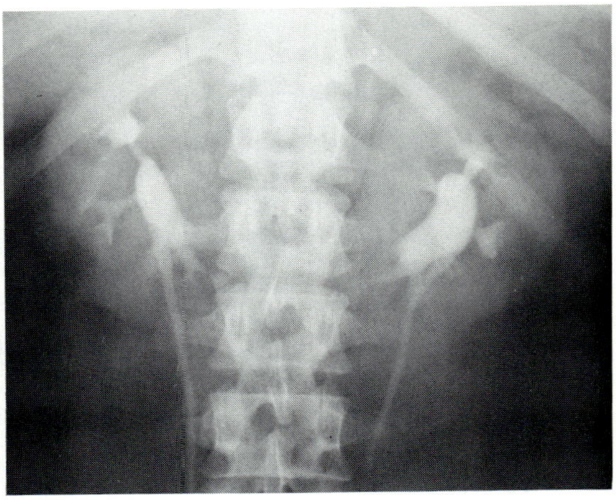

Figure 5-4. Horseshoe kidney. Urography shows reversal of the normal renal axis bilaterally (lower poles tilted medially). The margins of the lower poles can be seen aiming medially where they fuse over the spine. Note that the lower-pole calices project medially to their respective ureters; this is a typical finding.

While both kidneys may be ectopic to the true pelvis and not fused (Fig. 5-5A), it is more common to see fusion of the kidneys in such cases. This results in the so-called "lump" or "pancake" kidney (Fig. 5-5B). The large majority (95%) of crossed ectopic kidneys fuse with the contralateral kidney. This fusion is almost in-

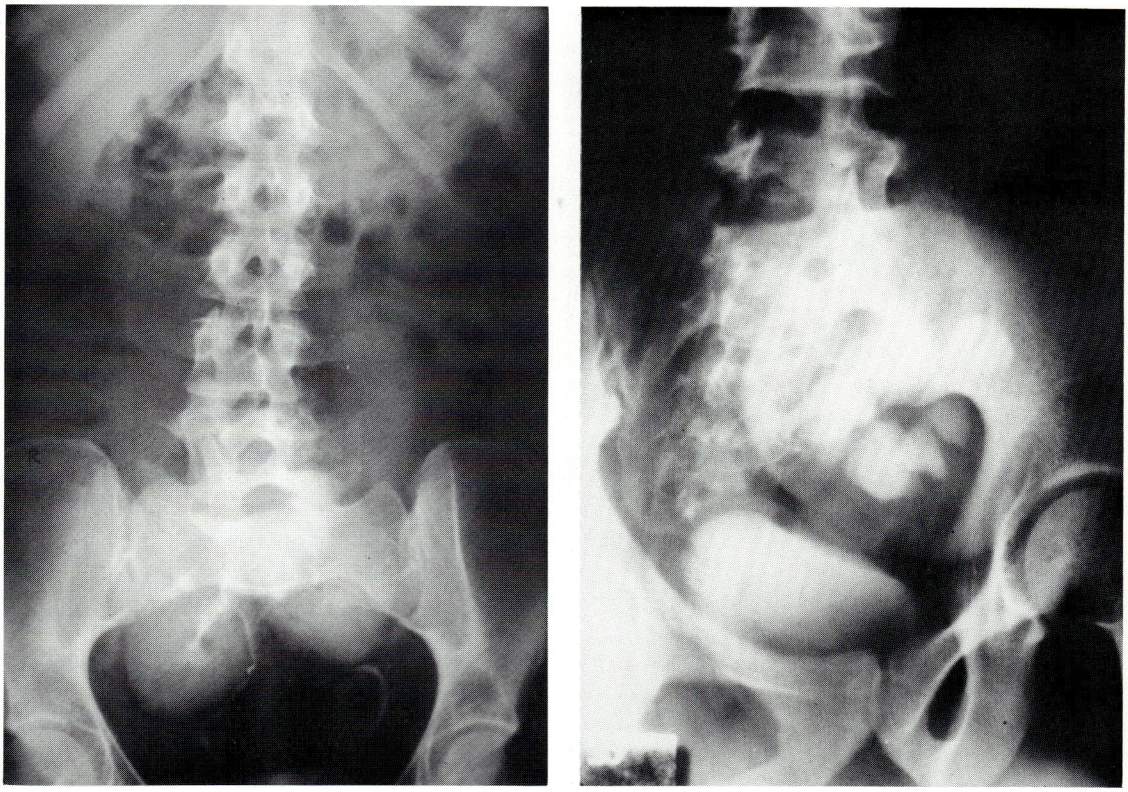

A B

Figure 5-5. Both kidneys ectopic to pelvis. A. Urography shows both kidneys in pelvis, but not fused. B. Urography depicts fusion of pelvic kidneys into a rounded "pancake" or "lump" kidney.

variably between the upper pole of the ectopic kidney and the lower pole of the other kidney (Fig. 5-6), and is commonly known as crossed fused renal ectopy. Generally speaking, ectopic and fused kidneys are more subject to trauma than are normally located kidneys.

UNIPAPILLARY KIDNEY/POLYCALICOSIS

The kidney of many mammals, including the rat, dog, sheep, rabbit, monkey, and cat, contain only a single renal papilla and its associated calix. This condition is rare in humans and, when present, is frequently associated with other significant urinary abnormalities. The unipapillary kidney, as this condition is called, is usually also hypoplastic. Abnormalities of the contralateral kidney are frequent and varied. Conversely, polycalicosis denotes a condition in which a larger than normal number of papillae and their adjacent calices are present. The normal kidney contains 10 to 14 papillae. Kidneys with polycalicosis are generally normal in size and exhibit normal function on urography.

ABERRANT RENAL PAPILLA

The aberrant renal papilla is of significance because it results in a filling defect within the collecting system that must be differentiated from pathologic conditions such as tumors or stones. The aberrant papilla protrudes into the side of an infundibulum or into any portion of the renal pelvis surrounded by renal parenchyma. There is no minor infundibulum or formed calix in such cases. The resultant finding on urography is a smooth round or oval lucent defect within the intrarenal collecting system. The smooth border usually distinguishes this lesion from a transitional cell carcinoma, and its fixed location is inconsistent with a free collecting system stone. Appropriate oblique views will

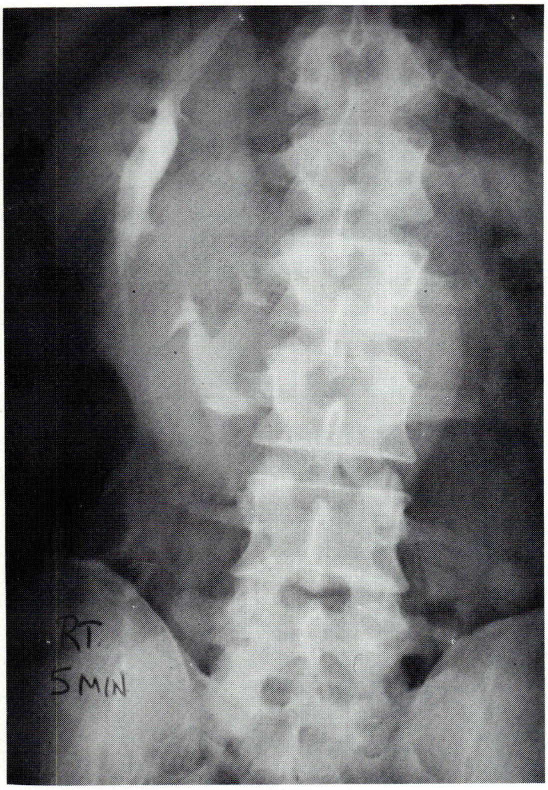

Figure 5-6. Crossed fused renal ectopy. Urography shows the ectopically crossed left kidney to be fused in its upper pole with the lower pole of the normally placed right kidney. Rotational changes are seen in both collecting systems.

allow confirmation of the diagnosis; when visualized in a tangential plane, the aberrant papilla can be seen to encroach on the collecting system from an extrinsic location, resulting in an indentation on the margin of the contrast-filled major infundibulum or renal pelvis.

CONGENITAL MEGACALICES

Congenital megacalices, also known as megacalicosis, is a condition in which the calices, usually unilaterally, are polygonally enlarged. There is no associated dilatation of the renal pelvis or ureter in such cases, nor is there a history of obstruction, pain, or infection. On urography there is prompt function. It has been postulated that this is a true congenital abnormality. However, some investigators feel that the large majority of kidneys with megacalices have been subjected to either obstruction or reflux at some time in the past, possibly even during fetal life.

URETER

CIRCUMCAVAL URETER

Most deviations of the ureter are acquired. However, one congenital anomaly, the circumcaval ureter, results in significant medial deviation of the right midureter with proximal obstruction. The inferior vena cava (IVC) develops embryologically from the posterior cardinal, subcardinal, and supracardinal veins. In normal individuals, the segment of the IVC above the renal veins is formed by the right subcardinal vein. The IVC below the renals is formed by the right supracardinal vein. Circumcaval ureter results when the infrarenal segment of the IVC is formed from a persistent right posterior cardinal vein rather than from the right supracardinal vein. The right ureter is carried medially as the posterior cardinal vein migrates in that direction to form the IVC. The autopsy incidence of circumcaval ureter is reported as 1:1,100; males are affected more frequently than females by a ratio of almost 3:1. Symptoms, which are not always present, are related to ureteral obstruction of varying degrees.

Urographically, in cases with mild degrees of obstruction, the proximal right ureter deviates medially, and the point of obstruction is at the region of the lateral wall of the IVC. With more significant obstruction, the dilated proximal right ureter becomes tortuous and usually exhibits a "reversed J" configuration before it descends medial to the ipsilateral lumbar pedicle, passing behind and around the anomalous inferior vena cava (Fig. 5-7). The diagnosis of circumcaval ureter can be confirmed by CT. This shows the ureter passing posterior and medial to the inferior vena cava [13]. This is an especially effective study if a ureteral catheter is placed prior to the CT examination. Symptomatic obstruction in cases of circumcaval ureter requires division of the ureter and reanastomosis lateral to the inferior vena cava.

URETEROPELVIC JUNCTION OBSTRUCTION AND MEGAURETER

Ureteropelvic junction obstruction and congenital megaureter will be discussed in detail in

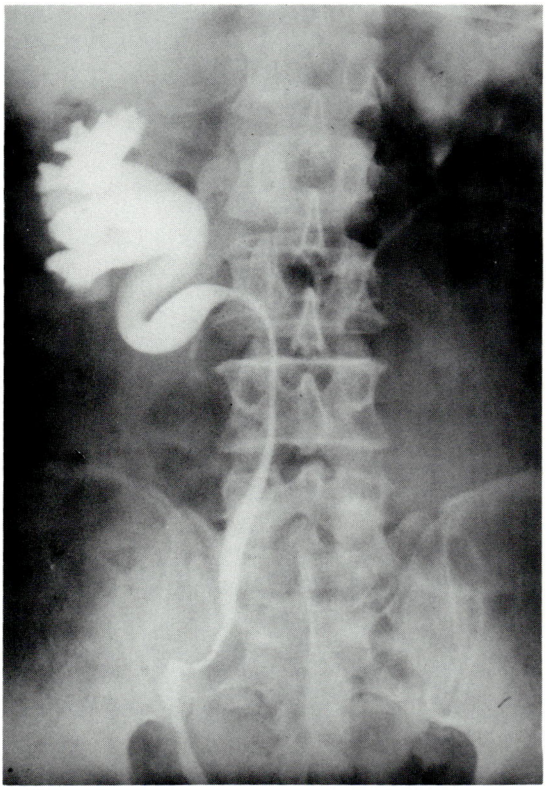

Figure 5-7. Retrocaval ureter. Retrograde pyelography shows the typical severe medial deviation of the right midureter. The collecting system and ureter proximal to the deviation are moderately dilated, and the proximal ureter shows the typical "reverse J" configuration.

Chap. 19. Generally speaking, both of these entities have a similar cause, which is derangement or deficiency of smooth muscle fibers and associated fibrosis, resulting in inability of the ureter to transmit a normal persistaltic wave. This obstruction is functional, as a ureteral catheter can be easily passed through either area of involvement. Of the two, the congenital ureteropelvic junction obstruction usually causes a more severe proximal hydronephrosis.

VALVES/STRICTURES/FOLDS OF THE URETER

Obstructive ureteral valves and congenital ureteral strictures are very rare entities. In the case of valves, a discrete diaphragm can occasionally be identified with secondary proximal dilation of the ureter. Congenital strictures may be of any length and smoothly taper at both ends. These strictures can occur anywhere throughout the ureter. Transverse ureteral folds are simply redundant mucosa extending into the ureteral lumen. These folds tend to disappear as the child matures and are not obstructive. Longitudinal folds, presenting as striations through the length of the ureter and extending into the renal pelvis, indicate a distensible ureter and are usually secondary to vesicoureteral reflex.

ECTOPIC URETERAL ORIFICES

The distal ureter in either single or duplicated systems can insert in a location other than the trigone, either near the bladder neck or extravesically. Ectopic insertion within the bladder does not usually result in significant pathology. Insertion into the posterior urethra in either males or females, however, may result in reflux during voiding and otherwise cause obstruction due to termination in a closed space. Likewise, ectopic insertion outside the urinary tract is usually obstructive in nature. Dysplasia of the kidney is more pronounced the more ectopically the ureter inserts, and it may be so severe that the kidney is essentially nonfunctional and forms only a few milliliters of fluid each day.

In males, the posterior urethra is the most common site of extravesical ureteral ectopy. The ureter may also end in the seminal vesicle, vas deferens, or ejaculatory duct. None of these locations is beyond the external urethral sphincter, so males do not present with urinary incontinence. Rather, a common clinical presentation is that of recurrent or chronic epididymitis. Men with ectopic insertion of the ureter into the genital tract will be found to have a nonfunctioning kidney on urography and dilated ipsilateral seminal vesicle on CT. This must be differentiated from a true seminal vesicle cyst associated with renal agenesis.

In females, ureteral ectopy to the vestibule, vagina, or cervix can occur. This results in continual dribbling incontinence of urine, which in a young girl beyond the age of toilet training should mandate radiographic evaluation of the urinary tract. The radiology of ureteral ectopy is discussed in detail in Chap. 18.

URETEROCELES

A ureterocele is a focal dilation of the submucosal portion of the distal ureter where it traverses the bladder wall. They can be classified as orthotopic (occurring in normal position on the trigone) or ectopic. Orthotopic ureteroceles, also known as "adult type" or "simple" ureteroceles, are typically found in association with nonduplicated ureters.

Urographically, the orthotopic ureterocele presents as a "cobra head" or "spring onion" deformity of the distal ureter in the region of the normally located ureterovesical junction (Fig. 5-8). If the ureter opacifies, the central portion of the ureterocele is filled with contrast in continuity with the remainder of the ureter and is surrounded by a lucent rim, which represents the bladder mucosa around the ureterocele as it protrudes into the bladder lumen. Orthotopic ureteroceles may be totally nonobstructive, or there may be varying degrees of proximal obstruction.

Of great importance is the acquired orthotopic ureterocele, or pseudoureterocele; this results from a bladder lesion, typically a transitional cell carcinoma, occluding the normal ureterovesical junction. Therefore, orthotopic ureteroceles detected in older patients require further evaluation. Several oblique views of the bladder phase of urography may demonstrate an irregular filling defect in the bladder immediately adjacent to the medial portion of the ureterocele.

Figure 5-8. Orthotopic ureterocele. Coned view of urogram shows mild dilation of the distal right ureter with a bulbous protrusion into the bladder (arrows). This is the "spring onion" or "cobra head" deformity of the distal ureter typical of this condition. The lucent rim surrounding the ureterocele is mucosa elevated by the intravesical portion of the dilated ureter.

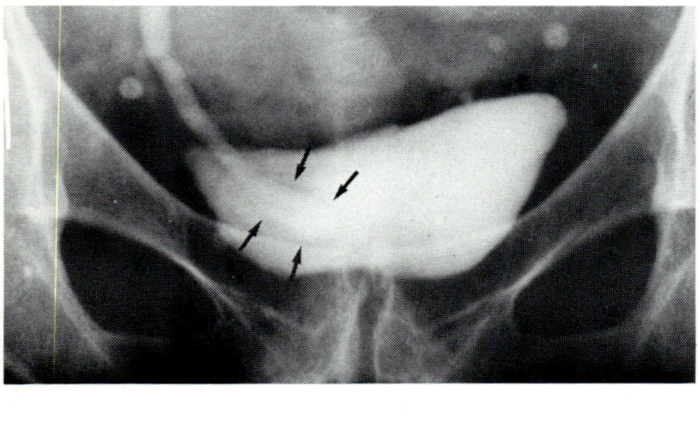

Ectopic ureteroceles are almost exclusively associated with ureteral duplications and will be discussed in detail in Chap. 18.

BLADDER

URACHAL ANOMALIES

The urachus is a fibrous cord that runs from the apex of the bladder to the umbilicus in the plane between the peritoneum and the transversalis fascia. Anomalies of the urachus result from incomplete obliteration of parts of this cord, which during embryonic development was a patent tube. If there has been no obliteration at all, a completely patent urachus persists, and urine may drain from the umbilicus. A urachal diverticulum is seen as a pocket projecting from the dome of the bladder and is the result of obliteration of the umbilical end of the urachal cord. These diverticula may be small or large and are usually asymptomatic. However, if they retain significant residual urine, they may be the site of stone or tumor formation. If the bladder end of the urachus obliterates, the result is a urachal sinus. This may be the site of recurrent infection or a frank abscess, either of which results in infected drainage from the umbilicus. Sinography usually delineates this inferiorly directed cavity. Finally, if both the umbilical and vesical ends of the urachus obliterate, a urachal cyst may develop in the nonobliterated, central portion of the urachus. These may be multiple or single and are usually asymptomatic unless, on rare occasions, they become infected. Ultrasound or CT (Fig. 5-9) will demonstrate a cystic mass (or masses) anteriorly in the region between the umbilicus and dome of the bladder in such cases.

BLADDER DUPLICATION AND SEPTATION

Bladder duplication and septation are extremely rare anomalies of the bladder. Complete duplication results in two bladders, one on either side of the midline. Each bladder receives a ureter and empties by a separate urethra. This duplication anomaly is often associated with duplication of other structures such as the penis, vagina, and rectum. Partial duplication of the bladder involves communication between the two sides and drainage via a single urethra.

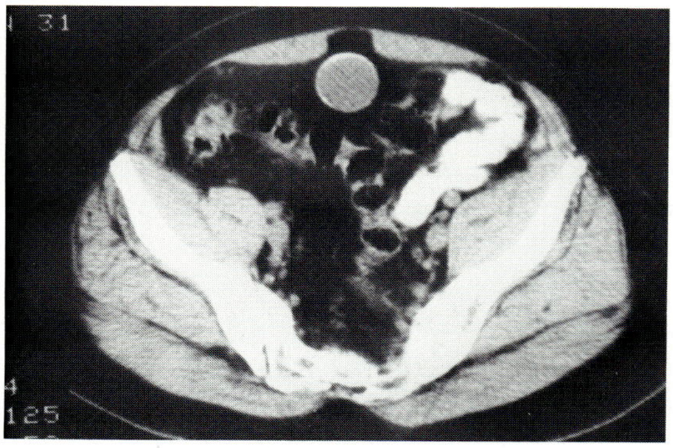

Figure 5-9. Urachal cyst. CT section immediately above bladder shows a cystic structure with calcified rim adjacent to the posterior surface of the anterior abdominal wall.

Another disorder of bladder compartmentalization is the division of a single bladder into two portions by either a sagittal or coronal septum that can be detected on urography or cystography. If incomplete, this type of septation causes no problems. If complete, with a ureter draining into the closed portion, the associated kidney will be dysplastic and nonfunctional.

CONGENITAL BLADDER DIVERTICULUM

Congenital diverticula of the bladder occur in close relation to the ureteral orifice. They usually lie slightly above and lateral to the orifice and have the potential of compromising the valve mechanism, thus resulting in vesicoureteral reflux. These are referred to as Hutch diverticula and may be quite variable in size. On rare occasions such diverticula may cause ureteral obstruction rather than reflux.

BLADDER EARS

Bladder ears are protrusions of the inferolateral portions of the urinary bladder bilaterally into the regions of the inguinal canals. They are seen in infants on either urography or voiding cystourethrography and are thought to be due to a close relation of the bladder to the inguinal rings in infants. They tend to disappear as the bladder fills and become less apparent as the child ages. This is a normal transient phenomenon in infants and should not be confused with true herniation of the bladder.

EXSTROPHY OF THE BLADDER

Exstrophy of the bladder results from failure of the midline mesodermal elements below the umbilicus to fuse [19]. In such patients, the rectus abdominis muscles are widely separated in the lower abdomen, and the bladder is seen open and everted on the lower abdominal wall. Around the bladder periphery the abdominal skin is continuous with the bladder mucosa. The trigone and ureteral orifices can be easily seen. The exposed bladder in true exstrophy is predisposed to epithelial metaplastic changes leading to adenocarcinomas. In the male, the penis is short and spadelike. The urethra is open along its dorsal surface as it extends to the opened bladder. Isolated epispadias, due to failure of dorsal fusion of the urethra, constitutes the lesser end of this spectrum. The incidence of exstrophy is approximately 1 in 30,000 births. The incidence in males as opposed to females is 3:1.

A plain film of the abdomen will reveal varying degrees of separation of the pubic symphysis (Fig. 5-10), which should never exceed 1 cm in normal cases. In full-blown exstrophy the pubes are widely separated. Early on, the upper tracts are normal on urography. The lower ends of the ureters make a wide lateral sweep and then pass medially and slightly upward to join the wall of the bladder in the region of the trigone. The dilated appearance of the distal ureters has been likened to that of

Figure 5-10. Exstropy. Plain film of pelvis reveals extremely wide separation of the pubes typical of severe exstrophy.

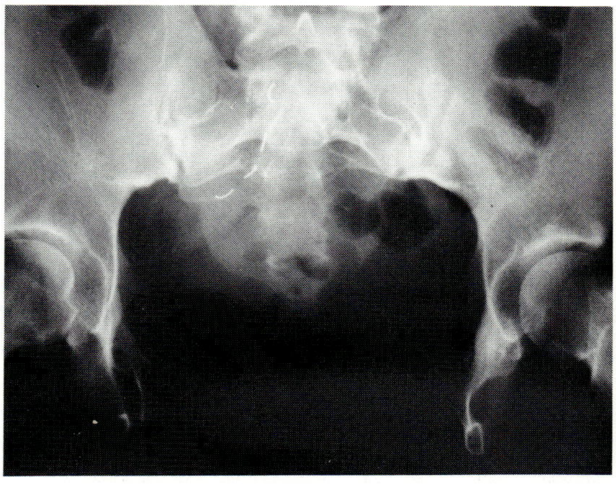

a "Hurley," the stick used in the traditional Irish game of Hurling.

While in some cases the bladder can be successfully closed primarily, many patients with exstrophy will require excision of the bladder and supravesical diversion of urine.

URETHRA

POSTERIOR URETHRAL VALVES

Posterior urethral valves are a common cause of congenital bladder outlet obstruction in male infants and young boys [14]. They can present in utero with bilateral hydronephrosis and urine ascites or be detected in the neonatal period. In some instances, valves can present in later childhood or even in an adult. Valves are congenital thick folds of mucous membrane occurring in the posterior urethra. They cause symptoms by obstructing the outflow of urine from the bladder. The urinary stream is frequently weak.

There are three types of posterior urethral valves (Fig. 5-11). Type I, the most common, are mucosal folds extending anteriorly and inferiorly from the distal verumontanum. Type II valves are mucosal folds seen near the bladder neck; these are very rare and are now considered an effect of bladder obstruction rather than a true congenital valve. The Type III valve, also rare, is an iris diaphragm usually located below the verumontanum and unrelated to it.

On voiding, the classic Type I posterior urethral valves capture the voided urine and billow out like sails, significantly obstructing the posterior urethra. As with any cause of bladder-outlet obstruction, the eventual result is hypertrophy of the bladder detrusor. The bladder neck also tends to hypertrophy and thus remains relatively narrow in relation to the dilated posterior urethra. The ureterovesical junctions may be obstructed because of thickening of the bladder wall or may permit massive bilateral vesicoureteral reflux. In either case, bilateral hydroureteronephrosis can be seen. The increased pressure in the pelvicaliceal system may result in leakage of urine into the perirenal space with formation of a urinoma, and if there is extravasation of significant amounts of urine, urine ascites or urothorax may result.

In cases of severely obstructing valves, urography reveals bilateral dilatation of the upper tracts either due to reflux or functional obstruction. During voiding cystourethrography, the urethral catheter can be passed in retrograde fashion easily into the bladder. However, during voiding, the posterior urethra is dilated with contrast medium, ballooning the saillike valves extending from the verumontanum distally (Fig. 5-12). The bladder neck is often narrowed and the urethra distal to the valves is

Figure 5-11. Diagram of posterior urethral valves in boys. Type I—These extend from the verumontanum distally and catch urine during voiding like a sail catches wind. Type II—Prominent tissue folds near the bladder neck. These are probably sequelae of bladder obstruction rather than a true valve. Type III—A diaphragm with small opening is found in the distal portion of the posterior urethra.

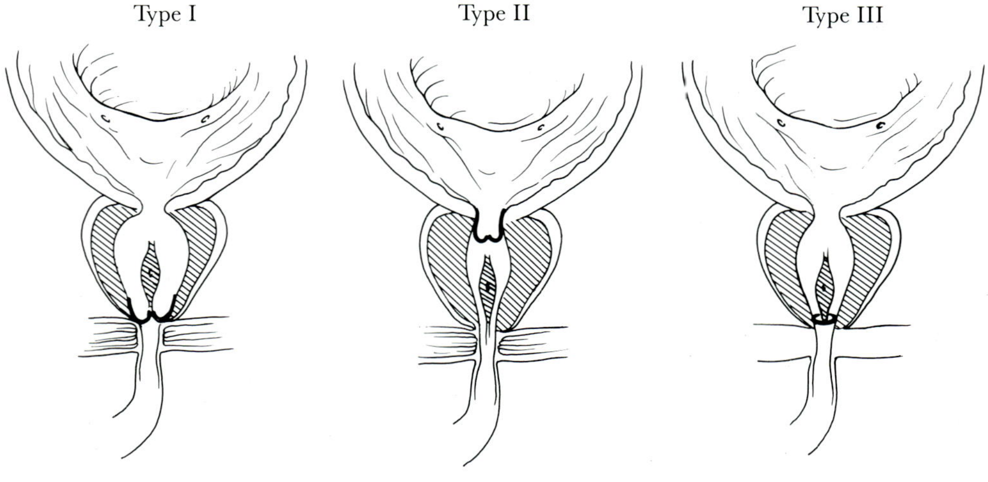

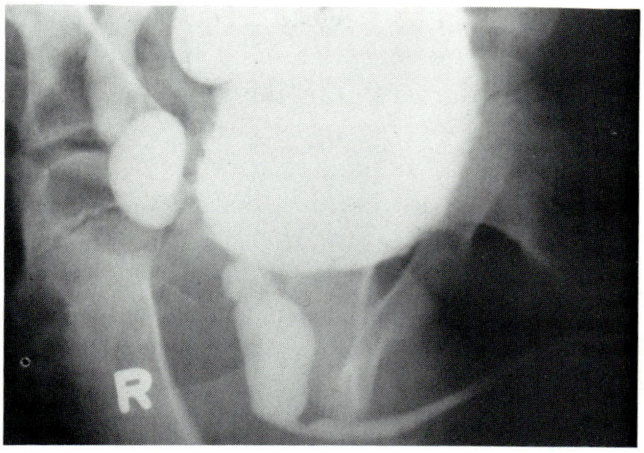

Figure 5-12. Posterior urethral valves, Type I. Voiding cystourethrography in young boy shows a dilated posterior urethra typical of this condition. The actual valves are not seen. Note trabeculated bladder with diverticula and reflux.

poorly distended. Vesicoureteral reflux is seen in about 50 percent of cases.

Treatment of posterior urethral valves is cystoscopic fulguration. However, temporary diversion of urine by vesicostomy or loop cutaneous ureterostomy is often necessary for decompression of the upper tracts.

ANTERIOR URETHRAL VALVES AND DIVERTICULA

Anterior urethral valves and saccular diverticula of the ventral anterior urethra are often difficult to differentiate [11]. Both are uncommon. Congenital diverticula are termed saccular or diffuse on the basis of their configuration. The diffuse type is a generalized dilatation of the entire anterior urethra, which has also been called megalourethra. The more typical saccular diverticulum has a rather characteristic appearance, with contrast material filling an oval-shaped structure on the ventral aspect of the anterior urethra during voiding cystourethrography. A saccular diverticulum may produce anterior urethral obstruction by a valvelike action of the distal lip of the diverticulum. As the diverticulum fills during the voiding phase, the thin distal lip is elevated against the roof of the urethra, producing a true obstruction. An anterior urethral valve can produce a very similar radiographic pattern but is differentiated by the proximal end of the urethral dilation forming an obtuse angle with the ventral floor of the urethra, unlike the saccular diverticulum, in which the proximal lip forms an acute angle (Fig. 5-13). In either case, stasis of urine in the region of the obstruction can result in retained stones and postvoid dribbling.

Dorsal urethral diverticula are very rare. These occur in the fossa navicularis (distal 2 cm of urethra) and are called lacuna magna. On voiding cystourethrography lacuna magna present as small rounded collections of contrast dorsal to the distal urethra, which often persist after voiding is complete.

Figure 5-13. Diagram of anterior urethral diverticulum and anterior urethral valve. While the radiographic appearance can be similar, note that the proximal lip of the diverticulum forms an acute angle with the floor of the urethra, while the valve results in a proximal obtuse angle.

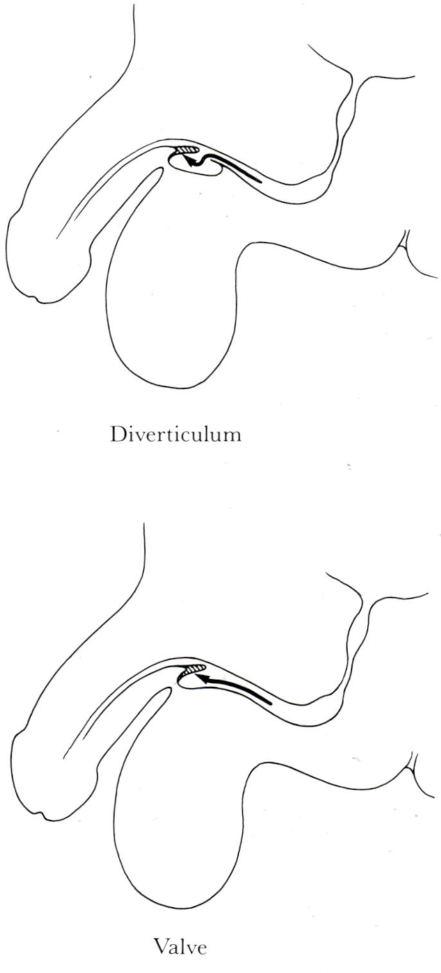

CONGENITAL URETHRAL POLYPS

Congenital urethral polyps are a rare cause of bladder outlet obstruction in boys [3]. These benign fibroepithelial structures originate from the verumontanum and are identical histopathologically to fibroepithelial polyps of the ureter, having a fibrovascular core covered with normal transitional epithelium. The majority of these polyps have a tendency to protrude toward the bladder from the posterior urethra and cause intermittent bladder neck obstruction. On voiding cystourethrography they appear as oval filling defects in the posterior urethra. Sonography demonstrates a soft-tissue polypoid mass projecting from the bladder neck into the bladder lumen.

CONGENITAL STENOSIS OF THE MALE URETHRA

Congenital urethral strictures, as opposed to posterior urethral valves, are quite rare in the male. These may involve the bulbous or penile urethra and are variable in length. Either retrograde or voiding urethrography demonstrates fixed areas of narrowing in the anterior urethra. Strictures or atresia of the female urethra also occur rarely.

COWPER'S DUCT CYSTS

Cysts of Cowper's ducts may be congenital in origin and on rare occasion may be large enough to present in the newborn as severe urethral obstruction due to encroachment on the lumen. Cowper's glands are paired and lie on either side of the membranous urethra. Their ducts course about 2 cm inferiorly before entering the bulbous urethra. A retention cyst in one of these ducts is seen by either voiding or retrograde urethrography as a rounded impression on the floor of the bulbous urethra. When symptomatic, treatment is by transurethral unroofing.

DUPLICATION OF THE URETHRA

As noted previously, urethral duplications can occur in association with bladder and penile duplications. However, those are to be differentiated from the duplications that exist within the single penis [4]. Radiographic evaluation is required in any patient who is referred with two meatal openings or with a double urinary stream. Urethral duplications can be either blind-ending or complete. The blind urethral duplication can open on the dorsal or ventral surface of the penis but does not communicate with the urethra or bladder. It can also originate from the normal urethral channel and end blindly in the periurethral tissue. In the complete variety, there can be two noncommunicating urethras arising independently from the bladder, each coursing to a separate meatus on the glans of the penis. Alternatively, a second urethra can arise from the main urethra and course independently to a second meatus on the penis. In yet another variety, two urethras can arise from the bladder and unite into a common channel distally (Fig. 5-14). The ventrally positioned urethral channel, regardless of the absolute position of its meatus, usually proves to

Figure 5-14. Duplication of the male urethra. Retrograde urethrography shows Foley balloon inflated in dilated common distal urethra. Two distinct channels are seen proximally, though the proximal origin of the ventral channel is not seen.

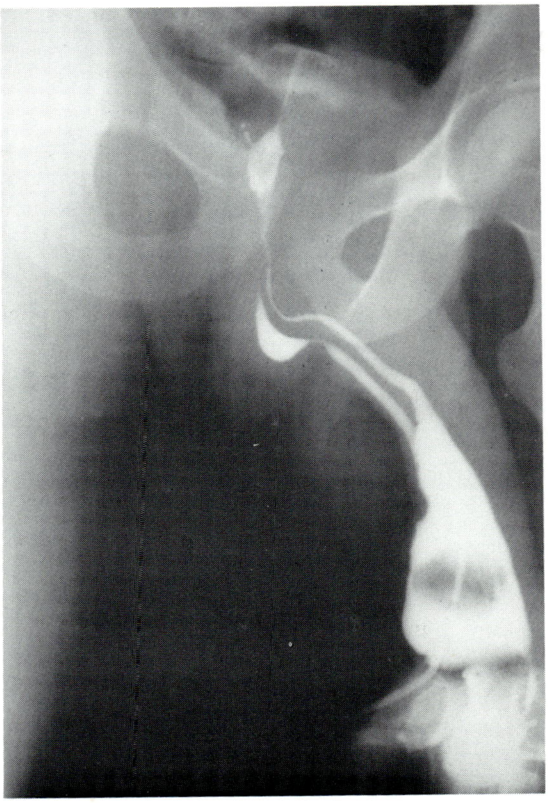

be the more functional channel. Radiographic evaluation usually requires both retrograde urethrography (often with two catheters) and voiding cystourethrography.

HYPOSPADIAS/EPISPADIAS

Epispadias has been discussed in relation to exstrophy of the bladder. This condition denotes a dorsal opening of the urethral meatus on the shaft of the penis. Conversely, hypospadias denotes a ventral location of the meatus proximal to its normal position on the glans penis. This abnormal location can be found anywhere from the corona to the perineum. With perineal hypospadias, there is frequently associated a fibrous band running the length of the ventral penis and resulting in a chordee, or ventral curvature of the penis. Stenosis of the meatus is not uncommon in hypospadias. The foreshortened urethra in either hypospadias or epispadias can be easily seen on voiding cystourethrography. Widening of the public symphysis is frequently seen with severe epispadias.

SEMINAL VESICLES, PROSTATE, AND TESTES

SEMINAL VESICLE CYSTS

Approximately two-thirds of seminal vesicle cysts are associated with ipsilateral agenesis of the kidney. This is due to the common origin of the seminal vesicle and the ureteral bud from the mesonephric duct. If there is simple failure of the ureteral bud, the end result is renal agenesis. However, if there is maldevelopment of the mesonephric duct, both the urinary and genital tracts are affected.

While the majority of seminal vesicle cysts are less than 5 cm in diameter, they can reach a size of 12 cm or more. The differential between seminal vesicle cyst with agenesis and ipsilateral ectopy of the ureter to the seminal vesicle is often difficult to make. Both result in cystic dilatation of the seminal vesicle and nonvisualization of the kidney. Nonfunction in the case of ectopic ureteral insertion is due to severe dysplasia of the kidney.

Further differential considerations in seminal vesical cysts include müllerian duct cyst, hydronephrotic pelvic kidney, pelvic abscess, cystic pelvic tumor, and anterior meningomyelocele. The last condition is usually associated with the "scimitar" sacral deformity: significant lateral deviation of an eroded sacrum away from the meningomyelocele.

Urographically, the bladder reveals extrinsic lateral compression in direct relation to the size of the cyst. While sonography can differentiate the cystic from the solid nature of the mass, CT is the definitive method for imaging these lesions and shows that the seminal vesicle is replaced by an associated thick-walled cystic structure that may on occasion appear solid because of hemorrhage within the cyst [8]. Needle puncture of the cystic structure will confirm the diagnosis if necessary, as only seminal vesicle cysts among the previously mentioned differentials contain spermatozoa [20].

The seminal vesicle can also, on rare occasion, be congenitally absent. This can be a unilateral or bilateral condition and may be associated with agenesis of the vasa deferentia. Unilateral absence of the vas deferens, when detected on physical examination, requires evaluation of the upper urinary tract; many of such cases are associated with ipsilateral renal agenesis.

DILATED UTRICLE

The utricle is a müllerian remnant that is normally present as a small cavity in the central portion of the verumontanum in males. It can be congenitally quite large. Dilated utricles are generally seen from infancy to adolescence. They are usually asymptomatic but may be associated with hypospadias or cryptorchidism. They can be demonstrated radiographically by voiding cystourethrography, which results in filling of the dilated utricle extending posteriorly from the prostatic urethra in the region of the verumontanum.

MÜLLERIAN DUCT CYSTS

Müllerian duct cysts occur in the midline in the location expected for a dilated utricle, though they do not communicate with the posterior urethra. They are most commonly detected during the third and fourth decades of life. They have varied clinical presentations, depending on the size of the cyst and whether or not it is infected. Symptoms include bladder outflow obstruction, lower urinary tract irritative symptoms, hematuria, suprapubic or rectal pain, and the presence of a midline pelvic mass palpable near the upper margin of the prostate on rectal examination. As with seminal vesicle cysts, ultrasound as well as CT and MRI have been useful in the imaging of müllerian cysts [18]. The diagnosis of müllerian duct cyst is usually confirmed by showing the anatomic relationship between the cyst and the verumontanum; the cyst lies posterior and superior to the prostate.

UNDESCENDED TESTIS

The undescended testis (cryptorchism, cryptorchidism) is a common anomaly in male infants. The incidence at birth is 3.5 percent, though this decreases to less than 1 percent by the age of 1 year because of spontaneous descent. The condition is bilateral in 10 percent of cases. The undescended testis is palpable in 80 percent of cases and impalpable in the remainder. In this last group, the testis is absent in 4 percent of cases. Cryptorchid testes may be found anywhere from the inguinal canal (80%) to the level of the kidneys.

This is a clinically significant condition, as the complications include infertility and an increased risk of malignancy in the abnormal testis. It has been estimated that men with an undescended testis have an almost 10-fold risk of dying from testicular malignancy as compared with men with normally decended testes. Orchiopexy is the treatment of choice and is usually performed at about the age of 1 year. In cryptorchid patients who are beyond the age of puberty, the undescended testis is usually removed because of the risk of malignancy.

The low-lying cryptorchid testis can usually be successfully imaged by gonadal venography, ultrasound, CT, or MRI. On the other hand, the high testis generally cannot be found. Since most urologists employ the same surgical approach for impalpable as for palpable testes and do not consider the procedure completed until the testis is found or proven absent, it has been suggested that diagnostic imaging in these cases will influence neither the decision to operate nor the surgical approach [5]. The imaging findings in undescended testes are discussed in Chap. 24.

PRUNE BELLY SYNDROME

The prune belly syndrome is a triad of findings consisting of congenital absence or deficiency of the abdominal wall musculature, anomalies of the urinary tract, and bilateral cryptorchidism. It is also known as the Eagle-Barrett syndrome and occurs in approximately 1 of 40,000 live births. The large majority occur in males, only 5 percent having been reported in female patients. It has been hypothesized that the entire complex of findings in this syndrome is secondary to urethral obstruction with subsequent distention of the bladder and abdominal laxity on the basis of this bladder distention. However, it is now thought that the prune belly syndrome is a multisystem disease complex whose cause is probably best explained by a mesodermal defect occurring in early embryological development [6].

Urinary tract abnormalities are the major prognostic factor in patients with prune belly syndrome. Twenty percent of patients are stillborn, 30 percent die of renal failure or urosepsis within 2 years of birth, and the remaining 50 percent usually exhibit varying degrees of urinary pathology. The most obvious clinical finding in patients with the syndrome is the shriveled prunelike appearance of the abdominal wall.

Radiographically, the abdomen is quite wide due to bulging of the flanks. At urography, approximately 80 percent of patients exhibit dilated, tortuous ureters that are more markedly widened in their distal portion (Fig. 5-15A). Vesicoureteral reflux is common. Involvement of the kidneys ranges from renal agenesis or hypoplasia, both of which are rare, to varying degrees of hydronephrosis; in many instances the kidneys are essentially normal. The bladder is generally enlarged, though without trabeculation in most cases. However, obstruction of the urethra occurs in a minority of cases, usually in infants who die early [2]. A patent urachus decompressing the bladder can occasionally be seen. There is frequently hypoplasia of the prostate, resulting in a characteristically wide

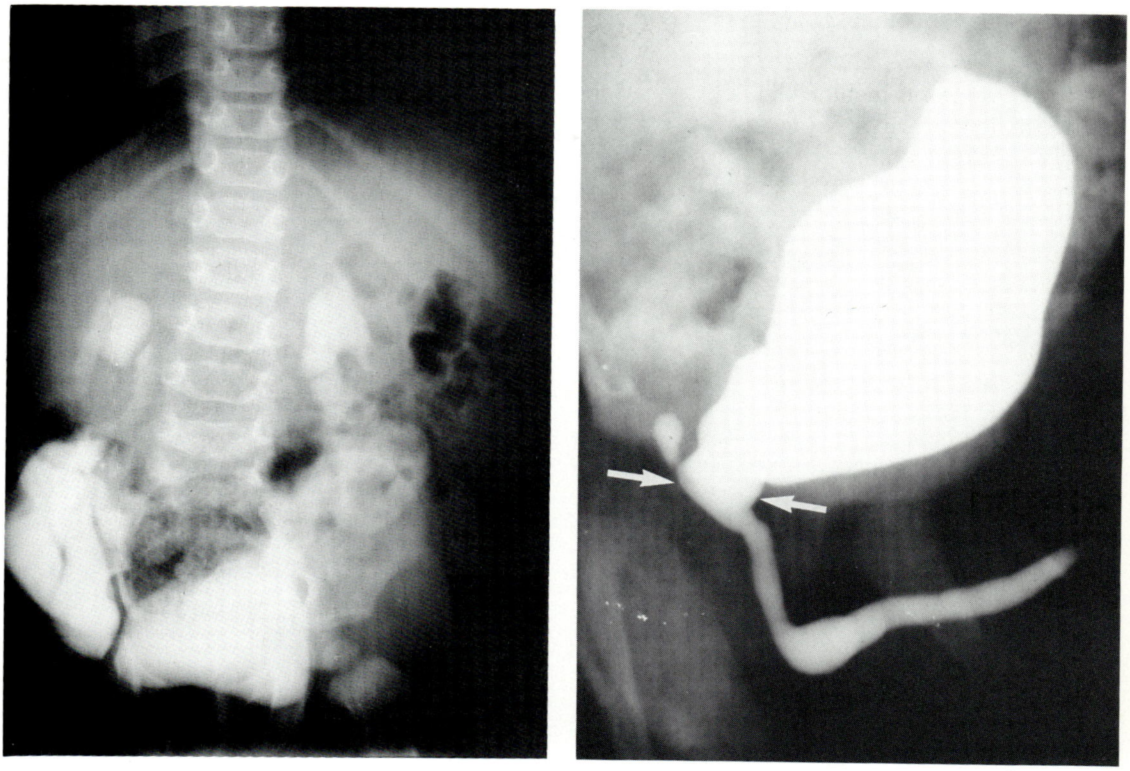

A B

Figure 5-15. Prune belly syndrome. A. Urography shows minimal dilation of the intrarenal collecting systems, though the ureters are dilated, tortuous, and laterally deviated. B. Voiding cystourethrography shows a widely dilated prostatic urethra (arrows) and a slightly dilated utricle extending posteriorly from the dilated urethra.

prostatic urethra tapering to the level of the urogenital diaphragm (Fig. 5-15B). On occasion, the anterior urethra may also be dilated throughout its length (megalourethra).

IN UTERO SONOGRAPHY FOR DETECTION OF CONGENITAL GENITOURINARY ABNORMALITIES

With recent improvements in sonographic equipment, it has become possible to evaluate the fetus accurately for genitourinary anomalies. The fetal kidneys and bladder can usually be imaged by 15 weeks of fetal age, and the adrenals can be seen at 16 to 18 weeks. At 20 to 25 weeks, the cortex and medulla of the kidney can usually be distinguished. It is now generally recognized that mild pyelectasis seen in the fetus is not unusual and is affected by the hydration status of the mother. Table 5-1 lists congenital

Table 5-1. Genitourinary anomalies detectable by fetal sonography

Agenesis of the kidney
Ectopic kidney
Multicystic dysplastic kidney
Polycystic kidney disease
Autosomal recessive
Autosomal dominant
Ureteropelvic junction (UPJ) obstruction
Ureterectasis
Reflux
Primary megaureter
Ureterocele
Patent urachus
Exstrophy of the bladder
Scrotal hydrocele
Mesoblastic nephroma

conditions of the genitourinary system that have been reported as effectively imaged by fetal ultrasound [7, 17]. Generally speaking, the sonographic appearance of each anomaly is similar to that encountered in the term infant after delivery. These findings have been discussed previously in this chapter or will be covered elsewhere in this book.

REFERENCES

1. Arant, B.S., Sotclo-Avila, C., and Berstein, J. Segmental "hypoplasia" of the kidney (Ask-Upmark). *J. Pediatr.* 95:931, 1979.
2. Berdon, W. E., et al. The radiologic and pathologic spectrum of the prune belly syndrome. *Radiol. Clin. North Am.* 15:83, 1977.
3. Caro, P.A., Rosenbery, H.K., and McCrum, H.S., III. Congenital urethral polyp. *A.J.R.* 147:1041, 1986.
4. Effmann, E.L., Lebowitz, R.L., and Colodny, A.H. Duplication of the urethra. *Radiology* 119: 179, 1976.
5. Friedland, G.W., and Chang, P. The role of imaging in the management of the impalpable undescended testis. *A.J.R.* 151:1107, 1988.
6. Greskovich, F.J., III, and Nyberg, L.M., Jr. The prune belly syndrome: A review of its etiology, defects, treatment and prognosis. *J. Urol.* 140: 707, 1988.
7. Hill, M.C., Lande, I.M., and Larsen, J.W., Jr. Prenatal diagnosis of fetal anomalies using ultrasound and MRI. *Radiol. Clin. North Am.* 26:287, 1988.
8. Kenney, P.J., and Leeson, M.D. Congenital anomalies of the seminal vesicles: Spectrum of computed tomographic findings. *Radiology* 149:247, 1983.
9. Kenney, P.J., et al. Adrenal glands in patients with congenital renal anomalies: CT appearance. *Radiology* 155:181, 1985.
10. Kenney, R.D., Flippo, J.L., and Black, E.B. Supernumerary nipples and renal anomalies in neonates. *Am. J. Dis. Child.* 141:987, 1987.
11. Kirks, D.R., and Grossman, H. Congenital saccular anterior urethral diverticulum. *Radiology* 140:367, 1981.
12. Kissane, J.M. Congenital Malformations. In R.H. Heptinstall (ed.), *Pathology of the Kidney.* Boston: Little, Brown, 1966.
13. Lautin, E.M., et al. CT diagnosis of circumcaval ureter. *A.J.R.* 150:591, 1988.
14. Macpherson, R.I., et al. Posterior urethral valves: An update and review. *RadioGraphics* 6:753, 1986.
15. Mascatello, V., and Lebowitz, R.L. Malposition of the colon in left renal agenesis and ectopia. *Radiology* 120:371, 1976.
16. Quan, L., et al. The VATER association. *Birth Defects* 8:75, 1972.
17. Rouse, G.A., et al. Current concepts in sonographic diagnosis of fetal renal disease. *RadioGraphics* 8:119, 1988.
18. Thurnher, S., Hricak, H., and Tanagho, E.A. Müllerian duct cyst: Diagnosis with MR imaging. *Radiology* 168:25, 1988.
19. White, P., and Lebowitz, R.L. Exstrophy of the bladder. *Radiol. Clin. North Am.* 15:93, 1977.
20. Yoder, I.C., and Pfister, R.C. Congenital anomalies of the adult bladder and urethra. *Semin. Roentgenol.* 18:267, 1983.

6

The Retroperitoneum

Three decades ago, the retroperitoneum was described, perhaps aptly, as a "hinterland of straggling mesenchyme, with vascular and nervous plexuses, weird embryonic rests and shadowy fascial boundaries" [12]. However, in recent years the evolution of cross-sectional imaging techniques has allowed clear delineation of the several spaces and potential spaces that make up the posterior abdomen. See Chap. 2 for a discussion of these compartmental boundaries.

Many pathologic conditions can occur in the retroperitoneum. Primary disease of the adrenals, kidneys, and ureters will be discussed in subsequent chapters. Other conditions, by virtue of their occurrence in the relatively confined retroperitoneal compartments, may directly affect the urinary tract by invading, surrounding, or displacing the kidneys and ureters. The retroperitoneal disease processes to be discussed in this chapter include fluid collections, retroperitoneal fibrosis, lymphadenopathy, primary retroperitoneal tumors, and chyluria.

FLUID COLLECTIONS

Various types of fluid collections can occur in the retroperitoneum. These include blood, urine, lymph, and pus. Urinomas can occur after rupture of the collecting system in infant boys with posterior urethral valves; these have already been discussed (Chap. 5). Blunt or penetrating abdominal trauma, with its resultant hemorrhage or urine extravasation, will be discussed in Chap. 25. The following section will deal with spontaneous hemorrhage, infected fluid collections, and lymphoceles in the retroperitoneum.

HEMORRHAGE

The most common cause of retroperitoneal hemorrhage other than trauma is rupture of an abdominal aortic aneurysm. Other sources of bleeding include diseases of the kidney or adrenal as well as any of the retroperitoneal vessels. Retroperitoneal hemorrhage can be life threatening, and its diagnosis, as well as the identification of its source, is necessary for institution of proper therapy

Abdominal aortic aneurysm, aortic diameter exceeding 3 cm, is a common condition that can result in catastrophic complications. An aneurysm less than 5 cm in maximal diameter has approximately a 5 percent chance of rupturing, while with aneurysms more than 7 cm in diameter the risk of rupture increases to over 75 percent [16]. All layers of the wall (intima, media, and adventitia) are involved in this dilation. Pseudoaneurysm results from a prior perforation of the aorta with subsequent resolution of the surrounding hematoma and formation of a cavity limited by adventitia only. Aneurysms are far more common in males than in females and in the large majority of cases are of atherosclerotic origin. Rarely, they can be secondary to prior trauma, syphilis, or mycotic infection or may be seen in conjunction with Marfan's syndrome. On occasion, an inflammatory process (perianeurysmal fibrosis), which may be difficult to differentiate from leakage of blood, can surround the aneurysm.

Radiographic evaluation of these aneurysms should include the following: craniocaudad extent, any involvement of the renal arteries or extension past the aortic bifurcation, maximum diameter, intraluminal thrombus, and any evidence of leakage. Several techniques are useful in imaging the aorta. Plain films of the abdomen will reveal calcifications in the wall of the aneurysm in up to 85 percent of cases. Sonography is a widely accepted method for screening patients with suspected aneurysms and for follow-up of enlargement when treatment is conservative. The aorta is seen in both longitudinal and transverse views as a tubular, echo-free structure in the left prevertebral area. Intramural thrombus can be seen as moderately echogenic soft tissue within the lumen. Using a longitudinal coronal–oblique plane of imaging with the liver as an acoustic window, the origin of the renal arteries can be seen in about half of patients [22]. However, sonography is not consistent in demonstrating the cephalad extent of an aneurysm in relation to the renal arteries; this is its major weakness.

Computerized tomography (CT) is currently the method of choice for evaluating aortic aneurysms. It is able to delineate their size and extent accurately and, by the use of intravenous contrast medium, can demonstrate compromise of the lumen by intraluminal thrombus. Peri-aneurysmal fibrosis is usually of lower attenuation than acute blood accumulation around the aneurysm during leakage. Furthermore, peri-aneurysmal fibrosis may be enhanced after administration of intravenous contrast medium, as opposed to hematoma, which is not. Involvement of the renal arteries and aortic bifurcation is usually detectable.

Angiography remains the gold standard for evaluating involvement of visceral branches of the aorta. However, in recent years magnetic resonance imaging (MRI) has also been shown to be effective in this regard [18]. The aorta and its major visceral branches appear as signal voids on spin–echo images, usually allowing their easy identification. When imaged in the transverse plane using a multislice technique, however, the most cranial slice of the imaged volume will often show a signal within the aorta due to a flow-related enhancement effect. Coronal and sagittal planes are useful for identifying involvement of the visceral branches from the aorta by an aneurysm. Unfortunately, the relatively long imaging time and the difficulty of monitoring patients while in the magnet usually preclude the use of MRI in evaluating a patient with suspected rupture of an aneurysm. A nonartifactual intraluminal signal can be caused by either slow flow of blood within the aneurysm or by intraluminal thrombus [10].

After aortic aneurysm, the most common causes of retroperitoneal hemorrhage are adrenal or renal pathology. While the term "spontaneous" implies the lack of observable injury, it is likely that in many instances the patient has suffered mild and unrecognized trauma [21]. In the adrenal, both primary and metastatic tumors can hemorrhage spontaneously. In the kidney, renal neoplasm is the most common cause of unprovoked bleeding. This is usually due to renal cell carcinoma or angiomyolipoma, but bleeding from almost all other renal neoplasms has been reported. Angiomyolipomas tend to be larger than 4 cm when they hemorrhage [Fig. 6-1A]. However, hemorrhage from renal cell carcinoma frequently occurs when the tumor is quite small—even in the range of a few

Figure 6-1. Spontaneous retroperitoneal bleeding due to renal lesions. A. Secondary to angiomyolipoma. Contrast-enhanced CT shows a fatty tumor at the lateral margin of the right kidney (arrow). The kidney is surrounded by blood in the perirenal space. B. Secondary to right renal cyst. Contrast-enhanced CT shows a cyst in the lateral margin of the right kidney. The kidney is compressed and distorted by a subcapsular hematoma (black arrows), and there is a collection of blood in the posterior portion of the perirenal space (white arrows) and strands of blood mixed with the perirenal fat in this area.

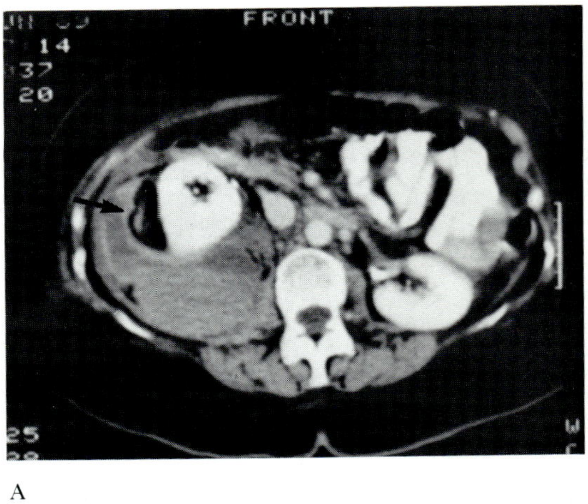

A

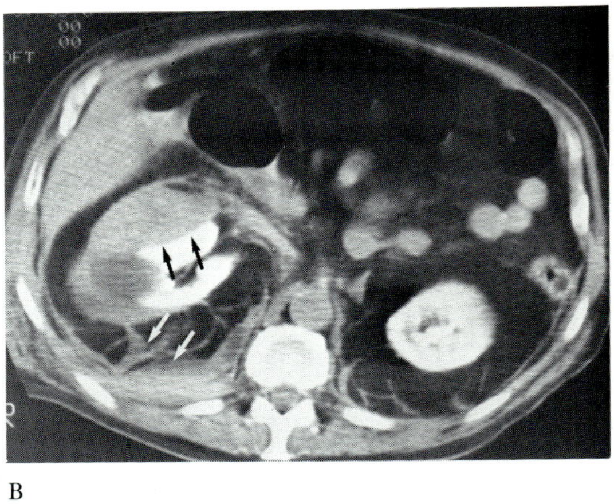

B

millimeters in diameter—and usually peripherally located. In these cases, detection of the responsible lesion is often quite difficult, particularly in light of the sometimes massive perinephric hematoma. In many cases, even CT or angiography reveals no abnormalities that can be specifically identified as the cause of the bleeding.

Other renal lesions that can result in spontaneous bleeding include bleeding diatheses (hemophilia, anticoagulation therapy), polyarteritis nodosa, renal arteriovenous malformations, inflammatory renal lesions (tuberculosis, abscess), hydroephrosis, and rupture of a renal cyst or vessel in the wall of a cyst (Fig. 6-1B). Retroperitoneal bleeding may also be idiopathic; the reported fraction of retroperitoneal hemorrhage for which no cause can be found 4 to 5 percent [1].

The majority of retroperitoneal hemorrhages, whether from an aortic aneurysm or renal–adrenal lesion, is seen in the perinephric space, though dissection into other retroperitoneal spaces is not uncommon. Hemorrhage confined to the anterior pararenal space may be due to duodenal or pancreatic trauma or hemorrhagic pancreatitis. Hemorrhage isolated in the posterior pararenal space, which does not contain any organs, is usually seen in patients on anticoagulant therapy. As in the case of aortic aneurysm, CT is the imaging method of choice in any patient with suspected retroperitoneal hemorrhage. This technique allows delineation of the extent and location of the bleeding. Acute hemorrhage is seen as soft tissue with an attenuation in the range of 40 to 60 Hounsfield units. If treated conservatively, the attenuation of the hematoma drops, approaching the density of water during the final stages of resolution. By MRI, acute hematomas generally exhibit low to medium signal intensities on T-1 weighted images; the signal intensity increases on T-2 weighted images. As the hematoma ages, the periphery (rim) has a higher signal intensity within a few days on T-1 weighted images and the collection then develops a more uniform high intensity in the chronic phase. The plain film and urographic findings of retroperitoneal hemorrhage are described in Chap. 25.

RETROPERITONEAL ABSCESS

Early symptoms of retroperitoneal abscesses can be nonspecific; they include nausea, vomiting, weight loss, fever, and anorexia. On occasion, there can be pain in the flank, or if the abscess is adjacent to or involves the psoas muscle, the patient may complain of pain referred to the ipsilateral hip that is exacerbated by extension or rotation of the thigh.

Over half of retroperitoneal abscesses occur in the anterior pararenal space; these are usually due to inflammatory disease of the pancreas. Those in the perirenal space are usually due to extension of inflammatory processes of the kidney. The rare abscess localized in the posterior pararenal space is most likely to be due to osteomyelitis of the adjacent spine or ribs [5]. Retroperitoneal abscesses may have a predominant fluid appearance, may have an appearance similar to a tumor with a necrotic center, may contain gas, or may be ill-defined with a diffuse inflammatory process extending into adjacent muscles.

Gallium scanning is an excellent method for screening patients with suspected retroperitoneal inflammatory disease, showing an area of increased radioactivity in the region of the abscess. As with retroperitoneal hemorrhage, CT is the best method for defining the extent and nature of this condition. A very small amount of gas within an abscess can easily be detected by CT. Purulent fluid will usually exhibit an attenuation slightly higher than that of water (10 to 20 Hounsfield units). Once the abscess has been defined CT is also useful in guiding diagnostic needle aspiration and catheter placement for percutaneous drainage.

The signal intensity of abscess fluid by MRI is variable and depends on the protein content of the abscess as well as on the amount of debris present within the lesion. On T1 weighted images abscess fluid commonly has a fairly low signal intensity; on T2 images abscesses are bright.

LYMPHOCELE

Lymphoceles are discrete collections of chylous fluid that occur as a complication of pelvic or retroperitoneal lymphadenectomy or renal transplant surgery because of inadequate ligation of disrupted lymphatic trunks. They may occur from several days to months after surgery, though an interval of several weeks is typical. If these lesions are large enough, they may cause venous obstruction, resulting in edema of the lower body and thromboembolism. Furthermore, they may cause painful abdominal distention and ureteral obstruction. On imaging, they are often difficult to distinguish from other retroperitoneal fluid collections.

Sonographic evaluation usually reveals a fluid-filled mass with absent or faint echoes and possibly septations, dependent debris, or both. These findings are also consistent with resolving hematoma or abscess, but the clinical history should be useful in reaching the correct diagnosis. CT is perhaps more definitive, as negative attenuation values of the fluid suggest fat content within a lymphocele. This finding would exclude abscess or hematoma. Percutaneous long-term catheter drainage is usually successful in treating large lymphoceles [24, 26]. On the other hand, small uninfected lymphoceles may be asymptomatic and may spontaneously resolve. Percutaneous aspiration is also useful in differentiating lymphoceles from other retroperitoneal fluid collections. These lymphatic collections, especially in the upper retroperitoneum, are characterized by contents with elevated triglyceride and protein levels.

RETROPERITONEAL FIBROSIS

Retroperitoneal fibrosis is a fibrotic process that becomes clinically significant when it produces ureteral obstruction. Although there are multiple causes of this condition, the majority (68%) of cases are considered to be idiopathic [20]. Idiopathic retroperitoneal fibrosis is known as Ormond's disease. Other causes include various drugs, retroperitoneal fluid collections, inflammatory disease of various intraabdominal organs, metastatic neoplasms, and previous surgery or radiation therapy. Table 6-1 expands on this list.

Grossly, retroperitoneal fibrosis is a nonencapsulated but reasonably well-delineated plaque of fibrous tissue with a woody consistency and gray-white color. On rare occasions this process can be found anywhere from the neck to the pelvic floor, but more commonly it is localized in the area of the lower aorta and common iliac arteries. It can extend laterally beyond the outer margins of the psoas muscles. Ureteral involvement by the plaque can be either unilateral or bilateral and usually occurs at the level of the common iliac arteries.

Table 6-1. Classification and causes of retroperitoneal fibrosis

Idiopathic (Ormond's disease)
Acquired (benign)
Drugs
Methysergide, ergotamine, methyldopa
Retroperitoneal fluid
Blood, urine, contrast medium
Inflammatory disease
Kidneys, pancreas, GI tract
Surgery
Radiation therapy
Acquired (malignant)
Desmoplastic reaction to various metastatic tumors

Idiopathic retroperitoneal fibrosis occurs predominantly in men, usually in the fifth and sixth decades of life. Only rarely has it been reported in children. Clinically, abdominal or back pain due to the fibrotic process itself may precede the flank pain that signals ureteral obstruction. In some instances the disease may be insidious and the ureteral obstruction found only during an evaluation for progressive renal failure of unknown cause.

As noted previously, various metastatic neoplasms may result in malignant retroperitoneal fibrosis. This condition is different from obstruction of the ureter by true retroperitoneal lymphadenopathy and is caused by a desmoplastic reaction that occurs in response to some tumors, notably Hodgkin's disease and other lymphomas, certain sarcomas, and various anaplastic carcinomas (breast, stomach, colon, prostate, lung, kidney). The radiographic findings in idiopathic or benign acquired retroperitoneal fibrosis can be identical to those produced by the malignant variety, resulting in the necessity for biopsy in some cases to establish the definitive diagnosis.

Radiographically, there are no plain-film findings to suggest retroperitoneal fibrosis. On urography, the typical findings are obstruction of one or both ureters by extrinsic compression;

bilateral involvement occurs in about half of cases. The degree of proximal obstruction depends on the extent and duration of ureteral involvement by the fibrous plaque. The point of obstruction is usually below the iliac crest, though virtually the entire ureter(s) may be involved. Older descriptions of the urographic appearance of the ureters in retroperitoneal fibrosis indicate medial deviation in the region of the plaque. However, recent evidence indicates that there is no significant deviation of the ureters from their normal course. Retrograde studies show a smoothly tapered narrowing of the ureter(s) in the region of involvement (Fig. 6-2A). With bilateral obstruction, one side may be more severely affected than the other.

Figure 6-2. Retroperitoneal fibrosis (idiopathic). A. Retrograde ureteropyelogram shows a smooth, tapered narrowing of the right ureter in the region of the upper sacrum (arrow) and hydronephrosis proximal to this narrowing. B. Sonogram of this area shows a relatively well defined hypoechoic plaque (arrows) just anterior to the sacrum (S). C. CT shows that the plaque envelops the calcified common iliac arteries. A stent has been placed in the right ureter (arrow) which is seen encapsulated in the right anterolateral margin of the plaque.

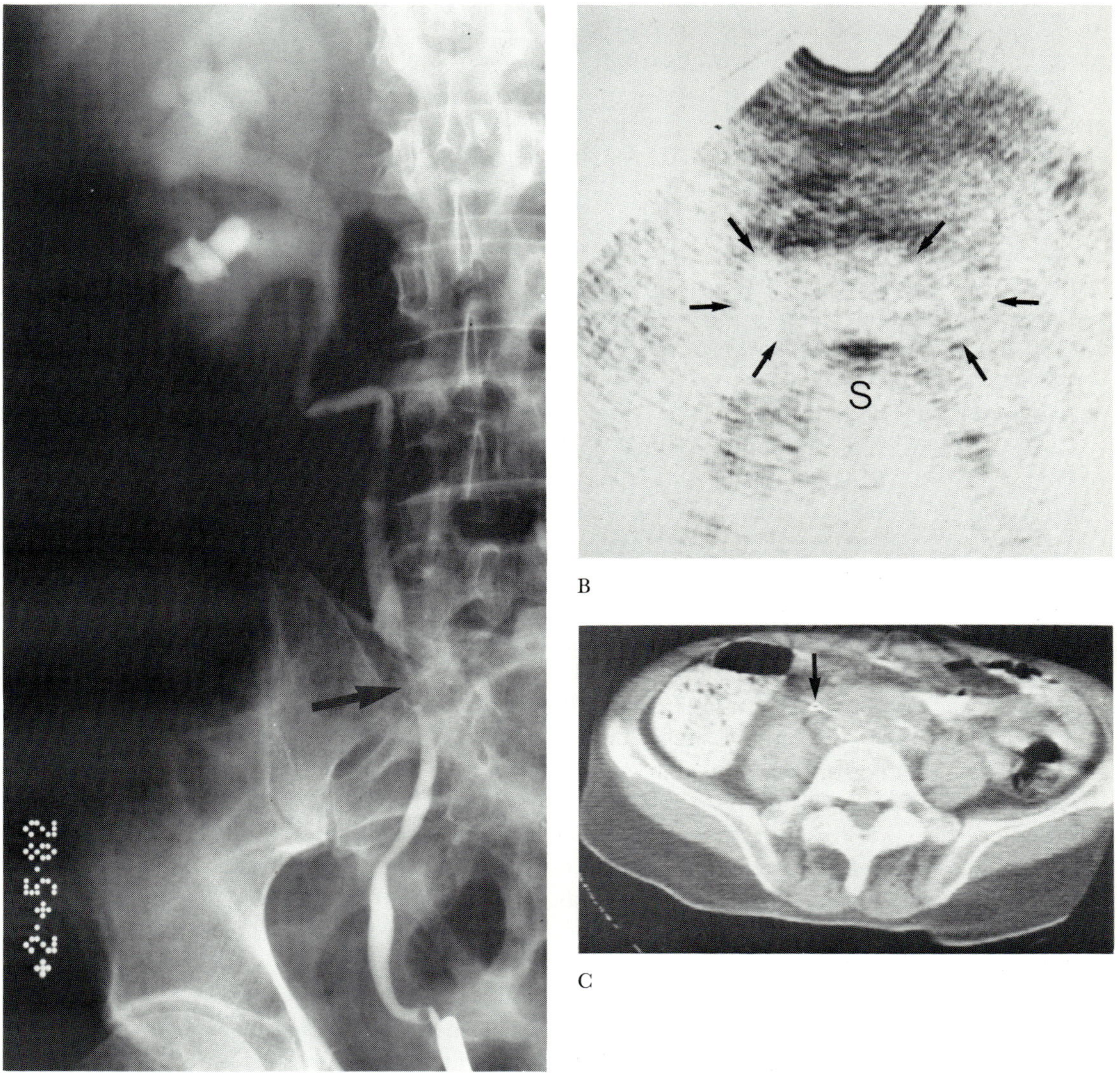

B

C

A

The sonographic appearance of retroperitoneal fibrosis is rather typical; a relatively echopenic, well-demarcated mass is usually seen anterior to the sacral promontory (Fig. 6-2B). However, CT is the more definitive method for evaluating this disease, although it may be difficult to differentiate the fibrotic plaque from true adenopathy in the region of the great vessels [4]. Generally speaking, retroperitoneal fibrosis is seen on CT as a plaque of tissue enveloping but not displacing the aorta, inferior vena cava, and ureters (Fig. 6-2C). The attenuation value of the plaque ranges between 30 and 50 Hounsfield units. After intravenous administration of contrast medium, this density may be seen to increase in some cases, indicating that the fibrotic process is vascularized. The ureters are usually seen lying anterolateral to the fibrotic mass and either adherent to it or completely enveloped for a short distance [7]. The obstruction of the upper urinary tract seen in patients whose ureters do not appear to be encapsulated by the mass may be secondary to an interference with ureteral peristaltic activity rather than true mechanical obstruction. It has been reported that retroperitoneal fibrosis does not result in anterior displacement of the aorta, while this finding is often seen with lymphadenopathy [9].

The diagnostic information provided by MRI regarding the extent of retroperitoneal fibrosis has been reported as similar to that derived from CT [13]. Furthermore, MRI is able to define the extent of constriction or obstruction of the aorta or inferior vena cava as their lumina exhibit signal voids during imaging—information that would require administration of an intravenous contrast agent on CT. MRI of retroperitoneal fibrosis reveals similar morphologic findings for both the benign and malignant varieties. On T2 weighted images, however, it has been reported that malignant retroperitoneal fibrosis exhibits a high signal intensity while the nonmalignant variety shows a low-signal intensity [2]. Furthermore, malignant retroperitoneal fibrosis tends to have a heterogeneous appearance while nonmalignant disease is uniformly homogeneous. Thus, MRI may prove to be superior to CT in its ability to differentiate malignant from benign retroperitoneal fibrosis.

When caused by drugs, retroperitoneal fibrosis may regress after cessation of drug therapy. Steroids have been useful in treating some cases of benign disease. Otherwise, progressive ureteral obstruction by benign retroperitoneal fibrosis usually requires freeing of the ureters from the fibrotic mass (ureterolysis) and transplantation of them into the peritoneal cavity to prevent recurrence. Percutaneous biopsy may be necessary in patients with no known primary malignancy in order to establish the true nature of the fibrotic process [14].

RETROPERITONEAL LYMPHADENOPATHY

The retroperitoneal lymph nodes lie adjacent to the aorta and inferior vena cava and their visceral branches. Metastatic involvement of these nodes can occur with the reticuloendothelial neoplasms as well as various sarcomas and carcinomas. The nodes may be discretely involved or conglomerate into large lymph-node masses in the retroperitoneum. Discrete lymph-node involvement by tumor is microscopic in the early stages, resulting in no change in the size of the nodes. As these metastatic lesions grow, the nodes enlarge, resulting in their detectability by various imaging methods. Normal lymph nodes range in size from 3 to 10 mm in diameter and are usually round or ovoid in shape. Abdominal lymph nodes are considered abnormal if they are larger than 1.5 cm in diameter [17]. The significance of an isolated retroperitoneal node measuring between 1.0 and 1.5 cm is equivocal, though visualizing a number of nodes in this size range should increase the suspicion of malignancy. As the metastatic process continues the end result may be conglomeration of multiple enlarged nodes, resulting in a large lobular retroperitoneal mass.

Lymphomas (both Hodgkin's and non-Hodgkin's varieties) and leukemias are related diseases. The lymphomas are thought to originate as a local disease of lymph nodes that exhibit predictable spread to become systemic. Leukemia, on the other hand, is thought to be a systemic disease from the onset [6]. Because of these differences, accurate staging is critical in lymphoma but rarely necessary in the evaluation of the leukemias. Of the lymphomas, 30 percent are Hodgkin's disease and the remainder are of the non-Hodgkin's variety. The non-Hodgkin's lymphomas and leukemia usually result in significantly enlarged nodes, while patients with Hodgkin's disease will often demonstrate more discrete involvement of individual nodes—a finding similar to that commonly seen with metastatic carcinomas. Most urologic tumors can result in metastatic retroperitoneal lymphadenopathy (Fig. 6-3A).

In the past pedal lymphangiography was a primary method for evaluating retroperitoneal nodes. This demonstrates that the enlarged nodes of non-Hodgkin's lymphoma and leukemia have a foamy internal architectural pattern.

Figure 6-3. Retroperitoneal adenopathy. A. CT demonstrates a discrete 3-cm node (arrow) in periaortic area (prostate cancer stage D2). B. CT shows a large, conglomerate node mass enveloping the calcified aorta (non-Hodgkin's lymphoma).

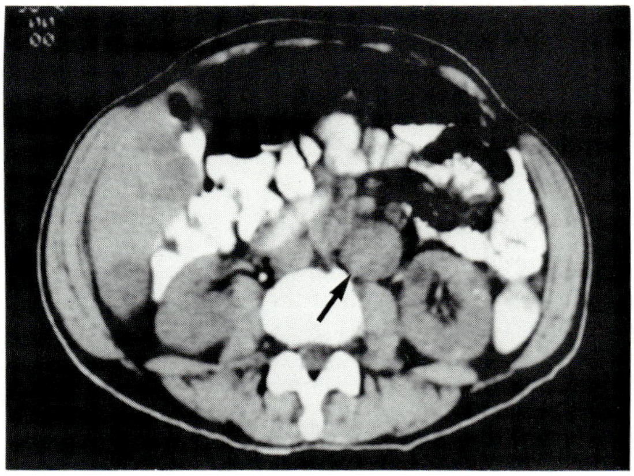

A

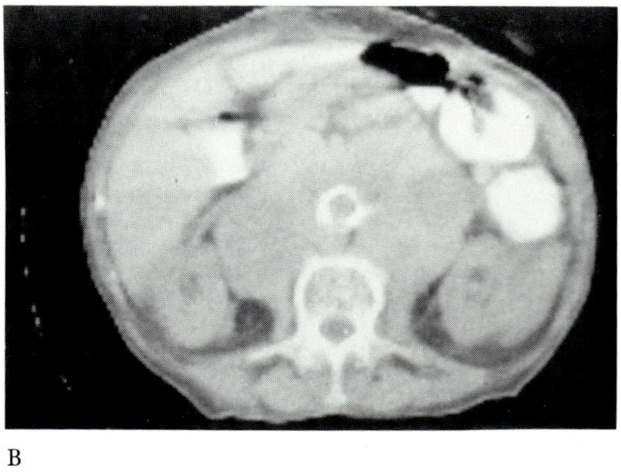

B

Typically, the Hodgkin's lymphoma and carcinoma patients are found to have discrete filling defects in nodes that might or might not be enlarged. However, this technique is not without complications and has essentially been replaced in many institutions by newer methods, notably CT and MRI. By CT, using the criteria for size previously discussed, enlarged nodes are seen as nonenhancing soft-tissue masses in the region of the great vessels. The major weakness of CT is its inability to detect microscopic metastatic foci in normal-sized nodes. Also contributing to the lack of specificity of CT is its inability to differentiate benign hyperplastic nodes from those enlarged because of malignant involvement. However, a benign hyperplastic node almost never exceeds 1.5 cm in diameter and is usually isolated. Furthermore, the shapes and locations of conglomerate node masses are similar in both lymphoma and metastatic disease from other tumors; this prevents their easy differentiation, though conglomerate lymph node masses 3 cm or greater in diameter are most commonly encountered with lymphoma (Fig. 6-3B).

With MRI, T1 weighted sequences provide optimal contrast between lymph nodes and surrounding fat; the signal intensity of nodes is medium in comparison with the high signal intensity of fat [19]. The sensitivity of MRI in detecting enlarged retroperitoneal lymph nodes appears to be similar to that of CT[11].

PRIMARY RETROPERITONEAL TUMORS

The term "primary retroperitoneal tumor" refers to neoplasms that originate independently in the retroperitoneum without primary connection to any of the retroperitoneal organs. The tissues in this area that are potential sources of such tumors include muscle, fascia, connective tissue, fatty tissue, blood vessels and lymphatics, remnants of the embryonic urogenital ridge, and nerves. It can therefore be appreciated that there is an immense variety of lesions that can be found in the retroperitoneum. Excluded from this discussion are the lymphomas, already covered in the section on lymphadenopathy.

As with retroperitoneal abscesses, primary retroperitoneal tumors grow slowly and produce vague, if any, symptoms before they reach significant size. For this reason, most primary retroperitoneal neoplasms are quite large when initially diagnosed, unless they are discovered inadvertently. Pain and mass are the most common presenting features.

Up to 90 percent of primary retroperitoneal tumors are malignant. The prognosis for cure is poor, since by the time they are detected they have usually widely infiltrated adjacent tissues. Hematogenous metastases are also common. Table 6-2 presents the various tumors that can be encountered in the retroperitoneum [3].

Aside from lymphoma arising in the retroperitoneal nodes, primary retroperitoneal neoplasms are rare. Liposarcoma is the most frequently found, followed by leiomyosarcoma [28]. Another relatively common lesion is malignant fibrous histiocytoma. These more common tumors usually present in older patients, and there is a male predominance. The remaining malignant neoplasms tend to occur in a younger age group as do the benign retroperitoneal neoplasms. The largest tumors found are the liposarcomas, which have an average diameter of 20 cm [15]. The other tumors tend to average 11 to 14 cm in size on detection.

To discuss the individual retroperitoneal tumors in detail would require far more space than can be allotted in an introductory textbook. Suffice it to say that while some of these lesions depict imaging findings that correlate with their cell type, in most instances the findings are nonspecific and needle biopsy is required to establish the definitive diagnosis.

On plain films retroperitoneal tumors are usually seen as large soft-tissue masses displacing bowel and other abdominal viscera; calcifications can occasionally be detected in these masses. On urography the ipsilateral kidney may be distorted or displaced and the ureter deviated (and possibly obstructed) by the retroperitoneal mass. Angiography still has a place in the evaluation of these lesions in that it can provide the surgeon with knowledge of the tumor's arterial supply and the degree of vascularity within the mass (Fig. 6-4A).

While sonography can provide some information regarding the tissue characteristics in retroperitoneal tumors, CT remains the method of choice for characterizing these lesions and determining the extent of their growth. Although CT is nonspecific in many instances, there are a number of features that may be used in diagnosis. Though calcification may occur in many of

Table 6.2. Primary retroperitoneal tumors

Mesodermal tumors
Fatty tissue
Lipoma
Liposarcoma
Smooth muscle
Leiomyoma
Leiomyosarcoma
Striated muscle
Rhabdomyoma
Rhabdomyosarcoma
Connective tissue
Fibroma
Fibrosarcoma
Lymphatics
Lymphangioma
Lymphangiosarcoma
Blood vessels
Hemangioma
Angiosarcoma
Hemangiopericytoma
Histiocytes
Malignant fibrous histiocytoma
Mixed tumors
Myxoma
Myxosarcoma
Mesenchymoma
Neurogenic tumors
Nerve sheath
Neurofibroma
Neurilemmoma
Malignant schwannoma
Sympathetic tissue
Ganglioneuroma
Neuroblastoma
Extraadrenal paraganglion system
Paraganglioma
Pheochromocytoma
Embryonic remnant tumors
Teratomas (benign and malignant)
Primary germ-cell tumors
Reticuloendothelial tumors
Lymph nodes
Lymphoma

Source: Adapted from M.A. Bosniak, S.S. Siegelman, and J.A. Evans. *The Adrenal, Retroperitoneum and Lower Urinary Tract*. Chicago: Yearbook, 1976, P. 234.

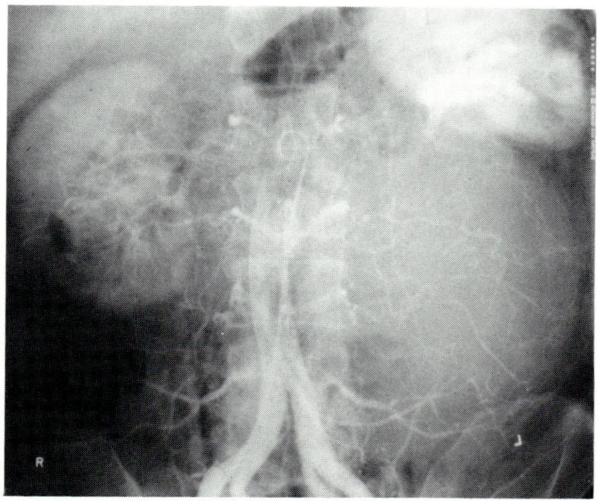

A

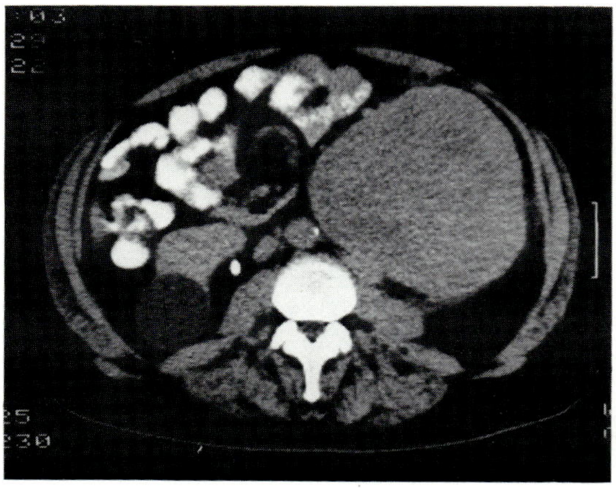

B

Figure 6-4. Malignant fibrous histiocytoma in retroperitoneum. A. Aortogram shows a large, somewhat vascular mass in the left retroperitoneum displacing the left kidney up and laterally and bowing the aorta to the right. B. CT demonstrates the homogeneous soft-tissue nature of mass, which enhanced after administration of intravenous contrast agent.

these lesions, its prevalence in malignant fibrous histiocytoma and mature teratoma should suggest these diagnoses. Large areas of necrosis in a tumor, also somewhat nonspecific, tend to be more frequent in leiomyosarcomas. Significant enhancement after administration of intravenous contrast medium is often found in the hemangiomatous tumors. However, leiomyosarcomas and malignant fibrous histiocytomas (Fig. 6-4B) also tend to enhance.

Lipomatous tumors of the retroperitoneum, because of their relative frequency of occurrence, deserve further mention. Fat-containing tumors comprise a spectrum from benign lipomas to highly undifferentiated liposarcomas. Simple lipomas are benign encapsulated lesions with a negative CT density similar to that of normal adipose tissue (−15 Hounsfield units or lower). Liposarcomas, on the other hand, may vary from well-differentiated tumors composed predominantly of fatty tissue to the pleomorphic variety, which exhibits a relative paucity of lipid [25]. The appearance of these lesions on CT correlates closely with their gross anatomical features. Liposarcomas, even though they may contain moderate to large amounts of fatty tissue, are usually easily differentiated from benign lipomas because of their soft-tissue components. On the other hand, most retroperitoneal liposarcomas are of the myxoid type, containing large amounts of connective tissue and relatively little lipid. On CT these myxoid tumors are of an intermediate density that on occasion can resemble a benign cyst or abscess. Furthermore, their density may occasionally be similar to that of muscle, making them impossible to differentiate from other soft-tissue retroperitoneal neoplasms. Pleomorphic, or highly undifferentiated, liposarcomas may have a relatively high soft-tissue density and also be indistinguishable from other solid retroperitoneal tumors.

Retroperitoneal teratomas, like the lipomatous tumors, may exhibit imaging characteristics that allow definitive diagnosis in some cases. These lesions, which can be found anywhere from the high retroperitoneum to the presacral area, typically occur within the first six months of life or in young adults. They are at least three times more common in females than in males. Less than 10 percent of these tumors undergo malignant degeneration. Radiographically, teratomas can present as predominantly cystic or solid masses or as complex lesions containing fat or sebum/fluid levels. Calcification in the form of amorphous deposits or prominent linear streaks can be seen in slightly less than half of cases [8].

Also noteworthy, the malignant fibrous histiocytoma is a pleomorphic tumor of the soft tissues possibly arising from histiocytes. The majority of histiocytic tumors are benign and only 12 to 14 percent involve the retroperitoneum. When retroperitoneal in origin they may be difficult to differentiate from other pleomorphic retroperitoneal sarcomas, including liposarcoma, rhabdomyosarcoma, or undifferentiated carcinoma [23]. The malignant variety of this tumor is quite aggressive and the prognosis is poor.

As opposed to determining the exact histology of a retroperitoneal tumor, perhaps the more important role of imaging is to define clearly its size, location, and any extension to adjacent structures or organs. This information is of particular use to the surgeon, who will probably excise or debulk the tumor regardless of the result of needle biopsy, or even if a biopsy procedure has not been performed. Since most of these tumors are highly malignant and tend to metastasize hematogenously, the exclusion of pulmonary, visceral, or bony metastases is another major task of the radiologist before curative surgery is undertaken.

At the time of this writing, no significant series of primary retroperitoneal tumors imaged by MRI has been reported. Given the multiplannar imaging capabilities of MRI, it is probably safe to say that this method will be able to define the size and location of these retroperitoneal lesions with an accuracy similar to that of CT. The real value of MRI may lie in its ability to determine whether the tumor has actually invaded adjacent retroperitoneal organs and structures.

CHYLURIA

Chyluria is the voiding of urine containing turbid-appearing chylous material ("white urine"). This condition is secondary to abnormal retrograde flow of lymph into rather than away from the kidney. The most common cause is filariasis. While this condition is rare in the United States, it is common in areas of the world in which filariasis is endemic, such as India, Japan, Southeast Asia, and various areas in Africa and South America. These patients are classified as having tropical chyluria as opposed to the nontropical variety, which can be secondary to a variety of causes, including retroperitoneal malignancy or infection, tuberculosis, trauma, surgery, and lymphangiomyomatosis [27]. The common factor in both tropical and nontropical chyluria is obstruction of the retroperitoneal lymphatics with subsequent collateralization of flow to the urinary tract.

While the only constant symptom of this disease is passage of a urine that is milky white, patients also occasionally complain of back pain and irritation of the lower urinary tract. Inspection of the urine, which can also be milky in patients with severe pyuria, reveals an absence of these inflammatory cells. When allowed to stand, fatty material in chylous urine rises to the top. Shaking the urine after addition of ether result in almost complete clearing.

Radiographically, the plain film and excretory urogram are usually normal. Pedal lymphangiography is the definitive study for evaluating chyluria since it can demonstrate the site of communication between the lymphatic system

Figure 6-5. Chyluria. Lymphangiography shows tortuous, dilated retroperitoneal lymphatics (arrow), absence of opacified nodes, and retrograde flow of contrast into the right renal lymphatics, which terminate in the pericaliceal areas.

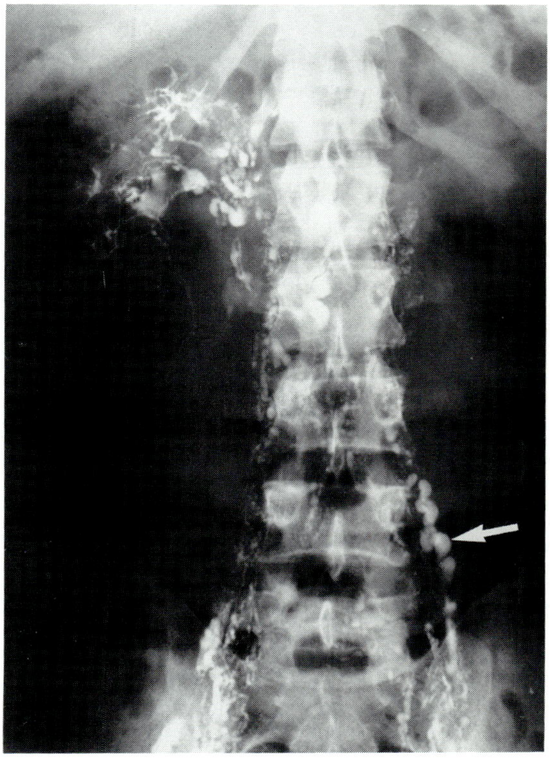

and the urinary tract. The typical findings on this study are an increase in the number, size, and tortuosity of retroperitoneal lymphatic vessels and the absence of opacification of the retroperitoneal nodes, which are usually replaced by fibrosis, tumor, granulation tissue, or in the case of lymphangiomyomatosis, muscle tissue. Unilateral or bilateral retrograde communications between the retroperitoneal and renal lymph vessels are the confirmatory findings in this disease. Lymphangiographic contrast material can be seen flowing in a retrograde direction into the renal lymphatics and eventually surrounding the collecting system, particularly in the region of the minor calices (Fig. 6-5). It is at this point that communication with the collecting system occurs; subsequently, lymphangiographic contrast material can be seen in the calices, renal pelvis, ureter, and bladder.

REFERENCES

1. Amis, E.S., Jr., and Pfister, R.C. Radiologic manifestations of urologic hemorrhage. In M.M. Bern (ed.), *Urinary Tract Bleeding: Diagnosis and Control by Medical, Radiologic, and Surgical Techniques*. Mount Kisco, N.Y.: Futura, 1985. Pp. 111–162.
2. Arrive, L., et al. Malignant versus nonmalignant retroperitoneal fibrosis: Differentiation with MR imaging. *Radiology* 172:139, 1989.
3. Bosniak, M.A., Siegelman, S.S., and Evans, J.A. *The Adrenal, Retroperitoneum and Lower Urinary Tract*. Chicago: Year Book, 1976. Pp. 231–335.
4. Brun, B., et al. CT in retroperitoneal fibrosis. *A.J.R.* 137:535, 1981.
5. Carter, B.L., and Wechsler, R.J. Computed tomography of the retroperitoneum and abdominal wall. *Semin. Roentgenol.* 13:201, 1978.
6. Castellino, R.A., Marglin, S., and Blank, N. Hodgkin disease, the non-Hodgkin lymphomas, and the leukemias in the retroperitoneum. *Semin. Roentgenol.* 15:288, 1980.
7. Dalla-Palma, L., et al. Computed tomography in the diagnosis of retroperitoneal fibrosis. *Urol. Radiol.* 3:77, 1981.
8. Davidson, A.J., Hartman, D.S., and Goldman, S.M. Mature teratoma of the retroperitoneum: Radiologic, pathologic, and clinical correlation. *Radiology* 172:421, 1989.
9. Degesys, G.E., et al. Retroperitoneal fibrosis: Use of CT in distinguishing among possible causes. *A.J.R.* 146:57, 1986.
10. Demas, B.E., and Hricak, H. Magnetic resonance imaging in the evaluation of the retroperitoneum. *Urol. Radiol.* 8:151, 1986.
11. Dooms, G.C., et al. Magnetic resonance imaging of the lymph nodes: Comparison with CT. *Radiology* 153:719, 1984.
12. Periureteric fibrosis. *Lancet* 2:780, 1957.
13. Hricak, H., Higgins, C.B., and Williams, R.D. Nuclear magnetic resonance imaging in retroperitoneal fibrosis. *A.J.R.* 141:35, 1983.
14. Lalli, A.F. Retroperitoneal fibrosis and inapparent obstructive uropathy. *Radiology* 122:339, 1977.
15. Lane, R.H., Stephens, D.H., and Reiman, H.M. Primary retroperitoneal neoplasms: CT findings in 90 cases with clinical and pathologic correlation. *A.J.R.* 152:83, 1989.
16. LaRoy, L.L., et al. Imaging of abdominal aortic aneurysms. *A.J.R.* 152:785,1989.
17. Lawson, T.L., et al. Magnetic resonance imaging of discrete and conglomerate retroperitoneal lymph node masses. *RadioGraphics* 5:971, 1985.
18. Lee, J.K.T. Magnetic resonance imaging of the retroperitoneum. *Urol. Radiol.* 10:48,1988.
19. Lee, J.K.T., et al. Magnetic resonance imaging of abdominal and pelvic lymphadenopathy. *Radiology* 153:181, 184.
20. Lepor, H., and Walsh, P.C. Idiopathic retroperitoneal fibrosis. *J. Urol.* 122:1, 1979.
21. McCort, J.J. Intraperitoneal and retroperitoneal hemorrhage. *Radiol. Clin. North Am.* 14:391, 1976.
22. Pardes, J.G., et al. The oblique coronal view in sonography of the retroperitoneum. *A.J.R.* 144:1241, 1985.
23. Usher, S.M., Beckley, S., and Merrin, C.E. Malignant fibrous histiocytoma of the retroperitoneum and genitourinary tract: A clinicopathological correlation and review of the literature. *J. Urol.* 122:105, 1979.
24. vanSonnenberg, E., et al. Lymphoceles: Imaging characteristics and percutaneous management. *Radiology* 161:593, 1986.
25. Waligore, M.P., et al. Lipomatous tumors of the abdominal cavity: CT appearance and pathology correlation. *A.J.R.* 137:539, 1981.
26. White, M., et al. Percutaneous drainage of postoperative abdominal and pelvic lymphoceles. *A.J.R.* 145:1065, 1985.
27. Witten, D.M., Myers, G.H., Jr., and Utz, D.C. *Emmett's Clinical Urography* (4th ed.). Philadelphia: Saunders, 1977. Pp. 2220-2228.
28. Yeh, H.C. Adrenal gland and nonrenal retroperitoneum. *Urol. Radiol.* 9:127, 1987.

7

The Adrenal

Prior to the invention of gray-scale ultrasonography and CT, most adrenal diseases were not amenable to investigation by radiologic techniques. Plain films of the abdomen and intravenous urography permitted the visualization of adrenal masses only if they were of considerable size or contained moderate to large amounts of calcification. The only other technique available for imaging the gland was angiography [35]. Arteriography of all adrenal vessels was time consuming and not without risk. Venography was a simpler method of investigating the gland, and during it sampling of adrenal effluent blood was possible for hormonal analysis, but the internal vasculature of the gland could not be identified. However, since the advent of high-quality ultrasonography and CT and the invention of MRI, adrenal imaging has progressed to the point at which screening for adrenal diseases is practical and differential diagnosis of certain adrenal conditions has become much easier [20]. In this chapter, adrenal medullary neoplasms will be dealt with first; a discussion of renal cortical tumors will follow; and adrenal dysfunctional states, differential diagnoses, and miscellaneous conditions will be presented as well.

MEDULLARY NEOPLASMS

PHEOCHROMOCYTOMA

Pheochromocytomas are relatively unusual tumors. They occur primarily in adults, most frequently in the fourth or fifth decade of life. In adults there is a slight female predominance, but there is a slight male predominance among children who acquire the tumors. Pheochromocytomas are thought to be the cause of hypertension in 0.1 to 0.5 percent of all hypertensive patients.

Ninety percent of pheochromocytomas arise in the adrenal medulla, but they also appear in the sympathetic ganglia in a number of sites. Their location is usually axial, and they may occur anywhere from the base of the skull to the floor of the pelvis. Most tumors appear within the abdomen or pelvis. Approximately 10 percent of adrenal pheochromocytomas are bilateral. In addition to the sympathetic ganglia, the tumor may appear in the organ of Zuckerkandl, which rests near the aortic bifurcation just inferior to the origin of the inferior mesenteric artery, and in the bladder [12]. Rare cases have appeared in the vagina and renal sinus. The tumors are made up of characteristic chromaffin cells; they may exhibit patchy central necrosis. Approximately 10 percent of the tumors are malignant.

Although most commonly pheochromocytomas appear as a single adrenal lesion not associated with other pathology, they form parts of several different syndromes and have a number of associated diseases. The multiple endocrine neoplasia type II (MEN-II) syndrome involves pheochromocytomas [10]. In MEN-IIA (Sipple's syndrome) pheochromocytomas are associated with medullary thyroid carcinoma and parathyroid hyperplasia or adenomas. In MEN-IIB (also occasionally called MEN-III) pheochromocytomas are associated with marfanoid facies and mucosal neuromas of the oral cavity as well. Patients with MEN-II syndrome may have adrenal medullary hyperplasia or multiple small pheochromocytomas. Sipple's syndrome is autosomal dominant; patients with characteristics that overlap those of MEN syndrome types I, II, and III are being reported. Pheochromocytomas are also occasionally encountered in patients who have the von Hippel–Lindau syndrome, in whom multiple renal cell carcinomas and cerebellar hemangiomas appear. Pheochromocytomas have also been encountered in patients with neurofibromatosis and in patients with renal artery stenosis [23] (the stenosis is sometimes intrinsic and sometimes has been caused by pressure from the adjacent tumor). There is a high incidence of gallstones in patients with pheochromocytomas.

Pheochromocytomas are usually hormonally active, but they need not be so; they excrete various combinations of epinephrine, norepinephrine, vanillylmandelic acid (VMA), normetanephrine, and metanephrine. These substances both produce the clinical signs and symptoms of the disease and permit screening by measuring their levels in urine or blood. Metanephrine and VMA levels are most useful in this regard.

The major sign produced by the tumor is hypertension, which may be paroxysmal. Symptoms include bouts of headache, palpitations, sweating, and apprehension; if the tumor exists in the bladder it may be associated with similar symptoms during bladder distention or micturition or with hematuria. Hyperglycemia may occur.

Histologically, pheochromocytomas have an appearance similar to that of the normal adrenal medulla. Although approximately 10 percent of the tumors may exhibit malignant biologic behavior, histologic distinction of malignant from benign tumors is difficult.

The tumors are multiple in approximately 10 percent of adult cases; in children they are multiple in at least a third of all cases. Distinction between multiple benign pheochromocytomas and metastases from a malignant tumor may be difficult. If all of the lesions appear in the adrenals or sites of sympathetic ganglia they are likely to be multiple benign ones; malignant tumors metastasize to bone, lung, liver, local nodes, and adjacent tissue. The tumors are frequently several centimeters in diameter; they have ranged in size from less than 1 to over 20 cm.

Radiography

Plain abdomen radiography usually does not reveal any evidence of pheochromocytoma. Although calcification may be seen in some of these tumors, its incidence is very low. Radiography may reveal evidence of metastatic disease in the lungs or bones; bony metastases tend to be lytic but may be mixed lytic and blastic; they are sometimes expansile. Skull, ribs, spine, and proximal femurs are common sites of bony metastasis.

Urography

Urography with nephrotomography may demonstrate adrenal pheochromocytomas by permitting direct visualization of the mass if the tumor is sufficiently large; clearly, the smaller the lesion the less likely it is to be visible. Larger tumors may displace the ipsilateral kidney inferiorly.

Ultrasonography

Gray-scale ultrasonography may demonstrate adrenal pheochromocytomas as masses of moderate echogenicity [6]. Their echotexture may be homogeneous or heterogeneous; central necrosis or hemorrhage may produce focal regions of very low echogenicity. Since ultrasonography may miss small lesions in patients who are difficult to examine, the technique cannot be used as a highly sensitive screening method.

Computed Tomography

CT [30, 40, 47, 49] has become the most commonly used method for visualizing pheochromocytomas (although some investigators have proposed that MRI or radionuclide scanning with ^{131}I-metaiodobenzylguanidine may successfully compete with CT for this role). CT is able to visualize most adrenals clearly, and hence almost all adrenal masses (missing only a few small lesions), and it is able to visualize most neck, mediastinal, retroperitoneal, and pelvic masses as well.

Pheochromocytomas usually appear as relatively homogeneous masses with attenuation values similar to that of kidney on CT scans without an intravenous contrast agent (Fig. 7-1). They may have internal regions of diminished attenuation if regions of necrosis have appeared. The lesions commonly enhance when an intravenous contrast agent is administered; lesions with central necrosis may demonstrate heterogeneous enhancement or reveal only a rim of viable enhancing tissue around the necrotic center.

In patients in whom CT reveals an adrenal pheochromocytoma the possibility of multiple lesions requires that scanning be continued at least throughout the abdomen and pelvis. Obviously, to discover all locations of extra-adrenal pheochromocytoma, the neck and entire chest need to be scanned as well, but this scanning protocol is time consuming and of relatively low yield. In patients who have a clinical syndrome that strongly suggests pheochromocy-

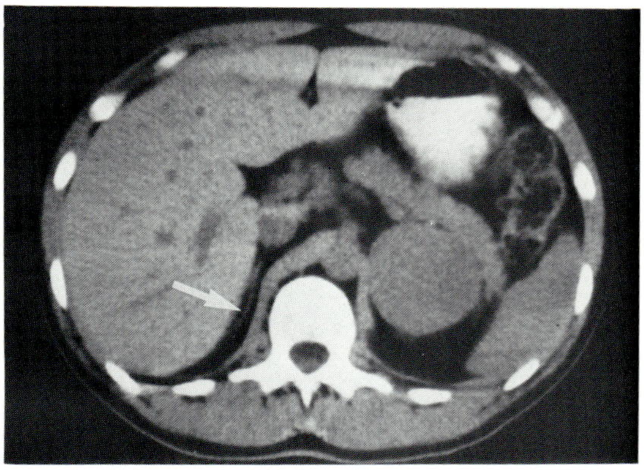

Figure 7-1. Left adrenal pheochromocytoma. CT reveals the left adrenal mass to be homogeneous and slightly less dense than liver. A limb of the normal right adrenal is seen (arrow).

toma but in whom the adrenals appear normal by CT, it becomes more important to scan the entirety of the remaining trunk and neck. CT may be used as a guide for percutaneous biopsy of these lesions.

Administration of an intravenous contrast agent [41] may cause the pheochromocytomas to secrete a pulse of hormones and produce a hypertensive crisis. Although many pheochromocytomas have been scanned using intravenous contrast medium without producing crises, treatment with a drug that provides alpha-adrenergic blockade is certainly worth considering. A good prophylactic regimen would include 20 to 100 mg of phenoxybenzamine by mouth twice a day until the patient becomes normotensive (which usually takes several days). If a patient should become acutely hypertensive after administration of a contrast agent, treatment with phentolamine (Regitine), 5 mg intravenously, should be given. Subsequently, 20 mg of the drug may be diluted in 500 ml of 5 percent dextrose solution and administered slowly by the intravenous route as blood pressure is monitored. Similar precautions and therapeutic maneuvers should apply during angiographic examination of lesions that may be pheochromocytomas and during percutaneous biopsies of these lesions [8]. Although it is currently rare for a patient to be referred for urography when he is known to have a pheochromocytoma, similar risks and treatments should be kept in mind.

Magnetic Resonance Imaging

MRI [9, 15, 21] has been shown to demonstrate nearly all pheochromocytomas; given the high tissue contrast that can be provided with T2 weighted MR images, MRI may have certain advantages over CT in screening for extra-adrenal tumors. However, MRI of large parts of the body is time consuming. Therefore total-body scanning with radionuclides may compete with MRI (and CT) for discovering extraadrenal tumors.

On T1 weighted images (Fig. 7-2A) the relatively long T1 of the lesions often causes them to be of slightly lower signal intensity than liver; they have signal intensities similar to renal

Figure 7-2. Left adrenal pheochromocytoma. A. T1 weighted MRI reveals the left adrenal mass to be slightly heterogeneous in intensity. B. T2 weighted MRI shows portions of the left adrenal to be extremely bright.

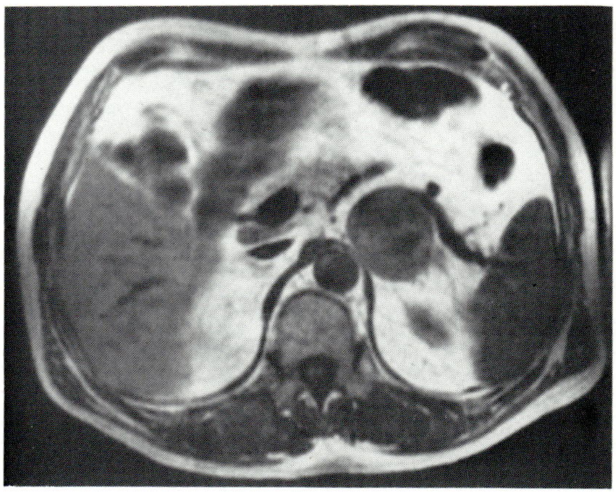

A

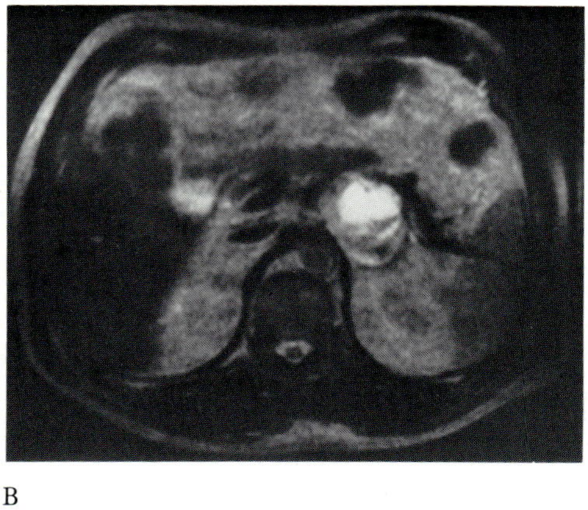

B

medulla and spleen. On T2 weighted images the lesions appear extremely intense: Of all the kinds of pathology that produce adrenal masses in adults, pheochromocytomas are, as a group, the brightest of all. The tumors may appear homogeneous or heterogeneous on T1 weighted images; their extreme brightness usually makes them look homogeneous on T2 weighted images, but occasionally they may look heterogeneous (Fig. 7-2B) if the image windows are adjusted correctly.

Radionuclide Studies

Imaging with cholesterol analogs does not permit visualization of adrenals containing pheochromocytomas, since the tumors are of medullary origin and compress or obliterate the cortex. Recently, ^{131}I- metaiodobenzylguanidine has been found to concentrate in pheochromocytomas [31, 40, 44] and to permit imaging of them [29] whether they are intraadrenal or extraadrenal. The method is nearly as sensitive as CT or MRI, allows differential diagnosis of pheochromocytomas from adrenal cortical tumors, and permits relatively rapid imaging of the entire body when it is necessary to search for metastatic disease.

Angiography

Pheochromocytomas may be well demonstrated arteriographically [11], although since the advent of CT the necessity to do so has diminished considerably. The multiple arteries that may supply each gland—and hence a tumor—may make visualization of the entire lesion tedious. The tumors are usually hypervascular (Fig. 7-3): The pattern of neovascularity varies but has been described in some patients as having a spoked-wheel configuration and in others as demonstrating a fine reticular pattern. The tumors commonly demonstrate a moderately intense stain in the tissue opacification phase; obviously, those with regions of necrosis or nearly complete necrosis will be hypovascular in the appropriate volumes. Tumors that are mostly necrotic may reveal only a perfused viable rim. It is possible to inject multiple vessels in an attempt to localize a pheochromocytoma whose site is not known; clearly, this is a time-consuming, sometimes dangerous, and not always successful process, and it should be avoided if at all possible.

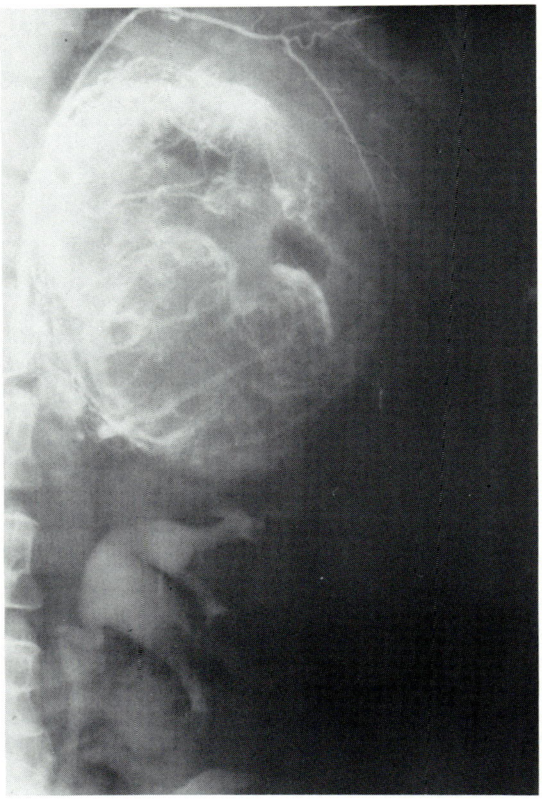

Figure 7-3. Left adrenal pheochromocytoma. Selective adrenal arteriography reveals the lesion to contain irregular neovascularity. The vascular pattern is similar to that which might be seen in an adrenal malignancy.

Venography of adrenal pheochromocytomas may be simpler than arteriography since each adrenal is drained by only one major vein. The commonest finding at adrenal venography is the displacement and stretching of intraadrenal veins. In patients who are strongly suspected of having a pheochromocytoma but in whom noninvasive imaging methods are unable to find the lesion, sampling of venous blood from the inferior and superior vena cava and the neck may provide a clue to the location of the lesion if each sample is analyzed for the hormonal products of the tumor. Again, this procedure is time consuming and not always accurate, and it should be avoided if noninvasive techniques can demonstrate the lesion.

NEUROBLASTOMA

Neuroblastoma is one of the most common malignancies of early childhood. It usually begins as a tumor of the adrenal medulla, but since it arises from cells originally stemming from neural crest ectoderm, it may also begin in the sympathetic chain anywhere in the trunk or neck. The tumors may be encountered as early in life as birth; approximately 28 percent appear in children less than 1 year of age, and at least 80 percent appear in children less than 5 years of age. The majority of the tumors appear in children prior to their third birthdays.

The tumors often present as palpable abdominal masses. Approximately 70 percent of the tumors arise in the adrenal and approximately 20 percent first appear in extraabdominal sites. Unfortunately, a majority of patients have fairly widespread tumor at the time of diagnosis, so that the disease may also present with symptoms due to distant disease; these may include pain from bony metastases, a variety of neurologic symptoms, and failure to thrive. Tumors in the pelvis have presented by producing bladder dysfunction. The lesions may secrete catecholamines; levels of these substances are often found to be elevated in the urine of patients with neuroblastoma.

The prognosis depends on the age of the patient at the time of diagnosis (the older the child, the worse the prognosis) and the stage. The staging of neuroblastoma is given in Table 7-1. Metastatic disease is most frequently found in the skeleton; in order of decreasing frequency, metastases are encountered in the skull, femurs, pelvis, ribs, tibia, vertebrae, mandible, and other bones. Radiologic staging is important in making treatment decisions: Only localized tumors that have not directly invaded vessels or other adjacent structures are amenable to surgery. Although neuroblastoma is often fatal, in some patients the tumor evolves from one that is histologically and biologically malignant to a benign ganglioneuroma; such changes have been seen both after partial excision and in untreated tumors.

Radiography

Plain radiography has largely been supplanted by ultrasonography for the diagnosis of adrenal neuroblastomas. Nevertheless, radiography often provides useful information: If it is large enough, a neuroblastoma anywhere in the abdomen will present as a soft-tissue mass that may be directly visible or may displace gut or solid viscera. At least half of all neuroblastomas will contain visible calcification. Plain radiography may also reveal bony metastases, which are usually lytic and poorly marginated; occasionally they may be mixed lytic and blastic. Signs of increased intracranial pressure on skull films may also be encountered. Urography may show that an adrenal neuroblastoma has displaced the ipsilateral kidney inferiorly.

Ultrasonography

Ultrasonography [50] is quite sensitive in demonstrating adrenal neuroblastomas (Fig. 7-4) and usually can demonstrate tumors elsewhere in the abdomen or pelvis unless they are very small. The tumors are moderately echogenic; they may contain regions of diminished echogenicity or lobules of increased echogenicity [2].

Figure 7-4. Adrenal neuroblastoma. Ultrasonography reveals an echogenic mass with acoustic shadowing.

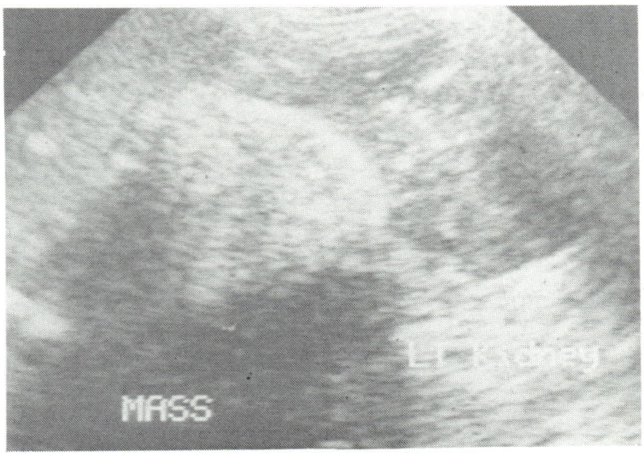

Table 7-1. Staging of neuroblastoma

Stage I	Tumor is limited to the organ or structure of origin.
Stage II	Tumor has extended beyond organ of origin but has not crossed the midline; local nodes may be involved.
Stage III	Tumor has extended directly across midline.
Stage IV	Tumor has remotely metastasized.

Foci of calcification, presenting as small regions of intense echogenicity with deep acoustic shadowing, may also be visualized.

Computed Tomography
CT virtually always demonstrates the lesion. Without intravenous contrast medium, it may show that the tumor has slightly less attenuation than adjacent soft tissues. The tumor may be either homogeneous or heterogeneous in attenuation; it usually enhances with contrast medium. CT is presumably slightly more sensitive than plain films in demonstrating calcification within the tumor. CT also usually demonstrates quite well the extent of the tumor, displays extension across the midline and extension into the perirenal, pararenal, and retrocrural spaces, and shows any displacement of the aorta or inferior vena cava or both. Clearly, CT (along with ultrasonography and MRI) is particularly useful in determining the operability of each lesion. Local and distant nodal metastases are visible as nodal enlargement; CT is presumably slightly more sensitive than plain films in demonstrating calcification within the tumor. Obviously, CT may demonstrate bony metastases when the portions of the skeleton containing the disease are examined; however, survey of the skeleton for metastatic disease is most easily accomplished by radionuclide scanning.

Magnetic Resonance Imaging
MRI is particularly efficacious in demonstrating the extent of neuroblastomas (Fig. 7-5) [13, 17]. On T1 weighted images the tumor tissue has a signal intensity roughly equivalent to that of the renal medulla or spleen; on T2 weighted images the tumor appears quite bright, with signal intensities similar to that of normal kidneys. When metastases to bones replace fatty marrow, the involved regions appear darker than normal marrow on T1 weighted images; the signal intensity on T2 weighted images of bony metastases may be similar to that of fatty marrow. MRI is particularly well suited to the exact delineation of the margins of the tumor. The flow void in the aorta and cava and other large vessels renders it relatively easy to determine the relation of the tumor to these vascular structures. The multiplanar capacity of MRI makes the technique superior to CT in determining the presence or absence of a plane between the tumor and adjacent structures. For example, distinguishing adrenal from upper-pole renal masses may be performed relatively accurately with coronal or sagittal MR images. MRI is

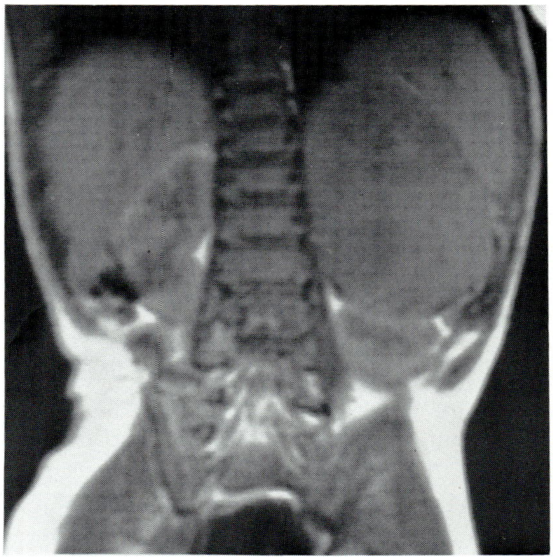

A

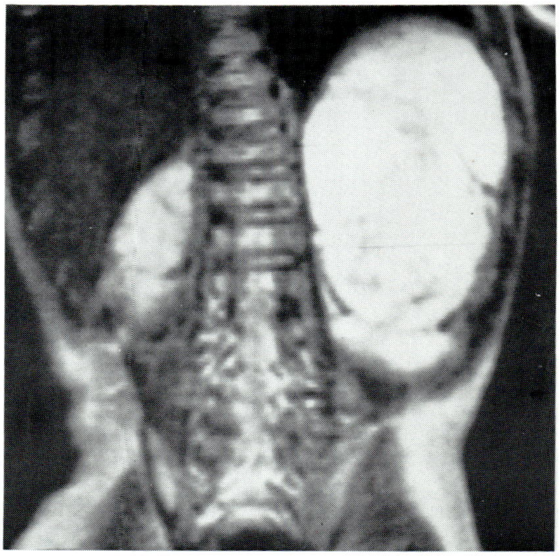

B

Figure 7-5. Adrenal neuroblastoma. A. T1 weighted coronal MRI reveals a left suprarenal mass whose signal intensity is slightly heterogeneous and similar to that of kidney. B. T2 weighted coronal MRI shows the mass as hyperintense and heterogeneous.

probably more sensitive than radiography in detecting skeletal metastases; its sensitivity vis-à-vis radionuclide scanning is not yet well established.

Radionuclide Studies
Radionuclide scans [24] are most useful in neuroblastoma in demonstrating the number and site of skeletal metastases. ^{99m}Tc-methylene-diphosphonate [45] or pyrophosphate images are relatively accurate in detecting metastatic disease and almost always reveal each metastatic deposit as a region of increased activity. The primary tumor, however, can also be imaged by uptake of ^{131}I metaiodobenzylguanidine.

Angiography
This technique currently has little clinical use in the evaluation of patients who have (or may have) a neuroblastoma. When performed, it shows the tumor to contain reticular neovascularity; there may be necrotic avascular regions within the tumor as well. If the cava or aorta or both have been displaced, angiograph obviously can demonstrate this fact; tumor thrombi within the cava are almost never encountered.

Differential Diagnosis
The entity that most frequently needs to be differentiated from neuroblastoma is Wilms' tumor. Although these tumors differ with regard to the ages at which they most commonly occur (Wilms' tumor patients are usually slightly older), the age ranges for appearance of the two tumors overlap considerably. If a tumor can be shown clearly to be arising from the adrenal it can be presumed to be a neuroblastoma, whereas tumors clearly of renal origin are usually Wilms' tumors. For lesions that do not permit this simple distinction, there are a number of useful features that can still be used. Calcification is more likely to appear in neuroblastoma. Neuroblastoma is more likely to produce retroperitoneal lymphadenopathy, vascular encasement, and aortic or caval displacement, although Wilms' tumor can produce any of these features. Retrocrural lymphadenopathy seems to be produced almost solely by neuroblastoma. Finally, neuroblastoma metastasizes most frequently to bone and, to a lesser extent, to liver, whereas Wilms' tumor usually metastasizes to pulmonary parenchyma.

CORTICAL NEOPLASMS

CARCINOMA OF THE ADRENAL

Primary carcinoma of the adrenal, or adrenocortical carcinoma, is an unusual malignancy. It may appear at any age, ranging from infancy to extreme old age; most commonly it appears in the fourth through sixth decades. The tumor arises in the cortex of the adrenal, is virtually always unilateral, and may reach 25 cm or more in diameter. The tumors, especially when large, often have focal regions of necrosis or hemorrhage or both; they are frequently calcified. Small tumors may be difficult to distinguish histologically from adenomas. The tumor is often discovered at a stage at which cure is unlikely; the lesions are classically large and advanced when diagnosed. The tumors may be nonfunctioning or may be hormonally active: Adrenogenital syndrome, feminization, virilization, Cushing's syndrome, and occasionally even Conn's syndrome may appear. Tumors that are hormonally active are likely to be diagnosed at a slightly smaller size (and therefore at a curable stage) than tumors that do not secrete a significant amount of hormones. Widespread tumors may present with constitutional symptoms such as weight loss and malaise; symptoms from metastases may be the first events to bring the tumor to clinical attention. The tumor may spread locally by directly invading the adjacent kidney, pancreas, liver, or diaphragm, and it may extend into the inferior vena cava, either as a tumor thrombus or directly through the wall of the vessel. Distant metastases are found in liver, lung, lymph nodes, peritoneal cavity, and brain. There is no particularly effective chemotherapy, and radiation therapy is rarely useful; surgery performed on early-stage tumors is the only hope for cure.

Radiography and Urography
If the tumor is large it may be seen as a soft-tissue mass, or it may display amorphous calcification. Rarely, bony metastases may be seen.

Urography may aid in the diagnosis since a mass of any size tends to displace the ipsilateral kidney downward; urography is not sufficiently sensitive to act as a screening test for adrenocortical carcinoma, however.

Ultrasonography
Ultrasonography is capable of imaging most primary adrenal carcinomas [22]; small tumors, however, especially in large or otherwise difficult-to-examine patients, may escape detection, so CT is the screening (and staging) technique of choice. When the tumors are visible on ultrasound examinations they tend to be of moderate echogenicity and relatively homogeneous when small; as the tumors enlarge they become heterogeneous in echo pattern, with regions of hypoechogenicity corresponding to liquefied regions of necrosis. In tumors that contain it, calcification is demonstrable by ultrasonography as it is in other tissues. The margins of the tumor are usually well delineated.

Computed Tomography
CT [14, 16] has been shown to be able to detect virtually all adrenal masses that ultimately turn out to be carcinomas (Fig. 7-6). When the lesions are small they have the CT characteristics of adenomas: They are relatively homogeneous in attenuation, may be slightly less dense than adjacent kidney or liver, and are round or ovoid

Figure 7-6. Primary carcinoma of left adrenal. Contrast-enhanced CT scan shows very large heterogeneous mass extending from adrenal area and occupying most of the left abdomen.

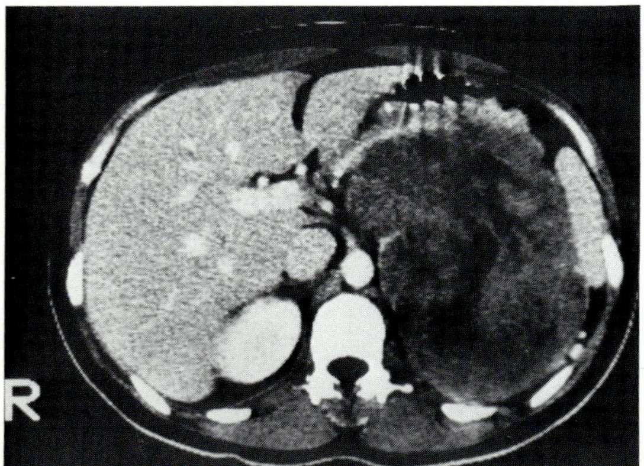

and smoothly marginated. As the tumors grow bigger, they may anteriorly displace the cava, splenic vessels, or pancreas. Larger tumors tend to be heterogeneous in attenuation; most adrenocortical carcinomas enhance irregularly with intravenous contrast medium, and a few may display rim enhancement. Calcification is easily detectable in tumors that contain it. Occasionally, anatomic differential diagnosis may be difficult by CT, especially vis-à-vis tumors that arise in the upper renal pole. If a patient with such a mass can be shown to have a normal adrenal gland clearly separated from the lesion an adrenocortical carcinoma is excluded. CT may reveal caval thrombosis in patients with large tumors; tumor thrombi may be difficult to distinguish from bland thrombi caused by caval compression by the tumor.

Magnetic Resonance Imaging
Adrenocortical carcinomas may look similar to adrenal metastases—that is, they may have signal strengths slightly lower than that of liver on T1 weighted images and considerably brighter than liver (but usually less bright than pheochromocytomas) on T2 weighted images. When the tumors are small, however, their signal characteristics may not be different from those of adenomas. Large heterogeneous tumors may reveal necrotic regions within them that have relatively low signal intensity on T1 weighted images and are quite bright on T2 weighted images; interstitial hemorrhage may alter the signal characteristics as well. Tumor thrombi produce a picture similar to that of tumor thrombi in other large venous structures. Coronal or sagittal views may help in the differential diagnosis between adrenocortical carcinomas and upper-pole renal carcinomas.

Angiography
Arteriography is usually not performed in the current workup of adrenocortical carcinomas but may occasionally provide useful information. Arteriography reveals that the adrenal artery supplying the tumor is enlarged; the tumor vascularity is usually fine and reticular, although occasionally coarse neovascularity may be seen. Arteriographic demonstration of

the artery supplying the lesion may be of value in distinguishing adrenocortical from renal cell carcinomas; also, as a group renal cell tumors tend to have coarser neovascularity than adrenal carcinomas, but the overlap in the neovascularity pattern is sufficient that this feature is not extremely reliable in differential diagnosis. Adrenal venography reveals the displacement and stretching of branches of the adrenal vein that are common to most adrenal tumors.

ADRENAL ADENOMAS

Benign adenomas of the adrenal gland are extremely common. Although usually nonfunctional, they may secrete sufficient hormones to produce Cushing's or Conn's syndrome. They may be solitary, but occasionally they may appear as two or three nodules in an individual patient; they may also appear as multiple small nodules, and this nodular hyperplasia may be difficult to distinguish from diffuse bilateral cortical hyperplasia. They have been estimated to occur at 2 to 8 percent of all autopsies; if an adenoma is defined in such a way as to include extremely small nodules, a much higher percentage of patients may harbor them. They are frequently encountered as incidental findings on CT [32] or MRI; when they are nonfunctioning these lesions have come to be known by some authors as "incidentalomas." There may be an increased incidence of adrenal adenomas in patients who have renal cell carcinoma [1].

Prior to the development of CT, nonfunctioning adrenal adenomas had little clinical significance since they neither produced disease nor could be diagnosed frequently by any technique other than exploratory surgery. But since large numbers of patients have been examined by CT, their frequent discovery has produced a common problem in that it is often difficult to distinguish them from adrenal metastases.

Radiography and Urography

Radiography and urography very rarely reveal adrenal adenomas since they are usually small (their average size is slightly less than 3 cm, and they are very rarely larger than 5 cm in diameter). Although CT reveals a very small percentage of them to contain small regions of calcification, the calcification is almost never visible on plain radiography.

Ultrasonography

Ultrasonography may reveal these lesions. Since they are small and usually asymptomatic, and since ultrasound demonstration of the adrenals is often difficult, the sensitivity of ultrasonography for detecting them is less than that of CT, at least for small lesions. When visualized, they are seen to be less echogenic than the surrounding fat; ultrasonographically demonstrable calcification is not a common feature.

Computed Tomography

CT [19, 25] reveals adrenal adenomas to be small solid masses (Fig. 7-7); in one series their size has been said to range from 1.2 to 5.0 cm, with an average of 2.9 cm. It is probably true that many cortical adenomas are considerably smaller than a centimeter in diameter and are not reliably visualized by CT. Their tissue attenuation is usually homogeneous; they are often seen to be of lower intensity than adjacent soft tissues such as liver or kidney [43] (although they are never as lucent as water or fat). They may contain tiny regions of calcification but usually do not. They are usually round or oval with sharp margins. They may be enhanced slightly with intravenous contrast medium; the enhancement is usually relatively homogeneous, but small punctate regions of greater enhancement may appear throughout the lesion [4].

Figure 7-7. Right adrenal adenoma. CT reveals an aldosterone-secreting tumor (arrows) to be small, ovoid, and relatively homogeneous. A normal left adrenal is seen.

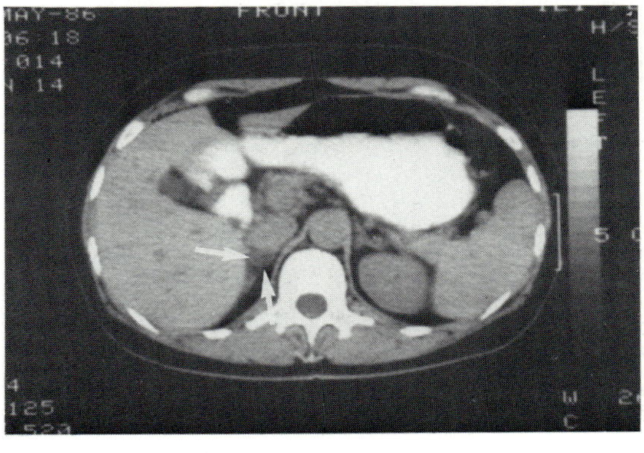

Magnetic Resonance Imaging
On T1 weighted images these lesions display an intensity similar to that of liver (Fig. 7-8A). On T2 weighted images the lesions also usually appear to be of approximately the same intensity as liver (Fig. 7-8B). Commonly, the signal intensity of adenomas is relatively homogeneous across the lesion; rarely, a focal area of necrosis or hemorrhage may cause a region of stronger signal intensity in T2 weighted images [9, 21].

Radionuclide Studies
^{131}I-19 iodocholesterol may accumulate in adrenal adenomas, producing concentrated activity that permits diagnosis of the lesions [27, 48].

Figure 7-8. Left adrenal adenoma. A. T1 weighted MRI reveals a small tumor (arrows) whose intensity is similar to that of liver. B. T2 weighted MRI reveals the same lesion (arrows) to be approximately isointense with liver again.

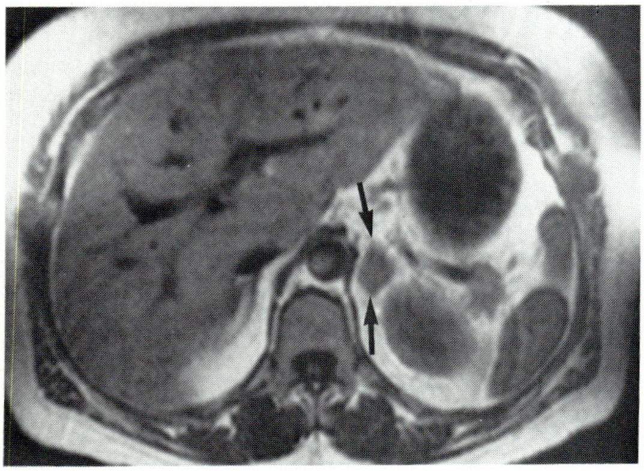

A

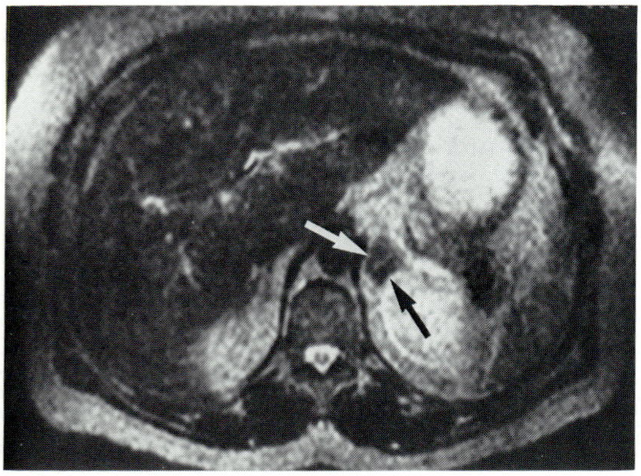

B

Angiography
Angiography is rarely performed on these lesions. If arteriography is performed, adenomas are frequently seen to be moderately vascular and to have a moderately intense capillary phase. The supplying arteries may enlarge.

OTHER NEOPLASMS

METASTASES TO THE ADRENAL GLAND

The adrenal glands are common sites for metastases from a number of primary malignancies. It has been estimated that one-fourth of all patients dying from malignancies have adrenal metastases, and that per gram of tissue the adrenals demonstrate more metastatic deposits than any other tissue in the body. Carcinoma of the breast and lung commonly metastasize to the adrenal, as does melanoma; many other tumors metastasize to the adrenal as well, including lymphoma and tumors of the kidney and ovary.

Diagnosis of adrenal metastases is particularly important since the adrenal may be the only site of metastasis and since diagnosis or exclusion of metastasis may determine the therapy of the primary tumor.

Radiography and Urography
Since metastases in the adrenal may be relatively small, radiography may not demonstrate them; large metastases may be seen as soft-tissue masses and may displace the kidneys inferiorly. They very rarely calcify.

Ultrasonography
Ultrasonography is somewhat less sensitive than CT in detecting metastases to the adrenals, at least when tumors are small. The metastases usually are moderately echogenic; they may contain areas of necrosis that appear to be of low echo intensity.

Computed Tomography
CT is probably the most sensitive examination for detecting adrenal metastases, although as MRI undergoes technical improvement the two methods may become equivalent in sensitivity. Sensitivity in CT is less than 100 percent; micro-

scopic metastases may exist within the adrenal gland without producing any morphologic changes detectable by CT [39]. Metastases in the adrenal usually appear solid (Fig. 7-9) and before administration of an intravenous contrast agent are often of equivalent density with adjacent renal tissue. They usually enhance when contrast medium is administered; enhancement may be heterogeneous. Infrequently, metastases may undergo hemorrhage; this hemorrhage, when acute, may appear slightly denser than adjacent soft tissue, or may resolve to appear as small fluid-filled areas. The borders of metastases may be irregular and extend small rows of strands into the adjacent fat. If sufficiently large, metastases in the adrenal may invade adjacent structures.

Magnetic Resonance Imaging

On T1 weighted images (Fig. 7-10A), the intensity of metastases is commonly equal to or slightly less in intensity than adjacent liver [9, 21]. They are classically considerably brighter than liver on T2 weighted images (Fig. 7-10B), although not as bright as the average pheochromocytoma. When the lesions are large enough so that uniformity of signal can be estimated they may demonstrate inhomogeneity of signal strength. Fluid or hemorrhage within them produce particularly bright images on a T2 weighted examination.

Figure 7-9. Metastasis to the left adrenal. CT reveals the lesion to be slightly lobular in outline (arrow). Another metastasis has destroyed portions of the lumbar vertebra.

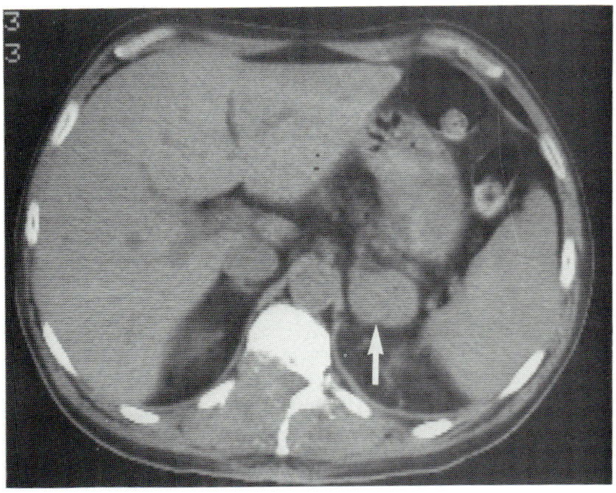

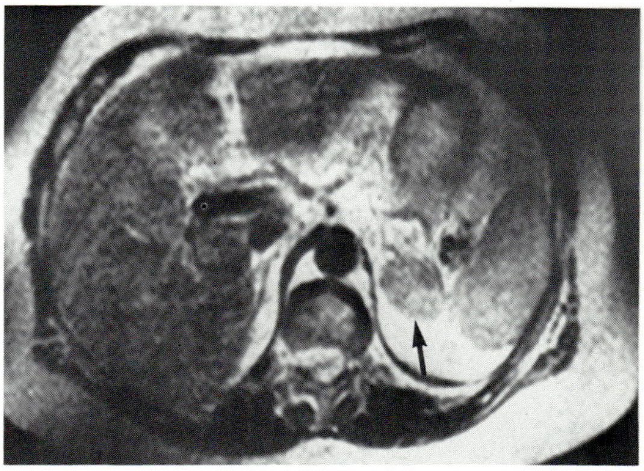

A

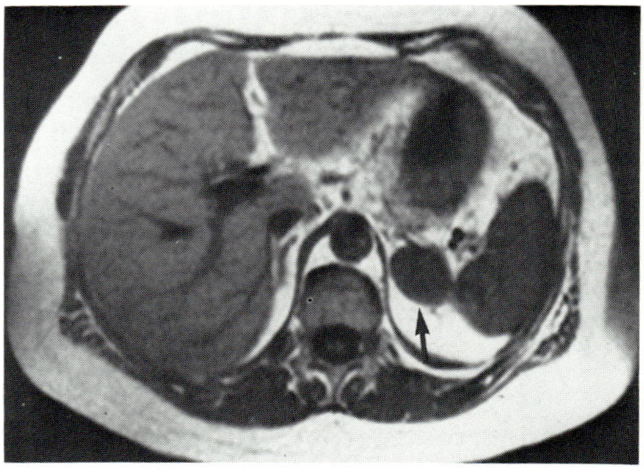

B

Figure 7-10. Metastasis to the left adrenal. A. T1 weighted MRI reveals the left adrenal mass (arrow) to be slightly less intense than liver and similar to spleen. B. T2 weighted MRI reveals the mass (arrow) to be brighter than liver and, again, similar in intensity to the spleen.

Angiography

Arteriography is rarely used in diagnosis of metastatic disease. Metastatic deposits usually reveal variable patterns of neovascularity and inhomogeneous tissue enhancement.

MYELOLIPOMA

Adrenal myelolipomas are rare, benign, nonfunctioning, and usually asymptomatic tumors. They appear throughout adult life but most frequently in the fourth through sixth decades. They consist of mixtures of bone marrow (myeloid) tissues and fat and occasionally contain foci of calcification. They do not metastasize and are not multiple. On the rare occasion when they produce symptoms (abdominal or flank discomfort), hemorrhage into the tumor or simply the size of the larger tumors are thought to be the causes.

Imaging

Radiography and urography may demonstrate calcifications in tumors that contain them; these studies usually do not show lucency in the fatty regions of the tumor, however. Ultrasonography usually reveals the tumors to be echogenic [3, 37], with either homogeneous or heterogeneous echotexture; calcification may produce the usual ultrasonographic findings. Since the tumors are usually surrounded by retroperitoneal fat, ultrasonography may fail to detect small fatty tumors; the echogenicity pattern is thought not to be sufficiently specific to permit a histologic diagnosis. CT [37] is the study that usually provides a definitive diagnosis: Classically, the tumors contain regions of tissue whose attenuation values are consistent with fat (Fig. 7-11) [3], measuring −20 Hounsfield units or even less. When tissue that is clearly fatty exists within an adrenal mass, the diagnosis of myelolipoma is sufficiently certain that resection is usually not required and biopsy may be omitted as well. Unfortunately, there may be a sufficiently high percentage of myeloid tissue or sufficient hemorrhage within the lesion that clearly fatty portions cannot be demonstrated; under these circumstances the CT diagnosis of a myelolipoma becomes less definite and histologic examination of tissue becomes necessary. Myelolipomas may enhance with administration of intravenous contrast medium and do so sufficiently that tissue that originally was clearly fatty may become sufficiently dense that its fatty nature is no longer clear; therefore it is important that these tumors be examined without a contrast agent if a specific diagnosis is to be made. Angiographic examination of these tumors usually reveals them to be relatively avascular. Reports of significant numbers of tumors examined by MRI are not yet available; however, anecdotal experience suggests that the fatty regions within the tumor may have the MRI characteristics of fat in other parts of the body.

Figure 7-11. A large right adrenal myelolipoma. CT reveals that most of the lesion (arrows) is composed of tissue whose density is similar to that of fat. (Courtesy of J. Farah, M.D., William Beaumont Hospital, Royal Oak, Michigan.)

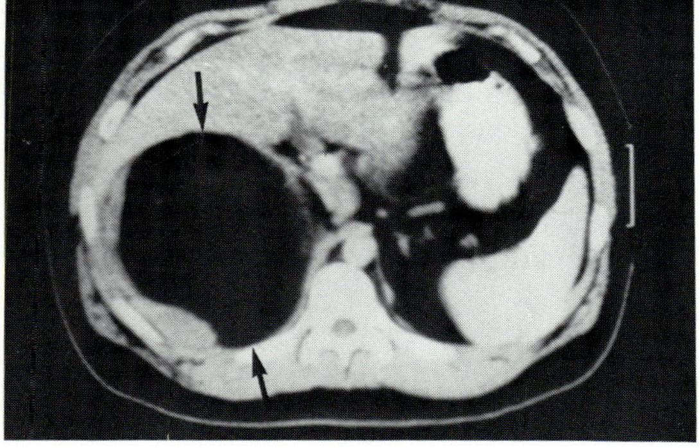

Occasionally, a differential diagnosis must be made. Differentiation of an adrenal myelolipoma from an upper-pole renal angiomyolipoma may rely on sagittal or coronal images (either ultrasonography or MRI) to search for a plane between the lesion and the kidney; alternatively, angiography may reveal a primary blood supply characteristic of one or the other of these tumors and may be helpful in that angiomyolipomas are characteristically vascular whereas myelolipomas are not. Certain benign adrenal cortical adenomas may be relatively low in CT attenuation values, and therefore raise the possibility of myelolipoma; demonstrating CT numbers of −20 Hounsfield units or below excludes adenomas for all practical purposes. Finally, a fatty adrenal tumor may be confused with a fatty primary retroperitoneal tumor such as lipoma or liposarcoma; when confusion persists resection may be required.

MISCELLANEOUS TUMORS

Mesenchymal or connective-tissue tumors of various histologies may appear in the adrenals; these are extremely rare. Occasionally, a hemangioma may be found; the diagnosis may be suggested if phleboliths are found within an adrenal mass.

MISCELLANEOUS CONDITIONS

ADRENAL CYSTS

Cysts of the adrenal gland are relatively rare. They have appeared in patients of all ages but usually are found in the third to fifth decades of life; there appears to be a female predominance. There are no characteristic symptoms; occasionally, if they are large, they may be palpated or produce a sensation of abdominal fullness. Cysts are divided by most investigators into four types: those of endothelial origin (angiomatous or lymphangiomatous), epithelial lesions, parasitic cysts (primarily echinococcal), and pseudocysts (thought to be usually the result of a remote hematoma).

On radiography and urography adrenal cysts may be invisible if they are small; large cysts may be seen as space-occupying lesions that displace the ipsilateral kidney inferiorly. Many adrenal cysts have linear or punctate calcification in the walls (Fig. 7-12).

Ultrasonography reveals findings similar to those encountered with renal cysts: The lesions are fluid filled and their walls have no appreciable thickness.

CT also reveals these cysts to have the same characteristics as renal cysts. They are thin-

Figure 7-12. Right adrenal cyst. Nephrotomography reveals a rim of calcification (arrow) in the inferior portion of the lesion.

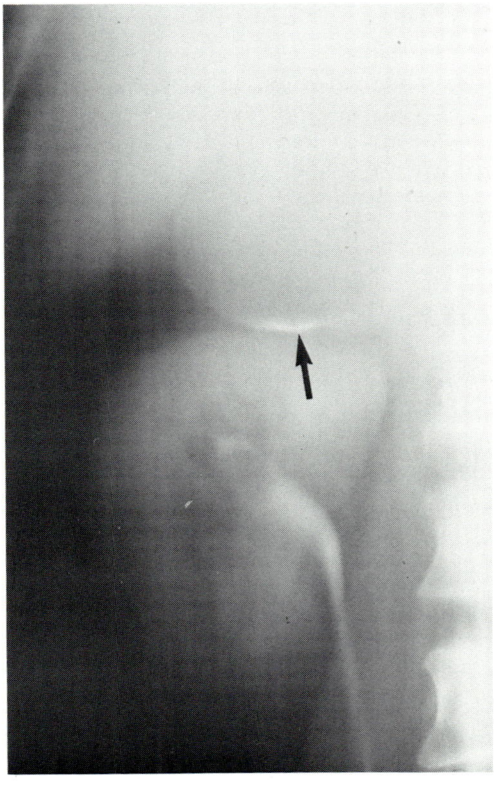

walled and usually contain material of fluid density; occasionally, the fluid might be slightly denser if the cyst is hemorrhagic.

MRI reveals the fluid of most cysts to be of low signal strength on T1 weighted images and high signal strength on T2 weighted images. Occasionally, hemorrhagic fluid may appear relatively bright on both T1 and T2 weighted images.

Angiography reveals the lesions to be completely avascular.

ADRENAL HEMORRHAGE

A number of circumstances may produce bleeding and hematoma formation within one or both of the adrenals. In neonates [29, 46] the adrenals are particularly large and apparently easy to injure. Hematomas may appear in them with some frequency; they are thought in most cases to be due to stressful delivery. In neonates anemia and jaundice may appear if the volume of the hematoma is large. At any age a number of factors may produce adrenal hematomas including surgery, severe sepsis, widespread burns, hypotension, coagulopathies, or trauma; meningococcemia may produce bilateral adrenal hemorrhage with acute adrenal insufficiency, which is known as the Waterhouse–Friderichsen syndrome. In neonates adrenal hemorrhage usually does not lead to adrenal insufficiency; bilateral severe adrenal hemorrhage later in life may do so, however.

Adrenal hematomas themselves rarely require specific therapy; obviously, acute adrenal insufficiency requires appropriate exogenous hormone treatment. The hematomas usually resolve spontaneously; the peripheral portions of the hematomas frequently calcify, sometimes as early as 2 to 4 weeks after birth. As the hematoma reabsorbs, the calcification may ultimately adopt the shape of a normal adrenal. Less frequently, a hemorrhagic pseudocyst will remain, which may or may not have a calcific rim.

Imaging

Adrenal calcification may be seen in the patterns described above during radiography or urography. Adrenal hematomas sufficiently large to depress the ipsilateral kidney are occasionally encountered; if they have reached the stage of forming a pseudocyst, the wall may be visibly enhanced by contrast medium.

Ultrasonography in neonatal acute adrenal hemorrhage reveals a mass in the adrenals (Fig. 7-13) in which few or no echoes may be seen [33]. But within the mass individual clots may be echogenic; with time the mass diminishes in size and the ultrasound images of the adrenal may revert toward normal. If the adrenals are calcified the calcification will be easy to detect by ultrasonography but often precludes the visualization of the parenchyma of the adrenal gland itself.

CT reveals masses in the region of the adrenal whose size correlates with the volume of the hemorrhage acutely; blood may be diverted into the periadrenal fatty tissues and cause strand-like densities on CT [36]. The attenuation values depend on the duration of the hematoma; acutely, contracted clots may appear denser than the adjacent renal parenchyma, whereas in the pseudocyst stage the fluid may be less dense than solid tissue. Most hematomas may be followed to resolution with CT.

MRI of adrenal hematomas [26] may reveal a variety of appearances (Fig. 7-14), depending on the age of the hematoma, the pulse sequence used, and the magnetic field strength. Very acute hematomas may appear of relatively low intensity on T1 weighted images and high intensity on T2 weighted images; later, the bulk of the hematoma may appear bright on both kinds of images. If the hematoma has been present for a sufficient time, a thin low-intensity rim may be seen at the periphery of the lesion, which presumably represents a ring of hemosiderin-laden macrophages. Within this rim a bright ring surrounding a lower-intensity center, characteristic of hematomas elsewhere, may be found.

Figure 7-13. Adrenal hemorrhage. Ultrasonography of the right adrenal reveals that the hematoma (arrows) has enlarged the gland but still retains a triangular shape. The hematoma is hypoechoic but not anechoic.

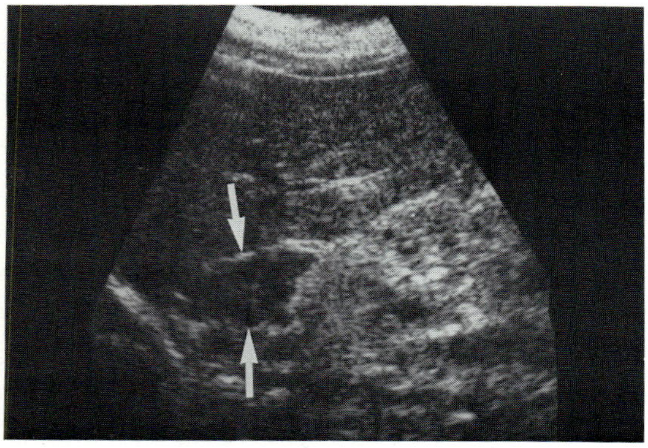

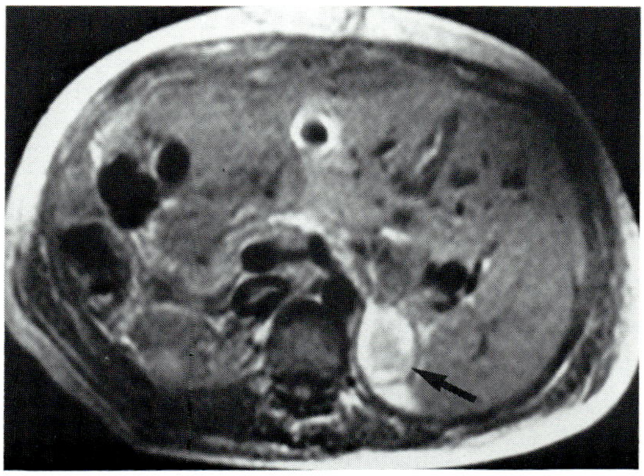

A

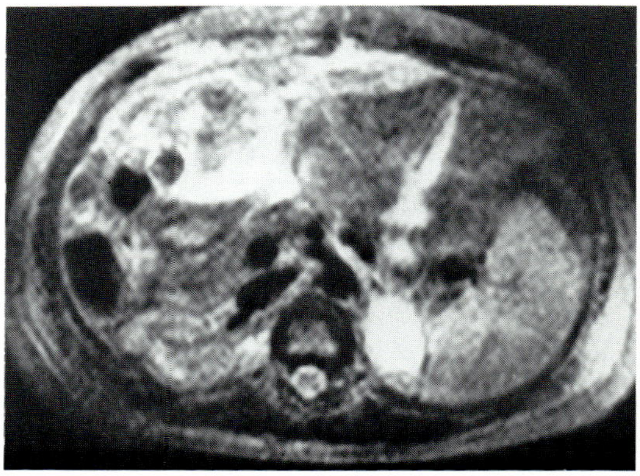

B

Figure 7-14. Left adrenal hematoma after blunt trauma. This patient had undergone a right hepatic lobectomy. A. T1 weighted MRI shows the hematoma (arrow) to contain a relatively bright ring around a center of medium intensity. B. T2 weighted MRI shows the hematoma to be uniformly bright throughout.

WOLMAN'S DISEASE

Wolman's disease is a very rare congenital syndrome characterized by the infiltration of multiple solid viscera with foam cells filled with cholesterol and triglycerides [51]. The patients present in early infancy with hepatosplenomegaly, multiple constitutional symptoms, and failure to thrive; progression to death is inevitable. The adrenals are enlarged but retain their normal shape and display multiple punctate calcifications, which can be easily visualized on radiography, CT, or ultrasonography.

GRANULOMATOUS DISEASES

Both tuberculosis and histoplasmosis may involve the adrenals. The glands may be slightly to moderately enlarged in acute or subacute cases and normal to diminished in size with punctate or amorphous calcifications in the chronic phase. Association with tuberculosis or histoplasmosis elsewhere in the body may help to establish the diagnosis; on occasion adrenal biopsy may be of value.

BECKWITH–WIEDEMANN SYNDROME

Beckwith–Wiedemann syndrome is a rare congenital syndrome characterized by gigantism, macroglossia, and umbilical hernia. Both cysts and cytomegaly are found in the adrenal cortices, producing enlargement of the adrenal glands.

ADRENAL VARICES

In patients with portal hypertension the left inferior phrenic and adrenal veins may communicate with the splenic vein, thus forming a portosystemic shunt. The enlarged left adrenal vein with its intraadrenal branches may simulate an adrenal mass. An adrenal-vein varix may also appear in the absence of portal hypertension.

MRI may demonstrate these veins, or CT (Fig. 7-15) may demonstrate that a space-occupying lesion within the adrenal is really a dilated vein if dynamic CT with a contrast

Figure 7-15. Left adrenal varix. CT reveals the varix (arrows), which resembles a small adrenal mass.

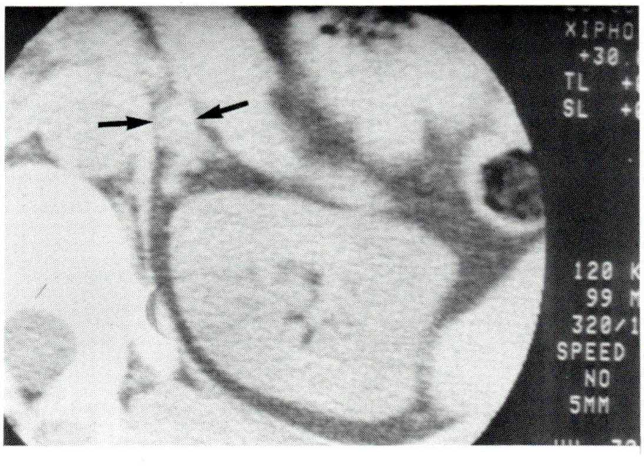

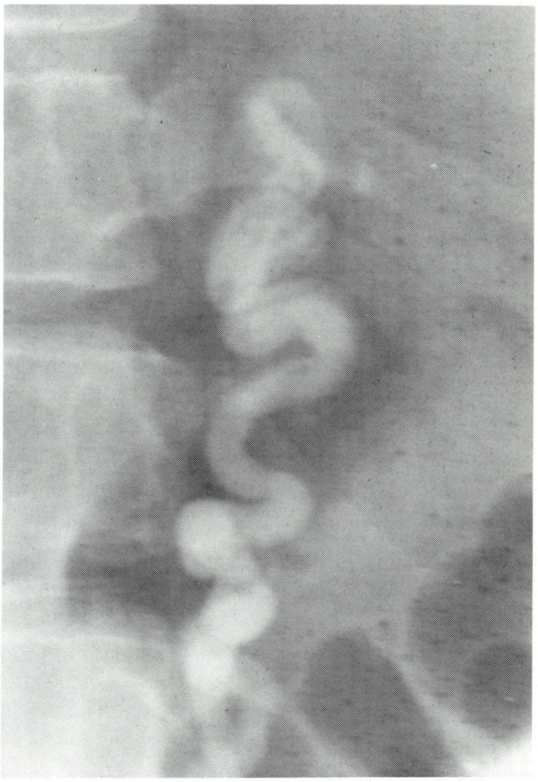

Figure 7-16. Left adrenal varix. Venography shows the vessel to be tortuous; it extends from the bed of the left adrenal to the left renal vein.

bolus is performed [7, 34]. Venography is usually not necessary but may be used to make a definitive diagnosis (Fig. 7-16).

IMAGING APPROACH TO ABNORMAL ADRENAL FUNCTIONAL STATES

Patients who have adrenocortical hypofunction (Addison's disease) may have a variety of adrenal abnormalities demonstrable by imaging. The adrenal glands may have been destroyed by any of several processes, including bilateral metastases or hemorrhage or subacute or chronic granulomatous disease; the manifestations of these are discussed elsewhere in this chapter. Alternatively, the adrenal glands may appear atrophic and display particularly thin limbs on CT images; the atrophy may be due to autoimmune processes.

Excessive production of adrenal hormones may produce any one of a variety of syndromes. Adrenal medullary hyperfunction should prompt a search for a pheochromocytoma. Cortical hyperfunction may produce Cushing's syndrome, hyperaldosteronism, or the adrenogenital syndrome.

Most patients with Cushing's syndrome have hyperplasia (Fig. 7-17) of the adrenal gland, which may not produce sufficient gross morphologic change to produce any abnormality on imaging techniques at all. If the syndrome is shown to be adrenocorticotropic hormone [ACTH] dependent, imaging workup of the pituitary should be performed, and if appropriate, searches for tumors that produce exogenous ACTH (including those of the lung, thymus, and pancreas) should also be made. Approximately 10 percent of patients with endogenous Cushing's syndrome have a functioning adrenal adenoma; these should be sought with CT. Occasionally, these adenomas may be sufficiently small to be missed by CT, and adrenal vein sampling may be necessary to localize the abnormality. About 5 percent of patients with Cushing's syndrome have primary adrenal carcinoma, the imaging characteristics of which are described elsewhere in this chapter.

Hyperaldosteronism (Conn's syndrome) may also appear as a reflection of primary adrenal disease. About 80 percent of these patients have a functioning adenoma; these tumors are often quite small, so that although they should initially be sought by CT, failure to demonstrate an abnormality by CT should lead to consideration of adrenal vein sampling. Most of the remainder of the patients have adrenal hyperplasia, which, as in the case of Cushing's syndrome, may appear as thickening of all adrenal limbs [18], but frequently produces no morphologic abnormality that can be detected by imaging. Patients with secondary hyperaldosteronism may have a number of primary diseases; at least two of these (renal artery stenosis and reninoma) require radiologic workup for exclusion.

Figure 7-17. Bilateral adrenal hyperplasia. CT reveals the limbs of both adrenals to be thickened (arrows). There is also metastatic disease of the liver.

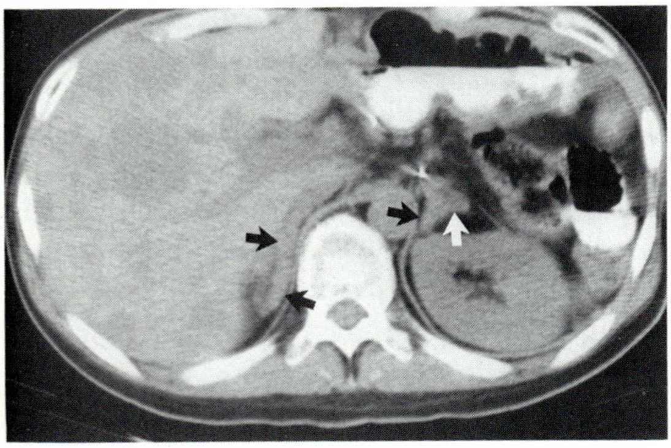

The adrenogenital syndrome may appear in children or adults. In congenital adrenogenital syndrome, the adrenals are often symmetrically enlarged. Rarely, this syndrome may be produced by an adrenal carcinoma or even an adenoma.

DIFFERENTIAL DIAGNOSIS OF ADRENAL MASSES

There are commonly occurring clinical situations in which differential diagnosis of a demonstrated adrenal mass is important. Under some circumstances a specific diagnosis is easy: A clearly fatty adrenal mass can be firmly diagnosed as a myelolipoma; benign adrenal cysts have ultrasound and CT characteristics that are unique; clinical and biochemical data usually identify adrenal masses that are pheochromocytomas; the age of the patient and location of the tumor almost always permits a firm diagnosis of neuroblastoma (chemical data and the progress of the lesion usually permit distinction of a neuroblastoma from an adrenal hemorrhage in babies in whom this becomes a problem); and appropriate biochemical studies permit the distinction of functioning from nonfunctioning adenomas. The average sizes of the lesions may be useful to know; Conn's adenomas are often quite small (<1.5 cm), whereas primary carcinomas are usually large (>6.0 cm) when discovered; unfortunately, adenomas, pheochromocytomas, and metastases have intermediate size ranges that overlap considerably.

Nonfunctioning adenomas and metastases may be more difficult to distinguish, and the need for a correct diagnosis is obvious [28]. The distinction is assisted first by considering the prevalence of the two diseases. In a population of patients examined by CT who are not known to have a primary malignancy, the prevalence of benign adenomas is many times greater than that of metastases from occult tumors. Even in populations of patients known to have specific tumors or in populations of patients drawn from an oncologic practice, adenomas may be somewhat more common than metastases [38]. CT permits further refinement of the differential diagnosis [4]: Adenomas are less likely to be multiple, are likely to have homogeneous tissue attenuation, often have tissue attenuation (without contrast) that is uniform and slightly less than adjacent soft tissues, and usually have sharp margins. Metastatic tumors are more likely to be heterogeneous in attenuation and to enhance heterogeneously with contrast medium. If they have regions of relatively low intensity, these have the configuration of focal necrotic regions. They are also more likely to be multiple and to have irregular margins.

MRI has been shown to aid in this differential diagnosis [42]. Metastatic tumors usually have slightly lesser intensity on T1 weighted images than do adenomas; on T2 weighted images metastatic lesions are, on average, considerably brighter than adenomas. There is some inevitable overlap, however, so that MRI may be inaccurate in about a fifth of cases; especially well-differentiated metastases may look like adenomas, whereas adenomas that have small regions of necrosis, edema, or hemorrhage may look like metastases. In addition, the exact intensities of each kind of lesion may vary from practice to practice as a function of different field strengths, pulse sequences, and comparison tissues. While MRI information is likely to make the probabilities of one diagnosis or another greater, it cannot be said to be accurate in all cases.

Percutaneous needle aspiration biopsy of these lesions is often of benefit; this can always be guided by CT [5] and, if the lesion is large enough, by ultrasonography. If a sample is recovered that clearly demonstrates signs of malignancy, a malignant tumor (either primary or metastatic) can be diagnosed with great confidence. The needle aspiration biopsy does not provide a 100 percent reliable answer in all cases: Errors may occur if the recovered sample is not from the lesion itself, if it is insufficient for analysis, or in cases in which metastatic carcinoma is present in the adrenal but is so well organized as to be difficult to distinguish from an adenoma. Despite these concerns, needle biopsy provides the correct diagnosis in most circumstances. Much less frequently, differential diagnosis of a primary adrenal carcinoma from a benign adrenal adenoma may be required. Both lesions may be functional or nonfunctional, so that biochemical studies are usually not conclusive. At the time of discovery, primary carcinomas of the adrenal are usually larger than adenomas and are much more likely to be heterogeneous and contain necrotic central regions and to contain calcification.

REFERENCES

1. Ambos, M.A., et al. Adrenal adenoma associated with renal cell carcinoma. *A.J.R.* 136:81, 1981.
2. Amundson, G.M., et al. Neuroblastoma: A specific sonographic tissue pattern. *A.J.R.* 148:943, 1987.
3. Behan, M., et al. Myelolipoma of the adrenal: Two cases with ultrasound and CT findings. *A.J.R.* 129:993, 1977.
4. Berland, L.L., et al. Differentiation between small benign and malignant adrenal masses with dynamic incremented CT. *A.J.R.* 151:95, 1988.
5. Bernardino, M.E., et al. CT-guided adrenal biopsy: Accuracy, safety, and indications. *A.J.R.* 144:67, 1985.
6. Bowerman, R.A., et al. Sonography of adrenal pheochromocytomas. *A.J.R.* 137:1227, 1987.
7. Brady, T.M., et al. Adrenal pseudomasses due to varices: Angiographic-CT-MRI-pathologic correlations. *A.J.R.* 145:301, 1985.
8. Casola, G., et al. Unsuspected pheochromocytoma: Risk of blood-pressure alterations during percutaneous adrenal biopsy. *Radiology* 159:733, 1986.
9. Chang, A., et al. Adrenal gland: MR imaging. *Radiology* 163:123, 1987.
10. Cho, K.J., et al. Adrenal medullary disease in multiple endocrine neoplasia type II. *A.J.R.* 134:23, 1980.
11. Christenson, R., Smith, C.W., and Burko, H. Arteriographic manifestations of pheochromocytoma. *A.J.R.* 126:567, 1976.
12. Das, S., Bulusu, N.V., and Lowe, P. Primary vesical pheochromocytoma. *Urology* 21:20, 1983.
13. Dietrich, R.B., et al. Neuroblastoma: The role of MR imaging: *A.J.R.* 148:937, 1987.
14. Dunnick, N.R., et al. CT appearance of adrenal cortical carcinoma. *J. Comput. Assist. Tomogr.*, 6:978, 1982.
15. Fink, I.J., et al. MR imaging of pheochromocytomas. *J. Comput. Assist. Tomogr.* 9:454,1985.

16. Fishman, E.K., et al. Primary adrenocortical carcinoma: CT evaluation with clinical correlation. *A.J.R.* 148:531, 1987.
17. Fletcher, B.D., et al. Abdominal neuroblastoma: Magnetic resonance imaging and tissue characterization. *Radiology* 155:699, 1985.
18. Francis, I.R., et al. Complementary roles of CT and 131I-MIBG scintigraphy in diagnosing pheochromocytoma. *A.J.R.* 141:719, 1983.
19. Geisinger, M.A., et al. Primary hyperaldosteronism: Comparison of CT, adrenal venography, and venous sampling. *A.J.R.* 141:299, 1983.
20. Glazer, G.M., Francis, I.R., and Quint, L.E. Imaging of the adrenal glands. *Invest. Radiol.* 23:3, 1988.
21. Glazer, G.M., et al. Adrenal tissue characterization using MR imaging. *Radiology* 158:73, 1986.
22. Hamper, U.M., et al. Primary adrenocortical carcinoma: Sonographic evaluation with clinical and pathologic correlation in 26 patients. *A.J.R.* 148:915, 1987.
23. Hill, F.S., et al. The coexistence of renal artery stenosis and pheochromocytoma. *Ann. Surg.*, 197, 484, 1983.
24. Howman-Giles, R.B., et al. Radionuclide skeletal survey in neuroblastoma. *Radiology* 131:497, 1979.
25. Huebener, K.H., and Treugut, H. Adrenal cortex dysfunction: CT findings. *Radiology* 150:195, 1984.
26. Itoh, K., et al. MR imaging of bilateral adrenal hemorrhage. *J. Comput. Assist. Tomogr.* 12:1054, 1988.
27. Jorgensen, H., Norman, N., and Sundsfjord, J.A. Scintigraphy with 131I-19-Iodocholesterol in adrenal disease. *Acta Med. Scand.* 197:345, 1975.
28. Katz, R.L., and Shirkhoda, A. Diagnostic approach to incidental adrenal nodules in the cancer patient. *Cancer* 55:1995, 1985.
29. Khuri, F.J., et al. Adrenal hemorrhage in neonates: Report of 5 cases and review of the literature. *J. Urol.* 124:684, 1980.
30. Laursen, K., and Damgaard-Pedersen, Karen. CT for pheochromocytoma diagnosis. *A.J.R.* 134:277, 1980.
31. Lynn, M.D., et al. Bone metastases in pheochromocytoma: Comparative studies of efficacy of imaging. *Radiology* 160:701, 1986.
32. Mitnick, J.S., et al. Nonfunctioning adrenal adenomas discovered incidentally on computed tomography. *Radiology* 148:495,1983.
33. Mittelstaedt, C.A., et al. The sonographic diagnosis of neonatal adrenal hemorrhage. *Radiology* 131:453, 1979.
34. Mitty, H.A., et al. Adrenal pseudotumors on CT due to dilated portosystemic veins. *A.J.R.* 141:727, 1983.
35. Mitty, H.A., and Yeh, H.-C. *Radiology of the Adrenals with Sonography and CT* (vol. 17 of Saunders Monographs in Clinical Radiology). Philadelphia: Saunders, 1982.
36. Murphy, B.J., Casillas, J., and Yrizarry, J.M. Traumatic adrenal hemorrhage: Radiologic findings. *Radiology* 169:701, 1988.
37. Musante, F., et al. Myelolipoma of the adrenal gland: Sonographic and CT features. *A.J.R.* 151:961,1988.
38. Oliver, T.W., Jr., et al. Isolated adrenal masses in non small-cell bronchogenic carcinoma. *Radiology* 153:217, 1984.
39. Pagani, J.J. Normal adrenal glands in small cell lung carcinoma: CT-guided biopsy. *A.J.R.* 140:949, 1983.
40. Quint, L.E., et al. Pheochromocytoma and paraganglioma: Comparison of MR imaging with CT and I-131 MIBG scintigraphy. *Radiology* 165:89, 1987.
41. Raisanen, J., et al. Plasma catecholamines in pheochromocytoma: Effect of urographic contrast media. *A.J.R.* 143:43, 1984.
42. Reinig, J.W., et al. Adrenal masses differentiated by MR. *Radiology* 158:81, 1986.
43. Schaner, E.G., et al. Adrenal cortical tumors with low attenuation coefficients: A pitfall in computed tomography diagnosis. *J. Comput. Assist. Tomogr.* 2:11, 1978.
44. Sisson, J.C., et al. Scintigraphic localization of pheochromocytoma. *N. Engl. J. Med.* 305:12, 1981.
45. Smith, F.W., et al. Primary neuroblastoma uptake of ^{99m}technetium methylene diphosphonate. *Radiology* 137:501, 1980.
46. Smith, J.A., Jr., and Middleton, R.G. Neonatal adrenal hemorrhage. *J. Urol.* 122:674, 1979.
47. Thomas, J.L., et al. CT of pheochromocytoma. *A.J.R.* 135:477, 1980.
48. Troncone, L., et al. Radioisotopic study of the adrenal glands using 131 I-19-iodocholesterol. *Br. J. Radiol.* 50:340, 1977.
49. Welch, T.J., et al. Pheochromocytoma: Value of computed tomography. *Radiology* 148:501, 1983.
50. White, S.J., et al. Sonography of neuroblastoma. *A.J.R.* 141:465, 1983.
51. Wolman, M., et al. Primary familial xanthomatosis with involvement and calcification of the adrenals. *Pediatrics* 28:742, 1961.

8

The Kidney: Cystic Disease

There are a large number of diseases that produce cystic pathology in the kidneys. These have been of particular interest to radiologists since the invention of urography. Many of them are common and most of them can be diagnosed only by imaging techniques. The differential diagnosis of certain manifestations of cystic disease continues to be an important problem in uroradiologic practice.

In this chapter a number of important diseases will be discussed (Table 8-1). Other cystic diseases—particularly those associated with multiple renal neoplasms and those due to infectious or inflammatory process—are discussed in the chapters on renal tumors and renal infections. There are numerous other entities in which renal cystic lesions appear but are extremely uncommon; these will not be described individually in this textbook.

A number of schemes have been proposed for the classification of renal cystic diseases. These include divisions of groups of diseases according to histologic characteristics established by microdissection studies, divisions according to appearance of the gross pathology or clinical images, and divisions according to cause. No system is perfect, and since in clinical practice we feel that knowledge of the pathology, presentation, imaging appearance, and differential diagnosis are the important issues with which to be familiar, we will not present a classification scheme; instead, the diseases listed in Table 8-1 will be dealt with individually, and their relation to each other will be discussed only in situations in which differential diagnosis among several cystic diseases is a clinically important problem.

SIMPLE RENAL CYSTS

Simple renal cysts are extremely common. Their prevelance increases with increasing age: More than half of all people over the age of 50 have at least one [44]. They are very uncommon in early adulthood, however, and are rare in children [26, 68, 70]. There is no sex predilection.

PATHOLOGY

Simple cysts are usually lined with a single layer of cuboidal epithelium; there may be a thin fibrous layer outside the epithelial lining. They contain light yellow, clear serous fluid. Thin septa may incompletely or completely traverse the lumen of the cyst. Renal cysts may be multilocular [4].

Simple cysts may range from a few millimeters to many centimeters in diameter. They may arise from the periphery of the kidney and extend outside the renal margins or may be partly or entirely surrounded by cortical or medullary parenchyma. When they arise relatively deep within the renal parenchyma, they may expand into the renal sinus (these cysts are called parapelvic cysts) [33, 53]. Occasionally, several small cysts may arise within the renal sinus; these are called peripelvic cysts.

CLINICAL COURSE

The vast majority of patients with simple cysts are completely without signs, symptoms, or any nonimaging laboratory abnormalities. On very rare occasions the cysts may be large enough to be palpable or to cause pain. Cysts have occasionally been thought to cause hematuria, but the hematuria is usually microscopic and occurs so rarely that another cause for bleeding must always be carefully excluded.

Complications are rare but do occur. Cysts may occasionally become infected [10] and produce pain, fever, and pyuria; it is often difficult to distinguish an infected cyst from a parenchymal abscess. Rarely, cysts may rupture [55] either into the perinephric space or collecting system and be associated with perinephric bleeding or hematuria; both spontaneous and posttraumatic rupture have been described.

Table 8-1. Cystic diseases of the kidney

Simple renal cysts
Autosomal dominant polycystic kidney disease
Autosomal recessive polycystic kidney disease
Acquired cystic disease of the kidney
Medullary sponge kidney
Juvenile nephronophthisis/medullary cystic disease
Multicystic dysplastic kidney
Pyelocaliceal diverticulum

Infrequently, cysts may compress an infundibulum, the renal pelvis, or the proximal ureter and cause partial obstruction of all or part of the kidney [34]. Rarely, an expanding cyst may compress renal parenchyma sufficiently to cause local ischemia, hyperreninemia, and systemic hypertension [39, 59].

IMAGING STUDIES

Most cysts produce no abnormalities on plain films. Occasionally, a large extrarenal cyst may be visible as a soft-tissue mass. One to two percent of benign cysts develop calcification in their walls. The calcification in the wall of a benign cyst is thin and curvilinear; thick, chunky, or amorphous calcification or calcification within the center of a lesion is more characteristic of renal cell carcinoma. Multicystic dysplastic renal disease may occasionally produce calcification within the rims of cystic lesions.

Simple renal cysts may produce a variety of appearances on urograms and nephrotomograms. Usually, they are seen as spherical or ovoid space-occupying lesions (Fig. 8-1). When they are within the kidney they appear relatively lucent as compared with the opacified parenchyma; however, when they are primarily outside the kidney and protrude into the perinephric fat, they may seem more dense because of the relative lucency of the surrounding fat. Small intrarenal lesions may produce no abnormalities of the renal outline or the shape of the collecting system. If they protrude outside the periphery of the kidney they may cause a local bulge in the renal outline; if they extend into the renal sinus they may displace portions of the renal collecting system, which are then indented or draped around the surface of a lesion. Reliable differentiation between a solid mass and a simple cyst is usually not possible on urograms without nephrotomography; if rigidly adhered to, certain nephrotomographic criteria may permit a reasonably certain diagnosis of a simple cyst. These criteria require that the lesion be homogeneously lucent, that its interface with normal renal parenchyma be sharp, and that any extrarenal portion of the lesion be bounded by a wall that is either paper thin or too thin to be seen at all; also, the lesion cannot contain chunky or central calcification and cannot invade the collecting system.

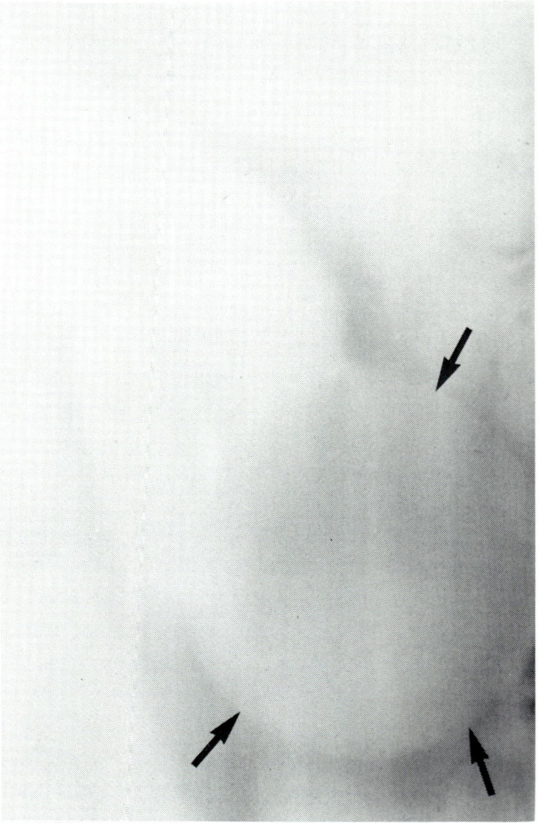

Figure 8-1. Simple renal cyst. Nephrotomography reveals the left lower pole cyst (arrows) to be lucent; it has no discernible wall.

Certain complications may be visible. Infundibular, pelvic, or ureteral compression with obstruction may be represented by clubbing of the obstructed calices; frequently, however, the calices may be distorted, stretched, or draped by the cyst and appear at first glance to be obstructed, whereas in fact they are merely distorted. Infection or hemorrhage into the cyst lumen is not detectable with urography. A cyst that has ruptured into the collecting system may be visible if its lumen is in continuity with the caliceal lumen and if both fill with contrast; differentiation between a ruptured cyst and a caliceal diverticulum may be difficult.

Most renal cysts first detected on urography require confirmation of their specific nature by ultrasonography; a small fraction of these will require CT or other procedures before a diagnosis can be established with certainty.

On ultrasonography [28] simple renal cysts have characteristics that, if strictly used as criteria, permit relatively reliable diagnosis. The lesions are spherical or ovoid fluid-filled regions. The lumina of the cysts are anechoic, the tissues deep to the cyst reveal evidence of enhanced through-transmission of sound, the deep wall of the cyst is well outlined by specular echoes, and there is no discernible thickness of any part of the cyst wall (Fig. 8-2). If there are echoes within the fluid or if the wall reveals focal or diffuse thickening or evidence of calcification, other cystic lesions, including abscesses, infected cysts, hematomas, and cystic necrotic carcinomas, must also be considered in the differential diagnosis [8]. If the center of the lesion is relatively hypoechoic but there is no enhanced through-transmission of sound evident deep to the lesion, solid but hypoechoic lesions such as lymphomas must enter the differential diagnosis as well. Of course, if even part of the lesion is seen to contain a mass, a simple cyst cannot be diagnosed.

Figure 8-2. Simple renal cyst. Ultrasonography reveals the cyst to be anechoic and to have dense echoes in its posterior wall. There is acoustic enhancement deep to the lesion.

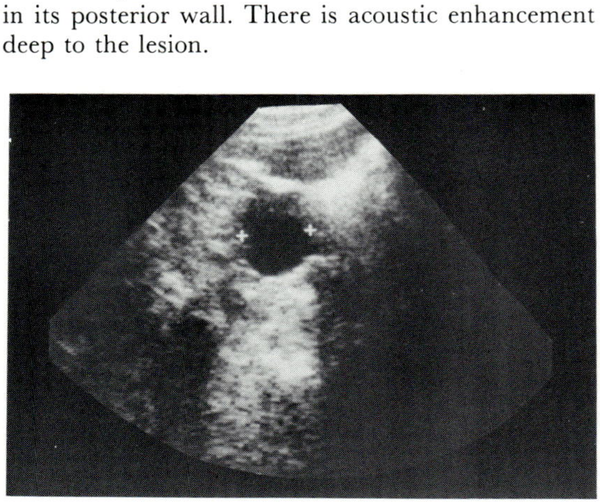

Focal hydronephrosis produced by an infundibular stricture or an obstructed duplicated upper-pole collecting system may occasionally mimic a simple cyst on ultrasonography. In addition, cystic lesions that arise outside the kidney but are closely related to it may occasionally be confused with simple renal cysts. Adrenal cysts may sometimes be difficult to distinguish from upper-pole cysts, pseudocysts may arise from the tail of the pancreas and be closely applied to the surface of the left kidney, and simple hepatic cysts that protrude from the inferior portion of the right lobe toward the right kidney may be confused with renal cysts.

Other renal lesions may occasionally be confused with simple cysts. Renal artery aneurysms may resemble parapelvic cysts, small multilocular cystic nephromas may occasionally mimic septated cysts, hydatid cysts may resemble septated simple cysts, and hematomas may look like cysts. In some cases CT or other examinations may be necessary.

The classic appearance of a simple cyst on CT is that of a spherical or ovoid lesion whose lumen appears homogeneous and has the approximate attenuation of water, varying no more than 10 Hounsfield units above or below zero (Fig. 8-3). The portion of the lesion that is intrarenal should have a sharp interface with the adjacent normal parenchyma, and any extrarenal portion should have a very thin or imperceptible wall. The lesion should not enhance when an intravenous contrast agent is administered. When these criteria are met, the lesion is virtually certain to be a simple renal cyst.

Many cystic lesions deviate from these classic appearances, however. Very small cysts may have their appearance altered by partial volume averaging with normal adjacent parenchyma so that even with thin CT slices the attenuation of the visualized abnormal region may be considerably higher than zero and may increase if an intravenous contrast agent is given. Obviously, some of these characteristics overlap with those of renal cell carcinomas, but since cysts vastly outnumber carcinomas these very small lesions are usually not worked up further when encountered on CT examinations.

The true density of renal cysts may also be considerably higher than zero; cysts have been

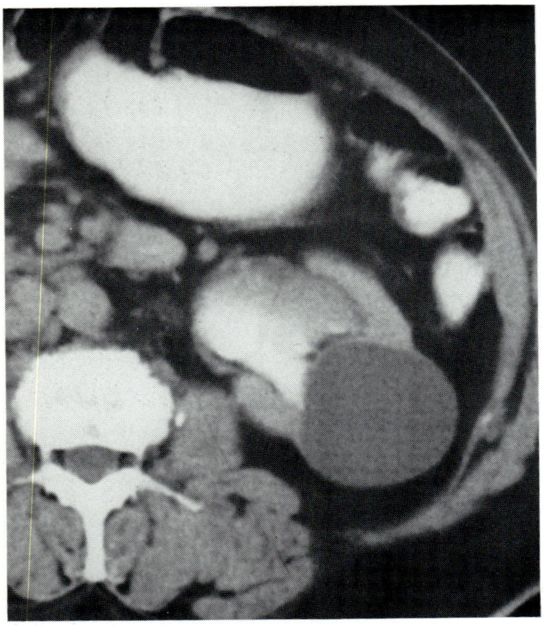

Figure 8-3. Simple renal cyst. CT reveals the cyst to have the density of water and to have a extremely thin wall. The collecting system is hydronephrotic and only partially filled with contrast.

reported with attenuations up to 90 Hounsfield units [16, 71, 75]. Most of these so-called hyperdense cysts have been presumed to be hemorrhagic since aspiration of them frequently yields fluid consistent with remote hemorrhage and since some cysts are found on MRI to have characteristics of hemorrhage. But hyperdense cysts have also been reported as containing pastelike calcified material or proteinaceous [18] but nonhemorrhagic fluid. If they are homogeneous, do not have thick walls or masses associated with them, and do not have thick or amorphous calcification, they can be safely presumed to be cysts. Nevertheless, it is wise to confirm the cystic nature of these lesions with ultrasound since occasional solid tumors may appear dense [13] by virtue of calcification within them and may not enhance very much when intravenous contrast medium is administered. Hyperdense cysts are discussed further in Chap. 10 on indeterminate renal masses.

There are other CT features that are useful to note. A simple renal cyst whose intrinsic wall is very thin may appear to have a thick wall on CT examination if the plane of the tomogram is such that a rim or beak of normal parenchyma is included in the slice and looks like a thick wall. As mentioned previously, the walls of benign cysts may occasionally calcify; if the calcification is thin and linear or curvilinear and does not extend into the central portion of the lesion and if the lesion does not enhance with administration of a contrast agent, it is still very much more likely to be a benign cyst than any other lesion. But if the calcification is associated with focal or diffuse wall thickening, with a solid mass, or with any enhancing tissue, the lesion cannot be assumed to be a cyst [14]. There are no CT features that always permit the distinction of infected from noninfected cysts. Infected cysts tend to have fluid with an attenuation slightly higher than that of water, but this is in no direct way different from dense fluid caused by previous hemorrhage. Also, although there may be other evidence of inflammation in the renal parenchyma adjacent to the cyst or in the fat at its periphery, these signs are not always encountered. Gas produced by gas-forming organisms is probably the only reliable sign, and lesions containing this feature can just as easily be abscesses as infected cysts. In the end, clinical findings, urinalysis, and analysis of aspirated fluid are usually necessary to distinguish infected from noninfected cysts.

On T1 weighted MR images [11, 25, 41] renal cysts usually appear as homogeneous low-intensity regions that are darker than any part of the renal parenchyma (Fig. 8-4). Some hemorrhagic cysts may appear bright on T1 weighted images (Fig. 8-5). T2 weighted images reveal cysts to be homogeneous and of relatively high intensity (Fig. 8-6). MRI is probably less sensitive than CT in demonstrating cysts and to date has not been as definitive as CT in distinguishing simple cysts from cystic neoplasms or other lesions.

The appearance of cysts on scintigraphy depends to a great extent on the size and location of the lesion [17]. A cyst that displaces normal renal cortical or medullary parenchyma will appear as a low-activity region on the normal scintigram [47] no matter what radioactive agent is used. A cyst that is entirely exophytic may displace little or no renal tissue and thus

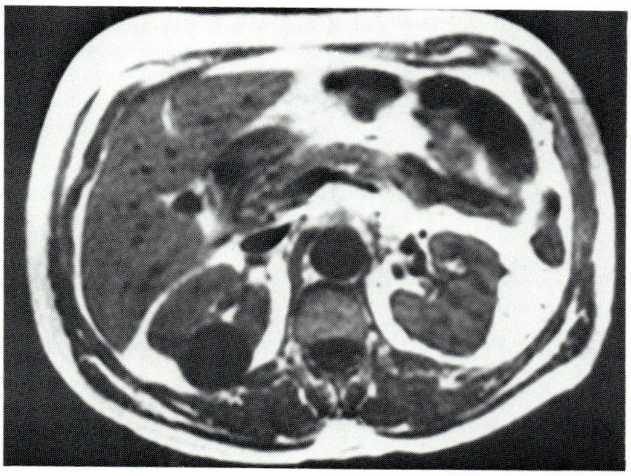

Figure 8-4. Simple renal cyst. T1 weighted MRI shows the cyst in the right kidney to be of low intensity and homogenous. The cortex and the medulla of the kidneys cannot be distinguished, which indicates renal parenchymal disease.

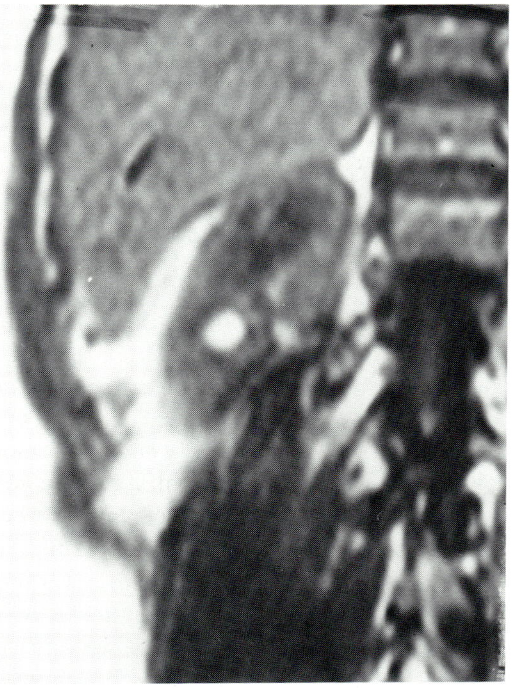

Figure 8-5. Hemorrhagic renal cyst. T1 weighted coronal MRI shows the hemorrhagic cyst to be an intense circular region, due to the paramagnetic properties of blood breakdown products.

produce no abnormalities on scintigraphy. Large peripelvic or parapelvic cysts may compress the collecting system and displace the parenchyma away from the center of the kidney;

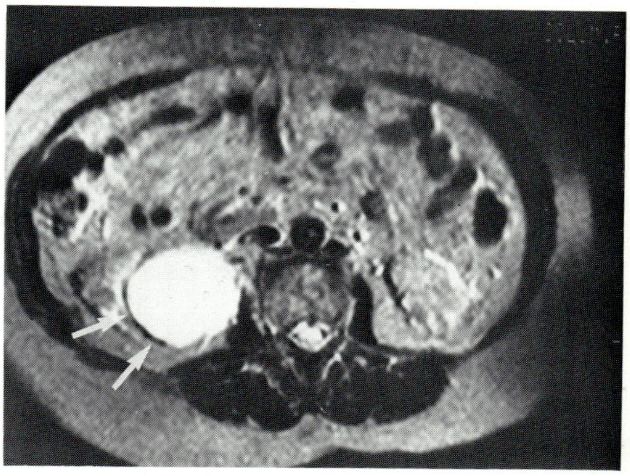

Figure 8-6. Simple renal cyst. T2 weighted MRI shows the cyst in the lower pole of the right kidney as an intense circular region. The dark rim adjacent to its lateral aspect (arrows) is a chemical shift artifact.

the low-activity region thus produced may mimic hydronephrosis in an otherwise normal kidney; appearance of activity in the ureter inferior to the kidney may provide a clue to the correct diagnosis, however.

Prior to the invention of high-quality ultrasonography and CT, angiography formed an essential part of the practice of distinguishing renal cysts from tumors, since most tumors contain neovascularity and cysts are avascular. Currently, arteriography plays almost no part in the distinction between cysts and solid tumors. However, if arteriography is performed on a kidney that contains a cyst, the usual finding is that of a spherical region in the renal parenchyma that contains no vessels whatsoever. The vessels in the surrounding tissue are draped or displaced around the lesion. Exophytic cysts may produce no displacement of the renal parenchymal vessels; occasionally a capsular artery or a vessel running in Gerota's fascia may be displaced by the cyst. If they are small, peripelvic or parapelvic cysts may produce no abnormalities whatsoever on arteriography.

Selective renal arteriography is thought to be less sensitive than high-quality CT or ultrasonography in demonstrating cysts. Occasionally, arteriography may be considered in making the differential diagnosis of lesions whose cause is not clear on CT; these are lesions that appear generally cystic but may have slightly thickened walls or regions of calcification that did raise the possibility of tumor. In some of these cases, the demonstration of tumor neovascularity in a small region of the lesion might suggest neoplasm. Unfortunately, small regions of vessels that look like tumor vessels may also be seen in inflammatory lesions so that a "positive" angiogram does not inevitably indicate neoplasm. Also, since these lesions usually have cystic necrotic carcinomas as part of their differential diagnosis, and since these tumors may be completely avascular, an angiogram that fails to show tumor neovascularity does not permit tumor to be excluded. Generally speaking, angiography has little use in the workup of cystic renal lesions.

Like angiography, in past years cyst puncture played a very important part in distinguishing simple cysts from tumors, but the part has shrunk considerably since the advent of ultrasonography and CT, so that cyst puncture is rarely necessary in current practice.

Demonstrating that a lesion is a simple cyst by cyst puncture requires both analysis of the aspirated fluid and radiography of the lesion after its cavity has been opacified with contrast medium [67]. The fluid in simple cysts is usually light yellow in color, without turbidity. Cytologic analysis of the fluid may reveal exfoliated cuboidal cells but no evidence of malignancy. The fluid is usually sterile. Routine analysis of aspirated fluid should include cytologic examination if the fluid is clear; if it is turbid it should also be cultured for infective organisms and antibiotic sensitivity tests should be performed.

Hemorrhagic cyst fluid poses a diagnostic dilemma [31]. The hemorrhage may have been caused by the needle puncture itself, may have been spontaneous in a benign cyst, or may represent the presence of a neoplasm. Unfortunately, significant amounts of either fresh or old blood in the aspirated fluid make it difficult to exclude neoplasms by cytologic means. It is this unfortunate limitation that has been one of the major reasons for a decline in the usefulness of cyst aspiration. Most cystic nonhemorrhagic lesions can be shown by CT to be simple cysts, whereas the lesions that after CT examination still may contain tumor are usually relatively dense on CT and therefore are usually thought to contain blood. Therefore, if failure to find malignant cells in bloody fluid does not exclude tumor, cyst puncture is often not useful. Examination of aspirated fluid from hemorrhagic lesions may, of course, indicate neoplasm if cytologic analysis shows unquestionable malignant cells, but a cytologically negative bloody aspirate often indicates that the lesion requires surgical resection in any case.

Radiography of the opacified interior of the cyst is an essential part of cyst puncture. After the lesion is punctured sufficient fluid should be removed for analysis, the aspirated fluid is replaced with an equal volume of soluble contrast agent, and the cyst is radiographed in several projections. The hallmark of a simple cyst is the smoothness of the interior wall. The shape of the interior of the cyst may be spherical or polyarcuate, and the interior may be traversed by one or several thin septa. Any nodule or irregularity of the wall should raise the suspicion of tumor; if feasible, the irregular portion of the wall or the nodule may be directly biopsied during the same examination.

AUTOSOMAL DOMINANT POLYCYSTIC KIDNEY DISEASE

Autosomal dominant polycystic kidney disease [66] is an inherited disorder that has been called polycystic renal disease, adult-type polycystic renal disease [32], autosomal dominant polycystic disease, and other names. Although attention is often focused on the renal pathology and on the effects the disease has on renal function, it is probably an inherited disorder with a large number of consequences, of which the renal changes are often the most striking.

The method of inheritance of the disease is straightforward: A child of someone with the disease has a 50 percent chance of having it, and any patient with the disease will always have a parent with it (although the disease may not be clinically evident in either parent, it can virtually always be found if sought). There is no sex predilection. Screening for the disease in the parents or children of patients who have it is entirely a matter of imaging: There are no physical or laboratory findings that can indicate the diagnosis with any certainty. Reports differ regarding which imaging technique is most sensitive in discovering the disease; careful nephrotomography, CT with contrast medium, and ultrasonography have all been advocated. Given its relative accuracy, inexpensiveness, and safety, ultrasonography of the kidneys and upper abdomen should be the screening technique of choice.

PATHOLOGY

The kidney contains innumerable cysts, which may form from any part of the nephron. The cysts are usually lined with a single layer of epithelium, but the epithelium may become hyperplastic and have several layers [27]; occasionally, even papillary growths may be found protruding into the lumina. Although the cysts are innumerable, they appear to form from only a small fraction of the nephrons; ultimate renal failure is presumed to be caused by compression of the remaining intrinsically normal nephrons by the enlarging cysts. The cysts vary in size from microscopic to many centimeters in diameter. The fluid within them may be clear, or it may contain evidence of recent or old hemorrhage. The cyst walls may calcify.

In the early stages of the disease, the affected kidneys may not be enlarged, but as the cysts increase in size, the overall kidney size increases. Once this occurs the outline of the kidney becomes abnormal: Multiple protruding cysts give it a bosselated or irregular appearance. For all practical purposes the disease may be assumed to involve both kidneys. Occasionally, a patient may be encountered early in the progression of the disease when only a few cysts in one kidney have enlarged; in this case the gross findings appear to be unilateral. More careful investigation will usually reveal disease in the other kidney, however. Case reports have appeared claiming that the disease may be truly unilateral, but most of these cases lack conclusive proof that the unilateral condition was not multicystic dysplastic kidney or multiple simple cysts in one kidney or bilateral disease with occult changes in the contralateral kidney.

In this disease, cysts are encountered in other organs as well. Cysts appear in the liver with a reported prevalence ranging from 40 to 90 percent. Pancreatic cysts have been reported in 5 to 10 percent of patients, and cysts have been described as occurring within the spleen, lung, brain, uterus, epididymis, esophagus, and thyroid.

The disease is accompanied by a greater-than-normal prevalence of other conditions as well; these include abnormalities of the mitral valve (specifically, mitral-valve prolapse), the aortic root, the aortic annulus, and the aortic valve [46]. Cerebral arterial aneurysms (Berry aneurysms) may appear in 10 to 36 percent of patients, and there is an increased incidence of colonic diverticulosis.

CLINICAL COURSE

Patients with the disease may have no clinical signs or symptoms and no laboratory evidence of disease. Indeed, many patients who have the condition—perhaps as many as half of them—may reach old age having suffered no consequences from it. But the classic description of the disease is of a group of abnormalities appearing in the third or fourth decade of life. These include flank or abdominal pain, gross or microscopic hematuria, palpable enlarged kidneys, systemic hypertension, and evidence of progressive chronic renal failure. The disease does not cause hepatic dysfunction. Occasionally, these patients may pass ureteral calculi and present with ureteral colic. The disease may present with signs and symptoms of a hemorrhagic stroke due to a ruptured intracerebral aneurysm. Patients with polycystic disease have a higher incidence of upper urinary tract infection than do those with normal kidneys. These infections appear primarily in female patients, are usually found to be due to enteric pathogens (suggesting that retrograde infection is the route), and may be very difficult to treat successfully, especially if the fluid within a cyst becomes infected, rather than just a focal region of renal parenchyma. Ultimately, the chronic renal failure may require dialysis, transplantation, or both, and the patients may suffer any of the complications of systemic hypertension as well.

The disease may be discovered as early as the prepartum period: Prenatal ultrasonography has been reported to show polycystic kidneys in some fetuses. Newborn babies may have enlarged palpable kidneys that on investigation turn out to be autosomal dominant polycystic renal disease. Or the disease may be discovered by imaging in asymptomatic patients at virtually any age [74]. Once the combination of the renal findings and a positive family history is seen, the diagnosis is reasonably certain. As described above, the signs and symptoms classically appear in the third or fourth decade but may show up at virtually any age. The long-term prognosis [12, 20] appears to depend, at least in part, on the severity of the disease when discovered: The patient with markedly enlarged kidneys, renal impairment, and hypertension in early or middle life virtually always faces progression of disease; the patient who in early middle age or later has an unmistakable diagnosis but has no hypertension, renal failure, or gross kidney enlargement may live for decades without clinical progression of the disease.

No direct cure is known. Occasionally attempts have been made to improve renal function by decompressing many of the cysts, but long-lasting or frequent success has not been reported. Appropriate treatment of the hypertension, chronic renal failure, and infection may be instituted as needed.

IMAGING STUDIES

Early in the course of the disease, plain films of the abdomen may reveal no abnormalities. If the kidneys are markedly enlarged, they may be directly visible; on rare occasions, faint calcification in cyst walls may be seen [42]. Stomach, duodenum, small bowel, and ascending and descending colon may be displaced by the enlarged kidneys

If the disease has not progressed, standard urography may reveal no abnormalities. In nonenlarged or slightly enlarged kidneys with multiple very small cysts, careful nephrotomography may be necessary to demonstrate the multiple small lucencies in the parenchyma; when they are demonstrable, there is no particular predilection for the cortex or the medulla. As the disease progresses, the kidneys enlarge and the lucencies of the cyst lumina may produce a mottled or "Swiss-cheese" appearance on the nephrogram. Enlarging cysts may protrude beyond the periphery of the kidney, and may distort the collecting system (Fig. 8-7), whose

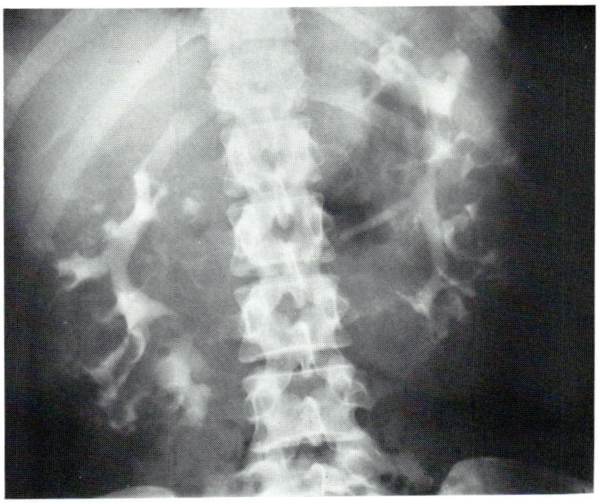

Figure 8-7. Autosomal dominant polycystic kidney disease. Urography reveals the kidneys to be enlarged; the collecting systems are distorted and the nephrogram is heterogeneous.

individual components may be compressed, draped, or even obstructed by the cysts. Hemorrhagic cysts are usually not distinguishable from uncomplicated ones. Occasionally, hepatic cysts may be seen. The collecting system may be normally or only faintly opacified. The overall length of the collecting system may be increased and the pelvis, infundibula, and calices may be stretched, indented, and distorted by the parenchymal cysts.

Ultrasound findings [28, 40, 45, 60] vary depending on the state of the disease. When the cysts are multiple and small, the only abnormality may be a generalized increase in the echogenicity of the renal parenchyma with a loss in the corticomedullary difference. As the cysts become larger they may become individually discernible as echolucent spherical regions (Fig. 8-8) that begin to replace the entirety of the parenchyma; normal parenchyma is often impossible to demonstrate. The renal sinus echoes become lost as the kidneys are distorted.

Ultrasonography may reveal spherical echo-free regions within the liver that represent the hepatic cysts and may demonstrate cysts in the pancreas as well.

Prior to administration of contrast medium, CT [45, 65] may demonstrate calcifications in the walls of some cysts.The density of the fluid in the cysts varies, even without calcification; nonhemorrhagic cysts have values approach-

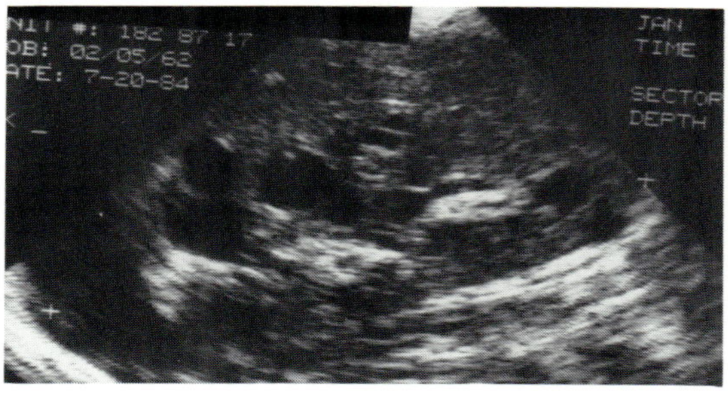

Figure 8-8. Autosomal dominant polycystic kidney disease. Ultrasonography reveals the kidney to be enlarged and to contain multiple anechoic cystic regions.

ing that of water, whereas hemorrhagic cysts increase in density [48, 52] and may display densities approaching 100 Hounsfield units (Fig. 8-9). Early in the disease, administration of a contrast agent reveals a mottled nephrogram in which innumerable small lucent regions are scattered throughout the cortex and medulla [60]. As the cysts enlarge, they distort the parenchyma more markedly, so that the remaining opacifying regions of renal cortex and medulla are completely riddled with lucencies (Fig. 8-10) and look like the cut surface of a sponge. Usually, sufficient function persists so that the calices may be opacified. As with ultrasonography, hepatic or pancreatic cysts, or both, may be demonstrated.

There is relatively little experience reported with regard to the radionuclide imaging of patients with this disease. If either a tubule-binding agent or an excreted agent is used, when

Figure 8-9. Autosomal dominant polycystic kidney disease. CT without an intravenous contrast agent shows the kidneys to be enlarged and virtually replaced by multiple cysts of various sizes and densities.

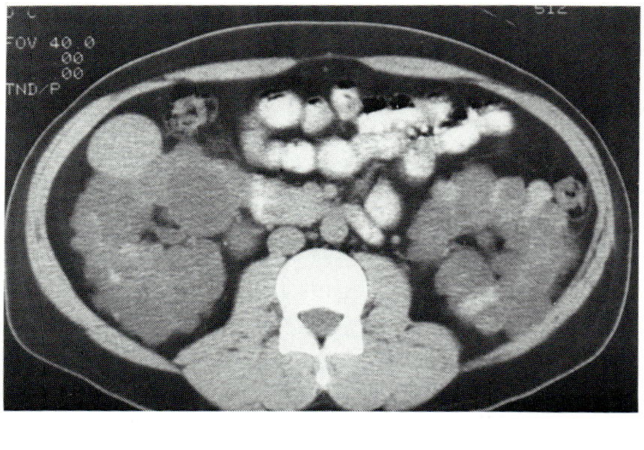

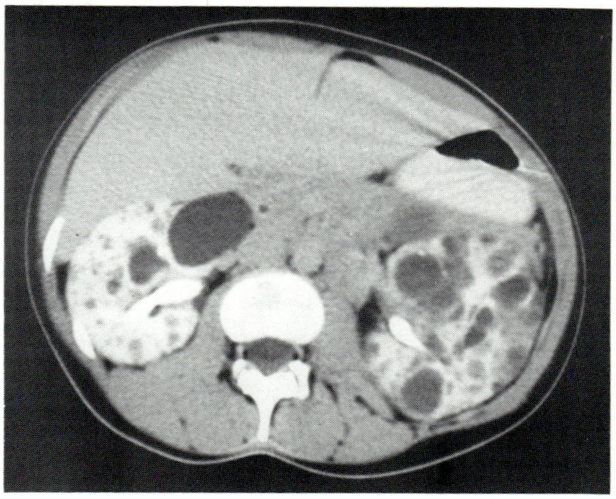

Figure 8-10. Autosomal dominant polycystic kidney disease. In this CT intravenous contrast medium has enhanced the renal parenchyma, which is riddled by innumerable cysts of various sizes.

the disease is advanced the kidneys are seen to be enlarged and the activity of the parenchyma is lessened and becomes inhomogeneous. If excreted agents are used the collecting system may appear to be elongated and distorted. Gallium scans reveal focal areas of increased activity in about half of all patients with adult polycystic disease and focal renal infection.

The morphology of the kidneys as demonstrated by MRI is similar to that revealed by CT. On T1 weighted images uncomplicated cysts are of low intensity and appear homogeneous. Hemorrhagic cysts may demonstrate higher signal levels from their fluid. In T2 weighted images, the cyst fluid is usually bright; as with T1 weighted images, hemorrhage within the fluid may cause some cysts to appear to be of different intensity from nonhemorrhagic cysts. Occasionally, particulate debris in hemorrhagic cysts may appear to be relatively low signal intensity on both T1 and T2 weighted images.

DIFFERENTIAL DIAGNOSIS

Multiple simple cysts may mimic the changes of autosomal dominant polycystic disease with most imaging techniques. With CT and nephrotomography, the distinction may be made by noting that with multiple simple cysts discrete regions of normal parenchyma can usually be found, whereas with polycystic disease innumerable smaller cysts fill the spaces between the large ones.

Occasionally, bilateral severe hydronephrosis may be initially confused with adult-type polycystic disease on ultrasonography. But the distinction can be made with considerable accuracy by noting that in polycystic disease the cysts are usually more numerous and vary more in size than do the dilated calices of hydronephrosis; also, with hydronephrosis the entire collecting system can often be demonstrated by ultrasonography to be continuous.

Occasionally, other conditions that produce multiple masslike lesions in the renal parenchyma may mimic polycystic disease on retrograde pyelography, intravenous urography, and occasionally even on nephrotomography. These might include tuberous sclerosis, in which multiple angiomyolipomas appear, and von Hippel–Lindau disease, in which multiple renal carcinomas appear; indeed, in both of these syndromes, multiple cysts may complicate the picture. Multifocal bilateral renal lymphoma or multiple metastases to the kidney from a primary carcinoma may occasionally produce caliceal abnormalities that mimic those seen in polycystic disease; careful ultrasonography or CT usually resolves the issue, however.

AUTOSOMAL RECESSIVE POLYCYSTIC KIDNEY DISEASE

Autosomal recessive polycystic kidney disease has been described by a number of phrases, including infantile polycystic disease, infantile sponge kidney, autosomal recessive polycystic disease, and many variants. It is really a condition with primary abnormalities in the liver as well as the kidney.

This is an unusual hereditary and congenital condition whose mode of transmission is autosomal recessive. The parents of children with the disease virtually never have manifestations of it, since it is exceedingly rare for anyone who is homozygous for the disease to reach reproductive age. The mode of inheritance ensures, however, that siblings of patients with the disease have a high chance of having it as well.

The considerable clinical variability of the disease has led to numerous attempts at classification of groups of patients. There is a wide range of ages of onset of certain symptoms, of ultimate severity of certain aspects of the disease, and of degrees to which renal or hepatic abnormalities will predominate. The disease has been classified into four groups: perinatal, neonatal, infantile, and juvenile. These groups contain patients whose ages at onset of serious symptoms increase in the same order. In general, the older the patient at the time of onset of serious disease, the more likely the hepatic, rather than the renal, components of the disease will predominate. In fact, a condition known as congenital hepatic fibrosis, which is often accompanied by mild urographic and pathologic abnormalities in the kidneys that are rarely of clinical significance, may represent the end of this clinical spectrum rather than a separate disease [69].

PATHOLOGY

The major renal abnormality is dilatation and hyperplasia of the collecting tubules of the kidney. These dilated tubules usually have lumina that are considerably smaller than the cysts seen in advanced adult-type polycystic disease; they often reach a maximum of only a few millimeters in diameter. The glomeruli and proximal tubules are usually normal; despite this, however, the dilated collecting tubules usually cause the kidneys to be enlarged. The enlargement may be marked, especially in infants, and is usually bilaterally symmetrical. If the patient survives a number of years, the radially oriented dilated collecting tubules may generate spherical cystic dilatations similar to the cysts seen in adult-type polycystic disease.

The severity of the renal changes, and the rate of their progression, is tremendously variable. At one extreme, it is probably true that only minimal dilatation of the collecting tubules may appear and may produce no significant functional abnormality. At the other extreme, virtually all of the collecting tubules may be severely dilated, the kidneys may be markedly enlarged, and renal function may be severely compromised. Although direct data about the natural history of the pathology in the kidney is limited (since successive renal biopsies are usually not performed), serial imaging studies and renal-function studies suggest that the course is variable; in some patients the changes in the collecting tubules may progress and in others may remain quite stable.

In the liver the primary pathology consists of

periportal fibrosis with hyperplasia and dilatation of the intrahepatic bile ducts. This is rarely severe at birth but is progressive throughout the life of any patient who has the disease. The changes do not produce hepatic failure but cause progressively severe portal venous hypertension; passive congestion of the spleen with progressive splenomegaly and evidence of variceal dilatation of all portosystemic anastomoses appear.

CLINICAL COURSE

The course of autosomal recessive polycystic kidney disease is very variable. It may be diagnosed in utero by ultrasonography [29]. The renal manifestations are most severe when it appears at birth or shortly thereafter. Markedly enlarged kidneys may be palpated at birth, with renal function abnormalities consisting of varying degrees of oliguria and failure of urinary concentration and acidification. There may be maternal oligohydramnios, and the infants may have pulmonary hypoplasia, pneumothoraces, or both. Death may be rapid because of either renal or respiratory failure. Evidence of hepatobiliary disease is rarely, if ever, apparent immediately after birth.

If the patient survives the immediate postpartum period the course of the renal disease may still be very variable [2]. Glomerular filtration rate may improve, remain unchanged, or slowly worsen, so that patients may experience anything from moderately rapid progression of renal failure to maintenance of good renal function that lasts for many years. Inevitably, however, the hepatic fibrosis and portal hypertension progress. The patients therefore may have no significant renal or direct hepatic dysfunction, but with progressive portal hypertension, the splenomegaly worsens and ultimately the varices bleed. Death from variceal hemorrhage is a common outcome and may occur anywhere from midchildhood years to early adulthood. When hepatic fibrosis and portal hypertension become apparent relatively late and there is no evidence of significant renal dysfunction, the disease is usually called congenital hepatic fibrosis rather than polycystic renal disease; it is possible—but not universally agreed—that the basic genetics and biochemistry of the patients are the same and only the variation and the severity of the renal abnormality determines whether the patients will live long enough for the hepatic disease to become manifest.

IMAGING STUDIES

In infants plain films show bilateral symmetrical flank masses, which represent the enlarged kidneys. These may be directly visible or may appear by virtue of displaced bowel gas. Later in life splenomegaly may become apparent on abdomen films and esophageal varices may be demonstrable on barium esophagography.

On urography the kidneys display varying degrees of enlargement and reveal an abnormal nephrogram (Fig. 8-11). If the renal disease is apparent early in life and renal dysfunction is severe, a homogeneous normal nephrogram never appears but is replaced by an inhomogeneous nephrogram consisting of radial striations ("sunburst" pattern) and whose most intense

Figure 8-11. Autosomal recessive (infantile) polycystic kidney disease. Urography reveals the kidneys to be markedly enlarged and to display a dense and inhomogeneous nephrogram ("sunburst" pattern).

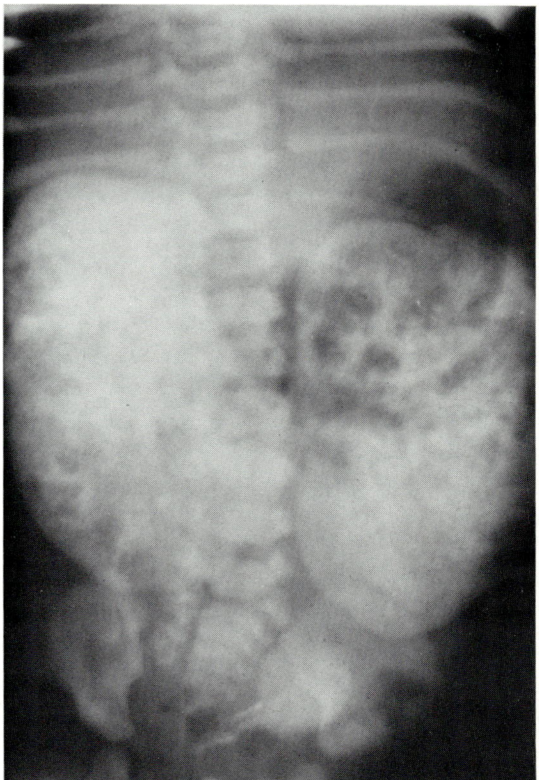

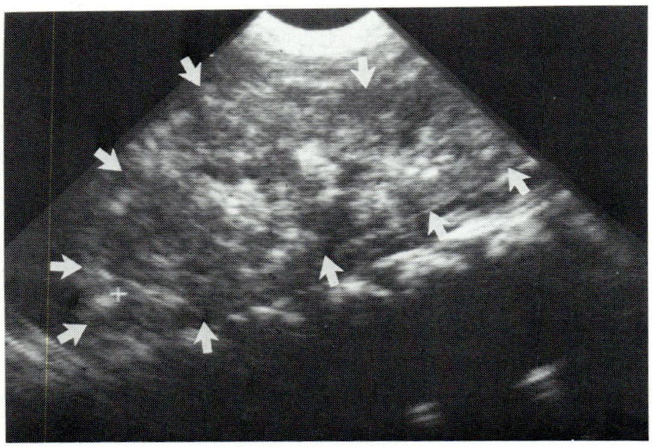

Figure 8-12. Autosomal recessive (infantile) polycystic kidney disease. The kidney (arrows) is enlarged. The echoes within it are disorganized; no clear corticomedullary differentiation can be seen.

period is delayed. Although small circular lucencies representing individual cysts may be seen, these are not a prominent feature of the disease, especially early on. The collecting system may be only very faintly opacified, even if opacified urine appears in the bladder. The nephrogram is often prolonged up to 24 hours or longer. CT findings parallel those seen at intravenous urography.

On ultrasonography [7, 28, 51] the kidneys appear enlarged (Fig. 8-12). The usual corticomedullary distinction is often lost, and the increased volume of renal parenchyma often obliterates the renal sinus echoes. The renal parenchyma appears abnormally echogenic, but the kidney does not appear to diminish the through-transmission of sound, so that structures deep to the kidney remain visible. The margin of the kidney may be amorphous. In some patients, the cortical mantle may appear less echogenic than the medullary pyramids.

The liver may or may nor appear abnormal; there may be a generalized diffuse increase in echogenicity. Splenomegaly and varices may be demonstrable.

ACQUIRED CYSTIC DISEASE OF THE KIDNEY

Acquired cystic disease of the kidney has also been known as acquired polycystic renal disease, uremic cystic renal disease [36], and cystic renal transformation in dialyzed patients. It has been subjected to considerable attention only since the advent of dialysis, but, in fact, it has been recognized for decades. It has been known since the past century that patients who have had chronic renal failure of certain types develop cysts in their kidneys. Many more patients have come to attention now that large numbers of them have been on dialysis for a number of years. It has even been suggested that the dialysis itself was responsible in some way for the cysts. What is more likely, however, is that the disease has an increasing incidence because dialysis results in increased duration of chronic renal failure.

Patients with chronic renal failure usually have marked diminution in renal parenchymal volume (except, of course, in conditions such as adult polycystic renal disease); they may have multiple small cysts prior to the onset of dialysis. When either peritoneal dialysis or hemodialysis begins, a diminution in renal size may be seen, and some of the cysts may decrease in size as well. As dialysis continues for a year or more, the kidneys again begin to increase in size as a result of the formation of innumerable small cysts. These cysts range in size from microscopic to 1 to 2 cm in diameter. The number and size of cysts and the size of the kidneys may continue to increase with increasing time on dialysis. If the dialysis continues for years, as many as 95 percent of patients will acquire the condition.

Successful renal transplantation seems, at least in part, to reduce the process of cyst formation [37, 72]. The size of the native kidneys may diminish again, and the number and size of detectable cysts may also decrease.

Acquired cystic disease seems to have a slight male predilection but no particular age range; it may appear whenever chronic renal failure is present and treated with long-term dialysis.

A common and unfortunate concomitant feature of acquired renal cystic disease is the development of renal neoplasms [22, 35]. These may be adenomas, carcinomas, or oncocytomas. The incidence of renal tumors rises with duration of dialysis; after many years of dialysis, tumors have been found in as many as 45 percent of patients.

PATHOLOGY

The cysts encountered in this disease are small and are often lined with a single layer of cuboidal epithelium. Frequently, however, the walls are thick and represent multiple layers of epithelium; the epithelium may even form papillary fronds that project into the interior of the cysts. The appearance of the cyst fluid is quite variable: It may be clear, yellow, or contain evidence of recent or old hemorrhage. Occasionally, a cyst may become infected and reveal inflammatory changes in the wall. Sometimes faint calcification may appear in the walls of the cysts; whether this has to do with the cyst wall itself or is due to secondary hyperparathyroidism caused by the initial renal disease is not clear.

CLINICAL COURSE

Most often acquired cystic disease is asymptomatic but the cysts may bleed. Sometimes the bleeding is silent and appears only within the cyst cavity, sometimes it causes what appears to be "spontaneous" retroperitoneal hemorrhage, and sometimes it may produce hematuria. Cases have been reported of abscesses forming from infected cysts; some patients have even passed stones. Tumors, when present, are usually silent when small, but if they metastasize, appropriate symptoms may appear.

IMAGING STUDIES

Since the patients virtually never have sufficient renal function to allow performance of intravenous urography, the findings of this disease on urography have not been described. At the time of writing, MRI and nuclear imaging findings have also not been described in any significant series.

Shrunken kidneys in patients with chronic renal failure are usually quite echogenic on ultrasonography, and they do not display a clear corticomedullary distinction. During the phase of the disease in which the cysts are very small, they are not individually recognized on ultrasound images and probably simply increase the degree of echogenicity of the entire parenchyma. As the cysts increase in size, the kidneys may increase in size on ultrasonography (Fig. 8-13), and the cysts may become individually apparent

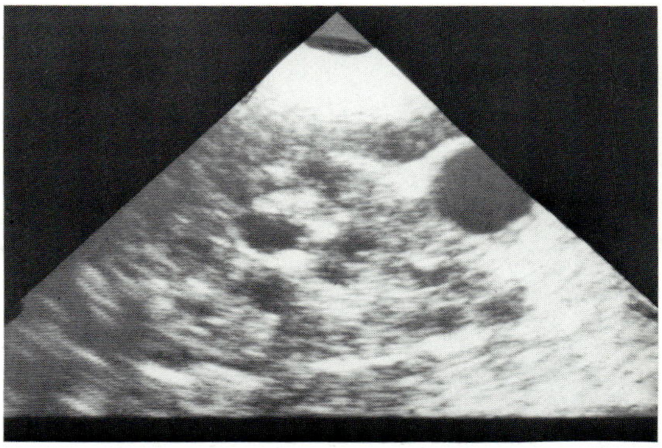

Figure 8-13. Acquired cystic disease. This patient had been on dialysis for many years; ultrasonography reveals the kidney to be echogenic and to contain multiple cysts.

as small spherical regions with few or no echoes. The faint calcification of the remaining renal parenchyma and of some of the cyst walls contributes to the overall echogenicity. Bleeding into some of the cysts may produce small echoes within the cyst lumina. This disease produces such alterations in echogenicity and kidney configuration that small neoplasms within the kidney may easily be missed; a growing renal carcinoma may be recognized if it reaches sufficient size.

CT examination [38, 49] shows that prior to the onset of dialysis the affected kidneys are usually uniformly shrunken. Small cysts may be visible. These may represent either uremic cystic disease or simple cysts that formed when the kidneys were healthier. As the patient spends a longer time on dialysis, the renal parenchyma increases in thickness and overall volume. At first individual cysts may not be visible; instead, only a fine mottling of the renal parenchyma may be visible. If the individual cysts become larger, lucencies appear within the parenchyma that are visible even without contrast enhancement (Fig. 8-14). Although there is some tendency for these cysts to appear at the interface between the cortex and the medulla, they often appear anywhere within the renal parenchyma and may involve the parenchyma more or less uniformly. The cysts tend to protrude neither from the renal surface nor into the renal sinus. The lumina of some cysts may be denser than others, presumably because of hemorrhage, and

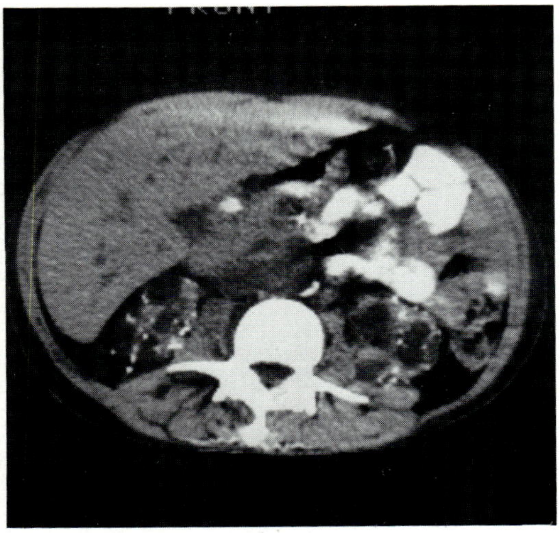

Figure 8-14. Acquired cystic disease. This is a long-term dialysis patient. CT without intravenous contrast reveals the kidneys to be of approximately normal size but to be distorted by multiple cysts. There are calcifications scattered throughout the kidneys as well.

faint calcification may be seen in the walls of the cysts or in the interstitium between them. Infection of the cysts may produce no signs whatsoever; only if an abscess with clear-cut gas bubbles appears may the diagnosis be made. Small tumors may be hard to detect; as in ultrasound images, CT may reveal parenchyma that is so distorted by the multiple cysts that the appearance of a small solid lesion may not be distinguishable from a hemorrhagic cyst. Only when the tumor reaches several centimeters in size may it be recognized. As with ultrasonography, the CT findings tend to regress is the patient receives a successful renal transplant.

MEDULLARY SPONGE KIDNEY

Medullary sponge kidney is an uncommon but by no means rare lesion characterized by focal cystic dilatations of the collecting ducts and sometimes by formation of small calculi within these dilated ducts. When the condition is mild and not associated with calcification, it is sometimes known as benign tubular estasia.

PATHOLOGY

The affected kidney or kidneys are usually of normal size. The abnormalities are more commonly bilateral but may be unilateral. They may affect all of the medullary pyramids of the kidneys or only a few. The changes may even be limited to one papilla. The primary abnormality is that of tubular or cystic focal dilatations of the collecting ducts in the medulla and papillae, although occasionally portions of the loops of Henle may be dilated as well. Small calcified concretions may form within the dilated regions; these calcifications are within the lumina of the ducts and are not calcification of the renal tissue itself.

CLINICAL COURSE

Medullary sponge kidney is usually seen in relatively young adults but may be encountered later in life or in childhood [56]. No significant numbers of cases have been reported in early childhood, and the condition is not known to be progressive. Most frequently, the disease is clinically silent and produces no measurable alteration in renal function. However, patients who have small stones within the dilated ducts may pass the stones into the lumina of the calices [61]; the stones may subsequently pass down the ureter and present with ureteral colic. Hence, pain and hematuria may be the presenting symptoms, and infection has been noted in a small fraction of the patients as well. The stones are not thought to form as a result of a metabolic abnormality but because of stasis of urine. The course is variable; the patients may be asymptomatic when the condition is discovered and may stay asymptomatic for many years. Alternatively, repeated bouts of ureteral colic may appear; long-term obstructive atrophy of the kidneys is rare. Cases have been described in which medullary sponge kidney is associated with hemihypertrophy of the body [30].

IMAGING STUDIES

On abdominal plain films small clusters of round or linear calcifications may be seen in the regions of the medullary pyramids. The numbers of calcifications are variable and may range from many dozen down to a single one or to none. Cortical nephrocalcinosis is not seen.

On urography the hallmark of the disease is a medullary nephrographic abnormality that represents filling of the dilated tubules with contrast (Fig. 8-15). The tubules may appear as fine

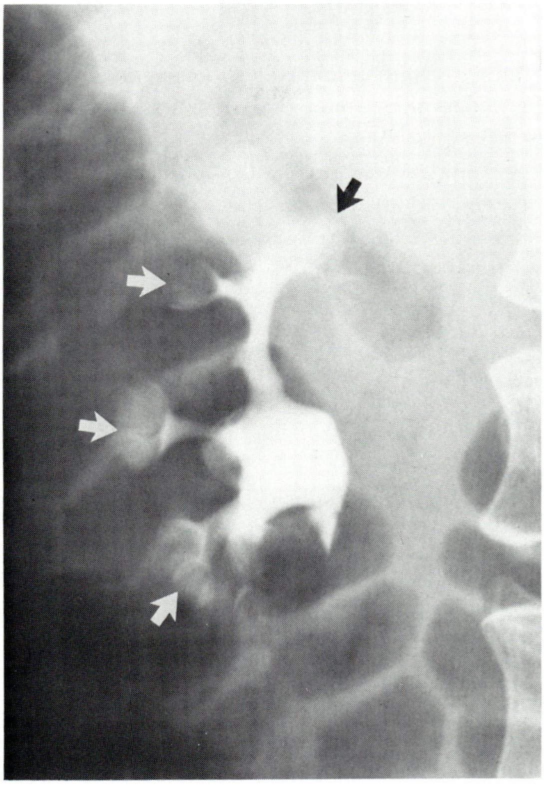

Figure 8-15. Benign tubular ectasia. Urography reveals a striated dense nephrogram (arrows) in the regions of the papillae. Medullary sponge kidney would appear similar except that the striations would be thicker and there might be medullary calcifications.

brushlike parallel striations in the papillae; alternatively, they may appear as considerably coarser striations, and may display focal cystic dilatation in which calcifications are present; the contrast medium appearing within the cystic dilatations obscures the calcifications. The cystic dilatations of the tubules are probably just below the level of resolution of CT, so that the nephrographic patterns are usually not recognizable at CT.

Care must be taken not to confuse a uniform nonstriated papillary blush with medullary sponge kidney; the former finding consists of a homogeneous papillary nephrogram that is denser than that seen in the outer medulla or cortex; it is a normal finding both on urography and contrast-enhanced CT. Differential diagnosis between medullary sponge kidney and infantile polycystic disease is usually not difficult. Although both may reveal parallel striations in the nephrogram of the medullary portions of the kidney, kidneys afflicted with infantile polycystic disease do not display medullary nephrocalcinosis. Also, in infantile polycystic kidney disease the kidneys are often enlarged, the striations often reach to the periphery of the kidney, and the patients in whom the disease is encountered are almost always much younger than the typical patient with medullary sponge kidney. Also, patients with infantile polycystic kidney disease almost always have ultrasound abnormalities in the kidney and eventually develop evidence of hepatic fibrosis and portal hypertension.

Differential diagnosis between medullary calcification caused by medullary sponge kidney and medullary nephrocalcinosis caused by any other condition is made by observing the dilated tubules or small contrast-filled cystic regions in medullary sponge kidney; these findings are not encountered with any other cause of medullary nephrocalcinosis.

Ultrasonography may reveal the medullary calcifications as very small hyperechoic foci that may or may not cast acoustic shadows; no ultrasound demonstration of the tubular dilatation has been described, and distinction between medullary sponge kidney calcifications and medullary nephrocalcinosis from other causes is usually impossible by ultrasonography.

JUVENILE NEPHRONOPHTHISIS/MEDULLARY CYSTIC DISEASE

Controversy exists over whether these are two distinct diseases or different manifestations of the same disease [23]. Both autosomal dominant and autosomal recessive modes of inheritance have been described [3]. The disease presents as polyuria, polydipsia, salt wasting, anemia, and renal failure clinically; the pathologic correlates are diminution in overall renal size with evidence of interstitial nephritis and medullary cysts. Cases of the disease have been described as appearing both in childhood and in early adulthood.

There is no extensive literature regarding the imaging findings. Since the kidneys are small, urography [9, 50], ultrasonography, and CT will reveal generalized diminution in corticomedullary volume; corticomedullary distinction on ultrasonography is usually not visible. When present, the medullary cysts are macroscopic but not very large; they are approximately 1 to 2 cm in diameter. They are not always visualized by urography but frequently may be demonstrated by ultrasonography [21]. CT, nuclear medicine, and MRI findings in these diseases have not been described.

MULTICYSTIC DYSPLASTIC KIDNEY

Multicystic dysplastic kidney is one name for a relatively uncommon condition that has also been known as cystic dysplastic kidney, unilateral polycystic kidney, cystic hypoplastic kidney, and a host of other names [15, 24, 43]. It is a congenital, but not hereditary, nonneoplastic lesion, which is usually unilateral but occasionally bilateral. The affected kidney does not function and is entirely replaced by cystic structures and primitive tissues that have given rise to its name.

PATHOLOGY

Grossly, the kidney is seen to consist of a collection of cysts of various sizes, ranging from less than a millimeter to several centimeters in diameter. There is neither normal parenchyma nor a normal renal pelvis or collecting system. The artery supplying it is usually extremely small. There is some degree of atresia of the ureter, ranging from stenosis and atresia of the most proximal portion through varieties of segmental atresia to complete absence of the ureter. The contralateral kidney is usually normal, but 10 to 30 percent of cases may display some sort of congenital anomaly; this is most frequently a ureteropelvic junction obstruction but may also be malrotation, horseshoe kidney, or even contralateral multicystic dysplastic kidney. The affected kidney, especially in infancy, may be considerably larger than the normal one but may diminish in size [57, 73]—or at least fail to grow—with normal development, so that in adulthood it usually is considerably smaller than the normal contralateral kidney.

Microscopically, the cysts are seen to consist of a layer of cuboidal epithelium. They usually contain clear fluid. In some cases, the lumina of the cysts do not communicate; in others, some or all of the cysts may communicate via primitive tubular structures (although not by virtue of being connected through a common clearly identifiable collecting system); this variant is known as the hydronephrotic type of multicystic dysplastic kidney. The central fibrous stroma may be abundant and contains nerves, blood vessels, and occasionally cartilage. There may be primitive tubular structures and primitive glomeruli, but no normal tubules or glomeruli are seen. Occasionally, the walls of the cysts may calcify; this calcification is usually seen in older patients

Rarely, the lesion may involve only part of an otherwise normal kidney.

CAUSE

The cause is not known with certainty, but probably consists of a failure of maturation of the ureteral bud. The ureteral bud forms part of the trigone, the entire ureter, the pelvis, infundibula and calices and also portions of the distal tubules. Normally, the ureteral bud grows cephalad to meet the metanephric blastema, which forms the glomeruli and proximal tubules. If the ureteral bud fails during embryogenesis to meet the metanephric blastema, when the more proximal tubules and glomeruli begin to develop and excrete fluid the individual obstruction of each proximal tubule might lead to the cystic transformation that ultimately produces a multicystic kidney.

CLINICAL COURSE

This lesion may be discovered at any time from fetal life [54] through late adulthood. In the fetus [19] ultrasonography has been the technique that demonstrates the lesion. It may be encountered as an isolated finding in an otherwise normal examination, or ultrasonography may reveal the oligohydramnios and bilateral renal dysplasia that constitute parts of Potter's syndrome. In early infancy the condition, if unilateral, may be encountered as a palpable flank or abdominal mass. It is one of the most common causes of palpable masses in the newborn; depending on the series reported, it may or may not be exceeded in frequency by the discovery of severe hydronephrosis secondary to congenital ureteropelvic junction obstruction. In the unusual cases in which the disease is bilateral, it is also accompanied by the typical Potter's facies, anuria, and fairly rapid demise. In adulthood [1] it is usually encountered as an incidental finding in some imaging study that visualizes the kidneys; these include urography, CT, ultrasonography, nuclear scintigraphy, and MRI. Although it is usually asymptomic in adults, it may be associated with pain, persistent infection, or hematuria. Other congenital abnormalities may be associated with the condition.

PROGNOSIS

When multicystic dysplastic kidney is bilateral, the prognosis is virtually certain death from uremia in the first few days after birth. When it is unilateral, the patient has an extremely good prognosis: Complications are unusual, and there is no definite increased incidence of malignant degeneration. Prognosis may be worsened by the presence of a lesion in the contralateral kidney that compromises its function.

In the past the lesion was often subjected to nephrectomy [6], although the rationale for this therapy had less to do with the avoidance of complications from the lesion than with the inability of imaging studies to exclude other lesions that would require resection. However, there has been a swing to conservative therapy in patients in whom the diagnosis can be established with certainty.

IMAGING STUDIES

In infants, a plain film of the abdomen may reveal indirect evidence of a unilateral flank or abdominal mass: Bowel and solid viscera may be displaced away from a unilateral soft-tissue density. In adults no specific mass may be visible, but on the affected side there is no normal renal outline. Occasionally, curvilinear calcification is seen in the walls of the cysts.

Intravenous urography reveals no evidence of excretion of opacified urine on the affected side. If a high dose of contrast agent is injected and careful tomography is done, thin rims of a faintly opacified tissue may be seen to represent the cyst walls. Retrograde pyelography may reveal varying degrees of atresia of the ureter: There may be complete stenosis of the most proximal ureter, several areas of more proximal partial ureteral stenoses, or a complete absence of the ureter. The cystoscopist may notice that the ipsilateral trigone is not present. In no case is a normal intrarenal collecting system seen.

Differential dignosis includes the "autonephrectomy" stage of tuberculosis, obstructive hydronephrosis without contrast excretion, and a multilocular cystic nephroma.

On ultrasonography [5, 28, 63] the lesion is represented as a collection of anechoic regions of various sizes (Fig. 8-16) [5]. No normal parenchyma is seen, nor is there evidence of renal sinus echoes. The walls of the anechoic regions may contain foci of calcification. Differentiation from severe hydronephrosis may be difficult, but certain signs may be useful [58, 62]. If the largest fluid-filled structure is central (that is, in the region of the renal pelvis) or if clear-cut communicating dilated infundibula can be shown to connect peripheral fluid-filled regions with a large central one, if a dilated ureter can be demonstrated, if the echogenic fat within the renal sinus can be seen around a dilated pelvis, or if renal parenchyma is seen, hydronephrosis is more likely to be present than is multicystic dysplastic kidney.

Radionuclide images show no evidence of parenchymal uptake or caliceal excretion of isotope. Failure of isotope to reach the affected

Figure 8-16. Multicystic dysplastic kidney. Ultrasonography shows multiple echolucent cysts in the renal bed without identifiable renal parenchyma.

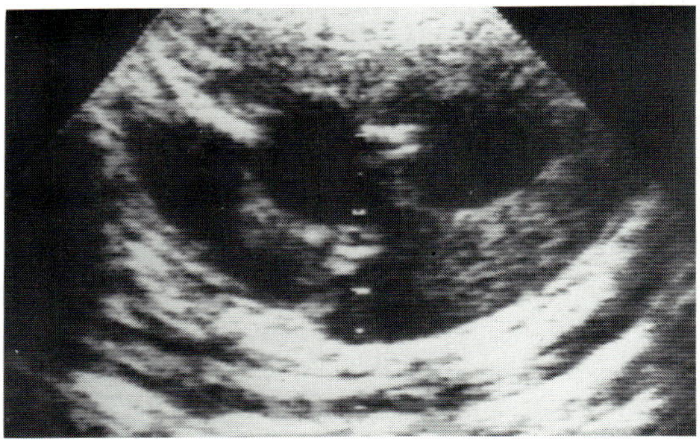

kidney maybe complete, so that a striking "cold spot" may be noted in the flank containing the affected kidney.

On CT the cysts of multicystic dysplastic kidney are displayed as circular regions with CT numbers equal to or slightly higher than that of water. The walls of the cysts and septa appear relatively thin (although they may be focally thickened) and may enhance slightly with the administration of contrast medium. If calcification is present it is seen in the cyst walls and appears curvilinear and relatively thin. Although the walls and fibrous stroma may enhance slightly with contrast agent, no excretion into the cyst cavities is seen in the majority of cases. But in the "hydronephrotic" variety of multicystic dysplastic kidney there may be a very faint increase in the density of the cysts.

In most cases needle puncture [64] of the cysts permits aspiration of clear yellow fluid. Injection of contrast usually reveals that the opacified cyst does not connect with other cysts. In a minority of cases, however, several cysts are seen to be continuous when contrast medium is injected; the connections between the two do not resemble a renal pelvis, however, and are either not clearly visualized or may appear as small tubular structures. If a dilated collecting system opacifies, of course, severe hydronephrosis rather than multicystic dysplastic kidney should be diagnosed. The interior of the cyst walls appears smooth.

Abdominal aortography may reveal no visible renal artery at all, or there may be a very small threadlike renal vessel. Branches of the vessel within the lesion are not seen, and there is no nephrogram.

PYELOCALICEAL DIVERTICULUM

While this entity is not a true cyst, it is probably more closely related to renal cystic disease, at least in structure, than it is to other renal pathology. Also known by names such as pyelogenic cyst and caliceal diverticulum, the term pyelocaliceal diverticulum is probably more appropriate, since these diverticula can arise anywhere from the renal pelvis to the fornix of a minor calix. They can range in size from a few millimeters to several centimeters in diameter, though their necks are always quite narrow. Clinically, these diverticula are usually asymptomatic, though occasionally they may be the source of urinary infection. They are rarely a cause of ureteral colic because of the inability of any contained stones to pass through the narrow neck. There are several theories regarding their origin, ranging from rupture of a cyst into the collecting system to developmental anomalies of the branching ureteral bud.

Radiographically, pyelocaliceal diverticula are seen on plain films only when they contain calculi. These calculi may be single or a collection of tiny stones; stones can be found in up to 50 percent of cases. On urography, the diverticula are usually visualized on later films as they fill in retrograde fashion from the opacified normal collecting system. On rare occasions, stone-containing diverticula may not fill with contrast medium during urography because of obstruction of their neck. In such cases, a stone or cluster of small stones found outside the collecting system should lead to the suspicion of an obstructed diverticulum. While pyelocaliceal diverticula are often peripherally located outside the normal topography of the calices, they may overlie the normal intrarenal collecting system when they extend anteriorly or posteriorly. They are usually single, but several diverticula may occur in the same kidney or they may be found bilaterally. Their configuration is usually round or ovoid. The narrow neck may or may not be seen to be filled with contrast medium. When sufficiently large, on sonography or CT they may be confused with an isolated hydrocalix. A stone-containing pyelocaliceal diverticulum is illustrated in Fig. 15–3.

REFERENCES

1. Ambrose, S.S., et al. Unilateral multicystic renal disease in adults. *J. Urol.* 128:366, 1982.
2. Anand, S.K., Chan, J.C., and Lieberman, E. Polycystic disease and hepatic fibrosis in children. *Am. J. Dis. Child.* 129:810, 1975.
3. Avasthi, P.S., Erickson, D.G., and Gardner, K.D. Hereditary renal-retinal dysplasia and the medullary cystic disease nephronophthisis complex. *Ann. Intern. Med.* 84:157, 1976.
4. Banner, M.P., et al. Multilocular renal cysts: Radiologic-pathologic correlation. *A.J.R.* 136: 239, 1981.

5. Bearman, S.B., Hine, P.L., and Sanders, R.C. Multicystic kidney: A sonographic pattern. *Radiology* 118:685, 1976.
6. Bloom, D.A., and Brosman, S. The multicystic kidney. *J. Urol.* 120:211, 1978.
7. Boal, D.K., and Teele, R.L. Sonography of infantile polycystic kidney disease. *A.J.R.* 135:575, 1980.
8. Bosniak, M.A. The current radiological approach to renal cysts. *Radiology* 158:1, 1986.
9. Burgener, F.A., and Spataro, R.F. Early medullary cystic disease: A urographic diagnosis? *Radiology* 130:321, 1979.
10. Cho, K.J., et al. Angiographic and ultrasonic findings in infected simple cysts of the kidney. *A.J.R.* 127:1015, 1975.
11. Choyke, P.L., et al. Focal renal masses: Magnetic resonance imaging. *Radiology* 152:471, 1984.
12. Churchill, D.N., et al. Progonsis of adult onset polycystic kidney disease re-evaluated. *Kidney Int.* 26:190, 1984.
13. Coleman, B.G., et al. Hyperdense renal masses: A computed tomographic dilemma. *A.J.R.* 143:291, 1984.
14. Curry, N.S., et al. An evaluation of the effectiveness of CT vs. other imaging modalities in the diagnosis of atypical renal masses. *Invest. Radiol.* 19:447, 1984.
15. De Klerk, D.P., Marshall, F.F., and Jeffs, R.D. Multicystic dysplastic kidney. *J. Urol.* 118:306, 1977.
16. Dunnick, N.R., et al Computed tomography of high density renal cysts. *J. Comput. Assist. Tomogr.* 8:458, 1984.
17. Elkin, M., and Bernstein J. Cystic diseases of the kidney: Radiological and pathological considerations. *Radiology* 20:65, 1969.
18. Fishman, M.C., et al. High protein content: Another cause of CT hyperdense benign renal cyst. *J. Comput. Assist. Tomogr.* 7:1103, 1983.
19. Fong, K.W., et al. Fetal renal cystic disease: Sonographic pathologic correlation. *A.J.R.* 146:767, 1986.
20. Gabow, P.A., Ikle, D.W., and Holmes, J.H. Polycystic kidney disease: Prospective analysis of nonazotemic patients and family members. *Ann. Intern. Med.* 101:238,1984.
21. Garel, L.A., et al. Juvenile nephronophthisis: Sonographic appearance in children with severe uremia. *Radiology* 151:93, 1984.
22. Gehrig, J.J., Jr., Gottheiner, T.I., and Swenson, R.S. Acquired cystic disease of the end-stage kidney. *Am.J. Med.* 79:609, 1985.
23. Giangiacomo, J., Monteleone, P.L., and Witzleben, C.L. Medullary cystic disease vs. nephronophthisis: A valid distinction? *J.A.M.A.* 232:629, 1975.
24. Gipson, T.G., Anderson, E., and Bradford, W.D. Multicystic renal dysplasia: Pathologic and clinical observations in 22 cases. *Clin. Pediatr.* 15:896, 1976.
25. Glazer, G.M. MR imaging of the liver, kidneys, and adrenal glands. *Radiology* 166:303, 1988.
26. Gordon, R.L., et al. Simple serous cysts of the kidney in children. *Radiology* 131:357, 1979.
27. Grantham, J.J., Geiser, J.L., and Evan, A.P. Cyst formation and growth in autosomal dominant polycystic kidney disease. *Kidney Int.* 31:1145, 1987.
28. Grossman, H., et al. Sonographic diagnosis of renal cystic diseases. *A.J.R.* 140:81, 1983.
29. Habif, D., Jr., Berdon, W.E., and Ming-Neng, Y. Infantile polycystic kidney disease: In utero sonographic diagnosis. *Radiology* 142:475, 1982.
30. Harris, R.E., Fuchs, E.F., and Kaempf, M.J. Medullary sponge kidney and congenital hemihypertrophy: Case report and literature review. *J. Urol.* 126:676, 1981.
31. Harris, R.D., Goergen, T.G., and Talner, L.B. The bloody renal cyst aspirate: A diagnostic dilemma. *J. Urol.* 114:832, 1975.
32. Hatfield, P.M., and Pfister, R.C. Adult polycystic disease of the kidneys (Potter type 3). *J.A.M.A.* 222:1527, 1972.
33. Hidalgo, H., et al. *A.J.R.* 138:667, 1982.
34. Hinman, F., Jr. Obstructive renal cysts. *J. Urol.* 119:651, 1978.
35. Hughson, M.D., Hennigar, G.R., and McManus, J.F.A. Atypical cysts, acquired renal cystic disease, and renal cell tumors in end stage dialysis kidneys. *Lab. Invest.* 42:475, 1980.
36. Ishikawa, I. Uremic acquired cystic disease of kidney. *Urology* 26:101, 1985.
37. Ishikawa, I., et al. Regression of acquired cystic disease of the kidney after successful renal transplantation. *Am. J. Nephrol.* 3:310, 1983.
38. Jabour, B.A., et al. Acquired cystic disease of the kidneys. *Invest. Radiol.* 22:728, 1987.
39. Kala, R., et al. Solitary renal cyst, hypertension and renin. *J. Urol.* 116:710, 1976.
40. Kelsey, J.A., and Bowie, J.D. Gray-scale ultrasonography in the diagnosis of polycystic kidney disease. *Radiology* 122:791, 1977.
41. Kulkarni, M.V., et al. Evaluation of renal masses by MR imaging. *J. Comput Assist. Tomogr.* 8:861, 1984.
42. Kutcher, R., Schneider, M., and Gordon, D.H. Calcification in polycystic disease. *Radiology* 122:77, 1977.
43. Kyaw, M. The radiological dignosis of congenital multicystic kidney, 'radiological triad.' *Clin. Radiol.* 25:45, 1974.
44. Laucks, S.P. Jr., and McLachlan, M.S.F. Aging and simple cysts of the kidney. *Br. J. Radiol.* 54:12, 1981.
45. Lawson, T.L., McClennan, B.L., and Shirkhoda, A. Adult polycystic kidney disease: Ultrasonographic and computed tomographic appearance. *J. Clin. Ultrasound* 6:297, 1978.
46. Leier, C.V., et al. Cardiovascular abnormalities associated with adult polycystic kidney disease. *Ann. Intern. Med.* 100:683, 1984.

47. Leonard, J.C., et al. Renal cortical imaging and the detection of renal mass lesions. *J. Nucl. Med.* 20:1018, 1979.
48. Levine, E., and Grantham, J.J. High-density renal cysts in autosomal dominant polycystic kidney disease demonstrated by CT. *Radiology* 154:477, 1985.
49. Levine, E., et al. CT of acquired cystic kidney disease and renal tumors in long-term dialysis patients. *A.J.R.* 142:125, 1984.
50. Link, D.P., Hansen, S., and Palmer, J. High dose excretory urography and medullary cystic disease of the kidney. *A.J.R.* 133:303, 1979.
51. Melson, G.L., et al. The spectrum of sonographic findings in infantile polycystic kidney disease with urographic and clinical correlations. *J. Clin. Ultrasound* 13:113, 1985.
52. Meziane, M.A., et al. Computed tomography of high density renal cysts in adult polycystic kidney disease. *J. Comput. Assist. Tomogr.* 10:767, 1986.
53. Morag, B., et al. Computed tomography in the diagnosis of renal parapelvic cysts. *J. Comput. Assist. Tomogr.* 7:833, 1983.
54. Older, R.A., et al. In utero diagnosis of multicystic kidney by gray scale ultrasonography. *A.J.R.* 133:130, 1979.
55. Papanicolaou, N., Pfister, R.C., and Yoder, I.C. Spontaneous and traumatic rupture of renal cysts: diagnosis and outcome. *Radiology* 160:99, 1986.
56. Patriquin, H.B., and O'Regan, S. Medullary sponge kidney in childhood. *A.J.R.* 145:315, 1985.
57. Pedicelli, G., et al. Multicystic dysplastic kidneys: spontaneous regression demonstrated with US. *Radiology* 160:23, 1986.
58. Ralls, P.W., et al. Severe hydronephrosis and severe renal cystic disease: Ultrasonic differentiation. *A.J.R.* 134:473, 1980.
59. Rose, H.J., and Pruitt, A.W. Hypertension, hyperreninemia and a solitary renal cyst in an adolescent. *Am. J. Med.* 61:579, 1976.
60. Rosenfield, A.T., et al. Ultrasonography and nephrotomography in the presymptomatic diagnosis of dominantly inherited (adult-onset) polycystic kidney disease. *Radiology* 135:423, 1980.
61. Sage, M.R., et al. Medullary sponge kidney and urolithiasis. *Clin. Radiol.* 33:435, 1982.
62. Sanders, R C., and Hartman, D.S. The sonographic distinction between neonatal multicystic kidney and hydronephrosis. *Radiology* 151:621, 1984.
63. Sanders, R.C., Nussbaum, A.R., and Solez, K. Renal dysplasia: Sonographic findings. *Radiology* 167:623, 1988.
64. Saxton, H.M., et al. Diagnostic puncture in renal cystic dysplasia (multicystic kidney): Evidence on the aetiology of the cysts. *Br. J. Radiol.* 54:555, 1981.
65. Segal, A.J., and Spataro, R.F. Computed tomography of adult polycystic disease. *J. Comput. Assist. Tomogr.* 6:777, 1982.
66. Segal, A.J., Spataro, R.F., and Barbaric, Z.L. Adult polycystic kidney disease: A review of 100 cases. *J. Urol.* 118:711, 1977.
67. Sherwood, T., and Trott, P.A. Needling renal cysts and tumors: Cytology and radiology. *Br. Med. J.* 27:755, 1975.
68. Siegel, M.J., and McAlister, W.H. Simple cysts of the kidney in children. *J. Urol.* 123:75, 1980.
69. Six, R., Oliphant, M., and Grossman, H. A spectrum of renal tubular ectasia and hepatic fibrosis. *Radiology* 117:117, 1975.
70. Steinhardt, G.F., Slovis, T.L., and Perlmutter, A.D. Simple renal cysts in infants. *Radiology* 155:349, 1985.
71. Sussman, S., et al. Hyperdense renal masses: A CT manifestation of hemorrhagic renal cysts. *Radiology* 150:207, 1984.
72. Vaziri, N.D., et al. Acquired renal cystic disease in renal transplant recipients. *Nephron* 37:203, 1984.
73. Vinocur, L., et al. Follow-up studies of multicystic dysplastic kidneys. *Radiology* 167:311, 1988.
74. Walker, F.C., Jr., et al. Diagnostic evaluation of adult polycystic kidney disease in childhood. *A.J.R.* 142:1273, 1984.
75. Zirinsky, K., et al. CT of the hyperdense renal cyst: Sonographic correlation. *A.J.R.* 143:151, 1984.

The Kidney: Tumors

Renal tumors have been variously characterized as benign or malignant; primary or secondary; epithelial or nonepithelial; arising from renal parenchyma, collecting-system structures, or the renal capsule; and histologically differentiated or undifferentiated. While many different types of tumors can involve the kidney, only a few make up the large majority seen in clinical practice. Table 9-1 classifies these lesions into benign and malignant categories.

The role of the radiologist in evaluating patients with a suspected renal lesion is threefold: to detect the lesion, characterize it as benign or malignant, and stage malignant lesions to determine proper therapy. Excretory urography with linear tomography is considered the primary screening examination in the evaluation of a suspected renal mass. The mass, if large enough, may result in a tumefactive bulging of the renal outline (seen best on nephrotomography) and effacement of adjacent calices or bowing of infundibula. Smaller masses may be entirely intrarenal in location and suspected only by their effect on the collecting system or by defects in the otherwise homogeneous nephrogram. When a mass is seen on the excretory urogram either ultrasound or CT is usually employed to define the nature of the lesion further. In most cases, when the excretory urogram is normal, further evaluation of the upper urinary tract is thought not to be necessary. However, exophytic renal masses protruding from either the anterior or posterior surface of the kidney can be easily missed even with linear tomography since they do not distort the collecting system or cause changes in the renal outline. By the same token, renal lesions, particularly those at the renal poles, can also be missed by CT because of the failure on axial scanning to recognize a lesion as separate from the normal polar parenchyma. It is therefore incumbent on the radiologist to recognize the limitations of the standard imaging methods used for detection of renal masses. Using CT as the standard, excretory urography with linear tomography can detect approximately 85 percent of lesions 3 cm or more in diameter [28]. Renal sonography has been shown to have a similar sensitivity for lesions of this size.

Currently, MRI does not appear to be as sensitive as CT in the detection of small renal masses. However, the ability of MRI to image in multiple planes has been found useful in determining the organ of origin of large masses when this was not clear on other studies. Furthermore, MRI has been shown to be accurate in staging renal malignancies. This will be discussed in more detail in subsequent sections.

Radioisotope renal scans, which are not normally used in detecting or staging kidney tumors, nonetheless exhibit a focal photon-deficient area corresponding to the location of the renal mass. This is a nonspecific finding consistent with either benign or malignant tumors. Renal cysts also produce this finding. However, radionuclide renal function studies may be employed to determine differential renal function in planning radical or partial nephrectomy for treatment of a renal tumor.

After detection of a renal mass, specific imaging characteristics are often useful in suggesting its cell type. Analyzing these imaging findings in conjunction with the clinical presentation often allows the preoperative determination of whether a lesion is malignant or benign. In this way, surgery can be tailored for maximal renal sparing. If a renal lesion is determined to be obviously malignant, accurate staging is of great importance in determining the surgical approach or the necessity for other types of therapy such as hormonal therapy, chemotherapy, or radiation.

BENIGN RENAL TUMORS

The great majority of benign renal tumors are quite small, originate from mesenchymal cells,

Table 9-1. Classification of renal tumors

Benign tumors
Angiomyolipoma (hamartoma)
Oncocytoma (proximal tubular adenoma)
Mesoblastic nephroma (fetal renal hamartoma)
Multilocular cystic nephroma (hamartoma)
Reninoma (juxtaglomerular-cell tumor)
Other benign primary tumors
Malignant tumors
Renal cell carcinoma
Wilms' tumor (nephroblastoma)
Tumors of intrarenal collecting system (transitional cell carcinoma, squamous cell carcinoma, mucinous adenocarcinoma)
Sarcomas
Secondary malignant tumors
Multisystem diseases associated with renal tumors
von Hippel–Lindau disease (renal cell) carcinomas)
Tuberous sclerosis (angiomyolipomas)

and are usually found incidentally at autopsy in up to 15 to 20 percent of cases. These include fibromas, myomas, lipomas, and angiomas or various combinations of these cell types. However, there are several benign tumors that can reach significant size and thus be detected on clinical examination or by imaging studies. There will be discussed individually in the sections to follow.

ANGIOMYOLIPOMA

Clinical Factors

The angiomyolipoma (AML) is considered a hamartoma of the kidney. For all practical purposes, however, it can also be defined as a benign renal tumor. It is composed of fat, smooth muscle, and abnormal blood vessels. These three tissues may vary tremendously in relative amounts from tumor to tumor. Grossly, the tumor is round or oval in configuration and well circumscribed, but without a true capsule. AMLs can range in size from a few millimeters to over 20 cm in diameter. In one series, the average size was approximately 9 cm [22].

Seventy-five percent of angiomyolipomas are found as a solitary renal mass, usually in middle-aged women. In about 20 percent of cases, angiomyolipomas are found to be associated with tuberous sclerosis. In these patients the tumors are usually multiple and bilateral. The remaining 5 percent of patients have multiple or bilateral angiomyolipomas but no other stigmata of tuberous sclerosis.

Symptoms include flank pain, flank mass, and hematuria. Hemorrhage into the tumor or into the perinephric space is not uncommon (see Fig. 6-1A). Such patients may present with hypotension. Although the tumor is benign, the risk of massive retroperitoneal hemorrhage usually prompts the consideration of surgical removal once the tumor has been discovered. This is particularly true when the angiomyolipoma is 4 cm in diameter or larger.

The differential diagnosis of AML includes simple lipomas, well-differentiated liposarcomas, teratomas, and atypical fat-containing Wilms' tumors. Furthermore, a fat-containing tumor thought to be in the upper pole of the kidney is difficult on occasion to differentiate from an adrenal myelolipoma. Most of these differentials are easy to resolve given the clinical setting and other radiographic features of the lesion. On rare occasions fat may not be found within an angiomyolipoma. This occurs when there is a predominance of muscular and vascular elements (angiomyoma) or when significant intratumoral hemorrhage obscures any fat that may be present.

Imaging Studies

Imaging of the angiomyolipoma can often result in the preoperative determination of the nature of the lesion. On urography AML is usually seen as a solid-appearing mass lesion, though on occasion, when there is a large amount of fat in the tumor, its radiolucent nature can be appreciated on the scout film or tomograms. However, because of the fat found in this lesion, sonography and CT are more definitive methods. Sonography usually identifies a highly echogenic mass due to this fat content (Fig. 9-1A). AML is the most echogenic of all the tumors that will be described in this chapter. However, in rare instances, other tumors can display an echogenicity approaching that of an angiomyolipoma. These include renal cell carcinoma, oncocytoma, and reninoma. The definitive diagnosis of AML is based on the detection of fat within the lesion by CT (Fig. 9-1B). The amount of fat may be minimal and require a careful search for its presence (Fig 9-1C). This can best be

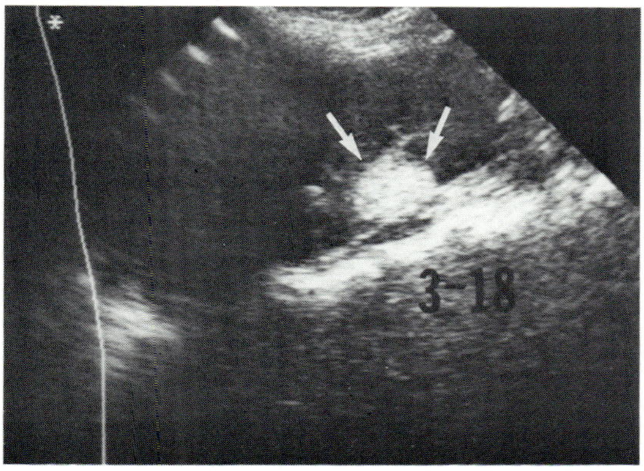

A

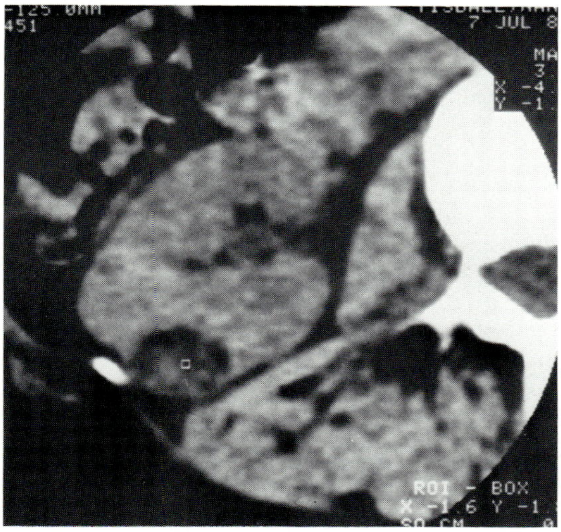

B

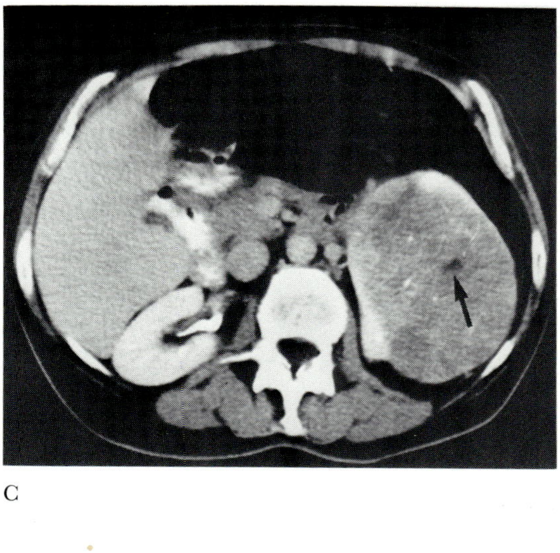

C

Figure 9-1. Angiomyolipoma. A. Right renal sonography demonstrates a highly echogenic mass in the posterior kidney (arrows). B. CT shows that this mass has fatty elements (Region of interest = −35 Hounsfield units). C. CT in another patient shows large tumor in left kidney. Thin sections were required to demonstrate the small amount of fat (arrow) necessary to differentiate the lesion from a renal cell carcinoma.

accomplished by the use of thin-section (5 mm) nonenhanced CT scans. Fat detected with this technique invariably measures −10 Hounsfield units or less [4].

With the high resolution of modern sonography, small echogenic nodules in the kidney are being found with increasing frequency in patients with unrelated problems. These are often less than 1 cm and usually prove to be AMLs when studied by CT. Tiny angiomyolipomas of the kidney are found in about 11 percent of autopsy cases. Therefore, highly echogenic lesions under 1 cm in diameter found incidentally in the kidneys probably do not require further imaging to confirm their true nature. However, for lesions over 1 cm, CT is recommended.

While MRI is not generally employed for imaging AML, the fatty component of these tumors can usually be readily demonstrated. The relaxation times of benign lipomatous tumors are in a range similar to that of normal subcutaneous fat. The fat in AML has a high signal intensity on T1 weighted images, and is of intermediate intensity with T2 weighting.

ONCOCYTOMA

Clinical Factors

The renal oncocytoma is a benign tumor arising from proximal tubular cells. This tumor is histologically categorized as Grade I or II, though the differences are subtle. The large majority are Grade I and have an excellent prognosis when treated by local resection. Grade II oncocytomas exhibit more aggressive behavior.

Oncocytomas are usually seen in middle and old age, with men being more commonly affected than women by a ratio of 1.7:1. They usually occur as single tumors and most are detected as incidental findings; however, they may be associated with pain or hematuria. Though they may reach over 20 cm in diameter, the typical oncocytoma is about 5 cm in diameter. They are usually round, well-defined, and reasonably homogeneous on cut section with the exception of a centrally located scar, which usually has a stellate configuration. There is no true capsule, their circumscribed appearance resulting from compression of the surrounding renal parenchyma into a pseudocapsule. Intratumoral necrosis and hemorrhage are uncommon, especially in the smaller tumors, and calcification is quite rare.

Imaging Studies

While the size of the tumor and its clinical presentation does not help in differentiating it from renal cell carcinoma, there are several imaging characteristics that allow the preoperative suggestion of its benign nature. On urography, the oncocytoma presents as a solid mass lesion of the kidney. As with other renal masses, its size and location determine the amount of collecting system distortion and focal abnormalities in the renal outline. On sonography most oncocytomas are homogeneous and relatively isoechoic with the surrounding renal parenchyma. A particularly important finding is the central scar, which can be hyperechoic or hypoechoic.

On CT oncocytomas appear as solid, enhancing mass lesions with smooth contours, distinct interfaces with adjoining renal parenchyma and homogeneous contrast enhancement. When present, the central stellate scar exhibits lower attenuation than the remainder of the tumor (Fig. 9-2A).

Angiographic evaluation of oncocytomas may show a spoke-wheel pattern (Fig. 9-2B) of the vasculature in about 25 percent of cases, though this is not specific for oncocytoma; 50 percent of tumors with this pattern are renal cell carcinomas. On later films in the angiogram the oncocytoma will usually exhibit a dense homogeneous blush, as opposed to the inhomogeneous tumor blush usually seen with renal cell carcinoma. Small intratumoral aneurysms have also been described with oncocytoma, though these can also be found in angiomyolipomas and renal cell carcinomas.

There are significant areas of overlap between the appearances of oncocytomas and renal cell carcinomas. Especially when they are small, re-

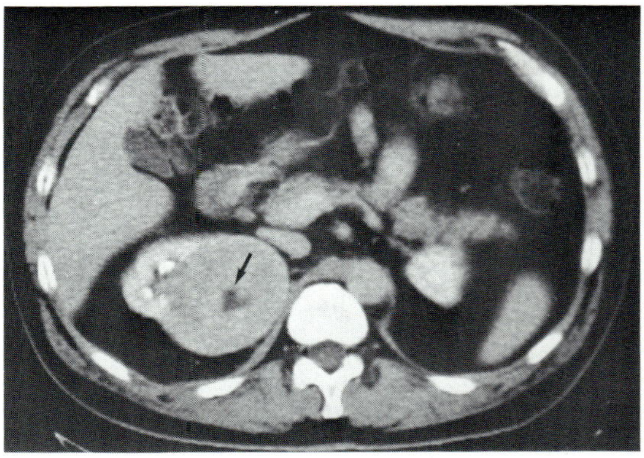

A

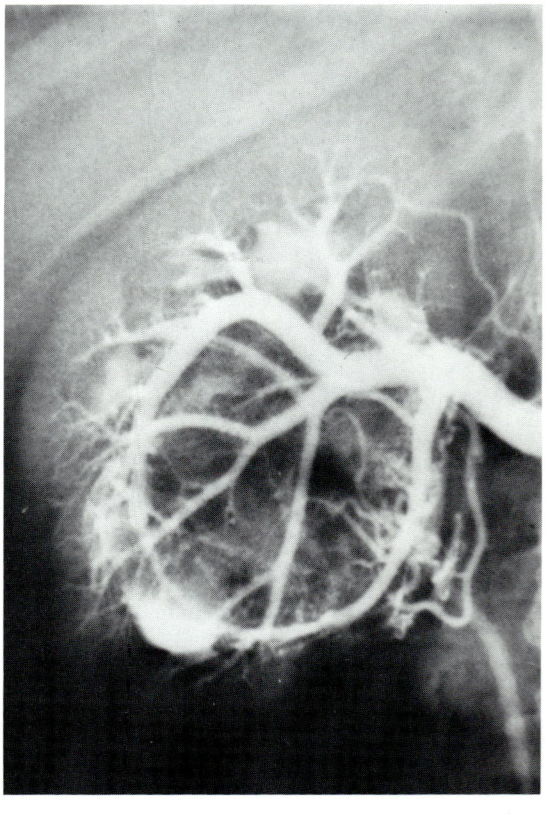

B

Figure 9-2. Oncocytoma. A. Contrast-enhanced CT section through right renal tumor shows homogeneous density with the exception of the central low-attenuation scar (arrow). B. Angiogram of tumor demonstrates a 'spoked-wheel'' pattern. (Courtesy of Alan J. Davidson, M.D. Armed Forces Institute of Pathology, Washington, D.C.)

nal cell carcinomas can be well defined and relatively homogeneous. However, in lesions over 3 cm in size, a relatively homogeneous appearance on ultrasonography or CT accompanied by a stellate central scar should lead the radiologist to suggest the diagnosis of oncocytoma [19].

MULTILOCULAR CYSTIC NEPHROMA

Clinical Factors

Multilocular cystic nephroma (MLCN), also called multilocular renal cyst, is a well-circumscribed, encapsulated mass that contains mutiple noncommunicating fluid-filled locules [16]. It is biphasic in its sex and age incidence. Boys with MLCN are almost always under the age of 4. In women, MLCN is likely to occur between the ages of 4 and 20 years of age or in the fifth and sixth decades of life. MLCN is usually solitary and occurs as an asymptomatic mass, though there may occasionally be associated hematuria. Septal calcifications are occasionally seen. The lesion may grow slowly or quite rapidly and is most commonly found in the lower pole of the kidney. On detection, the tumors range in size from 3 to 34 cm, with an average size of approximately 9 to 10 cm. Hematuria secondary to MLCN is often associated with herniation of the tumor into the renal pelvis.

Like angiomyolipomas, MLCN is viewed by some pathologists as a hamartoma [23]. On occasion, histologic examination of the tumor will reveal foci of cells that resemble renal cell carcinoma. However, the prognosis remains excellent with treatment by partial or total nephrectomy without adjuvant chemotherapy or radiotherapy.

The differential diagnosis of MLCN is extensive and includes cystic Wilms' tumor, septated cyst, segmental multicystic kidney, echinococcal cyst, segmental xanthogranulomatous pyelonephritis, and most importantly, renal cell carcinoma. The last can have a multilocular configuration in 5 percent of cases.

Imaging Studies

In patients with MLCN, plain films of the abdomen may show a mass, and calcification of a curvilinear variety is seen uncommonly in the periphery of the mass or in its septations. Excretory urography usually demonstrates a well-defined renal mass in an otherwise normal kidney. While tumor herniation into the renal pelvis can occasionally be seen during urography, it is usually best demonstrated by retrograde pyelography.

Ultrasound findings are determined by the composition of the mass, including the number and thickness of the septations and the size of the individual locules. Generally speaking, sonography usually demonstrates a cluster of echo-free masses separated by highly echogenic connective-tissue septae (Fig. 9-3A). If the locules are not sizable, sonography may demonstrate a nonspecific complex pattern.

CT similarly demonstrates a large, smoothly marginated, multilocular mass (Fig. 9-3B). After administration of an intravenous contrast agent the septa may enhance. The fluid contained within the locules will usually exhibit an attenuation value slightly higher than that of water, but does not enhance. Again, as with sonography, if the locules are small (1 cm or less) CT may demonstrate a complex mass indistinguishable from a malignant lesion. On MRI, the fluid in the locules shows very low signal intensity on T1 weighted images, but becomes very bright (high signal) with T2 weighting.

When studied by angiography, MLCN usually exhibits a hypovascular pattern, though with some tumor blush and neovascularity in the septae. On other occasions, MLCN may be avascular, with stretching and displacement of intrarenal vessels. There are no specific angiographic features to differentiate MLCN from renal cell carcinoma or Wilms' tumor.

RENINOMA (JUXTAGLOMERULAR TUMOR)

Clinical Factors

Reninomas are relatively rare renin-producing tumors arising from the juxtaglomerular cells of the kidney. They represent a curable cause of hypertension. Presenting symptoms, such as headache, often relate to the hypertension. The peripheral renin level is usually elevated, and there is evidence of secondary aldosteronism [7]. The reninoma is usually small, solitary, and located just beneath the renal capsule, often near one of the poles. The average tumor size is

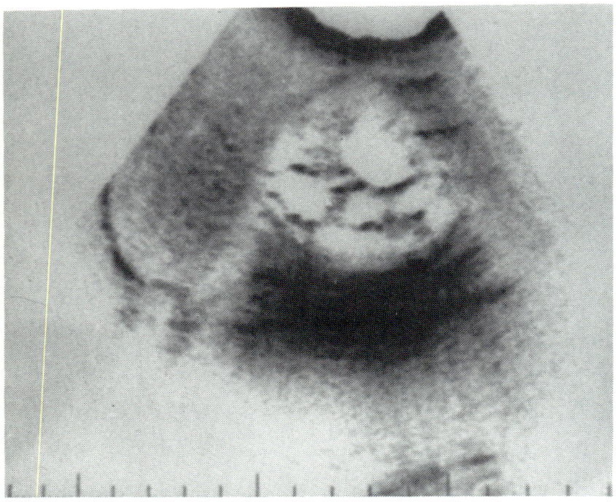

A

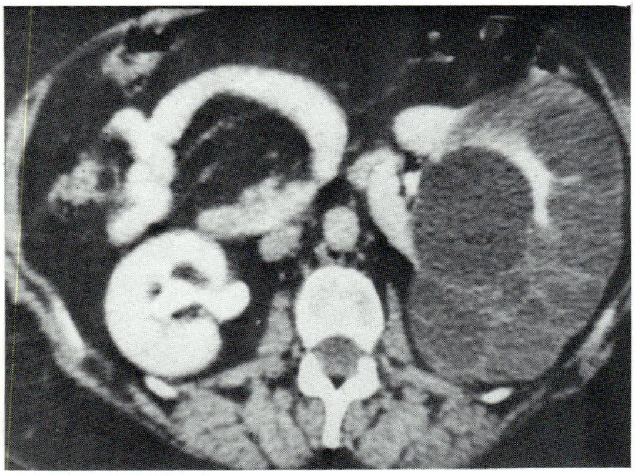

B

Figure 9-3. Multilocular cystic nephroma (MLCN). A. Sonography shows mass with echo-free areas separated by echogenic septae. (From E.S. Amis, Jr., and D.S. Hartman. Renal ultrasonography 1984: A practical overview. *Radiol. Clin. North Am.* 22(2):315, 1984.) B. CT section in another patient demonstrates a left renal mass with multiple fluid-density locules separated by septae, the largest of which is calcified.

2 to 3 cm. However, the tumor may be as small as several millimeters in diameter and not detectable by imaging studies or may reach a size of 6 cm or more. Most occur in younger women; the average age on presentation is about 30 years. Grossly, the reninoma is sharply marginated and surrounded by a pseudocapsule of compressed parenchyma. Small areas of intratumoral hemorrhage are common.

Excision of the tumor, either by wedge resection or partial nephrectomy, is curative and often accompanied by a dramatic relief of hypertension in the hours after surgery. The differential diagnosis for a patient with hypertension, hyperreninism, and secondary hyperaldosteronism should include reninoma, renal artery stenosis, renin secreting tumors of the lung, liver, or orbit, or other masses that may compress the renal artery or renal parenchyma.

Imaging Studies

Because of the small size of the tumor and absence of calcification, up to 75 percent of reninomas are not seen on urography. Sonographically, the tumor is usually echogenic, though usually not as much so as an angiomyolipoma (Fig. 9-4A). This echogenicity is due to numerous interfaces between the juxtaglomerular cells and the abundant small vascular channels within the tumor. If hemorrhage and necrosis have occurred, small hypoechoic areas can be seen within the mass.

On CT without contrast medium, the tumor is small and often isodense with the normal noncontrasted renal parenchyma. After administration of intravenous contrast medium, the tumor will usually be enhanced to some degree. The mass is usually hypovascular by angiography (Fig. 9-4B). Angiography is often helpful in eliminating renal artery stenosis as the cause of excess renin production.

MESOBLASTIC NEPHROMA

Clinical Factors

The mesoblastic nephroma, also known as a fetal renal hamartoma or congenital Wilms' tumor, is a benign renal tumor that is usually discovered as a palpable abdominal mass in the neonate. In the past it was believed that in neonates Wilms' tumor had a better prognosis than those occurring in older children. However, about 20 years ago it was realized that most of the renal tumors in the neonatal period were not Wilms' tumor but rather a distinct pathologic entity—the mesoblastic nephroma. This benign tumor consists mainly of connective tissue growing between the nephrons of the kidney and often replacing most of the renal parenchyma. The prognosis for a normal life after complete removal is excellent. Unlike Wilms' tumor, chemotherapy or radiation therapy after

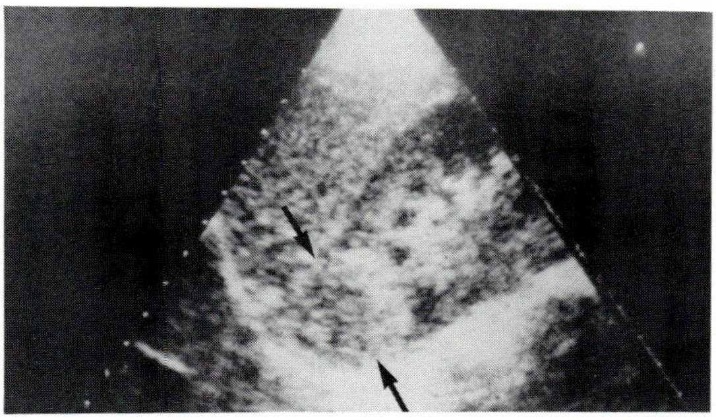

A

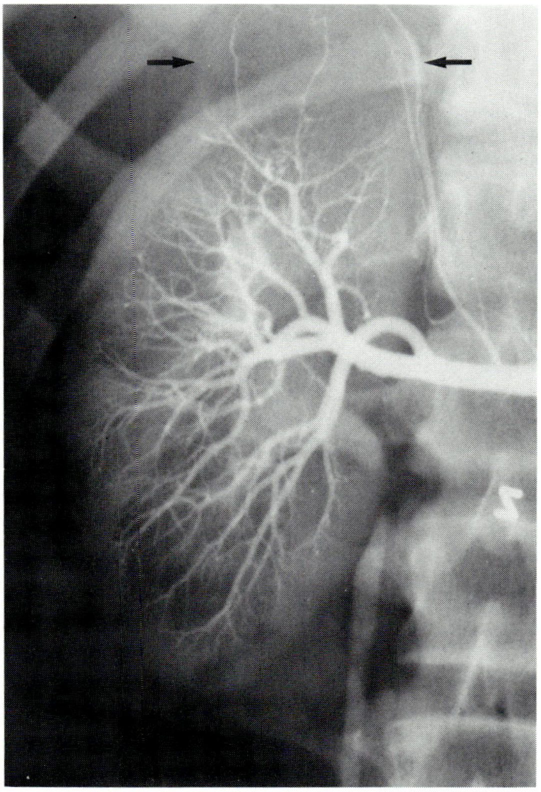

B

Figure 9-4. Reninoma (juxtaglomerular cell tumor). A. Sonography shows upper-pole mass with relatively high echogenicity (arrows). B. Right renal arteriography shows the upper-pole mass to be hypovascular (arrows).

surgery is not necessary. There is no race or sex predilection. Only on rare occasions is this tumor found beyond the neonatal period.

The tumor is not encapsulated and may measure between 8 and 30 cm in diameter [11]. Intratumoral hemorrhage and necrosis are uncommon, but if they occur they may result in cystic change within the tumor. Calcification in a mesoblastic nephroma is rare.

Imaging Studies

Urography will usually show a large renal mass with obvious distortion of the calices and renal outline. Renal sonography will either show a solid mass or, in the case with cystic degeneration, a complex pattern. The mesoblastic nephroma is the most common renal neoplasm during the first few months of life, and detection of a solid or complex renal mass in this age group usually leads directly to nephrectomy.

MALIGNANT RENAL TUMORS

Malignant renal tumors comprise about 2 percent of all malignant tumors. Of all primary renal malignancies renal cell carcinoma is by far the most common, comprising about 85 percent of this group, followed by tumors of the renal pelvis (transitional cell carcinoma, squamous cell carcinoma, mucinous adenocarcinoma) (7 to 8 percent), Wilms' tumor (5 to 6 percent), and renal sarcomas (3 percent). As with the benign tumors, the sections below will discuss both clinical and imaging findings of malignant renal tumors.

RENAL CELL CARCINOMA

Clinical Factors

Renal cell carcinoma (RCC), an epithelial malignancy of the renal parenchyma, has been variously called hypernephroma, nephrocarcinoma, Grawitz-cell tumor, and clear- or granular-cell carcinoma of the kidney. It occurs most frequently in the sixth decade and males are affected twice as commonly as females. Though uncommon in the pediatric age group, when it does occur the average age is about 9 years. As previously noted, RCC comprises the large majority (85 percent) of primary renal malignancies. The classical triad of gross hematuria, flank pain, and flank mass is found in only 10 to 15 percent of patients. In over a third of patients there are no presenting symptoms that can be traced to the primary tumor. Certainly, however, either microscopic or gross hematuria raises suspicion of malignancy of the urinary tract.

There are two broad histologic groups of RCC that may be defined on the basis of cellular architecture: papillary and nonpapillary [18]. Papillary RCCs, representing up to 15 percent of all RCCs, are composed of vascularized connective-tissue stalks lined by neoplastic cells in a single layer or with pseudostratification. The remainder of RCCs are nonpapillary and are characterized by cells arranged in tubules, cords, or spindle-shaped patterns. Papillary RCC is characterized by slower growth, lower stage at presentation and a better prognosis than nonpapillary RCC.

In the past, small renal tumors under 3 cm in diameter were traditionally called renal adenomas. These were considered benign because of their very low frequency of metastasis. However, there are no gross, histologic, immunologic, chromosomal, or ultrastructural features to distinguish adenoma from renal cell carcinoma [25]. It is therefore generally accepted that lesions less than 3 cm in diameter and indistinguishable from renal cell carcinoma are indeed early renal cell carcinomas and should be classified as such. While these lesions have low metastatic potential, there have been reports of metastases occurring with tumors smaller than 3 cm [5]. This classification is important because of the fact that more small renal tumors are being detected since the advent of CT and ultrasonography. One report indicates that only 5 percent of renal cell carcinomas found in the mid-1970s were less than 3 cm, while a decade later 25 percent were of this small size [25]. It is currently being debated whether these small, incidentally discovered tumors should be treated by partial nephrectomy or whether the patient should be subjected to the time-honored therapy of radical nephrectomy. In either case, the earlier detection of these small lesions will undoubtedly increase the cure rate for RCC.

RCC spreads by direct extension as well as by invasion of the venous and lymphatic systems. The lungs and bones are the most common sites of venous metastatic spread. Bone lesions are lytic and expansile because their hypervascular nature. Lymph node involvement has been estimated at 10 to 30 percent. Tumor thrombus in the renal vein and possibly extending into the inferior vena cava is found in 5 to 24 percent of cases [21]. Other metastatic sites include the liver, adrenal, and central nervous system. The opposite kidney is involved by synchronous lesions in up to 3.8 percent of cases.

Adrenal metastases from RCC occur in 18 to 25 percent of patients. They are usually not clinically apparent but are found incidentally at autopsy. These adrenal metastases must be differentiated from adrenal adenomas, which have been found to occur in 12 to 15 percent of patients with RCC as compared with 2 to 3 percent of the general population [1]. Awareness of this association is important in avoiding overdiagnosis of metastatic disease. As noted in Chap. 7, MRI is able to help differentiate between adrenal adenomas and metastatic lesions.

Grossly, RCC has ill-defined margins where it interfaces with the normal kidney. Intratumoral hemorrhage and necrosis are common, occurring in over half of cases. This may be so extensive that it leads to cystic degeneration of the tumor. At times cystic change can be so severe that it is difficult to differentiate the tumor from a complicated benign cyst. This cystic change will be discussed in more detail in the chapter on indeterminate renal masses. As previously noted, RCC can be virtually any size when initially diagnosed. Calcification, either central and punctate or peripheral and curvilinear, occurs in 10 to 20 percent of patients.

While many staging methods for RCC have been reported, Robson's modification of the Flocks and Kadesky staging method is generally accepted (Fig. 9-5). Survival has been shown to be directly related to the stage of tumor progression at the time of presentation. The overall 5-year survival for Stages I and II combined is 71 percent, as contrasted with 12 percent for Stages III and IV combined [12].

For Stage I and II disease, radical nephrectomy is the treatment of choice. When RCC has progressed beyond this stage, survival is very poor, since this tumor is not significantly amenable to other forms of therapy. Radical nephrectomy involves excision of the kidney encapsulated in Gerota's fascia. The ipsilateral

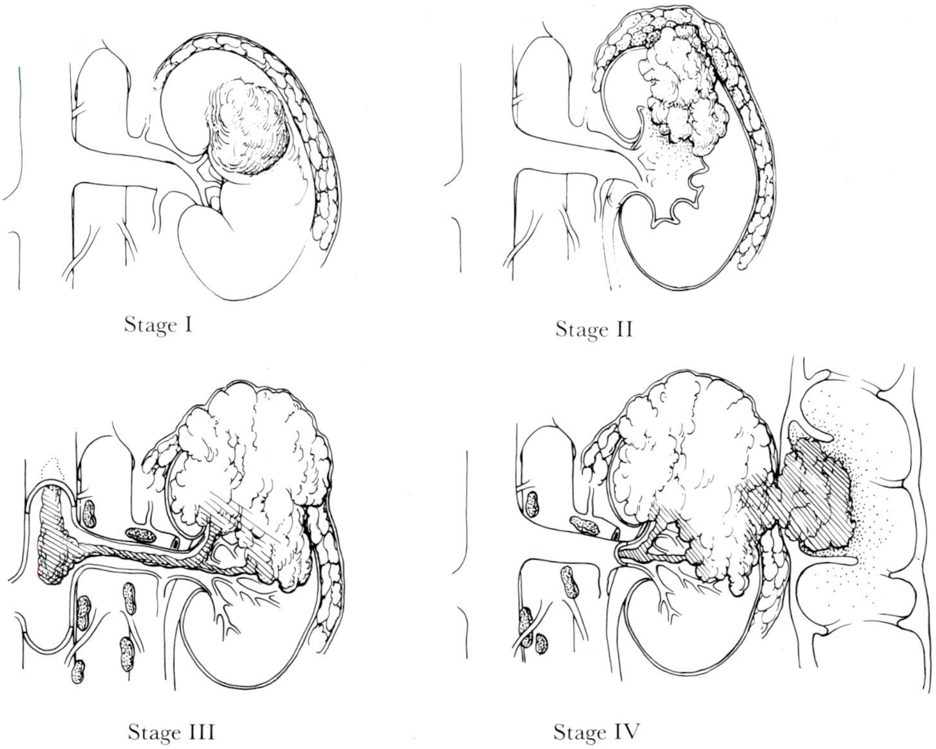

Figure 9-5. Staging of renal cell carcinoma. Stage I—Tumor confined inside renal capsule. Stage II—Tumor has invaded perinephric fat, but is confined within Gerota's fascia. Stage IIIA—Tumor thrombus in renal vein and may extend into inferior vena cava. Stage IIIB—Tumor involving hilar nodes. Stage IIIC—Tumor thrombus and nodal involvement. Stage IVA—Tumor invades adjacent organs. Stage IVB—Distant metastases.

adrenal is almost always removed en bloc with the specimen. Also performed as part of this surgery is dissection of the regional lymph nodes.

Imaging Studies

Plain films of the abdomen may reveal stippled, amorphous, or curvilinear calcifications in the region of the involved kidney, usually associated with a soft-tissue mass (Fig. 9-6A). Because of the high incidence of calcification in RCC, a calcified mass, even though only peripherally calcified, must be considered a malignancy until proven otherwise. Intravenous urography reveals mass effect distorting the collecting system or bulging the renal contour or both, depending on the size and location of the mass (Fig. 9-6B). The mass may be somewhat ill-defined or the margins clearly seen. When a mass that is presumably solid is detected on urography, the next imaging study should be CT. On the other hand, a mass that appears cystic on urography should be evaluated by sonography, which is cheaper and safer and often permits the diagnosis of simple cyst.

CT must always be performed before and after the administration of intravenous contrast media. Scanning before the administration of a contrast agent may allow identification of faint calcifications that were not appreciated on plain film radiography. After administration of contrast medium, RCC typically enhances in a quite irregular fashion. Areas of necrosis and hemorrhage, which may be centrally located or eccentric, can be easily appreciated (Fig. 9-6C). When these patterns are seen, RCC becomes the primary diagnosis.

The primary role of CT in staging RCC is to determine whether the tumor invades the perinephric fat, whether the renal vein (and inferior vena cava) are involved by tumor throm-

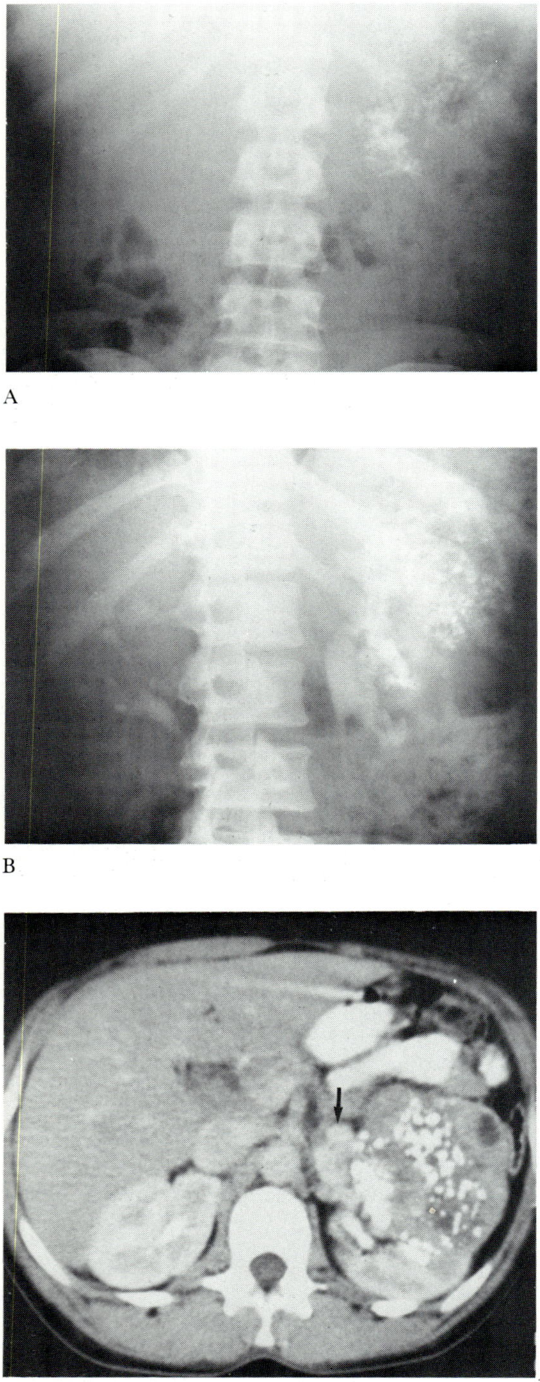

A

B

C

Figure 9-6. Renal-cell carcinoma with calcifications. A. Plain film of upper abdomen shows dense, stippled calcifications in region of left kidney. B. Urography shows renal mass in region of calcifications. C. Contrast-enchanced CT section through the mass shows the calcifications to be intratumoral. The mass enchances inhomogeneously and several small areas of fluid density represent necrosis. Enlarged nodes are seen in the left renal hilum (arrow), making this a Stage IIIB tumor.

bus, and whether enlarged nodes are present in the retroperitoneal area. CT is also useful in evaluation for pulmonary and hepatic metastases as well as for evaluating the adrenals. Perinephric invasion is the most troublesome CT area and accounts for more than half of all staging errors. Otherwise, CT is a reliable and accurate means of preoperatively staging RCC, with an overall accuracy of 91 percent [14]. The criteria for perinephric invasion by RCC include soft-tissue masses or strands extending into the perinephric fat (Fig. 9-7). However, perinephric soft-tissue masses are seen in only about half of the patients with proven Stage II disease, and perinephric stranding is a very nonspecific finding, being found in about half of patients with proven Stage I disease. Fortunately, both Stage I and Stage II tumors are treated by radical nephrectomy.

Metastatic adenopathy can be identified by CT with a sensitivity of more than 80 percent. The major difficulty here lies in the inability of CT to differentiate between benign enlarged nodes and those containing tumor. In one series, nodes between 1 and 2 cm in diameter were malignant in only slightly over half of cases [14]. However, all nodes over 2 cm in diameter contained tumor. Positive nodes are usually found first near the ipsilateral renal hilum. Stage IV disease is also difficult to assess when it is based on invasion of RCC into adjacent organs. Obliteration of the fat plane between RCC and the adjacent organ may occur without actual invasion in 15 percent of patients [14].

CT is also excellent for determining invasion of the renal vein and inferior vena cava by tumor thrombus. The renal veins can almost invariably be imaged. An enlarged ipsilateral renal vein without thrombus can be secondary to increased blood flow from arteriovenous shunting within the tumor. Dynamic thin-section CT scanning of the renal vein is recommended for the evaluation of possible tumor thrombus. After the level of the renal vein is determined, the patient is given an intravenous bolus of 75

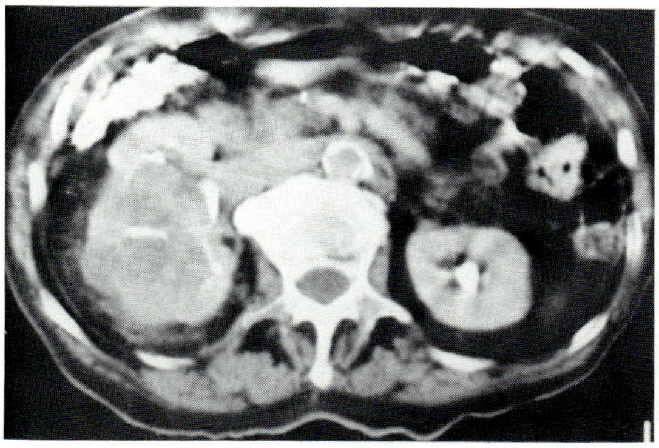

Figure 9-7. Renal cell carcinoma (Stage II). Contrast-enchanced CT section shows large, irregular right renal tumor with adjacent soft-tissue strands and small nodules extending into the perinephric fat.

to 100ml of contrast medium. Scanning is begun approximately 15 seconds after the initiation of the bolus administration, using 5-mm collimation and 5-mm table increments beginning slightly above the renal vein. Approximately 10 sections should be acquired as part of the dynamic sequence. Using this technique approximately 95 percent of tumor thrombi can be detected. The tumor thrombus within the renal vein or inferior vena cava usually presents as a lower attenuation defect (Fig. 9-8A), which on occasion may irregularly enhance [31]. At times, tumor involvement of the renal vein and inferior vena cava can be so gross that the diagnosis is obvious on CT without dynamic contrast studies (Fig. 9-9A).

Inferior vena cavography (Fig. 9-9B) and renal venography are often used when other imaging findings are equivocal regarding tumor thrombus involving the renal vein or inferior vena cava or when the extent of thrombus in the cava is in doubt. When the inferior vena cava is completely occluded, cavography may have to be performed from above and below to delineate the full length of the thrombus, which can, on occasion, extend into the right atrium.

Sonography has an accuracy roughly equivalent to that of CT in assessing the renal vein and inferior vena cava for tumor thrombi [21]. Venous tumor involvement is seen by sonography as an intravascular echogenic lesion (Fig. 9-8B). Sonography of the primary tumor shows a great deal of variability, including hypo-

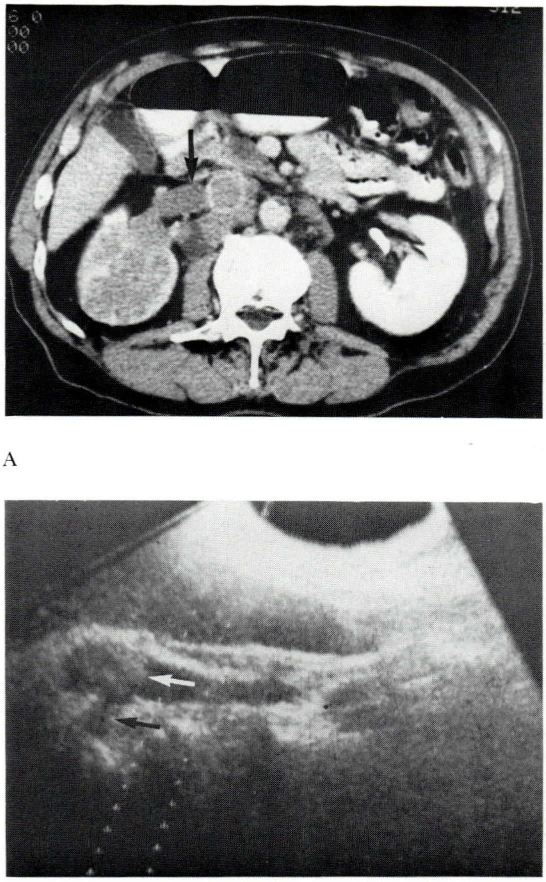

A

B

Figure 9-8. Renal cell carcinoma with tumor thrombus in renal vein and inferior vena cava (Stage III). A. Dynamic CT section at level of right renal vein shows tumor thrombus in renal vein (arrow) and extending into inferior vena cava. An enlarged retrocaval node in combination with the tumor thrombus makes this a Stage IIIC tumor. B. Sonography of inferior vena cava and right renal vein demonstrates tumor thrombus in the inferior vena cava (white arrow) extending from right renal vein (black arrow).

echoic, isoechoic, or hyperechoic solid lesions or a complex pattern (Fig. 9-10). Hyperechogenicity approaching that seen with angiomyolipoma is exhibited by approximately 5 percent of RCCs.

At present, MRI does not have the sensitivity demonstrated by CT for detecting small renal masses. Therefore it should not be used as a screening method for renal tumors. MRI of the primary tumor mass in RCC demonstrates

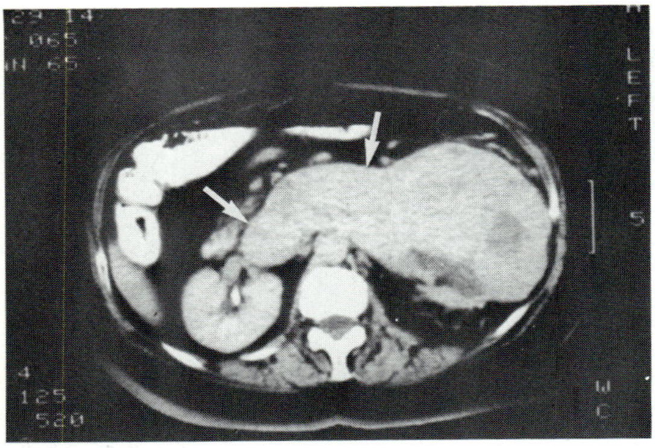

A

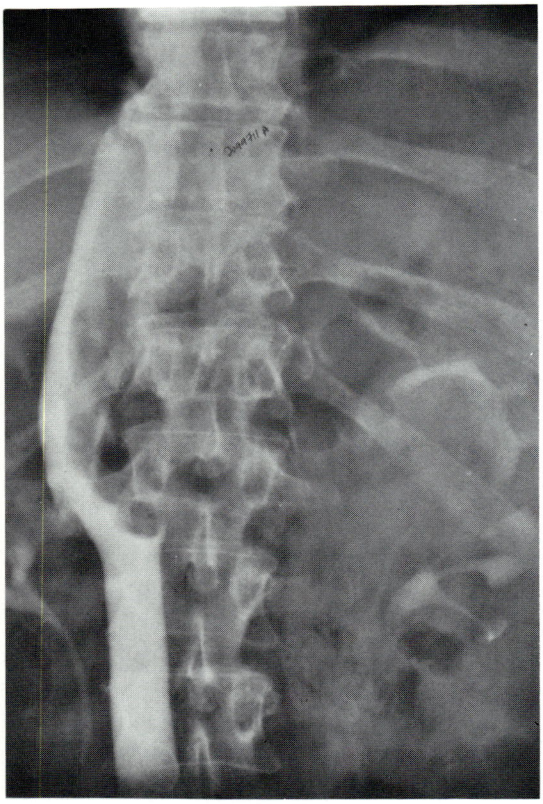

B

Figure 9-9. Renal cell carcinoma with massive tumor thrombus. A. Contrast-enchanced CT shows large left renal tumor growing through widened renal vein into cava (arrows). B. Inferior vena cavography shows a large intraluminal mass extending from the level of the renal veins to the diaphragm. C. Coronal T1 weighted MRI section at level of inferior vena cava also shows the tumor thrombus (T) outlined by lower-signal-flow void on the right (arrows). (Courtesy of Alan J. Davidson, M.D. Armed Forces Institute of Pathology, Washington, D.C.)

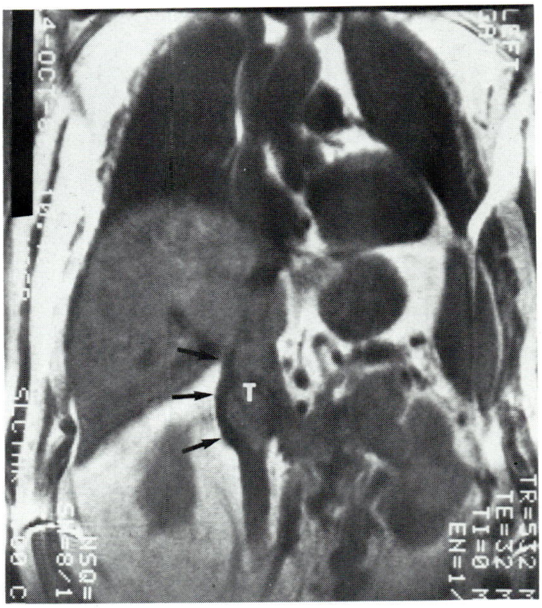

C

varied signal intensities, including isointensity with the normal renal parenchyma. The most common pattern is intermediate intensity on T1 weighted images, and a higher signal with T2 weighting (Fig. 9-11). These findings are nonspecific. However, it has been reported that the negative predictive value of MRI for the evaluation of tumor vascular extension is 98 percent and for tumor spread to adjacent structures, 99 percent [12]. The normal renal vein and inferior vena cava exhibit very low signal intensity because of flowing blood, while tumor thrombus in these vessels is seen as a mass with signal characteristics similar to the primary tumor (Fig. 9-9C). Therefore MRI has great potential as a staging modality. Like CT, MRI is not reliable in differentiating Stage I and II lesions or in determining the cause of slightly enlarged retroperitoneal lymph nodes. Current indications for staging of RCC with MRI include patients in whom the CT findings are equivocal and cases of inability to administer iodinated contrast media for CT scanning [8].

Renal arteriography is rarely used in patients with RCC. It has essentially no value in the detection, characterization, or staging of RCC as compared with the less invasive CT. Probably the only definite indication for preoperative

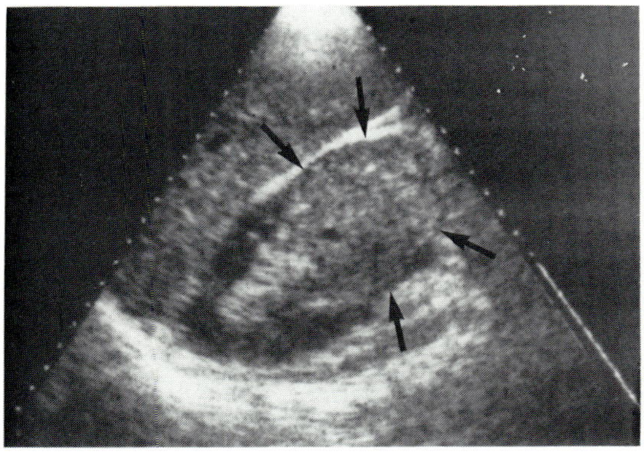

Figure 9-10. Sonography of renal cell carcinoma. In this case the tumor (arrows) involves the entire lower pole and is hyperechoic in relation to the normal renal parenchyma.

angiography is the need for vascular mapping (e.g., RCC occurring in a horseshoe kidney or prior to partial nephrectomy). When angiography is performed, the primary tumor exhibits a hypervascular pattern in approximately 75 percent of cases (Fig. 9-12), a hypovascular pattern in 20 percent, and an avascular pattern in the remaining 5 percent. The hypovascular and avascular tumors are more likely to be of the papillary histologic type.

WILMS' TUMOR

Clinical Factors

Wilms' tumor, also known as nephroblastoma, is the most common malignant abdominal tumor in children. Approximately 90 percent of children with this tumor will present with a palpable flank mass. The size of the tumor is usually quite large at the time of diagnosis, averaging 12 cm in diameter. There is a slight female predilection for the tumor. The peak age at which they are discovered is 2 years; 50 percent of all Wilms' tumors are discovered before the age of 3 and fully 75 percent before the age of 5. They are rare beyond the age of 10 but have been reported in young adults. Calcification is found in about 9 percent of cases. Symptoms include pain, malaise, fever, and weight loss. Microhematuria is common, though gross hematuria is not. An increased incidence of associated hypertension has been reported. Eighty-eight percent of Wilms' tumors are categorized as having favorable histology and 12 percent as having unfavorable histology.

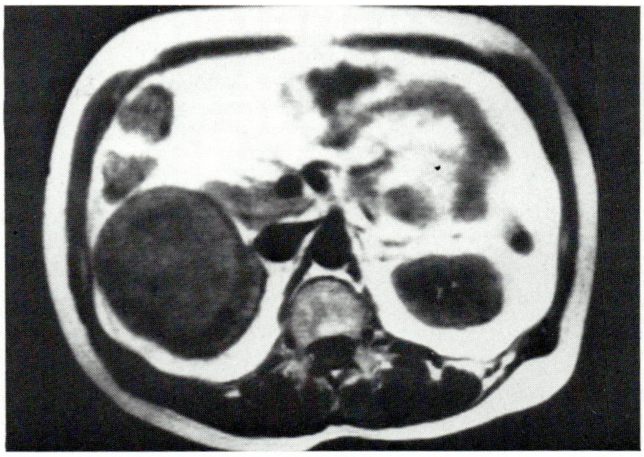

A

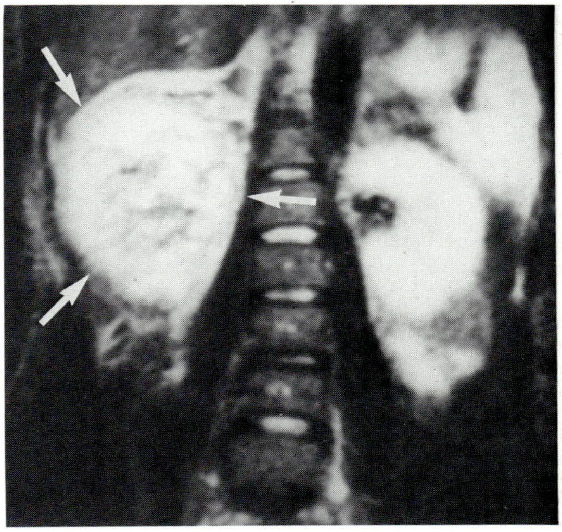

B

Figure 9-11. MRI of renal cell carcinoma. A. T1 weighted transverse section shows an inhomogeneous, moderately low signal intensity mass in the right kidney. Normal flow is seen in the aorta and cava. B. T2 weighted coronal section shows the tumor (arrows) to be of moderately high signal intensity and even more inhomogeneous.

Staging of Wilms' tumor is similar to that for renal cell carcinoma. These stages are given in Table 9-2. Renal vein or inferior vena cava involvement by tumor thrombus is found in 6 to 10 percent of patients. With current protocols combining surgical extirpation of the tumor, chemotherapy, and radiotherapy, the overall 5-year survival has reached 85 to 90 percent. For children with Stage I tumors, curability approaches 100 percent.

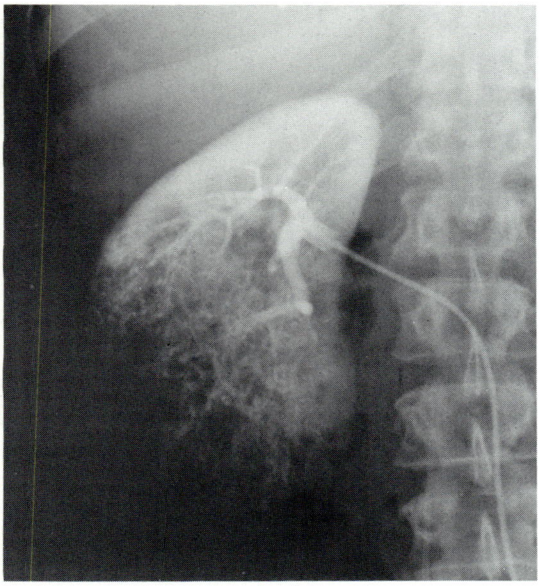

Figure 9-12. Typical hypervascularity of renal cell carcinoma. Right selective renal arteriogram shows a large, hypervascular, lower pole mass. Note the irregularity and tortuosity of the tumoral vessels.

Table 9.2. Staging of Wilms' tumor (nephroblastoma)

Stage I	No evidence of local spread
Stage II	Perinephric extension
Stage III	Lymph node involvement
Stage IV	Metastatic spread to liver, lung, or vena cava
Stage V	Bilateral tumors

Imaging Studies

On urography a Wilms' tumor presents as a large intrarenal mass distorting the collecting system (Fig. 9-13A). As with RCC, the major objective in staging a Wilms' tumor is the determination of the presence of local extension, venous or nodal involvement, and distant metastases. These are critical factors in assigning the patient to the proper treatment protocol. As would be expected, CT is excellent for staging this tumor; it provides the correct staging in 77 percent of patients [20]. CT findings in Wilms' tumor are similar to those already described for renal cell carcinoma (Fig. 9-13B).

Sonography of the primary tumor usually reveals a large size, sharp margination, and echogenic heterogeneity (Fig. 9-13C). Anechoic areas are frequently observed and are thought to correlate with hemorrhage and necrosis within the tumor. Mesoblastic nephroma, already discussed, appears to have similar sonographic features. The major differentiating factor between these lesions is the age of occurrence.

Reports have indicated that MRI has the potential for providing the same information as CT [3]. As with RCC, signal intensity of the primary tumor is highly variable and thus nonspecific in distinguishing Wilms' tumor from other solid tumors. Because it is noninvasive and does not employ ionizing radiation, MRI is thought to be well suited for pediatric imaging.

Nephroblastomatosis

No discussion of Wilms' tumor would be complete without mention of nephroblastomatosis. This condition is characterized by persistent metanephric blastema in the kidneys of infants and children. It is thought to occur as an arrest in normal nephrogenesis, resulting in persistence of residual blastema. Nephroblastomatosis is found in up to a third of kidneys with Wilms' tumor. In the normal term fetus, there is no remaining metanephric blastema.

Nephroblastomatosis may be either multifocal or diffuse [9]. In the multifocal type, involvement is usually microscopic but may manifest itself as Wilms' tumorlets, usually measuring less than 4 cm in diameter. In the less common diffuse variety the kidneys are significantly enlarged and sonography reveals multiple subcapsular and parenchymal hypoechoic areas. The nephromegaly and diminished parenchymal echogenicity in these cases can be mistaken for lymphoma sonographically. Patients with isolated nephroblastomatosis appear to be at risk for the subsequent development of Wilms' tumor, even though regression of the nephromegaly or nodules may occur.

TUMORS OF THE INTRARENAL COLLECTING SYSTEM

Clinical Factors

Transitional cell carcinoma (TCC) is the most common neoplasm of the renal collecting system and constitutes up to 7 to 8 percent of all malig-

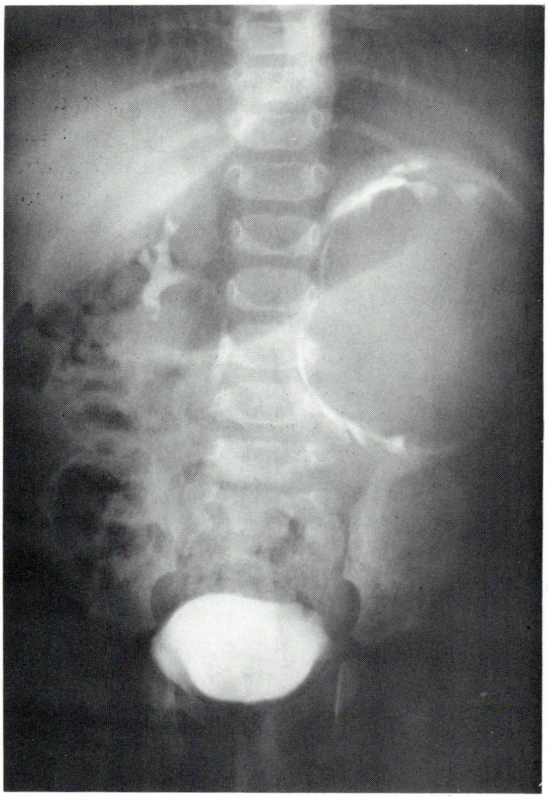

A

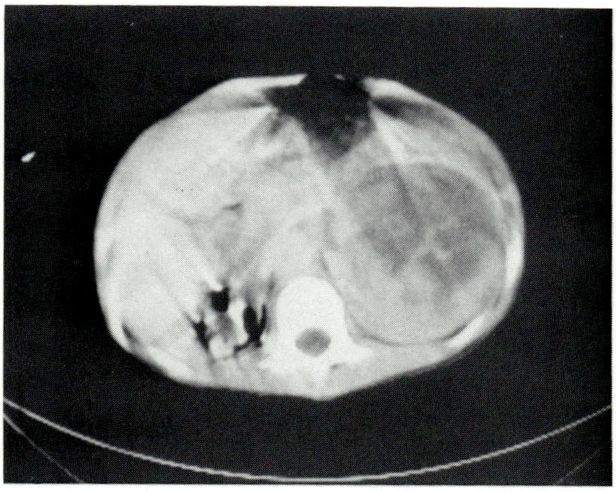

B

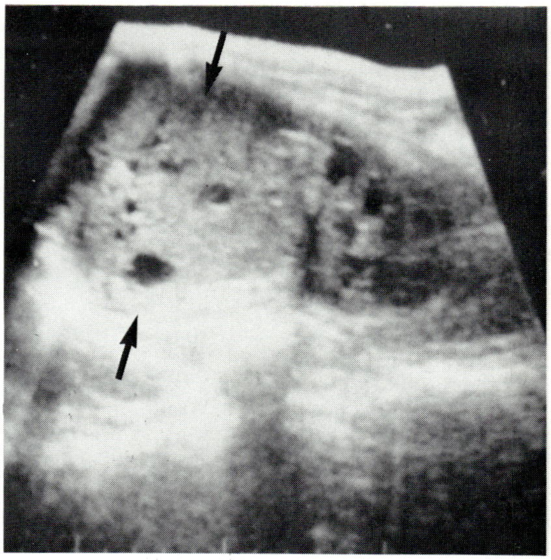

C

Figure 9-13. Wilm's tumor. A. Urography shows a large left intrarenal mass splaying the collecting system. B. CT section through mass reveals it to be inhomogeneous with lower-attenuation areas representing hemorrhage and necrosis. C. Sonography of the mass (arrows) shows it to be moderately echogenic with cystic areas of necrosis.

nant renal tumors. Squamous cell carcinoma, which may comprise up to 15 percent of malignant tumors occurring in the intrarenal collecting system, is usually associated with infection or stones. More debatable is its association with squamous metaplasia of the urothelium, which is also secondary to infection or irritation and typically results in mucosal plaques known as leukoplakia or sloughed keratin debris that forms a cholesteatoma (or "keratin ball") in the lumen of the collecting system. However, squamous cell carcinoma usually also presents as a plaque and is a highly lethal lesion. Even more rare is the mucinous adenocarcinoma that can occur in the collecting system. The remainder of this discussion will concern itself with transitional cell carcinoma.

TCC has a male sex predilection, men being affected three times more commonly than women. These tumors usually occur beyond age 60. Risk factors include analgesic abuse (predominantly phenacetin), exposure to aniline dyes or petroleum derivatives, heavy smoking, treatment with cyclophosphamide, and Balkan nephropathy. The reported incidence of bilateral synchronous TCC, metachronous upper tract TCC, or both ranges between 1 percent and 10 percent. Up to 40 percent of patients with renal TCC can be expected to present with bladder TCC between 15 and 48 months after discovery of the renal lesion [30]. Approximately 2 percent of TCC occurring in the intrarenal collecting system will calcify. Either microscopic or gross hematuria is common in patients with urothelial tumors.

Accurate staging, as with other tumors, is important in determining treatment regimen and prognosis. The stages of TCC are defined in Table 9-3. Tumor grade based on the degree of differentiation of the tumor histologically is also important in prognosis. Five-year survival for patients with Stage 0, A, or B disease is greater than 80 percent when treated by nephroureterectomy, which includes removal of a cuff of bladder in continuity with the distal ureter. The prognosis is much worse in the later stages of disease.

Imaging Studies

Even the few tumors that calcify are difficult to detect on plain films of the abdomen because of their small size. As previously noted, intravenous urography is the initial examination of choice for patients with suspected renal neoplasm. Moderate-sized transitional cell tumors are usually easy to detect as an irregular filling defect in the intrarenal collecting system (Fig. 9-14A). However, early lesions may be so subtle as to escape detection and large lesions, especially those in the renal pelvis near the ureteropelvic junction, may obstruct and prevent normal opacification of the collecting system. On occasion, an infundibular TCC may obstruct the infundibulum in which it lies and result in nonopacification of a portion of the intrarenal collecting system. In such cases it is important to ascertain whether the obstructing lesion is intraluminal (TCC) or whether it is a circumferential narrowing such as might occur with tuberculosis. This latter finding, however, can also occur with TCC.

Table 9-3. Staging of transitional cell carcinoma of intrarenal collecting system

Stage O	Tumor limited to mucosa
Stage A	Tumor invading lamina propria
Stage B	Tumor invading, but not beyond, the muscularis
Stage C	Tumor spreading beyond the muscularis into the sinus fat or renal parenchyma
Stage D	Distant metastases

Retrograde pyelography is usually indicated for better delineation of lesions suspected on urography, better opacification of a partially obstructed collecting system (Fig. 9-15A) and because it allows brushing of the lesion for more definitive histologic diagnosis. Urography and retrograde pyelography combined are about 95 percent accurate in detecting collecting-system malignancies; CT and ultrasonography are significantly less effective. However, CT is relatively effective in staging TCC in the collecting system. After administration of a contrast agent an intraluminal mass is usually identifiable in Stage 0, A, or B disease. While CT is not capable of detecting invasion of the muscular portion of the collecting system wall in these lower stage lesions, it usually shows the margins of the collecting system mass to be well defined (Fig. 9-14B). Scanning before the administration of contrast medium shows the tumor to be of soft-tissue density. Mild enhancement is noted after administration of a contrast agent in many patients. CT is usually capable of identifying Stage C disease when the mass has grown through the collecting system wall or infiltrated the kidney [2] (Fig. 9-15B). It is occasionally difficult to establish whether the lesion in the latter case is TCC growing into the kidney parenchyma or RCC growing into the collecting system.

The differential diagnosis for transitional cell carcinoma includes nonopaque urate stone, blood clot (in patients with gross hematuria), fungus ball, sloughed papilla, subepithelial hemorrhage, leukoplakia, cholesteatoma, and other collecting-system malignancies as previously discussed. CT is most effective in such cases in differentiating between urate stone and tumor. Urate stones will typically exhibit attenuation values of 300 or more Hounsfield units. Renal sonography has also been helpful in this regard since a urate stone will show a dense echogenic focus with acoustic shadowing. However, a similar finding can result when TCC is calcified [6]. Classically, sonography reveals a TCC in the collecting system as a solid mass causing separation of the central renal sinus echoes (Fig. 9-14C).

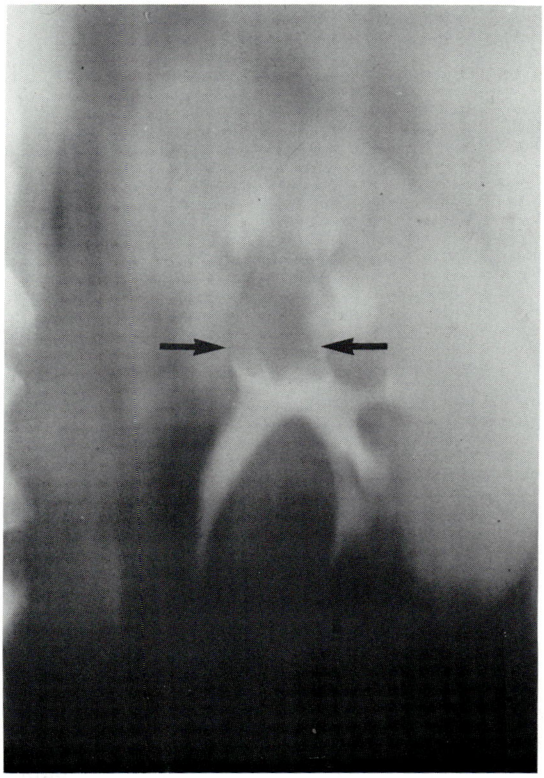

A

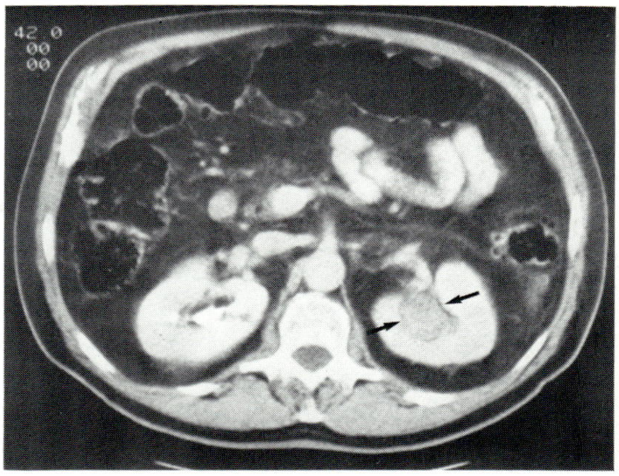

B

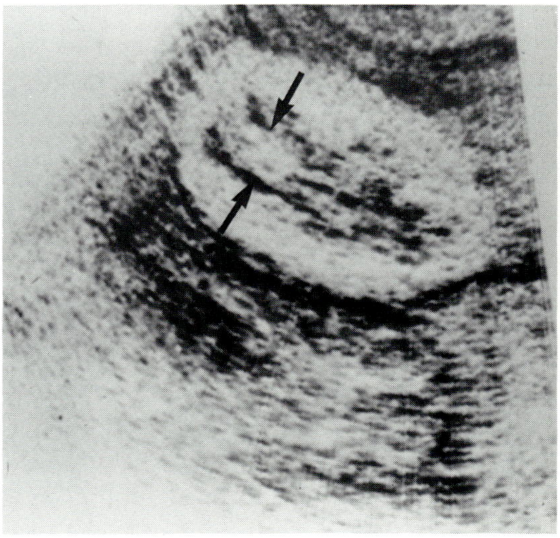

C

Figure 9-14. Transitional cell carcinoma of collecting system (Stage 0, A, or B). A. Nephrotomography shows filling defect (arrows) distending the upper-pole major infundibulum. The upper-pole calices are mildly dilated. B. CT shows a well-defined mass in the upper-pole collecting system of the left kidney (arrows). Sinus fat is intact. C. Sonography depicts the mass as a hypoechoic area "splitting" the sinus echoes in the upper pole (arrows).

RENAL SARCOMAS

Clinical Factors

Primary sarcomas of the kidney are relatively rare. The various mesenchymal cells found in the kidney provide a possibility for development of different histologic tumor types. The most common sarcomas seen in the kidney are leiomyosarcoma, fibrosarcoma, and liposarcoma [24]. Other sarcomas reported as involving the kidney include rhabdomyosarcoma, osteosarcoma, chondrosarcoma, malignant neurolemmoma, clear-cell sarcoma, angiosarcoma, and sarcomatoid carcinoma. Renal sarcomas usually occur in persons between the ages of 40 and 70 years. Men and women are approximately equally affected. Presenting symptoms include abdominal mass, pain, hematuria, and weight loss.

These tumors tend to arise from mesenchymal elements in the region of the renal sinus or in the renal capsule. They are usually well encapsulated. Sarcomas that originate in the renal parenchyma usually cannot be differentiated from RCC.

Imaging Studies

CT is useful in suggesting the diagnosis of renal sarcoma. In such cases, CT will typically

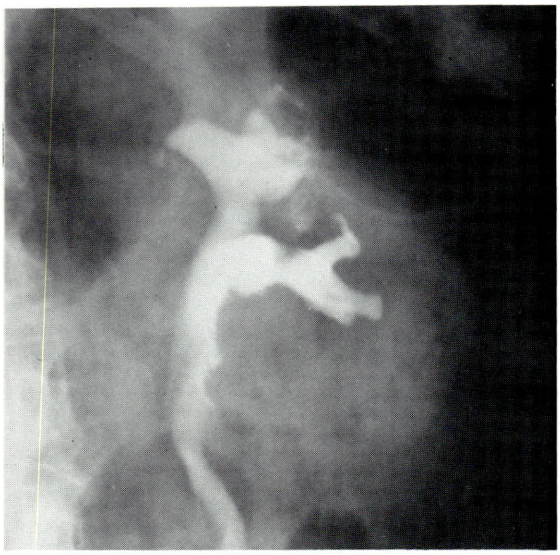

A

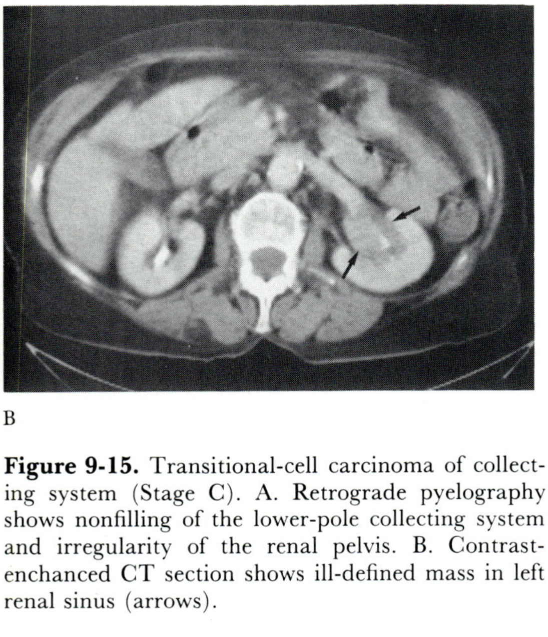

B

Figure 9-15. Transitional-cell carcinoma of collecting system (Stage C). A. Retrograde pyelography shows nonfilling of the lower-pole collecting system and irregularity of the renal pelvis. B. Contrast-enchanced CT section shows ill-defined mass in left renal sinus (arrows).

demonstrate a well-encapsulated neoplasm originating from the renal capsule, projecting into the perinephric space, and possibly indenting the underlying parenchyma. A lesion seen arising in the renal sinus, if not cystic, may also be considered of sarcomatous origin, though parenchymal tumors may also extend into the sinus. In cases of well-differentiated liposarcoma, the negative attenuation value of the fat within the tumor should suggest the diagnosis. Sarcomas do not usually involve the renal vein or the inferior vena cava. Angiography is nonspecific, usually showing an avascular or hypovascular mass with occasional areas of tumor neovascularity.

SECONDARY TUMORS OF THE KIDNEY

Metastatic tumors to the kidney are relatively common. However, they more frequently occur at the end stage of the neoplastic process and therefore are often not recognized until autopsy. Appoximately half of all metastases to the kidney are from the breast and lung. These are approximately equal in incidence. The kidney also represents one of the most common extranodal sites of metastatic lymphoma—only lung and breast tumors metastasize to the kidney more frequently [10]. Other metastatic lesions to the kidney include those from intestinal tumors and RCC of the opposite kidney. The kidneys may also be involved by leukemic infiltrates.

Metastatic foci in the kidney are usually clinically silent, but on occasion may cause pain or hematuria or both. Involvement may be by a solitary focal lesion, by multiple tumor foci, or by diffuse infiltration. In the case of a solitary metastasis, the major differential is that of a primary renal tumor. However, in patients with a known primary tumor outside the kidney, the presence of multiple solid renal masses should lead to the diagnosis of metastases. This can be confirmed by percutaneous aspiration biopsy if necessary.

On urography, one or more masses may be seen distorting the collecting system and the renal outline. In the cases with diffuse infiltration of the kidney, there may be renal enlargement with distortion of the collecting system or nonfunction. On ultrasonography the masses are usually hypoechoic or isoechoic as compared with the renal parenchyma. CT usually reveals one or more low attenuation masses that typically exhibit only mild enhancement after administration of intravenous contrast medium. If the metastatic process has diffusely infiltrated the kidney, CT will show a normal size or enlarged kidney with patchy, minimal, or no enhancement after intravenous contrast administration. The angiographic findings for metastatic lesions are usually similar to the vascular pattern of the primary tumor. These imaging findings, as described above, generally relate to metastases to the kidney from epithelial tumors.

The term *lymphoma* pertains to several distinct pathologic entities. However, the pathologic patterns of involvement of the kidney appear to be similar with these disease processes, though renal involvement is seen more frequently with non-Hodgkin's lymphoma than with Hodgkin's disease. Lymphoma to the kidney is usually secondary to hematogenous spread or direct extension of retroperitoneal lymphoma into the kidney. Renal involvement occurs in about a third of patients with lymphoma; bilateral involvement may occur in up to 75 percent of these cases [13]. As with the epithelial tumors, renal involvement may present as a solitary mass, multiple masses, or infiltration of the kidney by tumor. Involvement of the kidney by lymphoma is usually asymptomatic and is found late in the disease process after the diagnosis has been established.

Renal sonography often reveals the lymphomatous masses to be very hypoechoic. With multifocal lymphomatous lesions, the sonographic pattern may be confused with adult polycystic kidney disease (Fig. 9-16A). With careful technique, however, faint echoes can be seen within the nodular lesions, and poor through-transmission of sound can also be identified. CT is often helpful in identifying the lymphomatous origin of a focal or infiltrative renal process by demonstrating direct extension of the tumor from a retroperitoneal node mass (Fig. 9-16B).

American Burkitt's lymphoma, which also shows renal involvement in about one-third of cases, usually demonstrates a wider range of abnormalities. Burkitt's lymphoma is a type of non-Hodgkin's lymphoma occurring in Africa and North America forms. It is an aggressive neoplasm with a male preponderance, occurring in children around the age of 10 years. Renal sonography in these cases may reveal diffuse increase in renal cortical echogenicity, or focal masses, when present, may be hyperechoic or hypoechoic.

Leukemic cells can diffusely infiltrate the kidneys, resulting in enlargement and stretching,

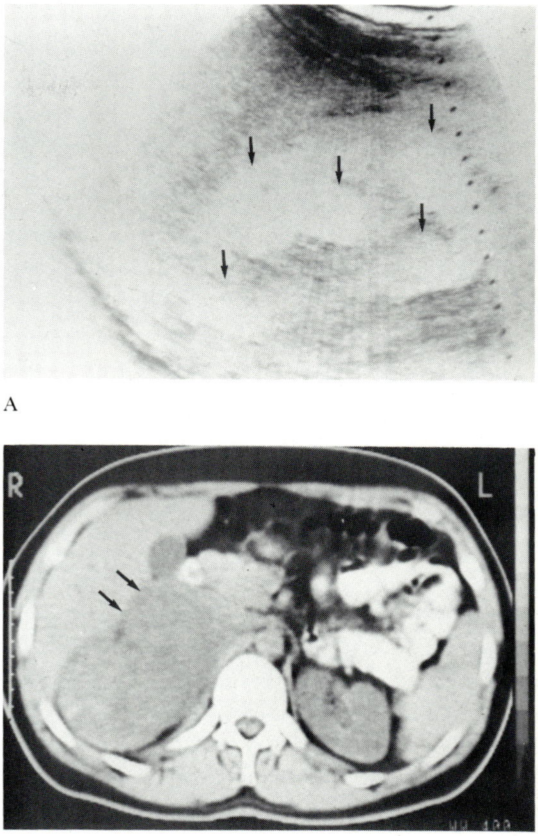

A

B

Figure 9-16. Lymphoma invading the kidney. A. Sonography shows multiple hypoechoic masses throughout kidney (arrows). The kidney is ill-defined. B. CT shows large retroperitoneal mass extending into kidney and enlarging it (arrows).

attenuation, or distortion of the collecting systems similar to that seen with polycystic disease or other infiltrative processes. During remission the kidneys return to normal.

MULTISYSTEM DISEASES ASSOCIATED WITH RENAL TUMORS

TUBEROUS SCLEROSIS

Tuberous sclerosis is an autosomal dominant hereditary disease characterized by mental retardation, adenoma sebaceum, and epilepsy. Multiple organs are usually involved, most commonly the brain and kidney. Renal hamartomas are the most common lesions after those of cerebral origin. These hamartomas, angiomyolipomas, occur in from 40 to 80 percent of patients with tuberous sclerosis. They are usually multiple and bilateral, usually appear before the age of 25 years, and tend to enlarge slowly.

Either single or multiple cysts also occur in 18 to 53 percent of patients with tuberous sclerosis [27]. This cystic involvement of the kidney may be so severe as to be confused with adult polycystic kidney disease [17]. There is also an uncommon association between tuberous sclerosis and RCC. Fortunately, RCCs occur in less than 5 percent of these patients, have a relatively benign nature, and tend not to metastasize. They are far more common in females and are bilateral in the majority of cases [29]. As with other renal cell carcinomas, calcification can occur in these tumors. Calcifications may also be seen in the walls of the renal cysts in tuberous sclerosis. Patients with tuberous sclerosis may be asymptomatic or have flank pain, palpable abdominal masses, hematuria, or even renal insufficiency.

CT or ultrasonography in patients with tuberous sclerosis will often reveal massively enlarged kidneys containing multiple cystic or solid lesions or both (Fig. 9-17A), or the kidneys may be normal in size with scattered cysts, tumors, or both (Fig. 9-17B). The angiomyolipomas will usually reveal the classic imaging characteristics previously described for that tumor. RCC can be suspected when solid lesions do not contain fat or are calcified.

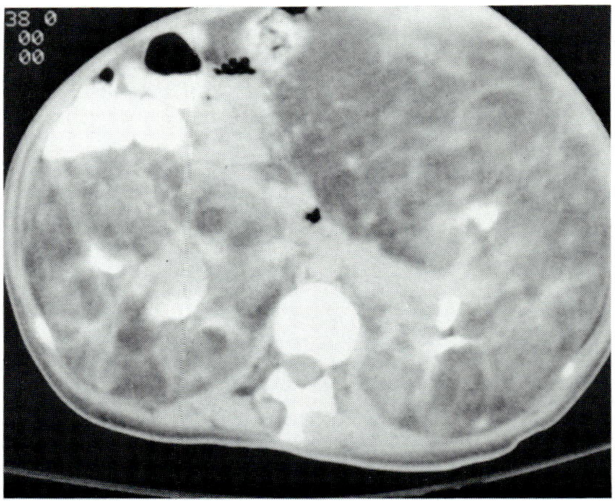

A

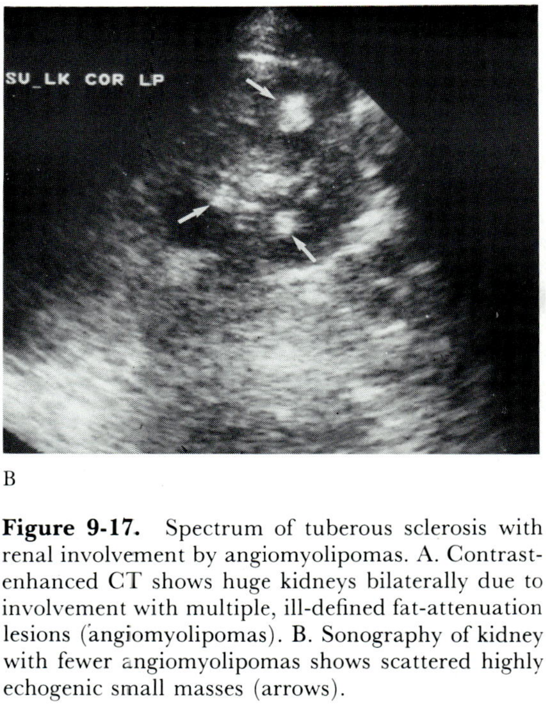

B

Figure 9-17. Spectrum of tuberous sclerosis with renal involvement by angiomyolipomas. A. Contrast-enhanced CT shows huge kidneys bilaterally due to involvement with multiple, ill-defined fat-attenuation lesions (angiomyolipomas). B. Sonography of kidney with fewer angiomyolipomas shows scattered highly echogenic small masses (arrows).

VON HIPPEL–LINDAU DISEASE

von Hippel–Lindau disease is a rare autosomal dominant disorder with variable penetrance associated with lesions in multiple systems. At least 25 distinct lesions have been described. The most frequently observed manifestations include retinal, cerebellar, and spinal hemangioblastomas, pheochromocytomas, pancreatic cysts, renal cysts, and RCCs [26]. RCCs occur in 38 to 55 percent of these patients; these tumors are often bilateral and multiple and tend to occur at an earlier age (usually about age 40) than sporadic RCCs in the general population. Unlike the renal cell carcinomas associated with tuberous sclerosis, these tumors have a well-recognized malignant potential. Simple renal cysts occur in up to 70 percent of von Hippel–Lindau patients. A few of these cysts have been reported to contain microscopic foci of RCC; this association is unrelated to cyst size.

Since RCC in von Hippel–Lindau disease exhibits virtually the same malignant potential as isolated RCC in adults, detection of these tumors when they are small is of great importance. They can be treated by local excision or simply by shelling out the lesion from the surrounding renal parenchyma.

Early RCCs complicating von Hippel–Lindau disease are difficult to detect by nephrotomography and sonography. Currently, CT of the abdomen appears to be the best screening method in family members at risk for this disease. This screening should begin around the age of 18 years and be conducted on an annual basis. Small renal cysts may be the earliest sign of von Hippel–Lindau disease detected during this screening regimen. The major roles of CT are to detect pheochromocytomas before patients are subjected to procedures such as angiography or cranial surgery and to detect RCC at an early stage, when it is amenable to local resection [15] (Fig. 9-18A). MRI is also useful in demonstrating the full extent of renal involvement (Fig. 9-18B) and in evaluating the adrenals in this disease. Patients with established von Hippel–Lindau disease clearly require annual study.

Figure 9-18. von Hippel–Lindau disease. A. Contrast-enhanced CT shows multiple simple cysts and renal cell carcinomas involving both kidneys. Note cystic change in the pancreatic head (arrow). B. Coronal T1 weighted MRI shows multiple cysts and tumors in the kidneys bilaterally.

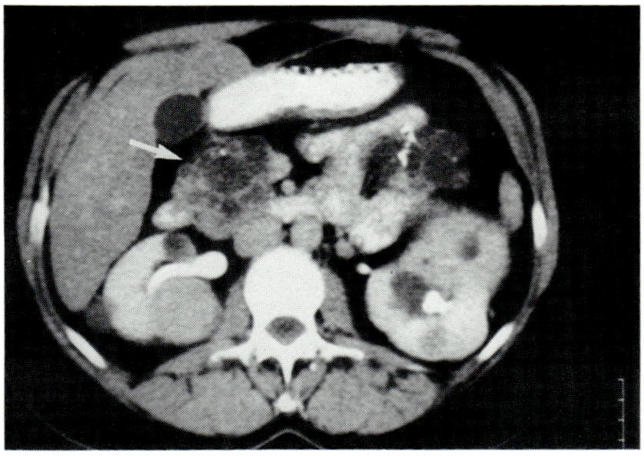

A

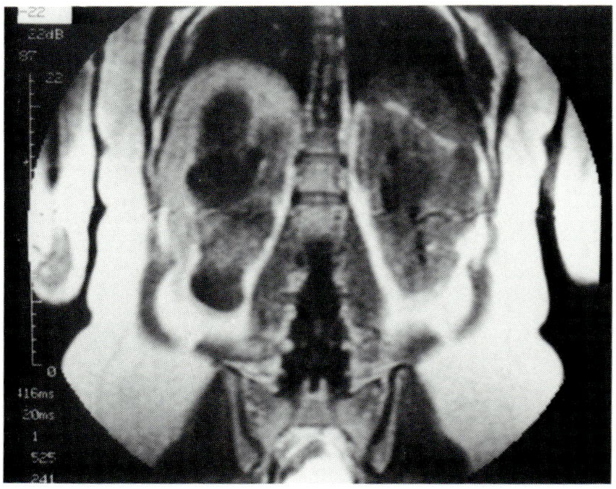

B

REFERENCES

1. Ambos, M.A., et al. Adrenal adenoma associated with renal cell carcinoma. *A.J.R.* 136:81, 1981.
2. Baron, R.L., et al. Computed tomography of transitional cell carcinoma of the renal pelvis and ureter. *Radiology* 1441:125, 1982.
3. Belt, T.G., et al. MRI of Wilm's tumor: Promise as the primary imaging method. *A.J.R.* 146:955, 1986.
4. Bosniak, M.A., et al. CT diagnosis of renal angiomyolipoma: The importance of detecting small amounts of fat. *A.J.R.* 151:497, 1988.
5. Curry, N.S., Schabel, S.I., and Betsill, W.L., Jr Small renal neoplasms: Diagnostic imaging, pathologic features, and clinical course. *Radiology* 158:113, 1986.
6 Dinsmore, B.J., Pollack, H.M., and Banner, M.P. Calcified transitional cell carcinoma of the renal pelvis. *Radiology* 167:401,1988.
7 Dunnick, N.R., et al. The radiology of juxtaglomerular tumors. *Radiology* 147:321, 1983.
8 Fein, A.B., et al. Diagnosis and staging of renal cell carcinoma: A comparison of MR imaging and CT. *A.J.R.* 148:749, 1987.
9 Franken, E.A., Jr., et al. Nephroblastomatosis: Clinicopathologic significance and imaging characteristics. *A.J.R.* 138:950, 1982.
10. Hartman, D.S., et al. Renal lymphoma: Radiologic-pathologic correlation of 21 cases. *Radiology* 144:759, 1982.
11. Hartman, D.S., et al. Mesoblastic nephroma: Radiologic-pathologic correlation of 20 cases. *A.J.R.* 136:69, 1981.
12. Hricak, H., et al. Detection and staging of renal neoplasms: A reassessment of MR imaging. *Radiology* 166:643, 1988.
13. Jafri, S.Z.H., et al. CT of renal and perirenal non-Hodgkin lymphoma. *A.J.R.* 138:1101, 1982.
14. Johnson, C.D., et al. Renal adenocarcinoma: CT staging of 100 tumors. *A.J.R.* 148:59, 1987.
15. Levine, E., et al. CT screening of abdomen in von Hippel-Lindau disease. *A.J.R.* 139:505,1982.
16. Madewell, J.E., et al. Multilocular cystic nephroma: A radiographic-pathologic correlation of 58 patients. *Radiology* 146:309, 1983.
17. Mitnick, J.S., et al. Cystic renal disease in tuberous sclerosis. *Radiology* 147:85, 1983.

18. Press, G.A., et al. Papillary renal cell carcinoma: CT and sonographic evaluation. *A.J.R.* 143:1005, 1984.
19. Quinn, M.J., et al. Renal oncocytoma: New observations. *Radiology* 153:49, 1984.
20. Reiman, T.A.H., Siegel, M.J., and Shackelford, G.D. Wilms tumors in children: Abdominal CT and US evaluation. *Radiology* 160:501, 1986.
21. Schwerk, W.B., Schwerk, W.N., and Rodeck, G. Venous renal tumor extension: A prospective US evaluation. *Radiology* 156:491, 1985.
22. Sherman, J.L., et al. Angiomyolipoma: Computed tomographic-pathologic correlation of 17 cases. *A.J.R.* 137:1221, 1981.
23. Sherman, M.E., et al. Multilocular renal cyst. *Arch. Pathol. Lab. Med.* 111:732, 1987.
24. Shirkhoda, A., and Lewis, E. Renal sarcoma and sarcomatoid renal cell carcinoma: CT and angiographic features. *Radiology* 162:353, 1987.
25. Smith, S.J., et al. Renal cell carcinoma: Earlier discovery and increased detection. *Radiology* 170:699, 1989.
26. Solomon, D., and Schwartz, A. Renal pathology in von Hippel-Lindau disease. *Hum. Pathol.* 19:1072, 1988.
27. Stillwell, J.T., Gomez, M.T., and Kelalis, P.P. Renal lesions in tuberous sclerosis. *J. Urol.* 138:477, 1987.
28. Warshauer, D.M., et al. Detection of renal masses: Sensitivities and specificities of excretory urography/linear tomography, US, and CT. *Radiology* 169:363, 1988.
29. Weinblatt, M.E., Kahn, E., and Kochen, J. Renal cell carcinoma in patients with tuberous sclerosis. *Pediatrics* 80:898, 1987.
30. Yousem, D.M., et al. Synchronous and metachronous transitional cell carcinoma of the urinary tract. Prevalence, incidence, and radiographic detection. *Radiology* 167:613, 1988.
31. Zeman, R.K., et al. Renal cell carcinoma: Dynamic thin-section CT assessment of vascular invasion and tumor vascularity. *Radiology* 167:393, 1988.

The Kidney: Indeterminate Masses

Simple renal cysts and renal cell carcinomas have been discussed in detail in Chaps. 8 and 9. In their classic presentations, there is usually no difficulty in differentiating these lesions by either sonography or CT if there is strict adherence to the criteria for diagnosing each lesion. However, benign renal cysts are not always simple and may exhibit characteristics suggestive of malignancy. Other benign cystic lesions in the kidney may also possess these characteristics. By the same token, renal cell carcinoma can undergo cystic degeneration or have a large cystic component and thus be indistinguishable from a complicated benign lesion. This spectrum between cyst and tumor will be discussed in this chapter.

EVOLUTION OF RENAL MASS EVALUATION

As recently as two decades ago, almost all renal masses detected on urography were surgically explored. After surgical determination of the nature of the lesion, malignancies were treated by radical nephrectomy and benign cysts were unroofed and their edges oversewn. Angiography, usually obtained preoperatively, was eventually found to have poor predictive capabilities in diagnosing the benign or malignant nature of avascular masses. With the advent of sonography in the mid-1970s, this method was used to characterize urographically discovered lesions. When the mass was seen to be cystic on nephrotomography, percutaneous needle punture was performed almost routinely. Cyst fluid was aspirated for cytology and fat stains—the latter usually thought to be positive in cases of cystic renal malignancies. With the needle still in place, the cyst cavity was opacified with contrast and "cystography" performed with imaging of the cyst wall in multiple planes to prove its smoothness. If these studies were all negative, the patient was presumed to have a benign cyst. After the development of CT, 100 percent accuracy was claimed in the diagnosis of a benign cyst [9]. It was suggested that renal cyst aspiration did not need to be performed when cystic lesions met all CT criteria for a benign cyst. CT thus became the gold standard for diagnosing renal cysts. Over the years, however, as technical advances were made with sonography, it too became highly accurate (98 percent) in diagnosing simple renal cysts [13]. Currently, the large majority of radiologists and urologists accept sonographic confirmation of the simple cysts seen on nephrotomography.

Since CT and ultrasonography have became more popular for evaluating multiple disease processes occurring within the abdomen, more and more incidental lesions have been discovered in the kidneys. Seven to nine percent of these renal masses are indeterminate [3, 17]. In such cases, the major clinical concern is the need for surgical exploration. Therefore, any subsequent evaluation must address this question.

NATURE OF INDETERMINATE RENAL MASSES

Before the imaging of indeterminate lesions can be discussed in any detail, it is necessary to define cystic changes that can be associated with renal cell carcinomas. The term *cystic degeneration of renal cell carcinoma* pertains to solid tumors that undergo central necrosis and hemorrhage due to the tumor outgrowing its blood supply. In such cases, less than 1 percent of the lesion's mass may be viable neoplastic tissue [11]. The necrotic areas within the tumor form pseudocystic lesions containing dark red or brown fluid consistent with old hemorrhage. On rare occasions the fluid may eventually become clear. As noted in Chap. 9, this type of cystic degeneration is common in renal cell carcinomas. On the other hand, a *cystic renal cell carcinoma* is a tumor that contains cystic elements not thought to be secondary to hemorrhage or necrosis; the fluid contained within the cystic structures is usually clear. Yet a third category is the *cystadenocarcinoma*, which is a primarily cystic lesion with a focus of renal cell carcinoma found within the wall or projecting into the lumen. The fluid in these lesions may be either clear or bloody. The postulated causes for this last category include a tumor nodule developing in the wall of a preexisting simple cyst, or a small renal cell carcinoma obstructing a tubule, resulting in the development of a cyst that eventually incorporates the primary tumor in its wall. Cytologic examination of the fluid in any of these lesions may be negative for malignant cells.

Complicated cysts, aside from those with idiopathic benign septations, usually result from hemorrhage or infection. Other benign lesions that occur in the indeterminate category include abscess, hematoma, pyocalix, infected pyelocaliceal diverticulum, and tuberculous cavity.

CATEGORIZATION OF INDETERMINATE RENAL MASSES

Bosniak [4] has categorized the spectrum of cystic renal masses seen on CT. He thought that it was important to set up criteria that would help to determine the best therapeutic approach to these lesions. Category I is a simple benign renal cyst meeting all criteria for benignity by both CT and ultrasonography as discussed in the chapter on renal cystic disease. Category II contains benign cystic lesions that are minimally complicated and for which experience is being accumulated that will hopefully allow the avoidance of surgery. Category III involves more complicated cystic lesions that exhibit some radiologic features seen in malignancy and therefore will most likely need surgical exploration. Category IV lesions include those that have a clearly malignant appearance and require surgery. Figure 10-1 diagrammatically depicts the spectrum of these lesions.

Within Category II, lesions exhibit imaging findings that cause concern: thin septations, rimlike wall calcifications, and high attenuation values on CT. The cystic lesions in Category III are more complicated. They exhibit radiologic findings suggestive of malignancy such as thicker or numerous septations, focal or diffuse thickening of the wall, and chunky or irregular wall calcifications. Some of these lesions will be benign and some will be malignant. Category IV lesions are clearly malignant by radiologic criteria even though they have large cystic components. These criteria include more centrally located calcifications, an obvious soft-tissue component of the mass, a discrete mural nodule, and some degree of enhancement after administration of contrast medium (Fig. 10-2). A few in this last category, however, will prove to be benign after surgical excision.

It must be emphasized that there are no significant reported series using the above classification on which recommendations to operate or not to operate can be based. In a small series at our institution, 22 primarily cystic lesions for which surgical proof existed were categorized based on CT findings without prior knowledge

Figure 10-1. Bosniak classification of cystic renal masses. Type I—Simple cyst. Type II—Thin "rim-like" calcification, thin septae, or hyperdense on CT. Type III—Thicker wall calcifications, thick septae, or thick wall. Type IV—Chunky calcification, thick, irregular wall, or eccentric cavity.

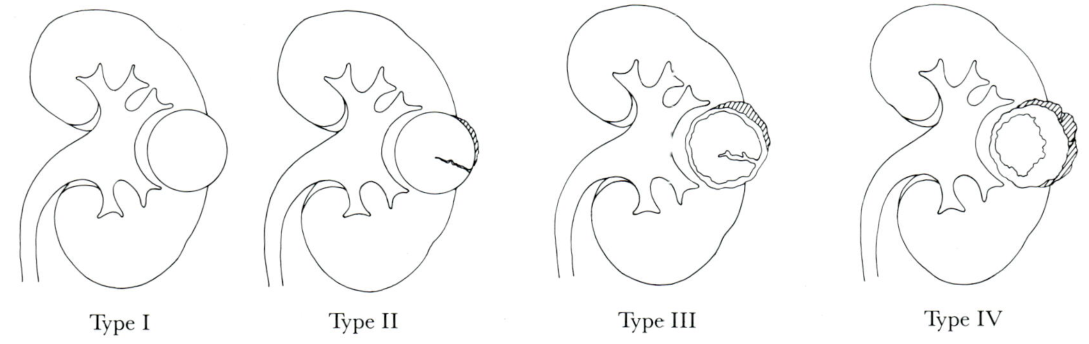

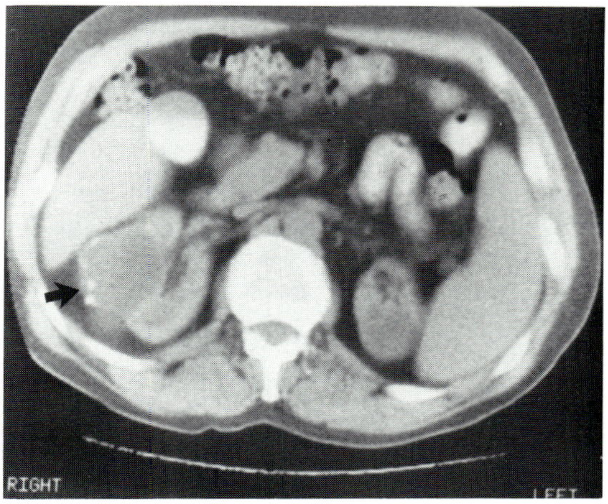

A

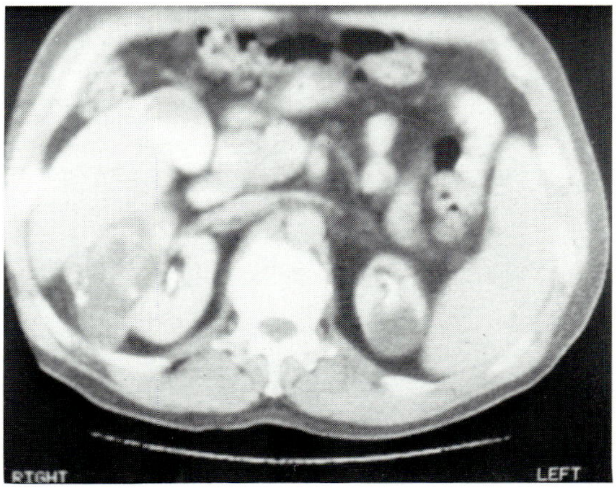

B

Figure 10-2. Enhancing soft-tissue component and calcification in cystic renal cell carcinoma (Bosniak Type IV). A. Precontrast CT shows chunky calcifications in wall of cystic right renal mass (arrow). Note simple cyst in left kidney. B. Postcontrast CT shows an enchancing soft-tissue component in the mass.

of their true cause. Of 4 lesions in Category II, the minimally complicated cyst, all were benign. Of 12 lesions assigned to Category III, 75 percent were benign, while the remaining 3 lesions were malignant. Of particular interest, of the 6 lesions placed in Category IV, 2 (33 percent) were found to be benign. It is obvious that histologic proof of the nature of a large number of indeterminate lesions will have to be gathered before definitive statements can be made about the need for surgery in a particular case as opposed to simple follow-up of a lesion that is presumed to be benign. The imaging findings suggestive of malignancy, such as septations, thick wall, hyperdensity, and calcification, will be discussed in more detail in the following section.

IMAGING FINDINGS SUGGESTIVE OF MALIGNANCY IN CYSTIC RENAL MASSES

SEPTATIONS

Fine septations are not uncommon in simple renal cysts. A cyst that meets all criteria for benignity by sonography or CT, with the addition of a thin septation and no other variation, can be considered benign [14]. The differential diagnostic considerations in such cases include simple cyst, inflammatory cyst, or hemorrhagic cyst. The septations in simple cysts are less than 1 mm in thickness, smooth, and are noted to attach to the wall of the cyst without associated thickening in that area (Fig. 10-3). When a mass contains multiple, irregular, or thick septations, or a thickening in the wall of the mass is noted at the point of attachment of the septa, these findings place the lesion in a higher category and probably mandate surgical exploration (Fig. 10-4). If septations within a lesion are numerous and irregular, a renal cell carcinoma becomes a possible diagnosis. The differential diagnosis in this case should also include multilocular cystic nephroma, which is a benign lesion.

WALL THICKENING

Thickening of the wall of a primarily cystic lesion has been recognized as a sign of potential malignancy since the early days of nephrotomography (Fig. 10-5). Even greater suspicion should be aroused when there is focal thickening or irregularity or a nodule seen at any point within the wall on CT or ultrasonography [10] (Fig. 10-6). Such lesions belong either in Category III or IV and usually require surgery. On occasion, the wall of a simple renal cyst may appear artificially thickened because of the location of the cyst near the renal margin; the thin layer of overlaying parenchyma in such

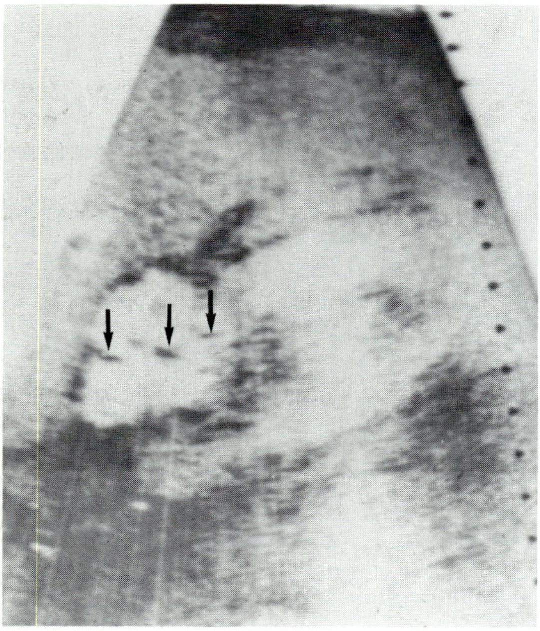

A

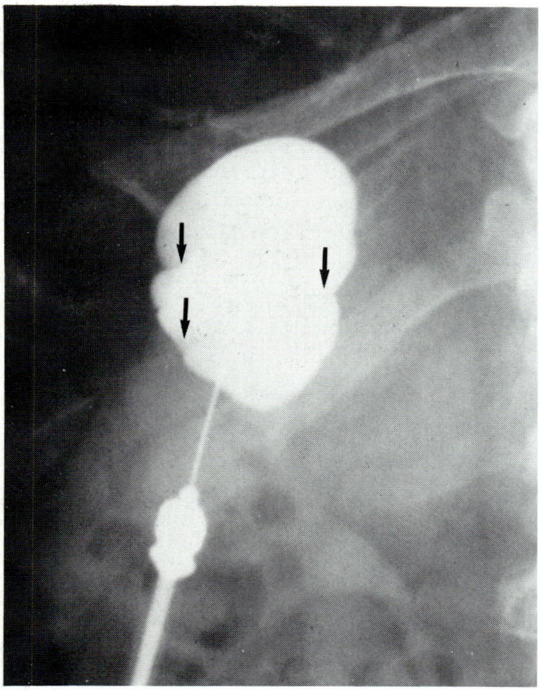

B

Figure 10-3. Septations in benign renal cyst (Bosniak Type II). A. Sonography of right kidney shows upper-pole mass to be cystic, though there are septations within the lumen (arrows). B. Percutaneous cyst puncture found clear cyst fluid with negative cytology. The septations are clearly seen (arrows). (From E.S. Amis Jr., J.J. Cronan, I.C. Yoder, R.C. Pfister, and J.H. Newhouse. Renal cysts: Curios and caveats. *Urol. Radiol.* 4:199, 1982.)

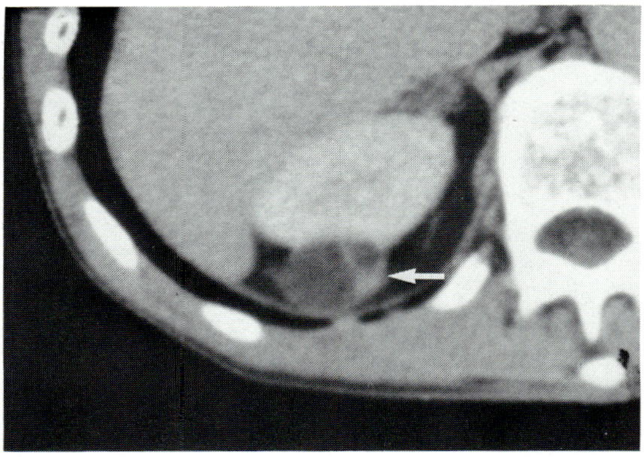

Figure 10-4. Septation in cystadenocarcinoma (Bosniak Type III). CT section shows predoninantly cystic mass in posterior right kidney. There is a single septation terminating in an area of nodular thickening of the wall (arrow).

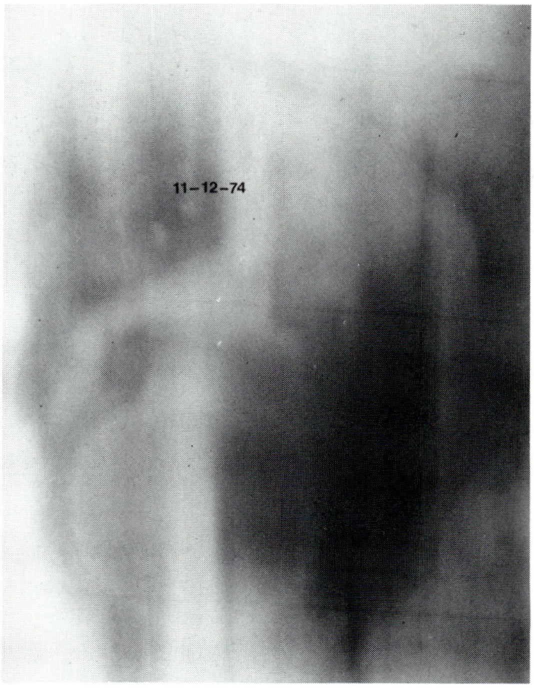

Figure 10-5. Thickening of wall in infected renal cyst. Nephrotomography shows a predominantly cystic mass in the lower pole of the left kidney. The wall is about 2 mm thick, as opposed to the paper-thin wall seen in uncomplicated simple cysts. Nephrotomography several months earlier had shown a normal thin wall, but the patient is now complaining of fever and left flank pain.

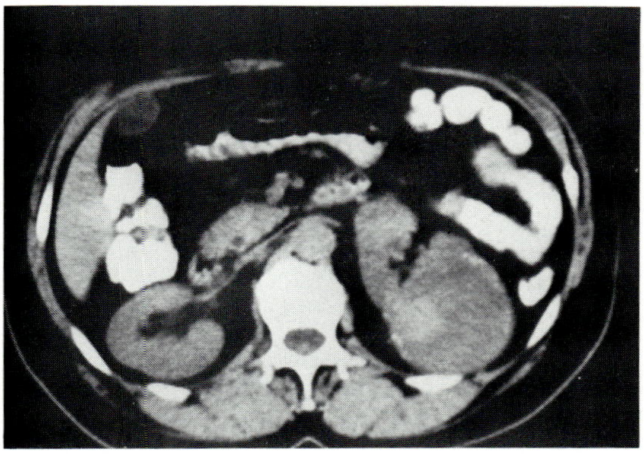

A

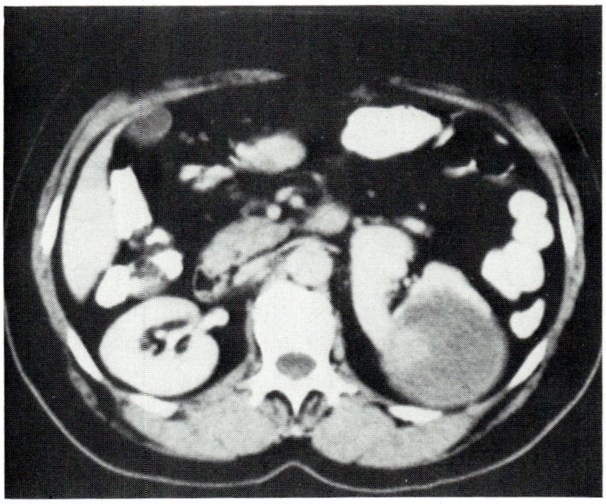

B

Figure 10-6. Mural nodule in cystadenocarcinoma (Bosniak Type IV). A. Precontrast CT shows a cystic mass in the left kidney with faint wall calcifications and a discrete 1.5-cm mural nodule. B. Post-contrast CT shows slight enhancement of the nodule.

cases should not be mistaken for the wall of the lesion [2] (Fig. 10-7).

CT HYPERDENSITY

High-density renal masses are unusual lesions detected by CT that represent a further diagnostic dilemma. The differential diagnosis is mainly between complicated benign cysts and malignant neoplasms. These masses are usually well-circumscribed and exceed the density of the adjacent renal parenchyma on CT scans without contrast medium (Fig. 10-8A). They tend to have attenuation values of 50 Hounsfield units or more [5]. They often measure 25 to 60 Hounsfield units greater than the adjacent

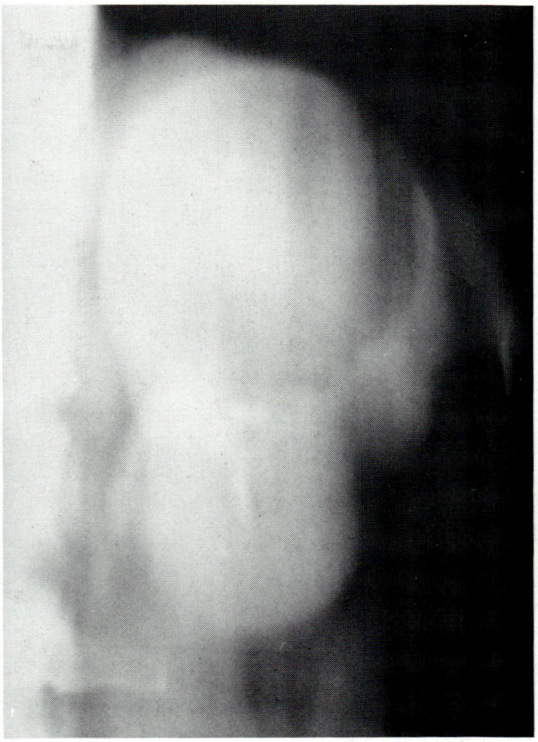

Figure 10-7. Pseudothick cyst wall. Nephrotomography shows cystic mass in the upper pole of left kidney. The thick appearance of the wall is due to compressed normal parenchyma surrounding the upper half of the cyst. Confirmed as benign by cyst puncture. (From E.S. Amis, Jr., J.J. Cronan, I.C. Yoder, R.C. Pfister, and J.H. Newhouse. Renal cysts: Curios and caveats. *Urol. Radiol.* 4:199, 1982.)

parenchyma and after the administration of intravenous contrast agent can be hypodense, isodense, or more dense in relation to the adjacent parenchyma. However, there is no significant enhancement of the lesion itself after administration of intravenous contrast medium.

Solid renal tumors may appear denser than unenhanced normal parenchyma on CT, but they are generally less dense relative to the kidney than are the true hyperdense cysts [18]. A solid renal tumor, usually a papillary renal cell carcinoma, may fail to enhance after the administration of intravenous contrast medium. However, the large majority of hyperdense lesions are complicated cysts, the hyperdensity in most cases being due to hemorrhage within a simple cyst. From 1 to 11.5 percent of all benign simple cysts are reported to be hemorrhagic

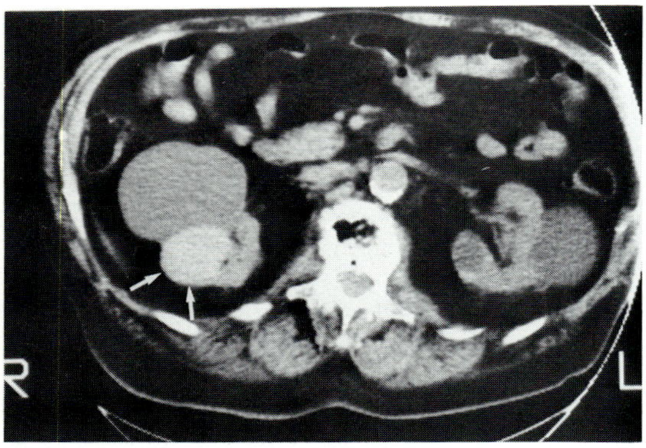

A

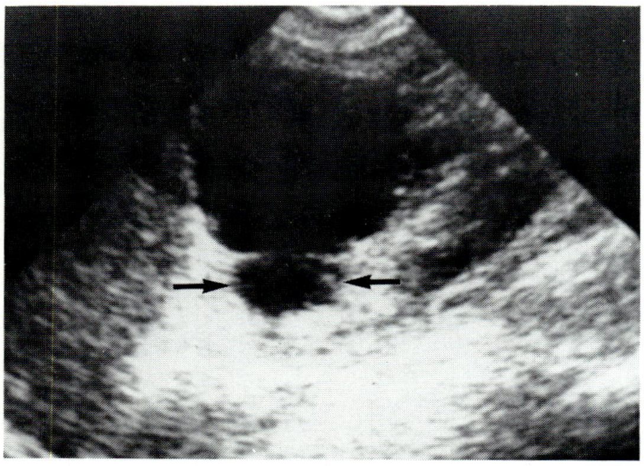

B

Figure 10-8. Hyperdense cyst (Bosniak Type II). A. Nonenhanced CT section shows multiple renal lesions. On the right, one mass (arrows) has a density higher than the adjacent normal renal parenchyma. The lesion did not enhance after administration of an intravenous contrast agent. B. Sonography shows the mass to be echo-free (arrows). The larger echo-free area anterior to the hyperdense cyst is the large cyst seen on CT.

[15]. The incidence appears to be even greater in patients with autosomal dominant polycystic disease of the kidney, at least one such dense hemorrhagic cyst being found in most patients with fully developed disease. The increased density of these cysts is probably due to the fact that clot retraction after hemorrhage concentrates the protein contents of the blood. It has also been postulated that an elevated iron content resulting from remote hemorrhage can result in this finding. Calcified debris has also been reported in some of these lesions. The cyst contents may be fluid or may be in the form of a firm coagulum that is impossible to aspirate. It is recommended that hyperdense lesions over 1.5 cm in diameter be studied by sonography. If the lesion fulfills all the sonographic criteria for benign cyst, it can be presumed to be a benign hemorrhagic cyst (Fig. 10-8B). However, old hemorrhage within a cyst may result in faint internal echoes and more attenuation of sound than would be seen with normal cyst fluid. In such cases, demonstration of the fluid nature of the mass is currently considered adequate criteria for recommending observation rather than surgery. Some reports have suggested that needle puncture of hyperdense cysts, if their contents are fluid, is indicated to confirm their benign nature.

CALCIFICATIONS

Calcification in both renal cysts and tumors has been mentioned in Chaps. 8 and 9 . Whenever calcification is seen in association with a renal mass, regardless of its configuration or location within the mass, the likelihood that the lesion is malignant is at least 50 percent. Calcification is usually categorized by pattern and location. Calcific patterns include amorphous, mottled, punctate, wavy, and curvilinear. The apparent location of the calcification, which is probably more meaningful than its pattern in differentiating cysts from tumor, can be peripheral or central. Calcification located centrally within a mass indicates a malignant lesion in over 90 percent of cases. Isolated peripheral rimlike calcification, while usually associated with benign simple cyst, still indicates a 20 percent risk of malignancy [7] (Fig. 10-9). On the other hand, benign cysts with more centrally located calcifications have been reported [8.]

When imaging calcified masses with CT, the most important factors in the determination of benign versus malignant lesions are a soft-tissue mass extending beyond the calcification (92 percent malignant) or a uniform nonenhancing water density center with calcification confined to the wall and no soft-tissue mass (approaching 100 percent benign) [2]. Since up to 70 percent of calcified renal cell carcinomas may be of the papillary type and therefore either hypovascular or avascular, enhancement on CT may not be seen [16]. Ultrasonography will be necessary

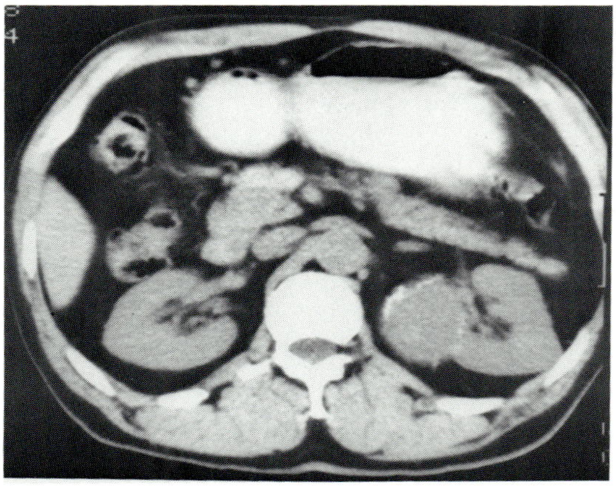

Figure 10-9. Peripheral calcifications in complicated cyst (Bosniak Type III). CT shows chunky rim calcifications in a nonenhancing cystic left renal mass. This proved to be a complicated benign cyst at surgical exploration.

in such cases to confirm the solid nature of the lesion. The calcified nonpapillary renal cell carcinomas, on the other hand, usually show inhomogeneous enhancement, unless there is a significant cystic component.

Aside from complicated cysts and calcified renal cell carcinomas, multiple other renal lesions may contain radiographically detectable calcification. Other tumors that can calcify include Wilms' tumor, transitional cell carcinoma, metastatic tumors to the kidney, angiomyolipomas, and very infrequently, oncocytomas. Benign lesions that can calcify include abscesses, tuberculous granulomas, hematomas, arteriovenous malformations, aneurysms of the renal artery, multilocular cystic nephromas, multicystic or polycystic kidneys, and echinococcal cysts. Most of these lesions have fairly typical radiographic characteristics that will allow them to be diagnosed with some degree of confidence, unlike the indeterminate lesions.

ADJUNCTIVE CYST PUNCTURE

After taking into account all of the imaging characteristics of an indeterminate renal mass as noted above, it is clear that even after evaluation with CT and sonography, a definitive diagnosis cannot always be reached. This is particularly true in Bosniak Categories II and III. Cyst puncture has been advocated in such cases as an adjunctive measure in increasing diagnostic accuracy. However, most radiologists believe that the information obtained by cyst puncture and opacification of the cystic lesion is available on ultrasonography and CT. Two surveys on the use of cyst puncture are of interest. In one, of 20 leading uroradiologists at large medical centers, 16 indicated that cyst puncture was performed in their institution less than 10 times per year. Most of the respondents indicated that the need for and use of the procedure has greatly decreased [4]. Another survey, this time of members of the Society of Uroradiology, indicated that the major indication for cyst puncture is conflicting results on two or more imaging methods [1]. Probably the major reason for this declining use of cyst puncture is the fact that clear fluid with negative cytology may occasionally be found in cases of cystic or necrotic renal cell carcinomas, as well as when renal cell carcinoma occurs in the wall of a cyst (cystadenocarcinoma). Conversely, false positive cytologies have been reported in benign renal cystic lesions. Furthermore, cystic malignancies with smooth walls have been reported [6]. Therefore, although the gross and laboratory characteristics of fluid aspirated from cystic renal masses in conjunction with the appearance of the wall can suggest the nature of the lesion, these findings are not always conclusively diagnostic. Thus, a negative aspirate in the face of imaging features suggesting malignancy should not change the decision to recommend surgical therapy.

RECOMMENDATIONS

Given the current status of imaging indeterminate renal masses, the philosophies of both the radiologist and referring physician concerning such lesions will vary from institution to institution, and it would be unwise to make a definitive statement regarding which lesions should be surgically explored. Certainly, benign simple cysts (Category I), once diagnosed, do not need follow-up or surgery. Category II lesions are probably benign and can probably be followed safely by imaging at regular intervals for 1 or 2 years to rule our growth or other change. Masses in Category III probably warrant surgical exploration based on a current knowledge. Category IV masses definitely require surgery, even though a few of these will be benign complicated cystic lesions.

Other parameters must, of course, be considered in the decision-making process. These in clude the age and overall physical condition of the patient at the time of discovery of the renal mass. In an elderly patient who is a poor surgical candidate, the natural history of a possibly malignant renal lesion, which can be slow growing, might not warrant a recommendation for surgery. On the other hand, the patient must be fully informed of the risk that a renal lesion might be malignant as compared with the risk inherent in surgical treatment. Once so informed, the final decision regarding treatment rests with the patient.

REFERENCES

1. Amis, E.S., Jr., Cronan, J.J., and Pfister, R.C. Needle puncture of cystic renal masses: A survey of the Society of Uroradiology. *A.J.R.* 148:297, 1987.
2. Amis, E.S., Jr., et al. Renal cysts: Curios and caveats. *Urol. Radiol.* 4:199, 1982.
3. Balfe, D.M., et al. Evaluation of renal masses considered indeterminate on computed tomography. *Radiology* 142:421, 1982.
4. Bosniak, M.A. The current radiological approach to renal cysts. *Radiology* 158:1, 1986.
5. Coleman, B.G., et al. Hyperdense renal masses: A computed tomographic dilemma. *A.J.R.* 143:291, 1984.
6. Curry, N.S., et al. An evaluation of the effectiveness of CT vs. other imaging modalities in the diagnosis of atypical renal masses. *Invest. Radiol.* 19:447, 1984.
7. Daniel, W.W., et al. Calcified renal masses: A review of ten years experience at the Mayo Clinic. *Radiology* 103:503, 1972.
8. Love, L., and Yedlicka, J. Computed tomography of internally calcified renal cysts. *A.J.R.* 145:1225, 1985.
9. McClennan, B.L., et al. CT of the renal cyst: Is cyst aspiration necessary? *A.J.R.* 133:671, 1979.
10. Novetsky, G.J., et al. CT diagnosis of renal cyst wall tumor *J. Comput. Assist. Tomogr.* 7:539, 1983.
11. Parienty, R.A., Pradel, J., and Parienty, I. Cystic renal cancers: CT characteristics. *Radiology* 157:741, 1985.
12. Patterson, J., et al. Calcified renal masses. *Urology* 29:353, 1987.
13. Pollack, H.M., et al. The accuracy of gray-scale renal ultrasonography in differentiating cystic neoplasms from benign cysts. *Radiology* 143:741, 1982.
14. Rosenberg, E.R., et al. The significance of septations in a renal cyst. *A.J.R.* 144:593, 1985.
15. Sussman, S., et al. Hyperdense renal masses: A CT manifestation of hemorrhagic renal cysts. *Radiology* 150:207, 1984.
16. Weyman, P.J., et al. CT of calcified renal masses. *A.J.R.* 138:1095, 1982.
17. Zeman, R.K., et al. Computed tomography of renal masses: Pitfalls and anatomic variants. *RadioGraphics* 6:351, 1986.
18. Zirinsky, K., et al. CT of the hyperdense renal cyst: Sonographic correlation. *A.J.R.* 143:151, 1984.

11

The Kidney: Inflammation

Inflammatory diseases of the kidney may have a variety of causes and may be associated with a number of abnormalities elsewhere in the urinary tract. This chapter will deal with the infectious diseases of the kidney that are important in urinary tract radiology and some infectious and inflammatory conditions that involve the collecting system and perinephric space. Inflammatory conditions that commonly involve only the ureters and lower urinary tract are dealt with in Chaps. 19 and 20.

BACTERIAL INFECTION OF THE KIDNEY AND URINARY TRACT

ETIOLOGIC AGENTS AND ROUTES OF INFECTION

The most common organisms to infect the urinary tract—at least in Western society—are gram-negative bowel flora, of which *Escherichia coli* is the most common [3]. Less frequently encountered, but still important, are species of proteus and klebsiella. The route of infection from bowel organisms is thought usually to be retrograde; perineal bacteria may traverse the urethra (especially the shorter female urethra) and infect bladder urine; retrograde infection of the upper tracts may follow. Less frequently, renal infection may be hematogenous in origin, with the offending bacteria originating from the skin or other foci of infection. Renal infection has also been postulated to occur sometimes by a lymphatic route, but compeling evidence for this is lacking.

Renal infection may appear in anatomically normal urinary tracts, but many abnormalities of both structure and function of the hollow urinary viscera may cause renal infection to appear more frequently and become more severe. Both upper- and lower-tract obstruction, no matter what the cause, may predispose to infection. Since ureteral peristalsis and periodic complete bladder emptying serve to wash out infecting bacteria in the normal urinary tract, obstruction that dilates the upper tract and interferes with peristalsis and prevents complete bladder emptying may slow the outward flow of urine and provide a constant reservoir for bacterial multiplication. Vesicoureteral reflux also promotes more severe infection: Clearly, infection may travel from the bladder urine to the calices and renal tubules much more easily if retrograde flow of urine occurs than if effective peristalsis causes the net flow of urine to be away from the kidney. Urinary stones, whether obstructing or not, may harbor bacteria in their interstices and thus continually recontaminate urine even if natural defense mechanisms or antibiotic therapy temporarily free the urine of pathogens. Also, certain renal parenchymal diseases, including those that involve focal renal scarring, may create local conditions in which both natural defenses and antibiotic therapy may be less able to eradicate infection from the affected portion of the renal parenchyma. Rarely, fistulae between the urinary tract and gut or foci of inflammation or abscesses adjacent to urinary structures may directly contaminate the urinary tract. Patients whose urinary tracts are intubated may undergo nearly constant urinary tract contamination from outside sources.

Systemic abnormalities may predispose to urinary infection as well. Both glycosuria and ineffective immune systems predispose diabetics to urinary infection; chronic granulomatous disease of childhood, acquired immune deficiency syndrome (AIDS), antineoplastic chemotherapy, or even extreme old age may make the urinary tract more vulnerable to infection.

SIGNS AND SYMPTOMS

The clinical diagnosis of urinary infection may be straightforward, especially in adults. Fever, flank pain, suprapubic discomfort, dysuria, urgency, frequency, and foul-smelling or cloudy urine may all suggest the diagnosis. In children too young to describe symptoms, the diagnosis may be more difficult; fever, failure to thrive, anemia, irritability, and other nonspecific systemic signs may be the only manifestations of urinary infection. Urinary infection may also be asymptomatic in both adults and children.

The laboratory diagnosis usually depends on recovery of significant numbers of bacteria from the urine, especially in samples collected by methods that minimize contamination. Pyuria is frequent; casts suggest involvement of the renal parenchyma.

GENERAL PRINCIPLES OF RADIOLOGIC EVALUATION

There is some controversy regarding which patients with urinary infection should be subjected to radiologic workup and exactly what that workup should be; these issues revolve around the prevalence of particular abnormalities in patients with urinary infection in particular age groups [2, 21, 33], and the sensitivity of the various techniques and methods for detecting these abnormalities.

In the newborn, urinary infection is at least as common in males as in females. Baby boys with urinary infection have a relatively high incidence of congenital urinary anomalies, particularly various combinations of posterior urethral valves and vesicoureteral reflux; all such babies should be investigated radiologically. Baby girls with urinary infection have a somewhat lower prevalence of anomalies requiring treatment, and their incidence of urinary infection is several times that of boys, especially as they become toddlers and reach school age. There has therefore been some controversy about whether a young girl with urinary infection should be investigated radiologically after a single urinary infection or whether workup should be withheld until the second or third infection.

There is also some controversy about the specific imaging examination to be used in young children with urinary infection. Since vesicoureteral reflux is commonly encountered in these children, voiding cystourethrography (VCUG) is an absolute necessity, whether performed fluoroscopically or as a radionuclide cystogram. In males, since the anatomic details of the urethra are particularly important, a radiographic VCUG should be performed. In girls the urethra is very rarely abnormal, so detection and quantification of reflux becomes the major task; for this, radionuclide cystography delivers a smaller radiation dose and may be slightly more sensitive than fluoroscopic cystourethrography and thus is preferred by some investigators [45]. In young children with urinary tract infection the upper tracts may be imaged [47] by intravenous urography, ultrasonography, or radionuclide scanning. Of these, intravenous urography carries the highest risk of adverse reaction and the highest radiation dose but probably provides the finest anatomic detail within the kidneys and calices. Sonography may fail to detect minor parenchymal scars but certainly will detect severely scarred or shrunken kidneys and should display any significant hydronephrosis or congenital renal anomaly. Radionuclide scanning, performed with agents handled either by glomerular filtration or tubular-cell uptake, may provide the most quantitative information about renal function but the least detailed anatomy. Authorities differ with regard to which should be used; there has been a trend to replace intravenous urography with urinary tract ultrasonography. For girls whose intravenous urograms are normal, some investigators suggest that studies to detect reflux may be omitted.

In adults the principles of designing radiologic workups differ [4, 13]. In young adult women, urinary tract infections are relatively common, with an incidence considerably higher than that found in young men, and there is an increased incidence associated with pregnancy. But the yield of abnormalities requiring treatment revealed by urography in young women—especially those who have had only one infection—is quite low and may not be very different from that which would be encountered in a randomly chosen sample of young women. Therefore there is no widespread conviction that urography should be performed on all young women—pregnant or not—after a first urinary infection. Multiple infections or infections particularly resistant to antibiotic therapy, however, may prompt radiologic workup, and in these women intravenous urography is still the most commonly performed examination, since the yield of ultrasonography and other imaging techniques in this population has not been widely investigated. An intermediate step might be to obtain a single film of the abdomen, since calcified stones may be seen in the small group of young women whose urinary infections are associated with anatomic abnormalities.

In older adults imaging investigation is usually withheld unless infections are numerous or resistant to therapy. In elderly men, associated symptoms suggesting prostatism may prompt imaging investigation even in patients whose urinary infections have not been a major problem.

ACUTE PYELONEPHRITIS

PATHOLOGY

The gross pathologic findings in acute pyelonephritis determine the imaging findings, so it is important to be familiar with them. Renal involvement may be unilateral or bilateral but is usually patchy; the involved areas are often wedge-shaped, with their apices in the papilla and their bases at the periphery of the kidneys. Infection very rarely involves the entirety of a kidney unless there is ureteral obstruction.

In mild cases, there may be no abnormalities other than a collection of polymorphonuclear leukocytes in the interstitium among the tubules. With more severe involvement, the density of the inflammatory cells increases, and there may be focal edema. Progression of the disease may produce small abscesses, within which the tubular anatomy is destroyed, but which usually spare the glomeruli, at least in the early stages. The abscesses may be microscopic; multiple small clusters of abscesses may coalesce to form a larger abscess. In general, the more severe forms of pathologic change are encountered much less frequently than the milder forms. When the infection is not accompanied by obstruction, reflux, or formation of macroscopic abscesses, successful treatment usually leads to resolution, with little, if any, scarring or significant loss of renal parenchymal volume.

It is rare for an infected kidney to cease functioning completely unless the infection is complicated by ureteral obstruction. Transient loss of concentrating ability is common, however.

Given the wide range of pathologic and imaging findings, it is not surprising that many names have been applied to acute bacterial infection of the kidney. Acute pyelonephritis, acute focal bacterial nephritis, renal preabscess, and lobar nephronia have all been used. We will use the term *acute pyelonephritis*; this phrase obviously refers to a spectrum of conditions and does not distinguish those involving only the parenchyma from those that actively involve the collecting system (a distinction that is neither possible by imaging techniques nor important in clinical management, at least in most cases).

IMAGING STUDIES

There is much literature regarding the findings in various kinds of images made from infected kidneys, but virtually all of the reported series involve groups of patients who have been thought by their physicians to be sufficiently sick to warrant radiologic investigation. Since there is no series that has subjected a group of consecutive patients with urinary infection to imaging, the true prevalence of each imaging findings is not known and is undoubtedly much lower than that reported in the available series. Probably, if all patients with urinary infection underwent any kind of radiologic examination, the large majority of the exams would be normal.

Intravenous Urography [7, 19, 43, 44]

Intravenous urography is often normal in patients with urinary infection. When abnormalities are found, they are restricted to the affected kidney and its collecting system. The kidney may appear slightly enlarged overall; there may be focal regions of parenchymal swelling, which may mimic masses. The nephrogram may be diminished in the swollen portions; occasionally, the nephrogram in the abnormal areas may appear striated or mottled. The collecting system may appear compressed or attenuated, presumably because of the edema of both the surrounding kidney and the caliceal walls. Rarely, opacification of the collecting system may be delayed and the concentration of contrast material in the urine from the abnormal kidney may be diminished. The combination of these findings may make the entire collecting system appear quite attenuated. In children there have been reports of dilatation of the collecting systems and ureters that drain infected kidneys [22]; this has been ascribed to ureteral ileus. The extent to which such findings may be due to vesicoureteral reflux is not entirely clear, however. Fine striations of the ureter have also been described. Again, these may be due either to inflammatory changes in the urothelium or to redundancy of the ureteral wall in ureters transiently dilated by reflux. The abnormalities of the infected kidney resolve on sucessful treatment of the infection. The appearance of new scars is rare in the absence of stones or vesicoureteral reflux [24], and although the kidneys have been described as diminishing in size with therapy [26, 27], they are probably returning to their original normal dimensions rather than becoming abnormally small.

Computed Tomography

Acute bacterial inflammation of the kidney produces CT findings (Fig. 11-1) that reflect those seen on intravenous urography, with the exception that CT is probably more sensitive to nephrogram abnormalities than urography [14, 23]. The affected kidney may be focally enlarged, and the nephrogram in the affected region may be mottled, striated, or absent; occasionally, there may be small regions of unusual intensity on the nephrogram, seen at the periphery of the lesion. In extreme cases, very small abscesses may appear as focal regions of diminished attenuation. Perinephric edema may appear as strands of material with the density of water extending outward from the kidney into the perinephric fat.

Ultrasonography

The findings of acute focal bacterial nephritis on ultrasonography reflect renal parenchymal changes [10, 32, 43]. When abnormal, the kidney may display regions of swollen parenchyma with diminished echogenicity and loss of the corticomedullary distinction (Fig. 11-2A). Rarely, echolucent areas adjacent to the kidney may be encountered, reflecting small perinephric effusions (Fig. 11-2B). On occasion, hemorrhage may occur in a region of focal bacterial nephritis resulting in an area of increased echogenicity (Fig. 11-2C) as opposed to the more typical echopenic lesion.

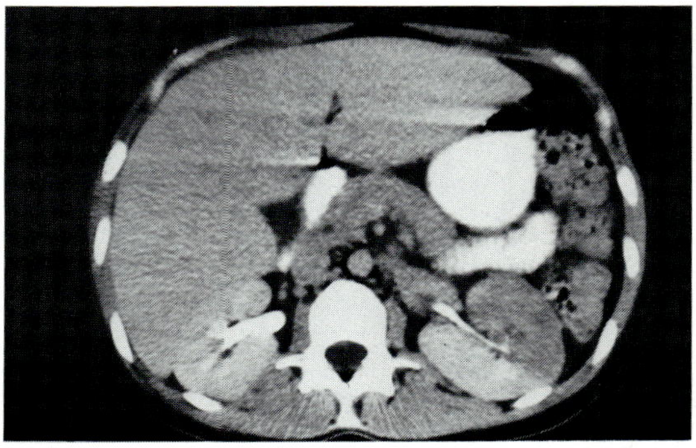

A

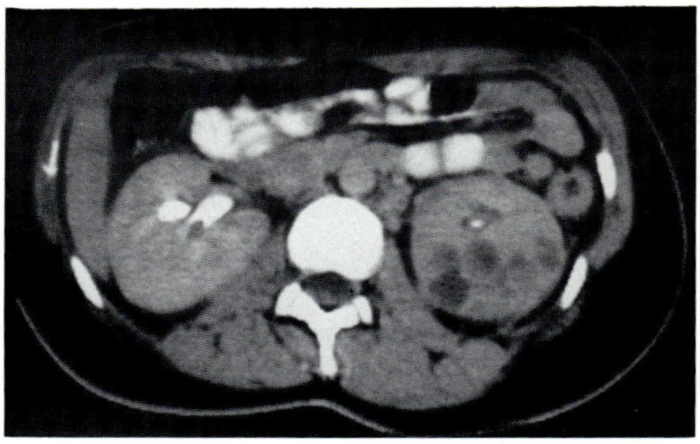

B

Figure 11-1. Acute bacterial nephritis. A. Contrast-enhanced CT reveals that the anterior portion of the left kidney is swollen and displays a diminished nephrogram. B. Contrast-enhanced CT in another case shows that the infected left kidney displays multiple relatively lucent regions; without therapy these might progress to frank abscesses.

Radionuclide Imaging

The findings on these examinations reflect the agent used for scanning. Technetium-labeled DTPA or glucoheptonate may reveal regions of diminished activity in the affected portions of the renal parenchyma; with gallium-labeled citrate, the infected portions may appear as focal areas of increased activity [18, 34, 49].

Angiography

Angiography is not used to work up urinary infections, but the findings may be encountered during angiographic studies done for other reasons [7, 25]. Arteriography may reveal the arteries to be stretched as they traverse the infected area; the nephrogram may be striated or

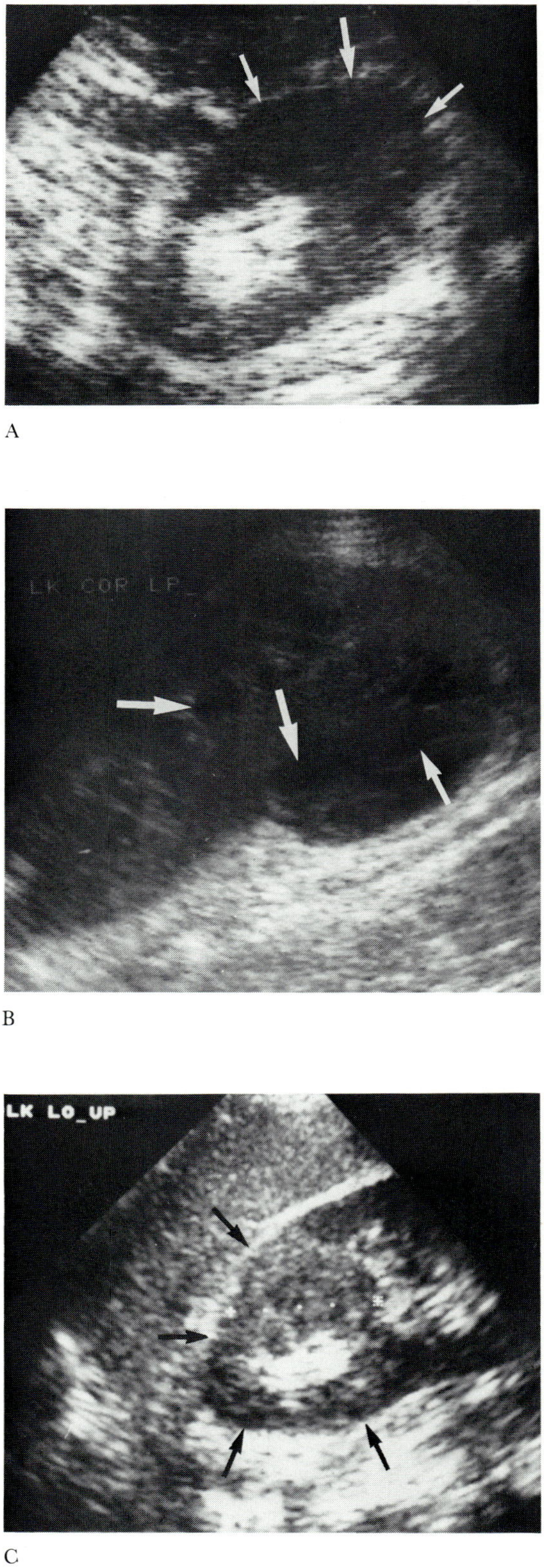

Figure 11-2. Acute bacterial nephritis. A. Ultrasonography reveals a region of focal parenchymal swelling with diminished echogenicity (arrows). B. In another case, ultrasonography reveals multiple anechoic regions (arrows). As in the case shown in Fig. 11-1B, these might ultimately coalesce if left untreated. C. In yet another patient, this one with hemorrhagic focal bacterial nephritis, ultrasonography shows the involved area in the upper pole of the left kidney (arrows) to be hyperechoic with respect to the rest of the kidney.

mottled, and there may be loss of the corticomedullary distinction. Epinephrine venography has revealed obstructed or stretched veins with segmental or diffuse attenuation.

EMPHYSEMATOUS PYELONEPHRITIS

CLINICAL FACTORS

Emphysematous pyelonephritis is an uncommon variant of acute pyelonephritis in which the infecting bacteria (typically E. coli) produce gas that is found in the renal parenchyma, collecting system, or perinephric space [11, 35]. Most patients who develop it have relatively severe diabetes mellitus. They tend to be acutely sick and may present with nausea, vomiting, abdominal or flank pain, fever, leukocytosis, pyuria, bacteriuria, and occasionally uremia; the mortality rate is high. Pathologic examination of the kidneys tends to reveal multiple small abscesses with gas in and around the renal tubules; these acute abnormalities are often superimposed on the chronic changes of diabetic nephropathy.

IMAGING STUDIES

The gas can usually be seen on a plain film of the abdomen (Fig. 11-3). If only emphysematous pyelitis is present, a collection of gas may be observed that conforms to the lumen of the collecting system. Gas within the kidney may be either mottled or display radial striations, and gas in the perinephric space may appear as mottled lucencies as well. Gas may extend widely throughout the retroperitoneal space. Intravenous urography may reveal various degrees of renal enlargement, diminished intensity of the nephrogram, and diminished opacification of

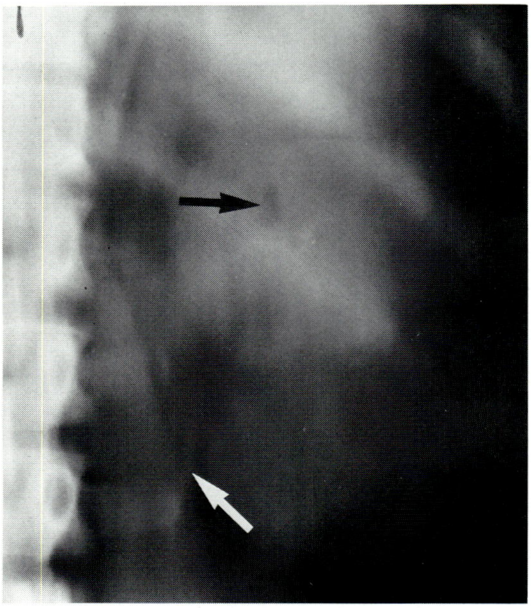

Figure 11-3. Emphysematous pyelonephritis. Nephrotomography reveals small collections of air (black arrow). Although a contrast agent has been administered, the collecting system is almost invisible; only a small amount of opacified urine is seen in the proximal ureter (white arrow).

the collecting system; the affected kidney may not function at all. CT reveals similar findings: The observed gas pattern is that described above for radiographs, and the kidneys may be enlarged with a diminished or absent nephrogram. Ultrasonography may reveal the gas bubbles as echogenic shadow-producing regions, but a significant number of cases have been reported in which the gas was not detected by ultrasonography.

RENAL ABSCESS

CLINICAL FACTORS

Frank abscesses in the renal parenchyma are not very common but appear with sufficient frequency to require familiarity with them. It should be obvious from the preceding discussion that focal regions of pyelonephritis may, when they become unusually severe, produce multiple small abscesses that ultimately coalesce to a single or loculated large abscess. This may occur in children [39] or adults, usually is caused by the same organisms that cause acute bacterial nephritis, and may occasionally be associated with ureteral obstruction or vesicoureteral reflux. In addition, however, renal abscesses may also appear after what is presumed to be hematogenous seeding of the renal parenchyma with bacteria. The offending organisms are often staphylococci or other gram-positive organisms that are thought to reach the kidney from infected sites on the skin or elsewhere. They originally are removed from the blood at the cortical capillaries and may form small microabscesses in the cortex, but they subsequently move to the medulla, where further small abscesses may form as well; the ultimate large abscess may occupy cortex or medulla.

The same clinical signs that occur with other kinds of renal infection may be present with renal abscesses; these include fever, abdominal or flank pain, local tenderness, palpable masses, leukocytosis, pyuria, and bacilluria. The disease may be indolent with minimal laboratory findings or the patients may be very sick; renal abscesses may even be fatal.

IMAGING STUDIES

On urography, a renal parenchymal abscess looks like a mass. It may obscure or enlarge the renal outline, may displace the kidney if it extends beyond the confines of the renal margin, and may displace and distort the caliceal system (Fig. 11-4). The center of a mature abscess is lucent; the edges of the abscess may enhance and appear either smooth or irregular. Rarely, gas may be seen within the abscess.

As might be expected, the CT findings are similar to those noted at intravenous urography [23]. The abscess is a rounded focal lesion whose center is of fluid density or slightly higher and does not enhance (Fig. 11-5); the periphery of the abscess may form a wall of variable thickness, which often enhances with administration of intravenous contrast material. Air bubbles may be seen within the abscess. The lesion may protrude beyond the border of the kidney and may be associated with CT evidence of edema in the perinephric fat.

Ultrasonography should visualize most, if not all, macroscopic abscesses. The center of the abscess is usually echo-poor (Fig. 11-6), but the appearance is variable: There may be very few

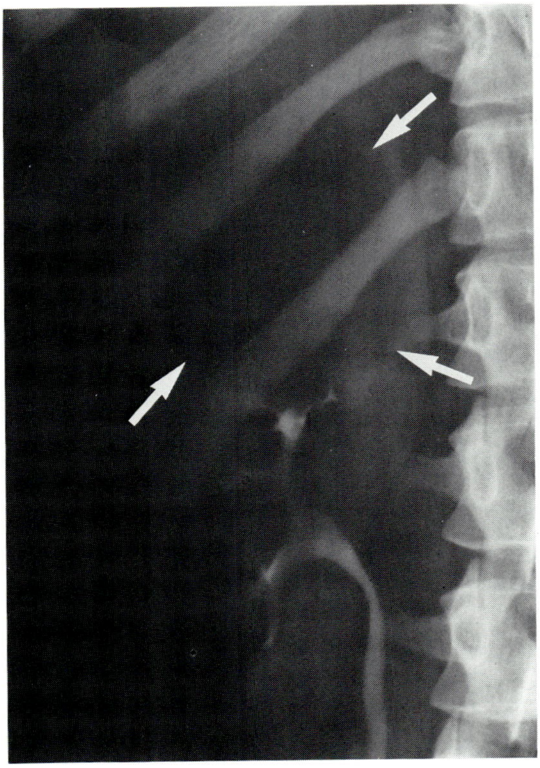

Figure 11-4. Renal abscess. Urography reveals a lucent region (arrows) in the upper-pole of the kidney, which expands the parenchyma.

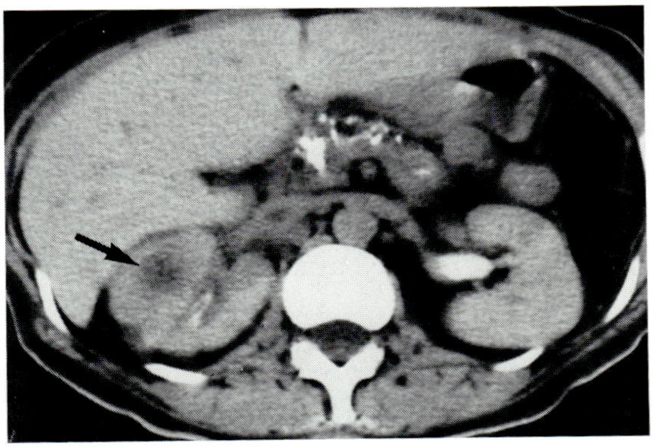

Figure 11-5. Renal abscess. CT reveals focal region of diminished enhancement (arrow) in the anterior aspect of the right kidney.

echoes, or a considerable number of echoes caused by debris floating within the central pus, or there may be a fluid-debris level as the solid material settles to the dependent portions of the lesion. The wall varies in thickness. There is

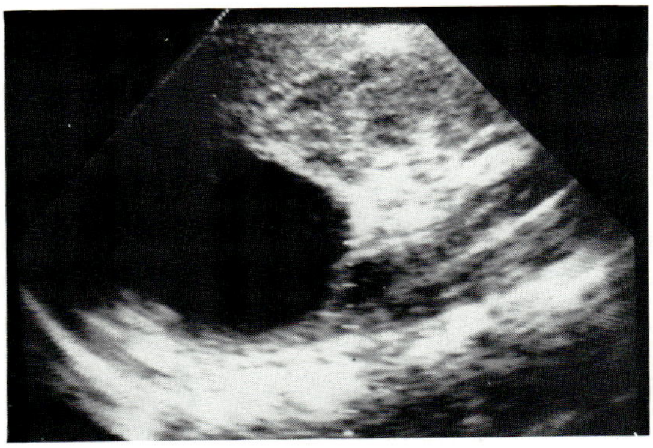

Figure 11-6. Renal abscess. Ultrasonography reveals a nearly anechoic region involving the upper renal pole.

often enhanced through-transmission of sound deep to the abscess.

Angiographic studies [25] are now rarely performed. They show displacement of arterial branches around the hypovascular lesion; the periphery of the lesion may appear quite vascular, however, and may have a relatively intense stain in the nephrogram phase. The vessels in the still-viable peripheral inflamed tissue may appear intrinsically abnormal.

As with acute focal bacterial nephritis, the nuclear imaging characteristics of renal abscess depends on the compound employed. Gallium-67 citrate usually shows a region of increased activity in the abscess [18]; technetium-labeled glucoheptonate or DTPA shows diminished activity in the center of an abscess.

Antibiotics are, of course, essential in the therapy of an abscess, but percutaneous treatment is usually very useful as well [6, 40]. Currently, percutaneous catheter drainage of an abscess, which is continued for as long as there is significant drainage of fluid from the cavity, is often performed. However, there have been reported cases of successful abscess therapy that involved needle aspiration and systemic antibiotics. Needle aspiration may need to be repeated before the pus inside the abscess is cleared, and gentle irrigation of the abscess cavity and possibly instillation of antibiotics through the needle have been recommended as well. Contrast medium injected through a needle into an active abscess (this should be done with caution, since extravasation of the pus within an abscess may cause acute septic shock) may reveal the inner surface of the wall to be smooth or irregular; the abscess cavity may be unilocular or multiloculated.

PERINEPHRIC ABSCESS

CLINICAL FACTORS

An abscess in the perinephric space may arise by simple extension across the renal capsule of a renal parenchymal abscess [42]. More commonly, however, it arises in patients with high-grade ureteral obstruction (usually from a stone) with an ipsilateral infected kidney. Presumably, extravasation of infected urine from a forniceal rupture allows the infection to spread into the perinephric space, where it may form an abscess; the abscess may then erode into the kidney parenchyma so that at the time of diagnosis it is not clear whether the intraparenchymal portion was primary or not. Less frequently, perinephric abscesses may arise from infections that were not originally within the urinary tract at all: Spinal tuberculosis may produce perinephric as well as psoas abscesses, diverticular abscesses may protrude into the perinephric space, duodenal perforations may become infected, pancreatic pseudocysts may become contaminated and erode into the perinephric space, and so forth. Despite this variety of potential routes of infection, acute pyelonephritis with an ipsilateral obstructing ureteral stone is the most commonly encountered predisposing condition. As with other types of severe renal infection, *E. coli*, proteus, and klebsiella are usually the offending organisms, and the patients are often diabetic. Clinical presentation is similar to that occurring with a renal abscess.

Perinephric abscesses may become large and erode or extend into other spaces. They may point at Petit's lumbar triangle or may dissect in the perinephric space inferiorly into the pelvis, ultimately to appear in the inguinal region, or may extend superiorly to the subphrenic space and even to the pleural space. They may also extend anteriorly and enter the peritoneal cavity.

IMAGING STUDIES

Perinephric abscesses display a wider range of imaging abnormalities than do renal abscesses. Abdominal radiograms may reveal air in the abscesses. The renal and psoas outlines may be obscured. Intravenous urography reveals a variety of abnormalities, including parenchymal and perinephric masses, regions of absent or diminished nephrogram, and occasionally a dense nephrogram at the border of the abscess. If the abscess is associated with ureteral obstruction, the collecting system usually does not opacify, and a ureteral stone is often visible. The collecting system may be distorted by any intrarenal portion of the abscess, and the kidney may be displaced. Ultrasound examination reveals that perirenal abscesses look much like intrarenal abscesses: The central portions are hypoechoic but may contain echoes from suspended debris, and there is usually enhanced through-transmission. On CT the central portions of the abscess are of fluid density and the peripheral portions may enhance with administration of intravenous contrast agent (Fig. 11-7). As described above, the anatomic extent of the abscess demonstrated on CT is extremely variable; occasionally, the organ of origin of the abscess may not be clear.

Gallium-67 citrate nuclear scans usually reveal regions of increased activity at the site of the abscess [18].

Ultrasound-guided or CT-guided needle aspiration may produce fluid whose purulent nature and specific bacteria distinguish perineph-

Figure 11-7. Perinephric abscess. CT reveals an inhomogeneous, relatively lucent region lateral to the left kidney and in the left psoas. The left kidney has been displaced anteriorly, and there is parenchymal inflammation, revealed as a region of diminished enhancement (arrow).

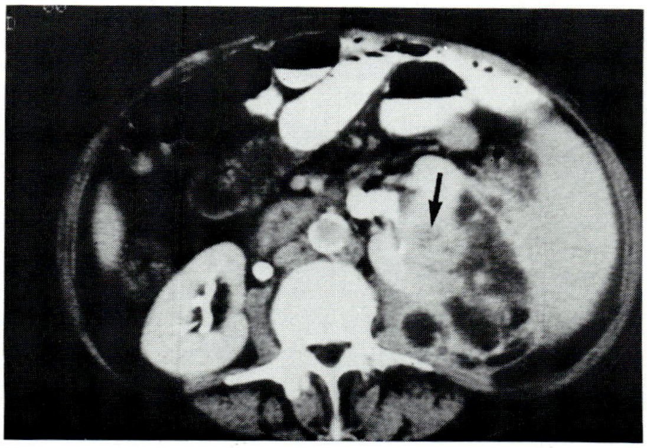

ric abscesses from other fluid-containing lesions (such as pancreatic pseudocysts). Percutaneous catheter drainage, along with antibiotic therapy, usually produces successful resolution of the abscess. The number and routes of the necessary catheters may vary considerably, depending on the anatomic extent and degree of loculation of the abscess.

PYONEPHROSIS

CLINICAL FACTORS

Pyonephrosis [50] is an unusual condition in which there is high-grade or complete obstruction of the ureter with infection in the kidney it drains, so that purulent urine or pus fills a distended collecting system. Any cause of ureteral obstruction may be associated with pyonephrosis, although stone disease is by far the most frequent offender. The condition varies in severity. There may be partial obstruction with an infected but anatomically nearly normal kidney that continues to produce urine, complete obstruction with severe renal dysfunction, or total nonfunction. The kidney may demonstrate anything from mild hydronephrosis to complete destruction of the renal parenchyma or replacement with xanthogranulomatous tissue. The collecting system may contain cloudy infected urine or frank pus.

The clinical presentation also varies. The symptoms may have been present for months or years or only a few days when the disease is diagnosed. There may be focal signs such as flank pain and tenderness; there are usually signs of urinary infection, including fever, pyuria, bacilluria, and lower-tract symptoms; and there may be systemic symptoms such as weight loss, anemia, nausea, and vomiting. The offending organisms are the same as those seen in less severe urinary infections. Pyonephrosis may be caused by fungal agents as well.

In the past, surgical resection and antibiotic therapy were the usual treatment. Since the development of percutaneous nephrostomy, many of these kidneys have been treated with antibiotics and drainage only. The drainage may be accomplished by retrograde ureteral stenting or percutaneous nephrostomy. Drainage is usually continued until the obstructing lesion has either resolved or been sucessfully treated; drainage also serves to permit the infection to be treated prior to surgical or other therapy of the obstructing lesion. The capacity of the affected kidney to regain function after therapy largely depends on the degree of parenchymal destruction present at the time of the diagnosis.

IMAGING STUDIES

Urographic signs vary. If the pyonephrosis is accompanied by considerable perinephric inflammation, there may be loss of the renal or psoas margins. The kidney may be enlarged. After administration of intravenous contrast medium, the appearance in the affected kidney is variable; there may be no nephrogram or pyelogram at all, there may be a nephrogram without a pyelogram, and, in a few cases, there may be faint opacification of the dilated upper tract. An acute "obstructive" nephrogram is only rarely seen when acute obstruction has been superimposed on more chronic partial ureteral occlusion. Since the obstruction is often caused by stones, however, urography frequently provides the primary diagnosis.

CT reveals evidence of hydronephrosis (Fig. 11-8). There are varying degrees of dilatation of the collecting system, thinning of the parenchyma, and enlargement of the kidney; there is often edematous infiltration of the

Figure 11-8. Obstructive pyonephrosis. The left kidney is hydronephrotic on CT and there is inflammation in the perinephric fat (arrows). Bubbles of gas are seen in the lateral aspect of the renal parenchyma and in the anterior portion of the distended intrarenal collecting system.

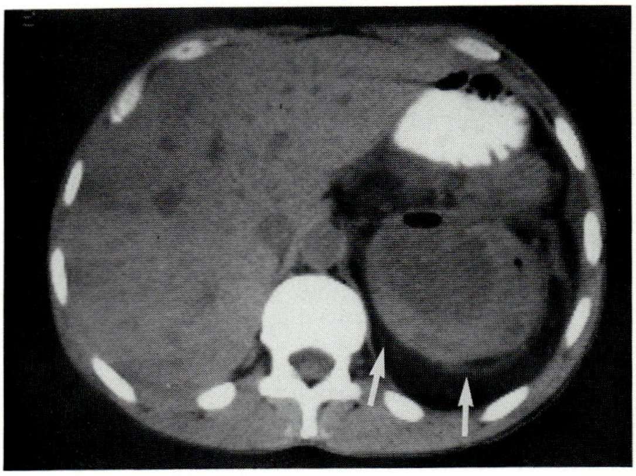

perinephric fat. The obstructing lesion is often directly demonstrated: Stones, as well as periureteral tumors or fibrosis, can be demonstrated even if they are not opaque on the plain films. There are no absolutely reliable CT signs for distinguishing pyonephrosis from uninfected hydronephrosis in all cases; demonstrating a dependent layer of debris in the collecting system or finding perinephric abscesses strongly suggest infection, and, of course, finding gas in the collecting system usually means infection. The nephrogram of the remaining parenchyma is variable and may be faint, inhomogeneous, or striated. Pyonephrosis and perinephric abscesses often coexist.

Ultrasonography [48] also reveals various degrees of hydronephrosis. Distinction of uninfected obstruction from pyonephrosis is often possible on ultrasonography by analyzing the echo pattern of the urine in the collecting system. Completely anechoic urine is usually (but not always) sterile. Finding fine scattered echoes throughout the urine suggests infection; finding coarse echoes from dependent debris (Fig. 11-9) or echoes from gas bubbles is quite reliable evidence that infection is present.

Figure 11-9. Obstructive pyonephrosis. Ultrasonography shows three dilated calices (black arrows) and a dilated renal pelvis (white arrow). There are multiple fine echoes within the spaces, presumably caused by debris suspended in pus.

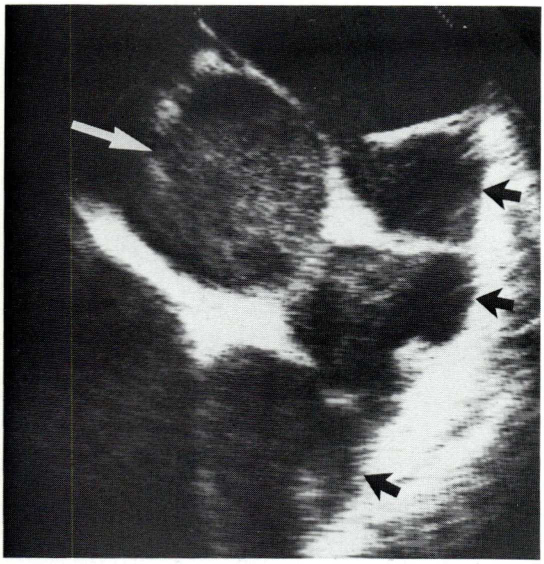

Radionuclide studies may assist in the diagnosis. Gallium-67 citrate examinations usually reveal increased activity in the infected kidney, although this finding may not permit the distinction among pyonephrosis, renal abscess, and perirenal abscess. Studies with glucoheptonate or DTPA reveal marked to complete absence of uptake and excretion in the affected kidney. After the condition has been treated with antibiotics and drainage, radionulide studies may help to estimate the amount of recovered function; these examinations, together with CT, ultrasonographic, or nephrotomographic estimates of the remaining volume of renal parenchyma, assist in deciding whether to resect the kidney.

Arteriography is rarely performed in patients with pyonephrosis. The findings include the stretching of the intrarenal branches of the artery characteristic of hydronephrosis and, in severe and longstanding cases, diminution of the diameter of the main renal artery and its branches. There may or may not be visible neovascularity; if it is present, small regions of fine neovascularity may be seen at the periphery of the dilated collecting system.

Antegrade pyelography is often extremely useful. A fine-gauge needle puncture of the affected collecting system permits aspiration of the urine; when pyonephrosis is present, observation of pus or foul-smelling cloudy urine may confirm the diagnosis immediately. Also, antegrade pyelography is particularly useful in outlining the collecting system so that definitive percutaneous nephrostomy can be performed [51]. Great care must be taken, however, both during antegrade puncture and placement of the nephrostomy tube, never to inject contrast agent into the collecting system except in smaller volumes than have already been aspirated from the collecting system; extravasation of pus caused either by overdistention or excessive manipulation of tubes or needles may severely and acutely exacerbate systemic sepsis. When a nephrostomy tube is used for therapy, it should be connected to a closed drainage system and allowed to remain until sterilization of the urine and stabilization of any recovered renal function permit definitive therapy of the lesion obstructing the ureter.

XANTHOGRANULOMATOUS PYELONEPHRITIS

CLINICAL FACTORS

Xanthogranulomatous pyelonephritis appears to be the end stage of longstanding obstructive pyonephrosis, focal obstructive pyonephrosis, renal abscess, or perirenal abscess [16, 30]. In this condition, the renal parenchyma is replaced by grossly yellow sheets of foamy lipid-laden macrophages, along with other inflammatory cells and fibrosis. Little or nothing remains of normal renal tubules or glomeruli, so the affected portions of the kidney have had their function permanently destroyed.

In adults, the lesion usually involves the entire kidney; over 70 percent of patients have an obstructing staghorn or ureteral calculus. But the disease may also be focal [41] and is more commonly so in children. Focal (tumefactive) xanthogranulomatous pyelonephritis may occur if there has been infundibular obstruction and infection or even if there has been a chronic renal parenchymal abscess without obstruction; occasionally, the lesion may extend outside the kidney and adopt the same morphology as a perinephric abscess.

The symptoms encountered are often those of a chronic renal infection and include fever, flank pain, pyuria and bacilluria, and a palpable mass; other systemic manifestations, such as weight loss, anemia, and nephrogenic hepatic dysfunction, have been encountered. Treatment almost always consists of surgical resection, although, since the lesion often has the appearance of hydronephrosis or abscess, some cases of xanthogranulomatous pyelonephritis may have been successfully treated with percutaneous catheter drainage without the specific diagnosis ever becoming apparent.

IMAGING STUDIES

Not surprisingly, the imaging characteristics of the lesion are often identical to those of chronic pyonephrosis with renal nonfunction or of a chronic renal or perirenal abscess. Plain films and urograms may reveal a mass. The mass is often accompanied by evidence of a ureteral or staghorn calculus; the mass itself may display fine mottled or stippled calcification, but this is unusual. Urography reveals a nonfunctioning kidney in cases in which the obstruction is at the level of the renal pelvis or lower; if there has been infundibular obstruction, urography may reveal a focal mass in which there is no excretion of opacified urine but which is accompanied by excretion of contrast material in the remainder of the kidney. Rarely, a parenchymal mass may be seen in a kidney in which the entire collecting system is opacified.

CT [15] reveals the features of an obstructive pyonephrosis or of an abscess (Fig. 11-10). The kidney is enlarged when it is involved in its entirety; the parenchyma is thinned and, although it may be enhanced somewhat with administration of an intravenous contrast agent, it is virtually never seen to excrete opacified urine. When the disease is focal, the same findings are limited to a portion of the kidney. Perinephric extension of xanthogranulomatous pyelonephritis produces the same CT appearance as a perinephric abscess, with a thick enhancing rim and a relatively lucent central portion. Gas has not been reported within xanthogranulomatous pyelonephritis; despite the lipid in the macrophages, tissue with the density of fat is not a CT feature of xanthogranulomatous pyelonephritis.

Ultrasonography also reveals findings of general or focal hydronephrosis or an abscess. The

Figure 11-10. Xanthogranulomatous pyelonephritis. CT shows multiple lucent regions involving the left kidney and extending beyond the renal border; there is an abscess in the left psoas as well. The kidney is displaced anteriorly. There are no imaging features in this case that permit absolute differentiation between intrarenal and perinephric abscesses.

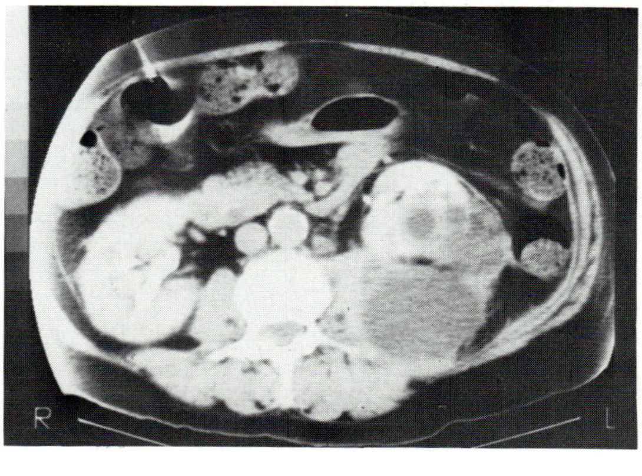

center of the lesion usually contains regions of relatively few echoes with enhanced through-transmission; if present, a staghorn calculus will appear as an echogenic shadowing structure. MRI reveals the features of hydronephrosis or abscess in patients with xanthogranulomatous pyelonephritis [36]: the pus-containing structures appear to be of relatively low intensity in T1 weighted images and relatively bright in T2 weighted images.

Glucoheptonate, dimercaptosuccinic acid (DMSA) or DTPA labeled with technetium reveal photopenic regions on renal scans. At angiography the central portions of the lesions are seen to be avascular; the peripheral portions usually do not contain neovascularity, but in a few cases there may be sparse inflammatory neovascularity visible.

As might be expected, differential diagnosis of xanthogranulomatous pyelonephritis from obstructive pyonephrosis or chronic abscess may be difficult. A lengthy clinical history, the complete absence of function of the affected kidney, (or portion thereof) and renal or ureteral stones may suggest the diagnosis, but often an exact diagnosis is permitted only by surgical examination of the resected specimen.

TUBERCULOSIS

CLINICAL FACTORS

Urinary tract tuberculosis is not very common in the United States, but the disease has certainly not been eradicated and may become a problem in patients with AIDS [38]. In many parts of the world, urinary tuberculosis is not an unusual disease, however; since its imaging manifestations virtually never resolve and since worldwide travel is becoming more prevalent, radiologists anywhere in the world should be familiar with its manifestations.

Tubercle bacilli have been demonstrated to reach the urinary tract by hematogenous dissemination from other foci of infection. The bacilli are initially disseminated throughout the cortices of both kidneys and may form microscopic granulomas. However, macroscopic progression of the disease is almost always unilateral. The bacilli descend along nephrons and form further granulomas within the medulla and papilla. These granulomas may coalesce and form cavities or cause parts of the papillae to become necrotic and slough. When the bacilli are shed into the urine they infect the walls of the calices, pelvis, and ureter, where they produce initial mucosal inflammation with ulceration, then granulomas, and ultimately fibrosis with strictures. Urinary obstruction from the strictures combines with direct caseation of the renal parenchyma to destroy all or parts of the kidney. The pattern of destruction depends on the relative rates of progression of parenchymal disease and hollow visceral obstruction. Obstruction may predominate, in which case massive hydronephrosis or hydrocalix may be the final stage. Alternatively, parenchymal caseation, necrosis, and calcification may predominate, which causes the kidney to be destroyed. Usually, however, both processes occur and may lead to a nonfunctioning, calcified kidney of any size; this process is called autonephrectomy. The bacilli also descend to the bladder, where processes similar to those that occur in the collecting system and ureter may cause obstruction, reflux, or both due to involvement of the ureteral orifices. In men the prostate, seminal vesicles, and epididymides may be involved, where caseating granulomas, abscesses, and calcification may ensue.

The clinical diagnosis of urinary tract tuberculosis is often difficult. Systemic symptoms such as fatigue, weight loss, and fever are nonspecific, and the urinary tract symptoms, which include flank, pain, hematuria, frequency, and epididymal abnormalities, are the same as those that are encountered in a variety of other inflammatory diseases. In some patients, the radiographic manifestations may be pathognomonic, but the absolute diagnosis of active tuberculosis can be made only by urine culture.

Therapy of urinary tract tuberculosis is almost entirely chemotherapeutic; surgery is only rarely used in resecting infected nonfunctioning kidneys. There is no simple correlation between the success of chemotherapy and imaging findings; the distinction between active and cured tuberculosis can only be made by multiple urine cultures. Unfortunately, in patients whose urothelium is involved with urinary tuberculosis successful chemotherapy may cause active inflammation to be replaced by scarring, so that strictures of the collecting system, ureter, and bladder may progress, with further compromise of renal function and exacerbation of lower tract symptoms.

IMAGING STUDIES

Although urinary tract tuberculosis is thought almost always to be accompanied by tuberculosis elsewhere, radiographic manifestations of extraurinary tuberculosis are by no means inevitable. Pulmonary tuberculosis may be visualized. In the abdomen, there may be calcification of the adrenals, lymph nodes, or psoas abscesses; calcified granulomata in the liver or spleen may appear. Renal and urinary tract calcifications are common; although they are unusual in the early stages of the disease, nearly every end-stage tuberculous kidney contains calcification. The calcification may take a variety of patterns. There may be linear or curvilinear streaks and mottled or amorphous calcification (Fig. 11-11). A characteristic appearance is for calcified caseous tissue to be very homogenous and only moderately dense, looking like ground glass; this has also been called a "putty kidney" (Fig. 11-12). The calcification is not bilaterally symmetrical and does ot have the pattern of cortical or medullary nephrocalcinosis described in Chap. 15. The calcification may extend along the ureter but only rarely is seen in the bladder. The prostate, seminal vesicles, and

Figure 11-11. Renal tuberculosis. The right kidney is small and nonfunctioning; it has undergone autonephrectomy. There are multiple curvilinear and amorphous regions of calcification within it.

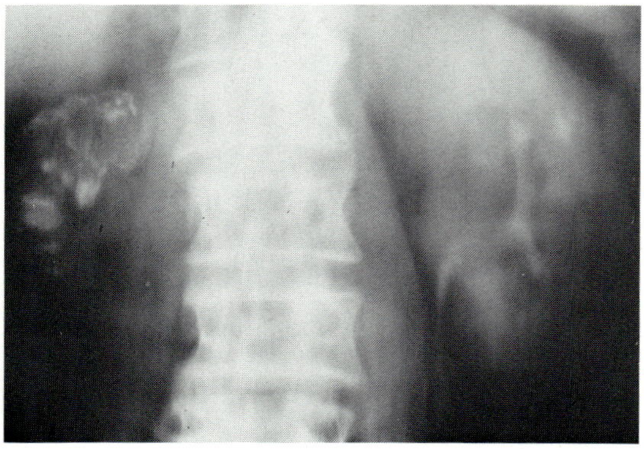

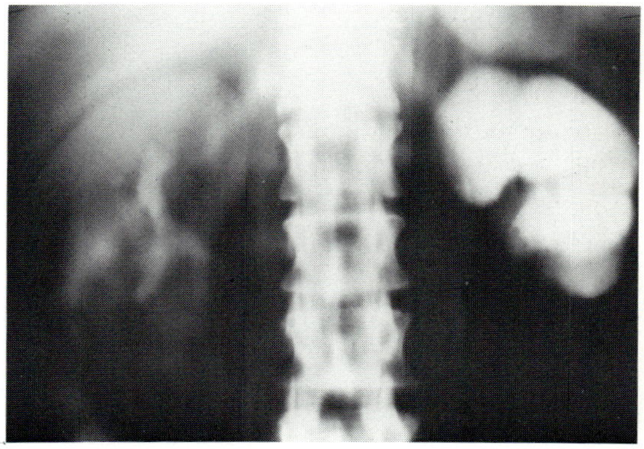

Figure 11-12. Renal tuberculosis. The dense opacity in the left renal fossa is calcification within caseous material that has filled the entirety of the hydronephrotic left kidney.

vasa deferentia may calcify, but the appearance of tuberculous calcification does not permit differentiation from other calcification in these organs.

Intravenous urography may display a variety of abnormalities depending on the stage of the disease. When there are only small cortical granulomata, the urogram may appear entirely normal. The earliest signs of medullary involvement are irregularity of the surface of the papilla, the small erosions of papillary necrosis, or even a completely sloughed papilla. Medullary cavities of various sizes may opacify. Individual infundibula or the renal pelvis or proximal ureter may reveal stenoses; these may produce dilatation of the calices when mild or focal or general hydronephrosis or a nonfunctioning kidney when severe. They may even completely occlude the pelvis or infundibulae so that antegrade or retrograde pyelography fail to cause contrast material to traverse the stenoses. A cicatricial or "purse-string" stenosis of the renal pelvis (Fig. 11-13) is highly suggestive of tuberculosis. The degree of opacification of the affected kidney ranges from normal to completely absent, depending on the severity of renal parenchymal destruction and collecting system obstruction.

The ureter may display single or multiple stenotic regions (Fig. 11-13) that have a predilection for the distal portions; alternatively, its wall may thicken and demonstrate multiple mild narrowings without functional obstruction.

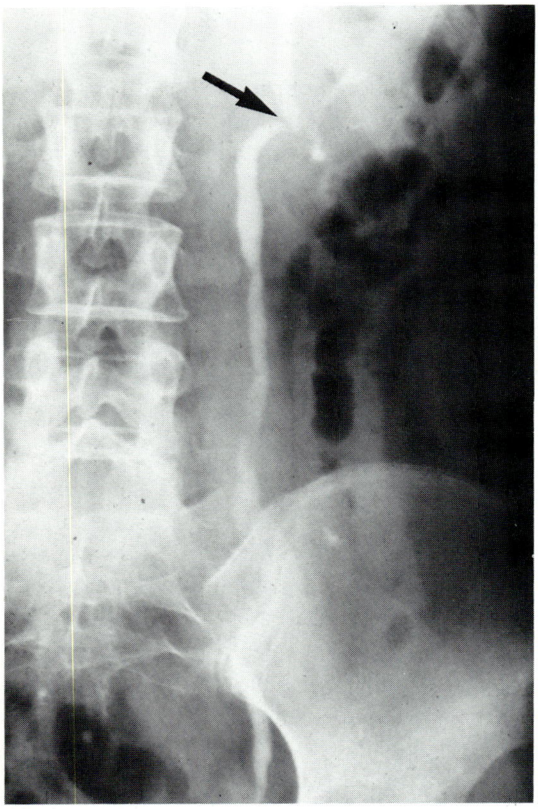

Figure 11-13. Urinary tract tuberculosis. Urography reveals a stenosis of the left renal pelvis (arrow) and multiple stenoses of the left ureter.

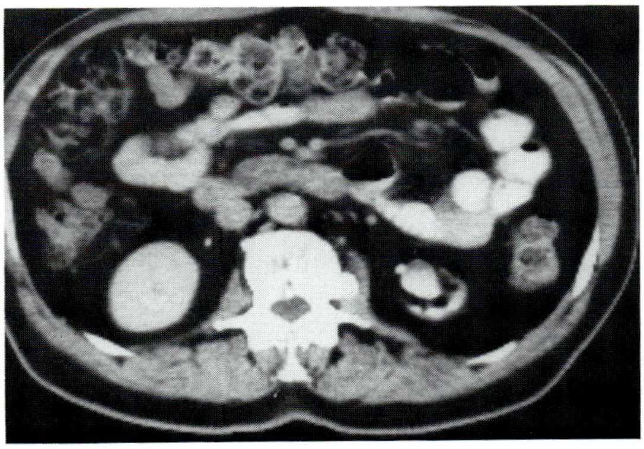

Figure 11-14. Renal tuberculosis. The left kidney is markedly shrunken. The opacity in the remaining renal parenchyma and renal pelvis is calcification; this kidney does not function at all.

Such a ureter may appear completely aperistaltic and relatively narrow, an appearance that has been called the "pipestem" ureter. The ureteral walls may calcify or puttylike faintly calcified material may be found within the lumen; parts of the ureter or its entirely may be involved. Tuberculous changes in the bladder are described in Chap. 20.

CT reveals renal changes very similar to those described for urography (Fig. 11-14). Occasionally, focal regions of noncalcified hydronephrotic kidney may be apparent on CT but invisible on urography; CT is more sensitive in detecting calcification.

Ultrasonographic images of the affected kidney are useful in a small number of cases. If the kidney is densely calcified, renal morphology may not be visible at all; only a dense shadowing calcified mass may be seen, and the differential diagnosis among end-stage tuberculosis, large staghorn calculi, and densely calcified tumors may be difficult to make. Various degrees of hydronephrosis may be demonstrable if they are not hidden by calcification.

Renal scintigraphy may be normal in early renal tuberculosis and reveal various degrees of diminished uptake and excretion as the disease progresses. The specific cause of the renal dysfunction is usually not distinguishable on scintigraphy, however.

Arteriography in early-stage renal tuberculosis would probably reveal no abnormalities. In a small autonephrectomized kidney, the main renal artery and its major branches are markedly diminished in diameter and the usual distribution of arcuate and interlobular arteries is totally destroyed. In cases in which the kidney has become severely hydronephrotic, the arteriographic pattern of severe hydronephrosis will be reproduced.

FUNGAL DISEASES

CLINICAL FACTORS

Fungus infection of the urinary tract [29, 37] is uncommon and usually appears in patients whose immune system has been compromised by such conditions as diabetes mellitus, advanced neoplasia, steroid therapy, long-term antibiotic treatment, immunosuppression after organ transplantation, and AIDS. Various species of candida, often *Candida albicans,* are probably the most commonly encountered agents of fungal infection in the western world. Cryptococcus and torulopsis species, aspergillosis and coccidioidomycosis may also be seen.

Any portion of the urinary tract, from the kidney parenchyma to the bladder, may be involved. Candida may infect the renal parenchyma and produce focal inflammation or multiple small abscesses; papillary necrosis and perinephric abscesses may also be seen.

IMAGING STUDIES

These may have the imaging features of focal inflammation or abscesses caused by any other species. A clump of hyphae may grow within the collecting system; this is usually known as a fungus ball (Fig. 11-15). It may be roughly spherical or adopt the shape of a collecting system in the same way that a staghorn calculus does. Candida, aspergillus, and nocardia may form such fungus balls. The imaging consequences of these mycetomas consist of varying degrees of hydronephrosis with radiolucent finding defects in the upper tract or bladder. Fungus balls are relatively echogenic on ultrasonography but do not produce shadows [46].

Figure 11-15. Candida fungus ball. Nephrotomography reveals several lucencies (arrows) within the right renal collecting system.

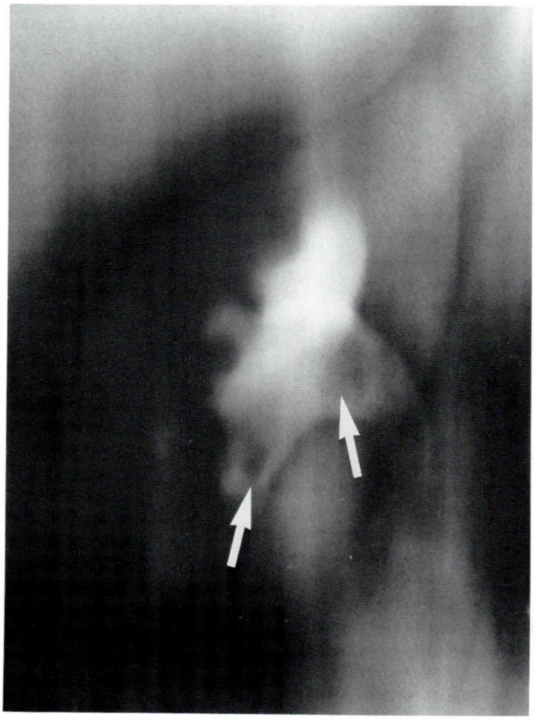

In addition to systemic antibiotic therapy, fungus balls are often treated with topical irrigation; radiologists may be involved in the treatment of these lesions since ureteral stents or percutaneous nephrostomy tubes may be placed for irrigation. Percutaneous extraction of fungus balls has been described as well [9].

ECHINOCOCCUS

CLINICAL FACTORS

Hydatid disease may be caused by *Echinococcus granulosus* or *E. multilocularis*; the former is more common [8, 17]. The distribution of the disease is worldwide; it is most often found in places where sheep or cattle are raised or in northern regions where caribou or deer are an important food source. The definitive hosts of the organism are dogs and wolves; the intermediate hosts are herbivores such as sheep, cattle, deer, and mice. The primary hosts acquire the disease by eating other infected animals; the intermediate hosts, including man, become infected by ingesting ova excreted in the feces of the intermediate hosts.

In man, the liver is the most common site of development of an echinococcal cyst. The kidneys are involved in only 2 to 5 percent of infected patients.

The renal cysts begin as unilocular structures whose walls have several microscopic layers. As they grow, daughter cysts may develop within the original cyst, and small capsules containing scolices may develop; the latter may accumulate in the dependent portions of the cysts to form what has been called hydatid sand. The cyst walls are usually not calcified during their early development but become progressively more calcified as they age.

IMAGING STUDIES

The imaging characteristics of the disease in the kidney are produced by the developing cyst. Urography may demonstrate a cystlike mass that, early in its development, may not differ very much in appearance from a simple cyst but that later usually demonstrates extensive calcification in the walls; as the wall collapses, the

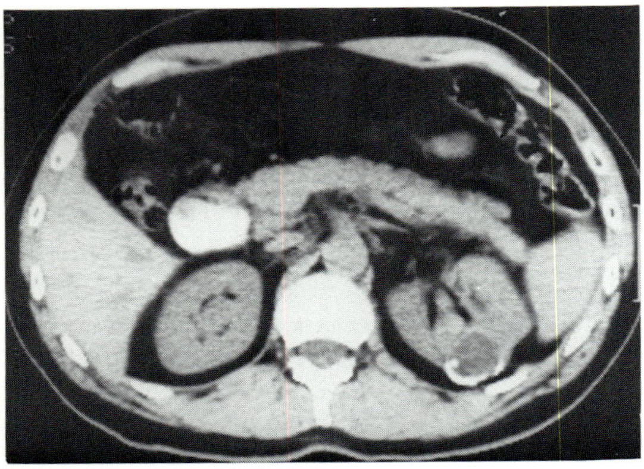

Figure 11-16. Echinococcal cyst. The cyst wall in the left kidney is irregularly calcified, and its posterolateral margin has collapsed slightly.

calcification may no longer be ringlike but may appear to be collapsed and amorphous. Rarely, the cyst may communicate with the collecting system and thus fill with opacified urine. CT reveals the same features (Fig. 11-16) and may additionally show individual daughter cysts within the major cyst. The ultrasonographic appearance varies; sometimes the walls of the daughter cysts may be demonstrable and hydatid sand may be seen collecting at the bottom of the cyst; a densely calcified lesion, however, may simply produce strong peripheral echoes and a dense shadow that obscures the internal structure. Arteriography reveals the cyst to be avascular. Needle aspiration of the cyst has been shown to permit successful diagnosis. Although considerable concern persists regarding the possibility of anaphylactic shock occurring if needle puncture causes cyst fluid to leak, this complication has not been found to be of practical importance in the small number of reported cases.

RENAL MALACOPLAKIA

CLINICAL FACTORS

Urinary tract malacoplakia occurs more frequently in the hollow viscera than in the kidney itself, but rare cases of renal parenchymal malacoplakia have been reported [20,31]. The disease may be unifocal or multifocal and may be unilateral or bilateral; occasionally, multifocal bilateral disease produces loss of renal function. The condition is most often encountered after multiple urinary tract infections, usually with *E. coli*. The histology of the parenchymal lesion is similar to that seen in the collecting system, ureter, and bladder. There are single or multiple tumorlike affected regions, which are yellow, brown, or gray and which contain large histiocytes called von Hanseman cells; these contain periodic acid-Schiff-positive cytoplasmic inclusions and small spherical calcified inclusions called Michaelis–Gutmann bodies.

IMAGING STUDIES

The imaging characteristics of this disease are extremely variable. Urography may show single or multiple space-occupying lesions of the renal parenchyma, with or without renal function. When the disease is multifocal the kidneys usually appear enlarged. The collecting systems may appear distorted by the parenchymal masses, and the hollow visceral manifestations of malacoplakia (which are described elsewhere) may also be encountered. On sonography, the kidney may be enlarged and the entire anatomy of cortex, medullary pyramids, and central sinus echoes completely distorted; a solitary mass is usually echogenic; the mass may extend from the periphery of the kidney. CT reveals a single mass or several masses within the kidney, which are usually not calcified. Angiography has been described; it reveals multiple hypovascular masses. However, neovascularity has been described in cases with solitary masses. Renal vein thrombosis may be found in association with renal malacoplakia [5].

CHRONIC GRANULOMATOUS DISEASE OF CHILDHOOD

Chronic granulomatous disease of childhood is quite rare. It is a hereditary abnormality in which there is a defect in the phagocytic function of leukocytes [12, 28]. It is associated with frequent purulent infections of the skin, lungs, bones, and abdominal viscera. A small number of cases have been reported with imaging abnormalities in the urinary tract; these most frequently include hydronephrosis (presumably due to scarring of the ureters or collecting systems), a thickened inflamed bladder wall with reduced bladder capacity, and acute renal inflammation or abscess formation.

REFERENCES

1. Allen, T.D. Pathogenesis of urinary-tract infections in children. *N. Engl. J. Med.* 273:1421, 1965.
2. Baker, R., and Barbaris, H.T. Comparative results of urological evaluation of children with initial and recurrent urinary tract infection. *J. Urol.* 116:503, 1976.
3. Bengtsson, C., Bengtsson, U., and Lincoln K. Bacteriuria in a population sample of women. *Acta Med. Scand.* 208:417, 1980.
4. Cameron, D.D., and Azimi, F. The value of excretory urography in the diagnosis of acute pyelonephritis. *J. Urol.* 112:546, 1974.
5. Clark, R.A., et al. Renal malakoplakia with renal vein thrombosis. *A.J.R.* 133:1170, 1979.
6. Cronan, J.J., Amis, E.S., Jr., and Dorfman, G.S. Percutaneous drainage of renal abscesses. *A.J.R.* 142:351, 1984.
7. Davidson, A.J., and Talner, L.B. Urographic and angiographic abnormalities in adult-onset acute bacterial nephritis. *Radiology* 106:249, 1973.
8. Diamond, H.M., et al. Echinococcal disease of the kidney. *J. Urol.* 115:742, 1976.
9. Doemeny, J.M., et al. Percutaneous extraction of renal fungus ball. *A.J.R.* 150:1331, 1988.
10. Edell, S.L., and Bonavita, J.A. The sonographic appearance of acute pyelonephritis. *Radiology* 132:683, 1979.
11. Evanoff, G.V., et al. Spectrum of gas within the kidney. *Am. J. Med.* 83:149, 1987.
12. Forbes, G.S., et al. Genitourinary involvement in chronic granulomatous disease of childhood. *A.J.R.* 127:683, 1976.
13. Fowler, J.E., Jr., and Pulaski E.T. Excretory urography, cystography and cystoscopy in the evaluation of women with urinary-tract infection. *N. Engl. J. Med.* 304:462, 1981.
14. Gold, R.P., McClennan, B.L., and Rottenberg, R.R. CT appearance of acute inflammatory disease of the renal interstitium. *A.J.R.* 141:343, 1983.
15. Goldman, S.M., et al. CT of xanthogranulomatous pyelonephritis: Radiologic-pathologic correlation. *A.J.R.* 141:963, 1984.
16. Goodman, M., Curry, T., and Russell, T. Xanthogranulomatous pyelonephritis (XGP): A local disease with systemic manifestations. *Medicine (Baltimore)* 58:171, 1979.
17. Haines, J.G., et al. Echinococcal cyst of the kidney. *J. Urol.* 117:788, 1977.
18. Hampel, N., Class, R.N., and Persky, L. Value of ^{67}gallium scintigraphy in the diagnosis of localized renal and perirenal inflammation. *J. Urol.* 124:311, 1980.
19. Harrison, R.B., and Shaffer, H.A., Jr. The roentgenographic findings in acute pyelonephritis. *J.A.M.A.* 241:1718, 1979.
20. Hartman, D.S., et al. Renal parenchymal malacoplakia. *Radiology* 136:33, 1980.
21. Hayden, C.K., Jr., et al. Urinary tract infections in childhood: A current imaging approach. *RadioGraphics* 6:1023, 1986.
22. Hellstrom, M., et al. Ureteral dilatation in children with febrile urinary tract infection or bacteriuria. *A.J.R.* 148:483, 1987.
23. Hoddick, W., et al. CT and sonography of severe renal and perirenal infections. *A.J.R.* 140:517, 1983.
24. Huland, H., Busch, R., and Riebel, T. Renal scarring after symptomatic and asymptomatic upper urinary tract infection: A prospective study. *J. Urol.* 128:682, 1982.
25. Jander, H.P., et al. Selective angiography in renal and peri-renal inflammatory lesions: Correlation with histopathology. *Br. J. Radiol.*, 52:536, 1979.
26. Johannson, B., Troell, S., and Berg, U. Urographic renal size in acute pyelonephritis in childhood. *Acta Radiol.* 29:155, 1988.
27. Johnson, C.E., et al. Renal ultrasound evaluation of urinary tract infections in children. *Pediatrics* 78:871, 1986.
28. Johnston, R.B., Jr., and Newman, S.L. Chronic granulomatous disease. *Pediatr. Clin. North Am.* 24:365, 1977.
29. Kintanar, C., et al. Neonatal renal candidiasis: Sonographic diagnosis. *A.J.R.* 147:801, 1986.
30. Klugo, R.C., et al. Xanthogranulomatous pyelonephritis in children. *J. Urol.* 117:350, 1977.
31. Lamb, G.H.R., and Ayers, A.B. Ultrasound findings in a case of renal malacoplakia. *Br. J. Radiol.* 50:753, 1977.
32. Lee, J.K.T., et al. Acute focal bacterial nephritis: Emphasis on gray scale sonography and computed tomography. *A.J.R.* 135:87, 1980.
33. McLachlan, M.S.F., et al. Urinary tract in schoolgirls with convert bacteriuria. *Arch. Dis. Child.* 50:253, 1975.
34. Mendez, G., Jr., Quencer, R.M., and Miale, A. Gallium-67 tomographic radionuclide imaging in pyelonephritis: A report of two cases. *J. Urol.* 120:613, 1978.
35. Michael, J., et al. Emphysematous pyelonephritis. *J. Urol.* 131:203, 1984.
36. Mulopulos, G.P., Patel, S.K., and Pessis, D. MR imaging of xanthogranulomatous pyelonephritis. *J. Comput. Assist. Tomogr.* 10:154, 1986.
37. Patriquin, H., et al. Neonatal candidiasis: Renal and pulmonary manifestations. *A.J.R.* 135:1205, 1980.
38. Premkumar, A. Genitourinary Tuberculosis and Schistosomiasis. In J. Taveras and J. Ferrucci (eds.), *Radiology: Diagnosis-Imaging-Intervention.* Philadelphia: Lippincott, 1989.
39. Rote, A.R., Bauer, S.B., and Retik, A.B. Renal abscess in children. *J. Urol.* 119:254, 1978.
40. Sacks, D., et al. Renal and related retroperitoneal abscesses: Percutaneous drainage. *Radiology* 167:447, 1988.
41. Shah, M., and Haaga, J.R. Focal xanthogranulo-

matous pyelonephritis simulating a renal tumor: CT characteristics. *J. Comput. Assist. Tomogr.* 13:712, 1989.
42. Sheinfeld, J., et al. Perinephric abscess: Current concepts. *J. Urol.* 137:191, 1987.
43. Siegel, M.J., and Glasier, C.M. Acute focal bacterial nephritis in children: Significance of ureteral reflux. *A.J.R.* 137:257, 1981.
44. Silver, T.M., et al. The radiological spectrum of acute pyelonephritis in adults and adolescents. *Radiology* 118:65, 1976.
45. Strife, J.L., et al. Nuclear cystography and renal sonography: Findings in girls with urinary tract infection. *A.J.R.* 153:115, 1989.
46. Stuck, K.J., et al. Sonographic demonstration of renal fungus balls. *Radiology* 142:473, 1981.
47. Sty, J.R., et al. Imaging in acute renal infection in children. *A.J.R.* 148:471, 1987.
48. Subramanyam, B.R., et al. Sonography of pyonephrosis: A prospective study. *A.J.R.* 140:991, 1983.
49. Traisman, E.S., et al. The localization of urinary tract infection with ^{99m}Tc glucoheptonate scintigraphy. *Pediatr. Radiol.* 16:403, 1986.
50. Watt, I., and Roylance, J. Pyonephrosis. *Clin. Radiol.* 27:513, 1975.
51. Yoder, I.C., et al. Pyonephrosis: Imaging and intervention. *A.J.R.* 141:735, 1983.

12

The Kidney: Vascular Disease

The kidney can be affected by systemic vascular disease, or, because of the high blood flow to the kidney and its homeostatic role in regulation of the body's blood volume, renal vascular disease can frequently have profound systemic effects. This chapter will address the various vascular problems that can involve the kidney, including their pertinent imaging findings.

RENOVASCULAR HYPERTENSION

Renovascular hypertension is elevation of the blood pressure resulting from renal ischemia usually related to stenotic lesions of the main renal arteries. Also, on occasion, it may be due to other renal lesions. For hypertension to be classified as renovascular in cause, by definition it must be improved or cured by correction of any renal abnormalities that are thought to be causative.

The role of the kidney in producing hypertension was clearly defined by Goldblatt and colleagues [13]. In 1934 they demonstrated in animal experiments that decreased renal perfusion caused hypertension and that restoration of normal blood flow to the kidney cured this hypertension.

INCIDENCE AND CLINICAL MANIFESTATIONS

The true incidence of renovascular hypertension is unknown. However, it has been reported to be responsible for approximately 1 to 5 percent of hypertension. Given that over 50 million people in the United States are hypertensive, the enormity of screening this population group for a renovascular cause can be appreciated.

Clinically, patients should be suspected of having a possible renovascular cause of their hypertension when onset occurs before age 30 or after age 50, when hypertension is malignant or has an abrupt onset, and when hypertension is refractory to medical therapy using multiple drugs. On occasion, a bruit can be detected over the renal artery when it is severely stenosed, but this is not normally the case, and absence of a bruit should not preclude further investigation.

MECHANISMS

The renin–angiotensin system has a central role in the control of blood pressure. Renin is an acid protease synthesized by the juxtaglomerular cells of the kidney and secreted in response to a variety of stimuli. The main factor in the stimulation of renin release is decreased pressure in the renal artery. Once released into the circulation, renin acts on angiotensinogen synthesized in the liver to generate angiotensin I. Angiotensin I is physiologically inactive; however, it is acted on by angiotensin-converting enzyme (ACE) to form angiotensin II. Angiotensin-converting enzyme is found in the lung and throughout the vascular system.

Angiotensin II is a potent arteriolar vasconstrictor and also stimulates the secretion of aldosterone by the adrenal gland. Aldosterone acts to retain sodium and thus increases the plasma volume. The combination of vasoconstriction and increased plasma volume leads to hypertension. The renin–angiotensin system as it relates to renovascular hypertension is depicted in Figure 12-1.

The renin–angiotensin system is a homeostatic regulatory loop [29]. In the normal kidney, decreased blood pressure such as might occur with hemorrhage or dehydration stimulates secretion of renin, which through the mechanism described above, results in a restoration of blood pressure.

CAUSES

More than 95 percent of cases of renovascular hypertension are secondary to involvement of the renal artery by artherosclerosis or one of the fibromuscular dysplasias [40]. In about two-thirds of patients, the cause of renovascular hypertension is atherosclerosis. The resultant renal artery stenosis typically involves the

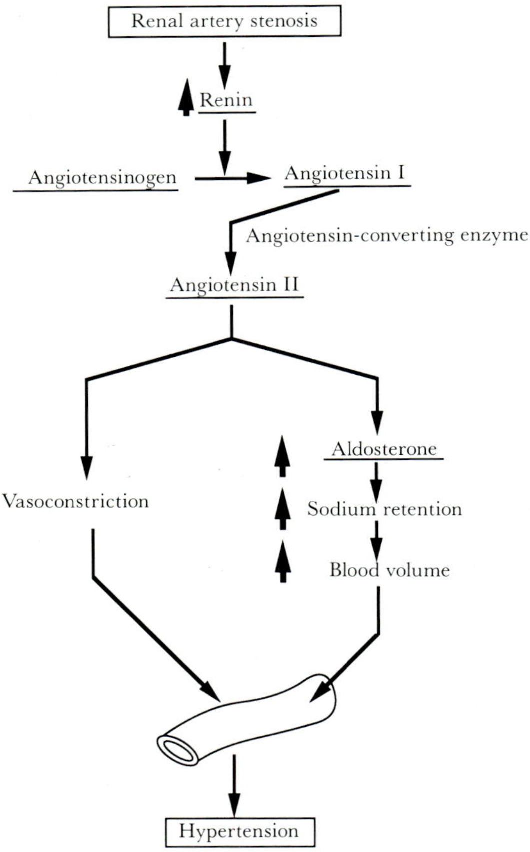

Figure 12-1. The renin–angiotensin system.

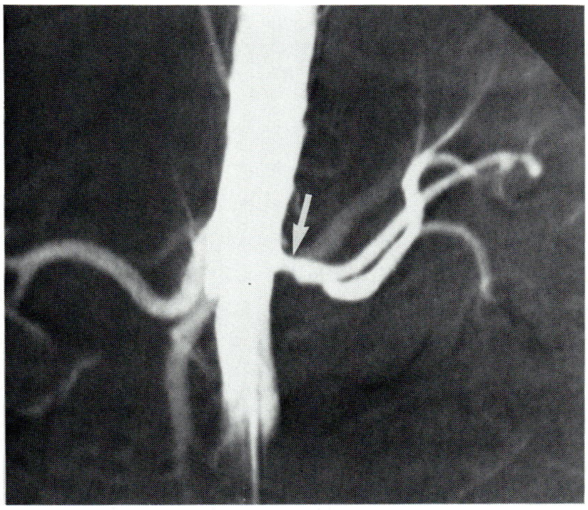

A

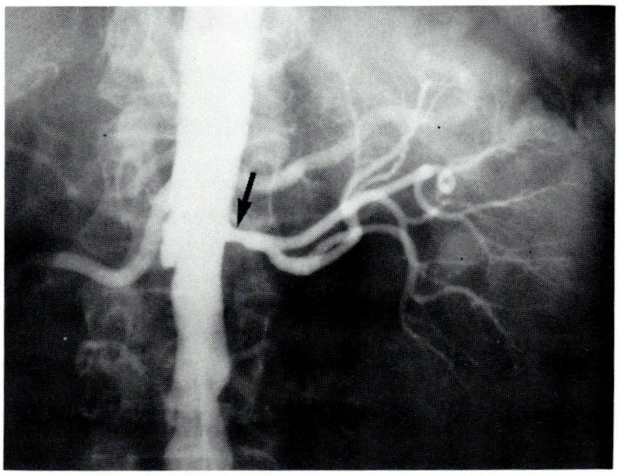

B

Figure 12-2. Atherosclerotic renal artery stenosis. A. Intraarterial digital subtraction aortography reveals a short area of stenosis in the left renal artery just distal to the ostium (arrow). B. Standard aortography confirms the lesion (arrow).

proximal third of the renal artery (Fig. 12-2) or may, with aortic involvement, include the ostium. This disease is typically seen in the aging male patient and is usually progressive. Complete vascular occlusion with renal infarction can result from dissection or thrombosis.

Various fibrodysplastic arterial conditions account for most of the remainder of cases of renovascular hypertension. These lesions are categorized on the basis of the layer of the renal artery wall involved. The most common of these conditions is medial fibroplasia, which represents approximately 75 percent of fibrodysplastic lesions [17]. This disease usually affects young women and results in a lesion involving the distal two-thirds of the main renal artery or extending into branch vessels. Alternating arterial stenoses and small aneurysms result in a typical "string of beads" arteriographic appearance (Fig. 12-3).

Intimal fibroplasia is rare but is the most common stenotic lesion when renovascular hypertension is seen in childhood. The resultant stenoses are long and irregular when studied angiographically. The other variants of fibromuscular dysplasia are also uncommon and include medial hyperplasia, perimedial fibroplasia, and medial dissection.

Other causes of occlusion of the main renal artery are rare and include trauma, embolization, aortic dissection, and impingement by a renal or adrenal mass. Renal artery aneurysms and arteriovenous communications have also

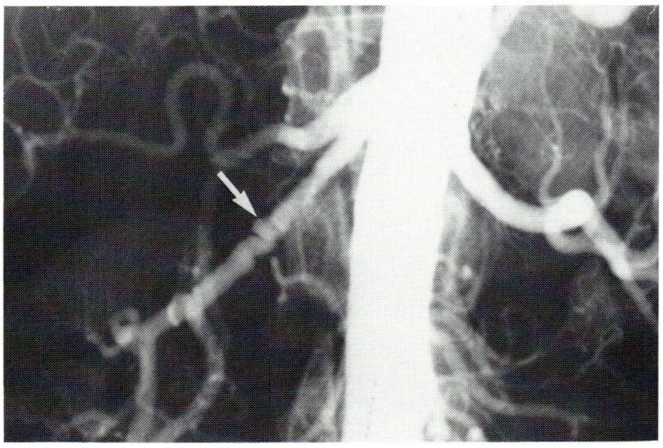

Figure 12-3. Medial fibroplasia renal artery stenosis. Aortography reveals alternating stenoses and small aneurysms of the right renal artery resulting in the typical "string of beads" appearance (arrow). Compare with the normal left renal artery.

been associated with renovascular hypertension, usually as a result of ischemic change in the tissues whose vascular supply is affected by the abnormality.

Renovascular hypertension may also be caused by disease of the small vessels of the kidney. These conditions are called vasculitides and will be discussed more thoroughly in a subsequent section. Renal parenchymal disease, such as chronic atrophic pyelonephritis, may also secondarily affect circulation in the small vessels of the kidney and result in hypertension. Likewise, renal masses (cysts or tumors) may impinge on the renal vasculature at virtually any level of the renal vascular tree and result in hypertension, though in cases of renal cell carcinoma, the tumor may also secrete a reninlike substance [17]. Reninoma, already discussed in Chap. 9, causes hypertension by the elaboration of true renin.

A final condition that can result in renovascular hypertension—the Page kidney—deserves to be discussed. The Page kidney results when fluid, either blood or urine, contained within the subcapsular or perirenal space, exerts pressure on the kidney and produces ischemia [34]. The large majority of these cases involve young males with a history of blunt trauma causing injury to the kidney. Subsequent hemorrhage (85 percent) or urine extravasation (15 percent) results in either a subcapsular or perirenal mass compressing the kidney; the volume of these collections usually exceeds 500 ml. The interval between a presumed traumatic event and the discovery of hypertension varies from days to years but is generally less than 1 year. While many of these will spontaneously resolve, percutaneous or surgical decompression may be necessary when hypertension is unrelenting.

IMAGING

In the past multiple imaging techniques have been advocated for screening the hypertensive population at risk for renovascular hypertension. These studies include hypertensive urography, radioisotope renography, selective renal vein renins, and digital subtraction angiography. Hypertensive urography, discussed in Chap. 3, is considered positive if there is delayed appearance time of contrast in the calices, relatively smaller renal size, and delayed washout of contrast material on the involved side (Fig. 12-4). A radioisotope renal scan demonstrating a unilateral decrease of renal perfusion, size, or intensity of uptake is generally considered a positive screening test (Fig. 12-5). However, a review of multiple series of patients studied with hypertensive urography or radioisotope renography indicates that the overall sensitivity of each of these two examinations is only about 75 percent [16]. Furthermore, these studies do not provide anatomic information about the responsible lesion, and correlation of therapeutic results with definitive treatment has been poor. Accordingly, most authorities no longer recommend these techniques for the evaluation of renovascular hypertension.

A renal vein renin ratio (ratio of renin produced by the involved kidney over that of the uninvolved contralateral kidney) of 1.5 or greater is generally considered a positive lateralizing sign and predictive of renovascular hypertension. Using this ratio, a favorable response to correction of a renal artery lesion can be predicted in as many as 90 percent of patients [40]. However, a nonlateralizing result is not nearly as specific, and false negative ratios can occur in up to half of patients with renovascular hypertension. Furthermore, as with the other studies that rely on functional data rather than direct demonstration of renal artery anatomy, asymmetric bilateral involvement may be easily missed.

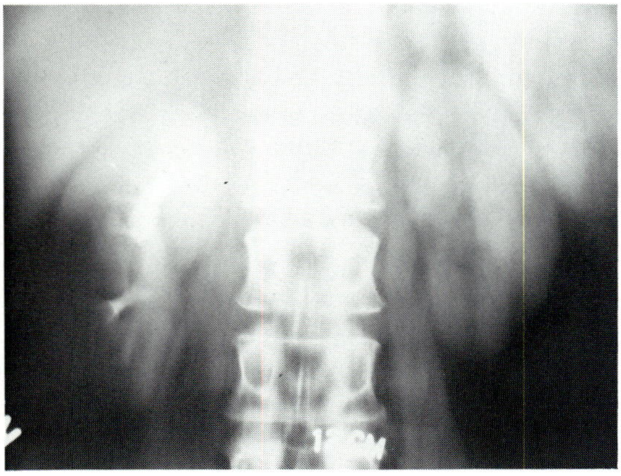

A

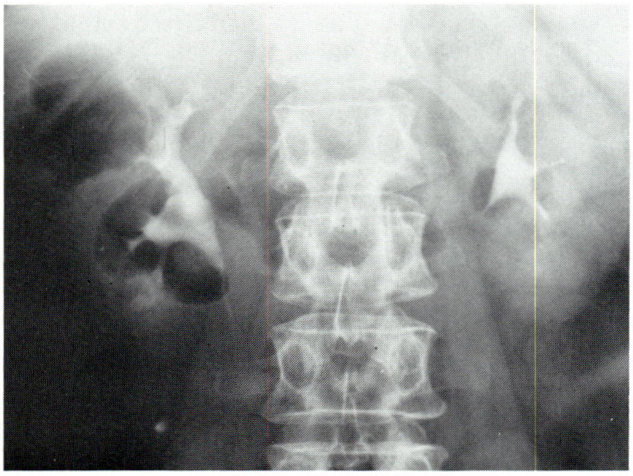

B

Figure 12-4. Urographic findings suggestive of renovascular hypertension. A. Three-minute film shows normal function on the right, while the left kidney is somewhat smaller than the right and has no contrast in the collecting system. B. Fifteen-minute film shows a normal pyelogram bilaterally. This pattern is consistent with diminished blood flow to the left kidney.

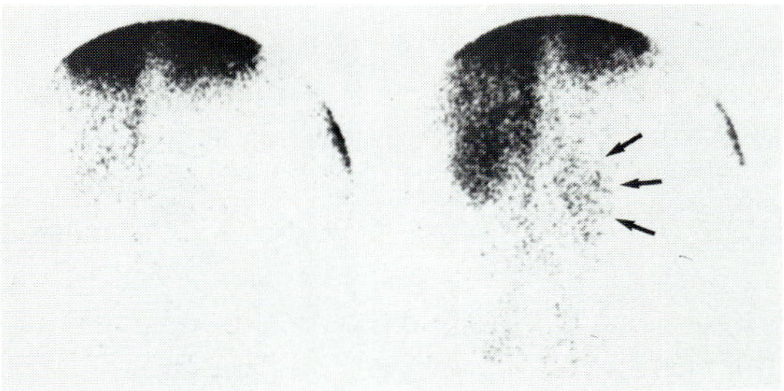

A

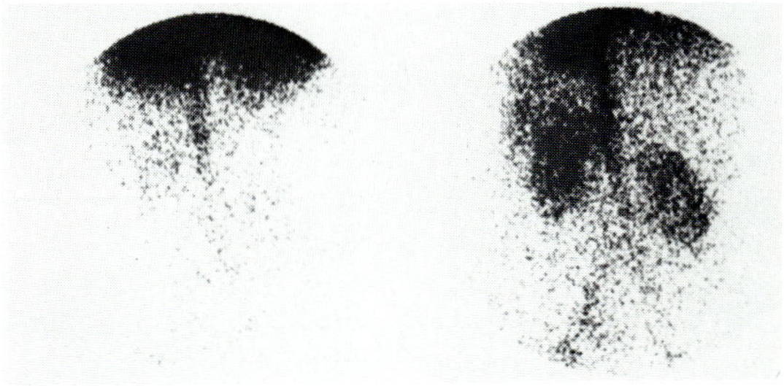

B

Figure 12-5. Isotope renogram suggestive of renovascular hypertension. A. Technetium-99m-DTPA flow study shows significantly delayed perfusion of the right kidney on this posterior view (arrows). The left kidney is normally perfused. B. Repeat study 8 days after successful percutaneous transluminal right renal angioplasty shows good perfusion of both kidneys.

Renal intravenous digital subtraction angiography involves intravenous injection of contrast material, after which image intensification is used to record the vascular system of the kidney. Computer assistance is then used to allow enhanced visualization of the abdominal aorta and renal arteries. This technique is susceptible to motion artifacts, and decreased spatial resolution limits its scope to visualization of arterial lesions in the main renal artery or its immediate branches. Furthermore, it has been reported to overestimate the degree of stenosis in some atherosclerotic lesions and to underestimate stenosis in fibromuscular dysplasia in up to a third of cases [39]. While this examination is still used effectively as a screening tool for renovascular hypertension by some institutions, it is not generally recommended in this regard.

Renal arteriography remains the gold standard for diagnosing lesions that may be responsible for renovascular hypertension; furthermore, this study is necessary before percutaneous or surgical treatment of indentified lesions is undertaken. However, preliminary outpatient screening of patients at risk for this disease can be accomplished by intraarterial digital subtraction angiography, in which small amounts of contrast medium are injected intraarterially via a 4 French catheter. If a renal arterial lesion that may be responsible for renovascular hypertension is identified (see Fig. 12-12A), confirmatory standard angiography and subsequent percutaneous transluminal angioplasty can then be performed by transferring catheters over a guide wire using the same puncture site. Some practitioners now perform percutaneous angioplasty based simply on the demonstration of a renal artery stenosis.

As previously noted, atherosclerotic stenoses are usually found in the proximal third of the renal artery. These may be smooth or irregular, their length is variable, and the lumen may be narrowed eccentrically or circumferentially. Complete occlusion is seen as a tapered stump with no filling of the renal arterial tree distally. With medial fibroplasia, the small aneurysms often overlap the interspersed stenoses and thus make it difficult to evaluate the true degree of narrowing. With stenosis of any cause, the measurement of pressure gradients across the lesion is helpful in determining its clinical significance.

Several newer technologies have also been applied to the evaluation of renovascular hypertension. These include captopril renography, Doppler sonography, and magnetic resonance imaging. Captopril renography involves performing a base-line isotope renogram using DTPA or iodohippurate (Hippuran), followed by the oral administration of captopril (25 mg) and then a repeat study. Captopril blocks the action of angiotensin-converting enzyme and results in a reduction in the circulating level of angiotensin II. It further blocks the efferent arteriolar constriction that takes place in the glomerulus and that has a significant role in the maintenance of glomerular filtration in the patient with renovascular disease [2]. Because of the profound effect of captopril in lowering glomerular filtration on the affected side, there is a dramatic change in the captopril renogram in patients with renovascular hypertension. This is seen as a decreased uptake of the administered radiopharmaceutical by the abnormal kidney. Furthermore, the rate of washout of radioactivity from the involved kidney is significantly reduced. In patients who are not hypertensive on the basis of renovascular disease, no change is noted on the renogram after captopril administration. While this techniqiue holds considerable promise, much additional work is necessary to determine its appropriate use, specificity, and sensitivity.

Initial reports of the use of duplex Doppler ultrasonography in the diagnosis of renal artery stenosis indicate promising results. In one study, correlation with angiography was 93 percent [36]. This technique compares the peak velocity in the renal artery to that in the adjacent abdominal aorta. It has been shown that if this value exceeds 3.5, it is likely to be associated with a greater than 60 percent diameter-reducing renal artery stenosis. However, this technique has a steep learning curve, requires a lengthy examination time, and is limited in cases of patient obesity or in cases in which excessive abdominal gas is present.

The evaluation of differential renal blood flow by magnetic resonance imaging using contrast agents and the possibility of high resolution depiction of the renal arterial vasculature by various magnetic resonance techniques are potentially useful screening examinations for the future.

TREATMENT

It has been conclusively demonstrated that surgical correction of renovascular hypertension is superior to drug therapy [18]. However, surgery requires general anesthesia, and many patients are poor risks for surgical intervention. Therefore, percutaneous transluminal renal angioplasty (PTRA) has become the treatment of choice for many demonstrated renal artery stenoses and has proved to be a successful technique for correcting these conditions [38].

An in-depth discussion of the technique of PTRA is beyond the scope of this book. Generally speaking, a balloon diameter of approximately the size of the normal renal artery or slightly larger is recommended. With atheromatous lesions, as the balloon is inflated the vessel wall is stretched and splitting of the plaque and intima occurs; there is also stretching or splitting of a portion of the media as well as the adventitia. The disrupted arterial layers heal by fibrosis and the pressure of flowing blood maintains the patency of the lumen (Fig. 12-6). Nonatheromatous dysplastic lesions are even more amenable to PTRA, the lesions being stretched or split or both.

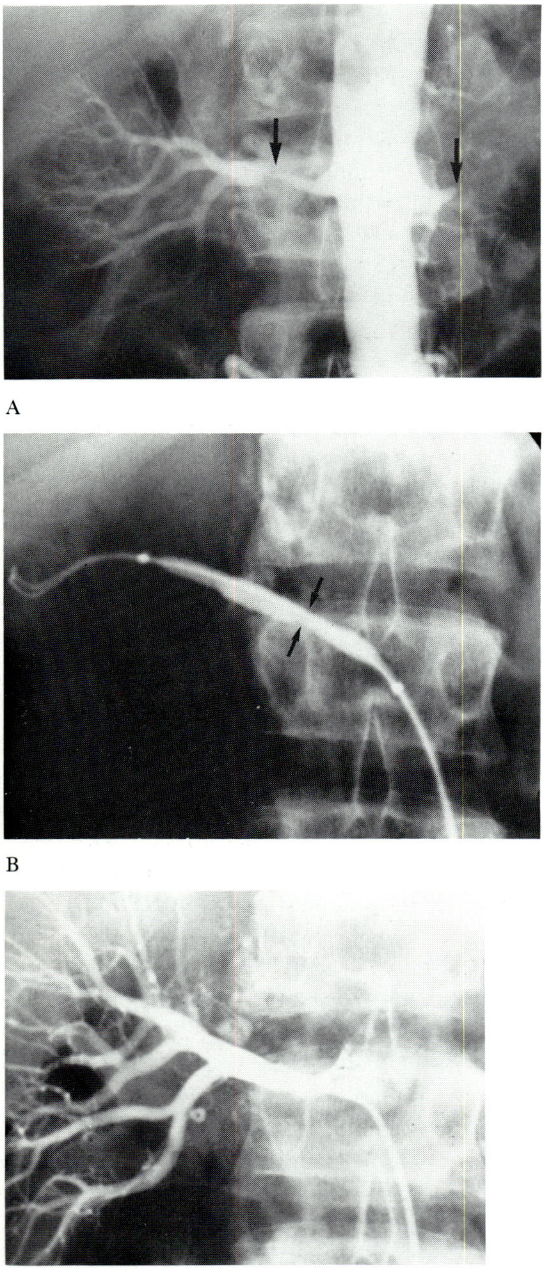

A

B

C

Figure 12-6. Percutaneous transluminal renal angioplasty (PTRA). A. Standard aortography shows severe atherosclerotic disease involving both renal arteries. The left is completely occluded (arrow) and there is severe narrowing on the right (arrow). B. PTRA with balloon inflated. Note the "waist" in the region of the stenosis (arrows). C. Selective right renal arteriography after PTRA shows normal diameter of the renal artery.

The overall technical success rate of PTRA is reported as 80 to 90 percent [20, 37]. Generally, patients with fibromuscular dysplasia have almost uniformly good response to PTRA, with over a half being cured and most of the remainder significantly improved [40]. Of patients with atherosclerotic plaques, PTRA will result in cure in less than one-fourth of patients and improvement in about half [40]. Cure is defined as a return to normotensive status without the necessity of adjunctive drug therapy. However, since PTRA is a relatively new technique, most follow-up studies are for 4 years or less; therefore the durability of the reported results over the long term has yet to be determined.

Generally speaking, PTRA appears to be as effective as, and possibly superior to, surgical bypass for fibromuscular dysplasia [26]. For atherosclerotic lesions, the optimal therapy appears more complicated and is related to the anatomic location of the lesion. For lesions involving only the renal artery, angioplasty is superior to bypass procedures. For lesions involving the ostium of the renal artery, surgical bypass appears slightly more effective. Major complications of PTRA occur in about 5 percent of patients and include renal artery dissection, disruption, or thrombosis. The mortality rate associated with transluminal angioplasty is 1 to 2 percent.

NEPHROSCLEROSIS

Nephrosclerosis (hardening of the kidney) is the term used to describe the alterations of the renal vasculature seen in essential hypertension. Similar lesions may result from atherosclerotic disease. In most cases there is narrowing of small branches of the renal arterial tree secondary to thickening of the wall or atheroma formation, resulting in renal ischemia and overall diminished renal function [32]. In advanced cases, the kidneys are uniformly decreased in weight, and the capsule is adherent to the cortical surface. There is decreased cortical thickness with occasional well-defined scarring involving the cortex between calices.

Urography shows bilaterally small kidneys with poor function. Focal scars, as noted above, may occasionally be seen. Sonographically, the renal cortex is usually isoechoic or hyperechoic as compared with the echogenicity of the liver. With significant parenchymal thinning, increased fat deposition is noted in the renal sinus; this can be detected by sonography as an increase in size and echogenicity of the central renal complex and can also be easily identified by CT or MRI. Angiographic findings are dependent on the distribution of arterial abnormalities.Generally speaking, there is narrowing of the arcuate and interlobular arteries that is almost impossible to detect without magnification. On late films, the cortical nephrogram may be somewhat diminished and irregular.

RENAL INFARCT

Infarction of the kidney can result from various causes, including renal artery thrombosis or embolism, vasculitis, shock, or trauma [41]. The most common cause is embolism secondary to cardiac disease. Infarcts can be focal or global.

Clinically, acute infarctions of the kidney result in sudden onset of flank pain associated with fever and nausea and vomiting; however, this symptom complex only occurs in about 50 percent of patients. On occasion the pain may resemble renal colic. In some patients, hypertension is seen. Laboratory results include leukocytosis, proteinuria, and hematuria. These findings relate to the degree of infarction, and with small infarcts, the patient may remain entirely asymptomatic.

IMAGING

Global renal infarcts characteristically result in nonvisualization of the affected kidney on intravenous urography. In such cases the retrograde pyelogram is usually normal. With smaller infarcts, the urogram may reveal only a relative absence of contrast material in the ischemic areas of the kidney during the nephrogram phase with failure of adjacent caliceal filling during the pyelographic phase. On occasion, the urogram may be normal. Radionuclide scanning appears to be more sensitive than urography in detecting segmental infarcts. In these cases, it reveals segmental areas of decreased radioisotope uptake that correspond to the areas of infarction [24].

The cortical rim sign refers to a thin rimlike nephrogram in the peripheral renal cortex of an otherwise nonfunctioning infarcted kidney studied by urography [15]. It can also occur in renal vein thrombosis and acute tubular necrosis. The rim of remaining functioning kidney seen on the nephrogram probably represents visble subcapsular renal cortex about 2 to 4 mm in thickness that has retained its function because of perfusion by the capsular collateral circulation.

On sonography, acute renal infarcts are typically seen as hypoechoic regions. However, focal renal infarctions have also been reported as echogenic and tumefactive in nature [8].

Segmental renal infarcts have a relatively characteristic CT appearance. These appear as well-defined areas of low attenuation that are usually wedge-shaped on contrast-enhanced scans (Fig. 12-7A), though without a contrast agent there is no appreciable difference between ischemic and normal kidney [11]. Global infarcts are seen as nonfunction of the involved kidney on contrast-enhanced scans or faint patchy opacification of the parenchyma (Fig. 12-7B). Acutely, the kidney may be enlarged, though later shrinkage occurs. The cortical rim sign can be seen in association with infarct by CT as well as by nephrotomography; in one report, it occurred in 50 percent of cases studied by CT [14]. Other findings associated with renal infarct include subcapsular hematomas and mass effect in the region of infarction. The mass effect is most likely due to edema.

The CT differential diagnosis of acute renal infarct primarily involves pyelonephritis, since this entity can produce multiple areas of low attenuation within the kidney, and its clinical presentation may be similar to that of renal infarct. The cortical rim sign would be highly suggestive of infarct since it has not been described in patients with pyelonephritis.

As segmental infarcts heal, they typically result in focal cortical scarring. These scars are seen during imaging as well-defined indentations of the renal contour between calices, as opposed to the scarring adjacent to clubbed calices seen in chronic atrophic pyelonephritis.

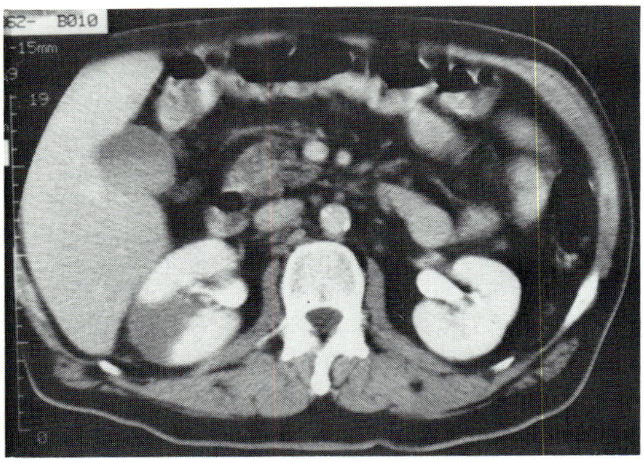

A

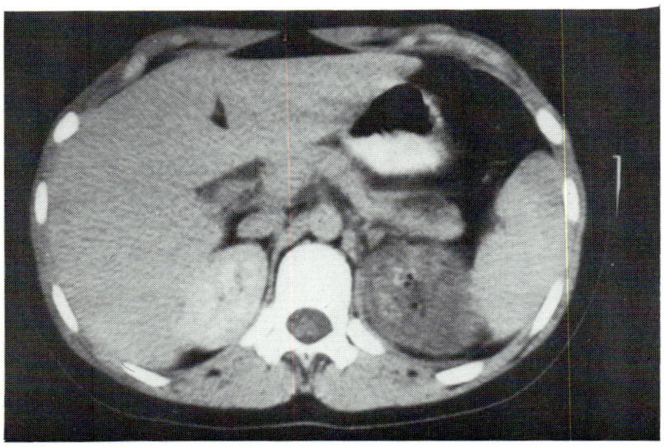

B

Figure 12-7. Renal infarct (CT findings). A. Segmental infarct. Contrast-enhanced CT scan reveals a well-demarcated wedged-shaped area of low attenuation posterolaterally in the right kidney. (Courtesy of Greg Carsen, M.D., Booth Memorial Hospital, Flushing, NY.) B. Global infarct. Contrast-enchanced CT scan shows only minimal patchy opacification of the left kidney.

VASCULITIDES

Renal vasculitides are characterized by a focal necrotizing inflammation of the medium-sized and small renal arteries. This results in the formation of multiple small intrarenal aneurysms and vascular narrowings or occlusions. Renal infarction and hemorrhage may complicate the picture. Polyarteritis nodosa is the most well-described of the various aneurysm-forming vasculitides. However, the differential diagnosis of multiple intrarenal aneurysms has gradually been expanded: Systemic lupus erythematosus, Wegener's granulomatosis, scleroderma, intravenous drug abuse, and metastatic atrial myxoma have all been shown angiographically to mimic the aneurysm formation seen in polyarteritis nodosa [6]. The remainder of this discussion will be confined to the radiographic findings in polyarteritis nodosa, the archetype of the necrotizing vasculitides.

Polyarteritis nodosa is a collagen disease usually affecting young to middle-aged men. The kidneys are involved in more than 80 percent of cases, the liver in 60 percent, and the spleen in about 45 percent. The typical aneurysms seen in polyarteritis nodosa arise from the interlobar and arcuate arteries and range in size from 1 to 10 mm in diameter; they may range in number from two to innumerable. Clinically, patients with polyarteritis nodosa may develop hypertension secondary to ischemic infarct or may hemorrhage from rupture of the small intrarenal aneurysms. This hemorrhage may oc-

Figure 12-8. Polyarteritis nodosa with perirenal hemorrhage. Selective right renal arteriography shows multiple small aneurysms primarily involving the interlobar arteries. The kidney is displaced inferiorly by a perirenal hemorrhage.

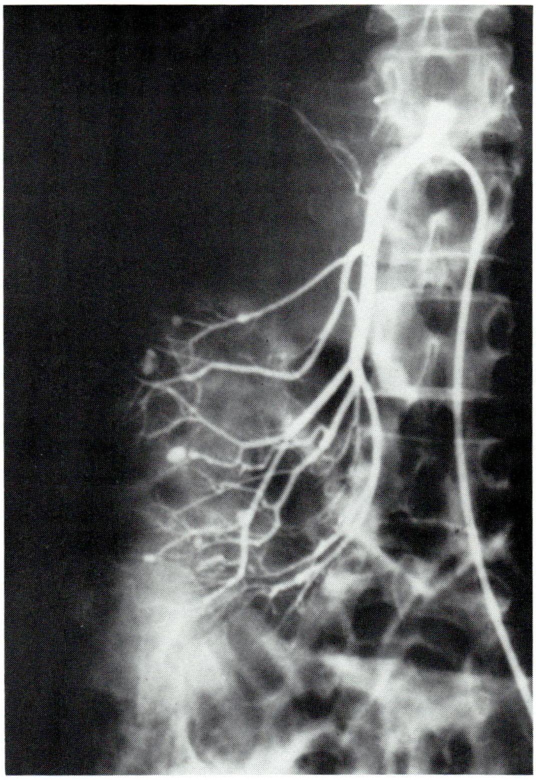

cur intrarenally or, more commonly, into the perirenal space. Once hemorrhage has occurred urography may reveal little or no function of the kidney in question, an enlarged renal shadow, or a poorly defined flank mass. Retrograde pyelography may reveal ureteral deviation or attenuation of the caliceal system due to the perirenal hematoma. Angiography remains the definitive study for demonstrating the intrarenal aneurysms (Fig. 12-8) and can often identify the point of bleeding Ref [27]. CT and ultrasonography are useful in defining the extent of perirenal hemorrhage once it occurs.

OBSTRUCTIVE VASCULAR CROSSINGS

Clinically unimportant vascular impressions are visible on intravenous urography in up to 20 percent of adults and 3 percent of children [35]. These are most common in the region of the superior infundibulum and renal pelvis and are usually seen as linear or nodular extrinsic impressions on films when abdominal compression has not been applied. After the application of compression, the defects disappear or become less apparent.

On occasion, vascular impingement can cause obstruction of the superior infundibulum or the ureteropelvic junction. These specific instances will be discussed below.

FRALEY'S SYNDROME

While upper-pole infundibular stenosis is a common complication of diseases such as renal tuberculosis or transitional cell carcinoma, clinically significant obstruction due to vascular compression can also occur (Fig. 12-9). When this condition is associated with ipsilateral flank pain, it is known as Fraley's syndrome [9]. In such cases, the infundibulum can be compressed between an artery and a vein, between two arteries, or between an artery and the renal parenchyma. Before surgery is considered, impaired drainage of the upper-pole major calix should be confirmed by studies such as delayed films obtained during urography or by isotope renography. Arteriography has also been advocated to demonstrate the vascular impingement on the infundibulum. Therapy is surgical and involves either infundibuloplasty or partial nephrectomy.

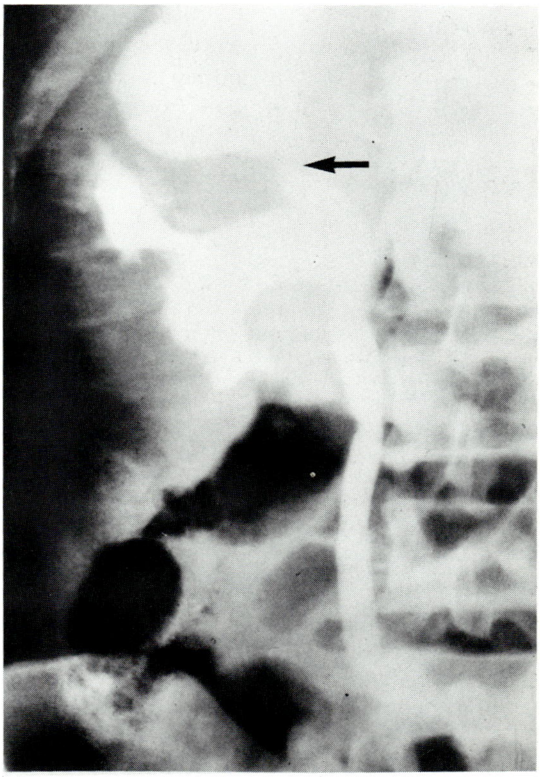

Figure 12-9. Fraley's syndrome. Urography shows an extrinsic bandlike obstruction of the right-upper-pole infundibulum (arrow) and an associated dilatation of the upper-pole major calix in a patient with intermittent right flank pain. Vascular impingement on the upper-pole infundibulum found at surgery; partial nephrectomy performed.

VASCULAR URETEROPELVIC JUNCTION OBSTRUCTION

The large majority of ureteropelvic junction obstructions are due to deficiency or derangement of smooth muscle in this region. However, in up to 10 percent of cases an artery crossing the ureteropelvic junction has been shown to be the cause of obstruction. This artery may be an accessory renal artery arising from the aorta or a branch of the main renal artery that loops inferiorly across the ureteropelvic junction. This type of obstruction is frequently associated with intermittent symptoms. Standard imaging studies reveal pyelocaliceal dilatation with a typical rounded appearance of the extrarenal portion of

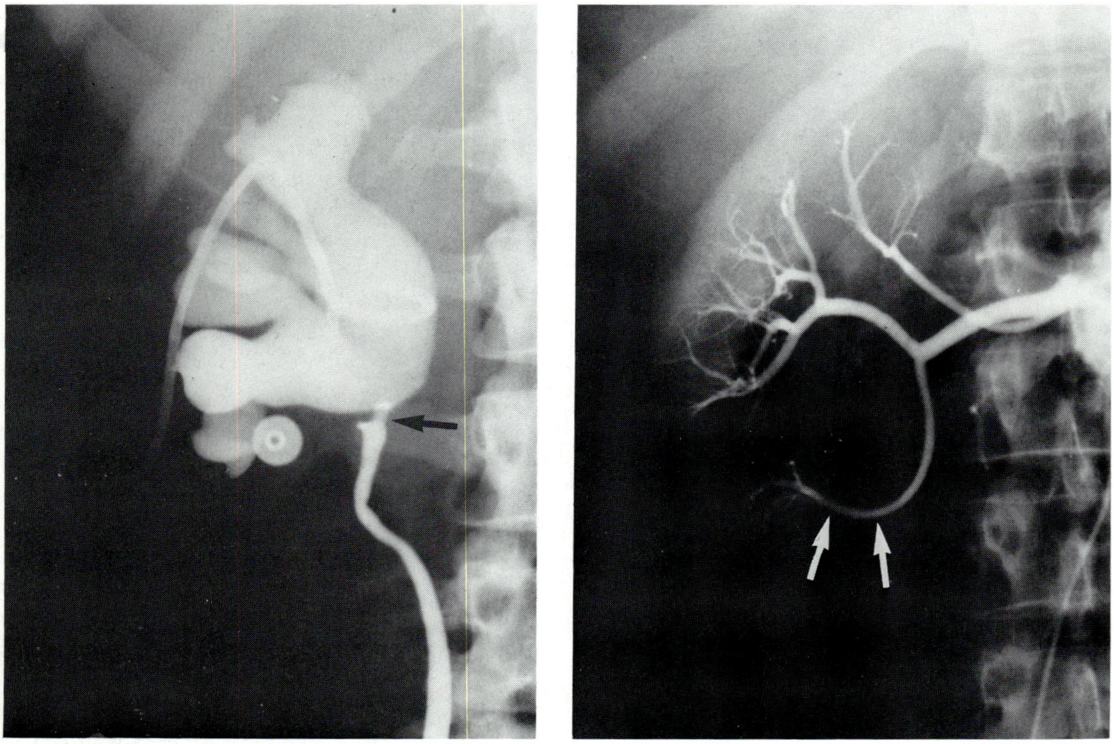

A B

Figure 12-10. Ureteropelvic junction obstruction secondary to crossing vessel. A. Nephrostography performed via a percutaneous nephrostomy shows moderate right hydronephrosis secondary to extrinsic compression (arrow) at the ureteropelvic junction. B. Selective right renal arteriography shows a branch of the main renal artery looping inferiorly across the region of the ureteropelvic junction (arrows).

the renal pelvis. Antegrade or retrograde studies may reveal an extrinsic linear impression at the ureteropelvic junction that is suggestive of the vascular cause of the obstruction (Fig. 12-10A). Angiography is the preferred technique for anatomically demonstrating the relation of the offending vessel to the ureteropelvic junction (Fig. 12-10B).

In some cases, the vascular crossing may have only a partial role in the obstructive process. If there is an associated intrinsic narrowing of the ureteropelvic junction, the renal pelvis may balloon over an aberrant renal artery as it dilates, with the resulting angulation worsening the obstruction.

RENAL ARTERY ANEURYSM

Renal artery aneurysm, as discussed in this section, is to be differentiated from the multiple small main or branch renal artery aneurysms associated with fibromuscular dysplasia and from the multiple small intrarenal aneurysms associated with the vasculitides. There are several types of these isolated renal artery aneurysms, and they are often incidental findings during angiography or other imaging studies. The most common is the saccular aneurysm that usually occurs at the bifurcation of the main renal artery [28]. Postulated causes include congenital arterial wall defects, trauma, and atherosclerosis. A thin-walled bulge develops, which may remain small or gradually increase in size to 4 to 5 cm in diameter. Atherosclerotic changes may develop in the aneurysm wall and become calcified, making the aneurysm visible on abdominal plain films as a ringlike shadow near the hilus of the kidney and usually above the renal pelvis (Fig. 12-11). Small saccular aneurysms are typically asymptomatic.

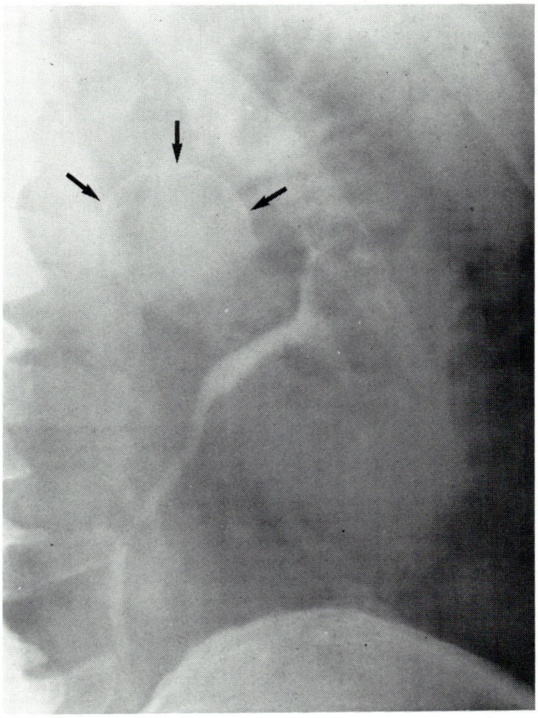

A

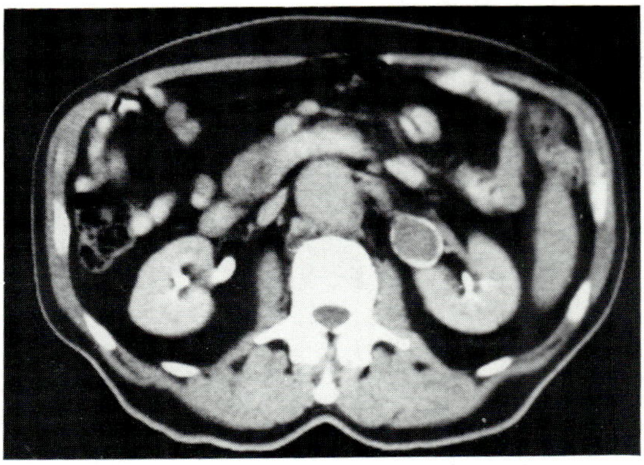

B

Figure 12-11. Renal artery aneurysm. A. Urography shows an incomplete 3-cm-diameter rim of calcification (arrows) above the left renal pelvis. B. Contrast-enchanced CT shows the aneurysm to be completely calcified and filled with nonenhancing clot.

When they are less than about 2 cm is diameter and well calcified, surgical intervention is usually not recommended. However, when they are larger or when calcification is incomplete, the likelihood of rupture is increased and surgical intervention may be necessary.

Another type of renal artery aneurysm is the fusiform, poststenotic dilation distal to the focal stenosis of fibromuscular dysplasia in young patients. These aneurysms may be three or four times the diameter of the normal renal artery and be up to 2.5 cm in length. In such cases, surgical repair will be necessary as opposed to transluminal angioplasty, which is usually the treatment of choice for uncomplicated fibromuscular dysplastic stenoses.

The most devastating type of renal artery aneurysm is one that dissects and presents clinically with the sudden onset of pain that may resemble renal colic. In such cases, urography will often show a nonvisualizing or poorly functioning kidney. Hypertension may be an etiologic mechanism or may develop secondary to the dissection.

On rare occasions, renal artery aneurysms may be mycotic in nature. This presumes an infectious process involving the renal arterial wall, either by a lodgment of septic emboli from bacterial endocarditis, by lodgment of bacteria in diseased intima (atherosclerotic plaque), or by injury to an artery with concomitant contamination [5]. Mycotic aneurysms have a great tendency to rupture, and they can harbor virulent organisms despite adequate antibiotic treatment. Typically, arteriography reveals a small solitary aneurysm of a branch of the main renal artery with occlusion of the artery distal to the aneurysm.

ARTERIOVENOUS MALFORMATIONS AND FISTULAS

Arteriovenous communications in the kidney, when congenital, should be referred to as arteriovenous malformations. Seventy-five percent of arteriovenous communications are acquired [21] and should be referred to as arteriovenous fistulas. In this latter group, the most common cause is penetrating trauma or needle biopsy; other causes include neoplasm, blunt trauma, and surgery [30].

The congenital malformations exist from birth and may enlarge gradually to produce signs and symptoms. Common symptoms include hematuria and hypertension. Less often encountered are an abdominal bruit, flank pain,

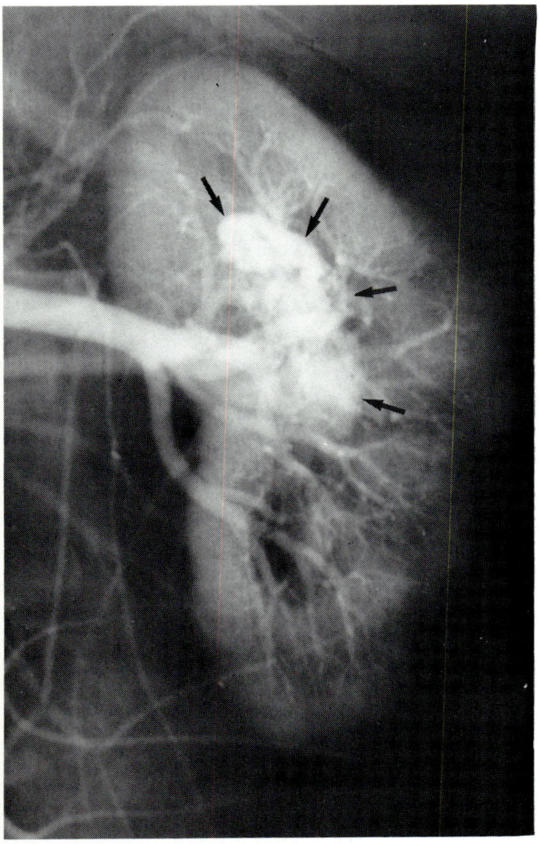

A

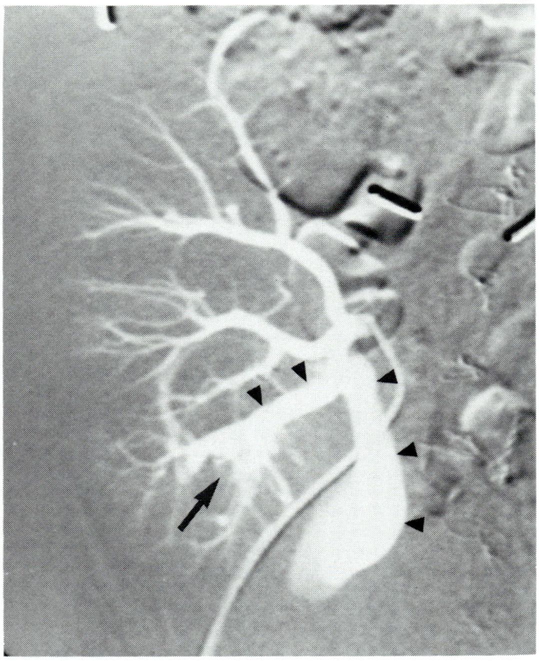

B

Figure 12-12. Arteriovenous communications. A. Selective left renal arteriography shows dense opacification of a cirsoid congenital arteriovenous malformation (arrows). B. Selective intraarterial digital subtraction renal arteriography of transplanted kidney demonstrates an arteriovenous fistula (arrow) at site of recent needle biopsy. Instantaneous filling of the renal and iliac veins is seen (arrowheads)

or high-output cardiac failure. These congenital lesions are usually referred to as cirsoid, indicating multiple vascular communications (Fig. 12-12A). On the other hand, traumatic fistulas are usually fed by only one or a few arteries and are drained by a similar small number of veins (Fig. 12-12B).

Urography is usually nondiagnostic. In the cirsoid type, sonography reveals multiple anechoic tubular structures feeding the malformation as well as an enlarged main renal artery and vein [33]. Sonography of the acquired fistula usually shows an anechoic intarenal tubular structure that may contain echogenic intraluminal thrombus. Flow within these lesions can be easily identified with Doppler studies. Arteriography or digital subtraction techniques can provide a definitive diagnosis and also demonstrate venous filling during the early arterial phase due to the rapid shunting through the lesion. MRI or contrast-enhanced CT can also demonstrate the nature of these vascular lesions.

Traumatic arteriovenous fistulas can often be treated successfully percutaneously using a variety of occluding agents. Congenital malformations, on the other hand, because of the multiplicity of feeding vessels, are more difficult to embolize. Small arteriovenous fistulas secondary to needle biopsy, which account for up to half of all acquired lesions, frequently require no treatment because spontaneous closure is common.

RENAL VEIN VARIX

Varices of the renal vein are rare and are usually incidental findings. It is unclear whether these lesions cause hematuria. They may be congenital in origin or secondary to thrombotic

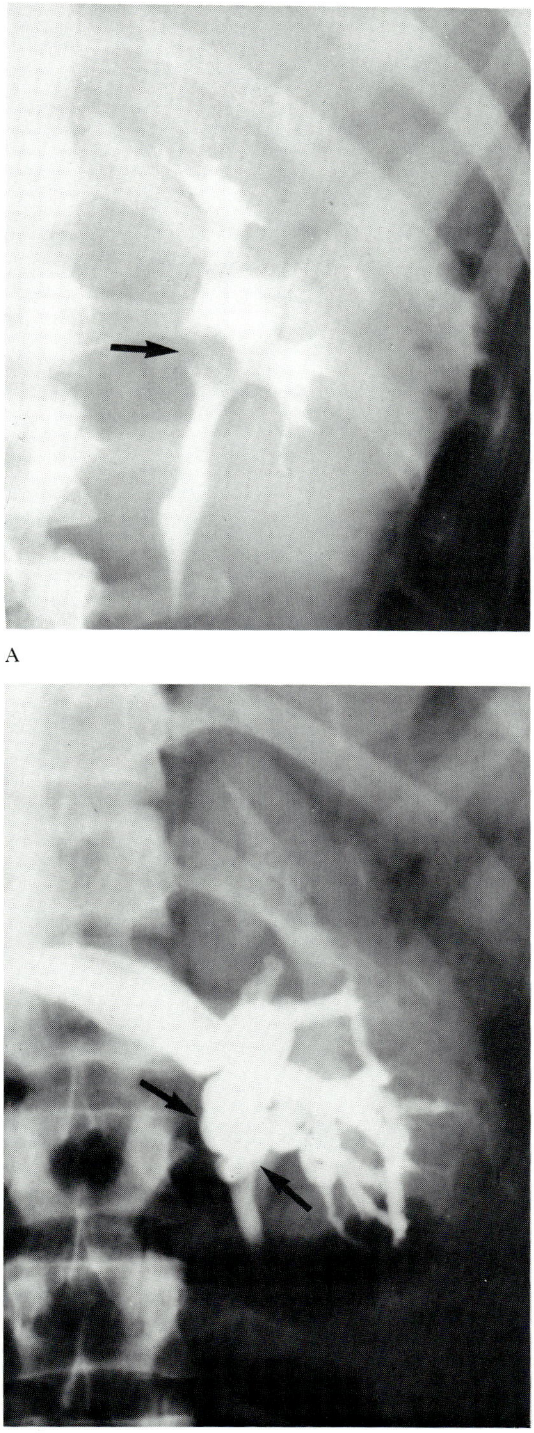

A

B

Figure 12-13. Renal vein varix. A. Urography shows a defect in the left renal pelvis (arrow), which appears extrinsic in origin. B. Selective left renal venogram shows the tortuous renal vein varix (arrows).

occlusion of the renal vein by tumor or bland thrombus, portal hypertension, or abnormalities of the renal vein or inferior vena cava [3]. Since renal vein varices are more common on the left than on the right, one cause may be compression of the left renal vein between the superior mesenteric artery and abdominal aorta (the nutcracker effect) [1].

The urogram may be normal, or there may be extrinsic notching of the renal pelvis or proximal ureter (Fig. 12-13A). While the varices can occasionally be identified by sonography, contrast-enhanced CT, or MRI, selective phlebography remains the definitive examination for demonstrating the venous ectasia (Fig. 12-13B).

PAPILLARY NECROSIS

Renal papillary necrosis, while not a disease entity per se, is a distinct clinicopathologic syndrome that is found in association with several systemic diseases affecting the kidney. It is generally believed that these diseases affect the medullary vasculature, resulting in focal ischemic necrosis of the papillary portions of the medullary pyramids [7].

Papillary necrosis may present as part of an acute fulminating illness that progresses to rapid demise of the patient, may exhibit a more prolonged course extending over many years with exacerbations of symptoms at varying intervals, or may be completely asymptomatic. The diagnosis of papillary necrosis is usually established by urography, by histologic examination of the kidney at autopsy, or by fragments of necrotic papillae passed in the urine.

Multiple underlying disorders can result in papillary necrosis (Table 12-1). The leading

Table 12-1. Causes of papillary necrosis*

Pyelonephritis
Obstruction
Sickle-cell hemoglobinopathies
Tuberculosis
Cirrhosis of the liver
Analgesic abuse
Renal vein thrombosis
Diabetes mellitus

*Note that the first letters of these entities form a mnemonic device—the acronym POSTCARD.

causes are diabetes mellitus, analgesic abuse (especially phenacetin), and sickle-cell hemoglobinopathies (both homozygous and heterozygous patients).

Clinically, the passage of a sloughed papilla may result in ureteral colic that is indistinguishable from that seen with ureteral calculi. Hematuria is also common during the acute phase and may be massive at times. Other symptoms and findings are usually related to the underlying primary disease process. The incidence of transitional cell carcinoma in the collecting system is increased 10-fold in patients with papillary necrosis secondary to analgesic abuse.

Radiographically, the changes secondary to papillary necrosis are best demonstrated by intravenous urography or retrograde pyelography. There are several caliceal changes consistent with papillary necrosis, as shown in Figure 12-14. Streaks or ovoid collections of contrast material can extend obliquely from the caliceal fornix either on one or both sides of the papilla, indicating early necrotic change. Alternatively, contrast material may extend into the central portion of the papilla, the so-called medullary type of papillary necrosis (Fig. 12-15A); as the necrotic process continues, contrast medium can be seen extending from both fornices curving around the papilla in the medullary pyramid, resulting in a "lobster claw" deformity (Fig. 12-15B). When the necrosis is complete the sloughed papilla may be retained in the calix, resulting in a ring sign, or be passed in the urine, leaving a rounded calix without benefit of the normal conical papillary impression. If the detached necrotic papilla is retained in the calix for a prolonged time, it may calcify in a rimlike fashion [23]. The various radiographic patterns of papillary necrosis are nonspecific in that no particular type is typical for a given cause.

With papillary necrosis, unlike chronic atrophic pyelonephritis in which the calices may also have a rounded appearance , there is usually no parenchymal scarring. Furthermore, the kidney generally maintains its normal size and shape in most instances of papillary necrosis. However, if papillary necrosis occurs secondary to infections such as fulminating pyelonephritis or tuberculosis, focal parenchymal scarring may eventually be found. Also, if papillary necrosis occurs with severe diabetic or analgesic nephropathy, the kidneys typically shrink as they approach end-stage renal failure.

When occurring as a sequela of systemic disease, papillary necrosis may be unilateral or bilateral. Obviously, when secondary to unilateral infection or obstruction, it is seen only on the involved side.

Differential diagnostic considerations include small caliceal diverticula or medullary sponge kidney, either of which can result in small collections of contrast medium in the region of the papilla adjacent to the calix [22].

Figure 12-14. Patterns of papillary necrosis. A. Normal calix and papilla. B. Central erosion of papilla (medullary type). C. Streaky erosion extending from caliceal fornix. D. "Lobster claw" deformity resulting from bilateral forniceal erosions into the medullary pyramid above the papilla. E. Necrotic papilla retained in calix after sloughing. If retained long enough, rimlike calcification of the papilla can occur. F. Rounded calix after passage of sloughed papilla. While this is radiographically similar to the clubbed calix found in chronic atrophic pyelonephritis, there is usually no adjacent parenchymal scarring.

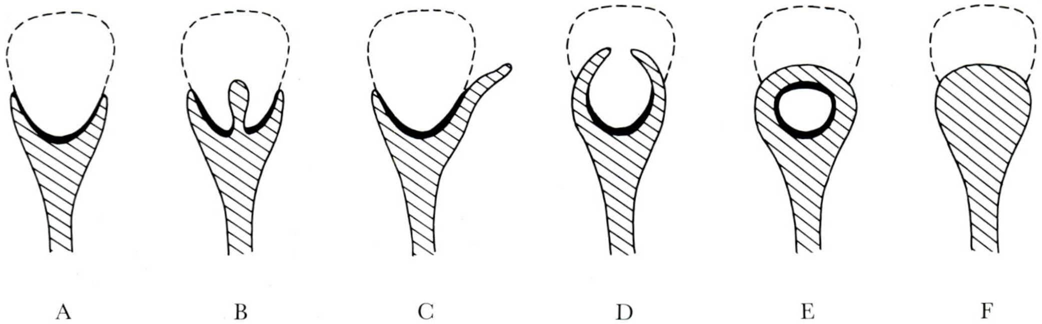

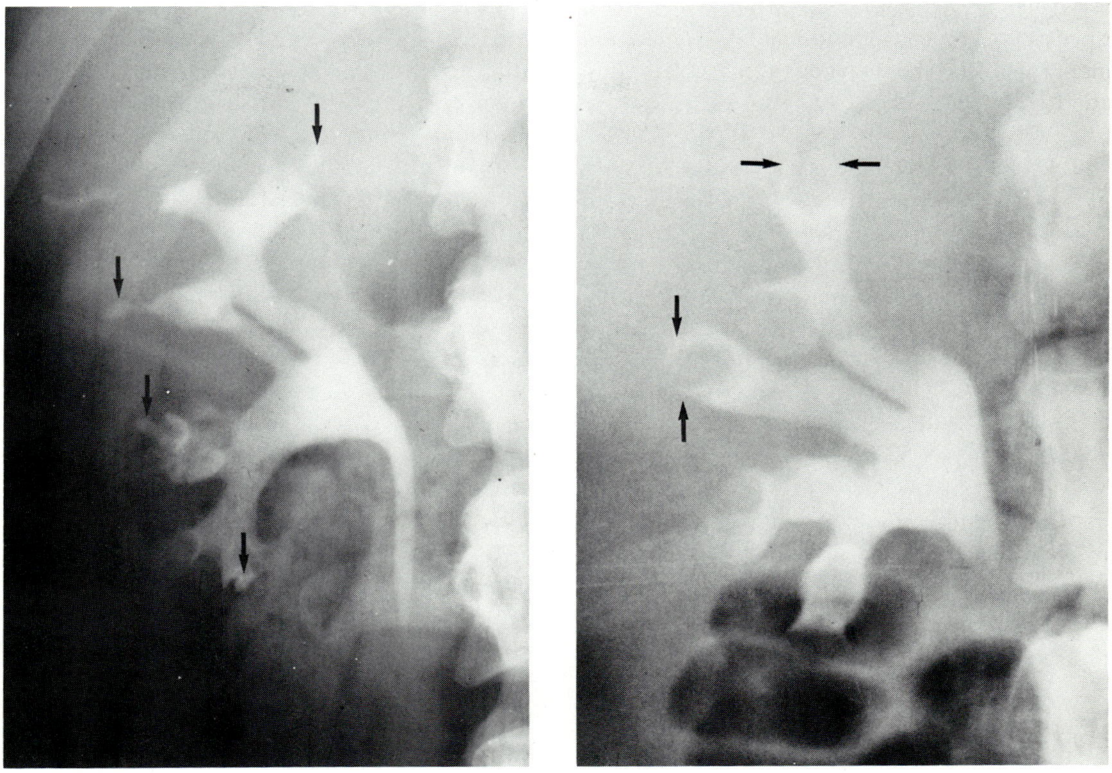

A B

Figure 12-15. Urographic findings in papillary necrosis. A. Medullary type—Small ovoid collections of contrast medium are seen extending into the papillae (arrows). B. "Lobster-claw" type (arrows).

RENAL VEIN THROMBOSIS

Until recently, renal vein thrombosis was discovered only at autopsy. It is perhaps still underdiagnosed because of its variable clinical and radiographic presentations. The exact incidence of the entity is unknown since patients are often relatively asymptomatic and recovery can occur spontaneously.

CAUSES

Up to 40 percent of all cases of renal vein thrombosis occur in infants, usually in association with either dehydration or maternal diabetes mellitus [4]. Pediatric cases typically occur during the first 2 weeks of life and nearly all patients in this group are less than 2 years old. In adults, renal vein thrombosis usually occurs in association with underlying renal disease rather than as a primary lesion. It occurs most commonly in association with membranous glomerulonephropathies, glomerulonephritis, systemic lupus erythematosus, papillary necrosis, and diabetes mellitus. In patients with the nephrotic syndrome, a frequent accompaniment of glomerular disease, the incidence of renal vein thrombosis approaches 50 percent. Less commonly, renal vein thrombosis is seen in association with trauma, pregnancy, burns, or intraabdominal surgery as well as secondary to extrinsic compression of the renal vasculature by tumor, hematoma, or aneurysm [19]. While thrombosis of the inferior vena cava usually does not extend to the level of the renal veins, in cases in which renal blood flow is compromised (severe renal disease, hypotension) clot can extend into the renal veins.

PATHOPHYSIOLOGY

The degree to which renal vein thrombosis will affect the kidney depends on the anatomy of the renal veins. On the left, the main renal vein is joined by the ipsilateral ureteral, gonadal, and adrenal veins. These collateral pathways allow the left kidney more resiliency than the right during an occlusion. In comparison, the right renal vein is joined only by the right ureteral vein.

After acute complete occlusion of a renal vein, the kidney swells and becomes tense and cyanotic. Because of the increased renal venous pressure, arterial blood flow diminishes by up to 75 percent. If the venous obstruction is not relieved, the kidney increases in size during the first week and then progressively decreases in size during the following 2 months, ultimately resulting in a small atrophic kidney.

With acute partial occlusion, the changes previously described occur in proportion to the degree of obstruction, and the kidney may return to near normal size if collateral flow has occurred. If occlusion is gradual, collateral circulation almost always evolves, and the kidney may remain essentially unchanged.

SYMPTOMS AND SIGNS

In the neonatal period the infant with renal vein thrombosis is usually extremely ill and has vomiting. Adults usually complain of severe lumbar or abdominal pain. At any age, one or both kidneys may be palpable and tender. Initial gross hematuria is common, followed by persistent microscopic hematuria or even anuria. Laboratory tests may reveal a progressive azotemia and proteinuria. If obstruction is incomplete, symptomatology and signs are less severe and often nonspecific. With slowly progressive thrombosis, patients typically are asymptomic.

IMAGING

Intravenous urography is often the initial examination performed in these patients. The involved kidney (or kidneys) generally exhibits poor or absent opacification. During the pyelographic phase, the intrarenal collecting system is stretched and compressed by the parenchymal edema, exhibiting an appearance not unlike autosomal dominant polycystic kidney disease.

Sonography of renal vein thrombosis shows an enlarged kidney with decreased cortical echogenicity during the early phase [31]. After a week or so, there is an increase in cortical echogenicity with preservation of corticomedullary definition. After several weeks, decreased renal size and increased cortical echogenicity are seen along with loss of corticomedullary definition. Duplex Doppler ultrasonography can suggest renal vein thrombosis only in cases of complete occlusion [14]. Unfortunately, partial or segmental thrombosis usually goes undetected as the residual venous flow can still produce a Doppler signal.

CT can occasionally directly demonstrate a low-attenuation thrombus in the renal vein or can result in other findings suggestive of the disease, including renal vein enlargement, the presence of perirenal collateral vessels, and a prolonged period of corticomedullary distinction in the involved kidney [12] (Fig. 12-16). Inhomogeneous, delayed, or persistent parenchymal opacification and delayed or absent pyelocaliceal visualization may also occur [10].

The scintigraphic pattern of renal vein thrombosis includes delayed blood flow to a relatively large kidney and delayed accumulation of tracer. This is somewhat nonspecific but should suggest acute renal vein thrombosis in the appropriate clinical setting [25]. MRI, with its ability to image flowing blood in the renal vein, may also be of use in diagnosing this condition.

Renal venography with direct selective catheterization remains the definitive procedure to establish the diagnosis (Fig. 12-17). If occlusion is incomplete, a radiolucent area in the main

Figure 12-16. Renal vein thrombosis. Contrast-enhanced CT scan shows a poor nephrogram on the right and clot in the renal vein (arrow).

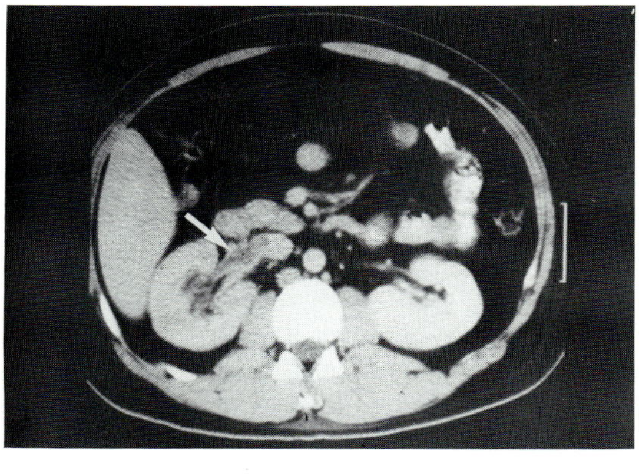

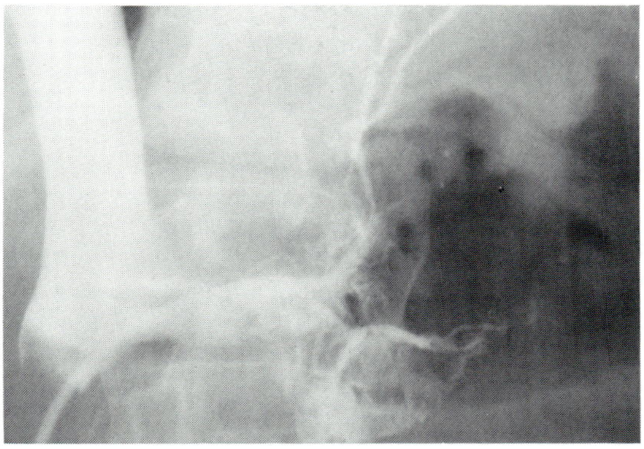

Figure 12-17. Renal vein thrombosis. Selective left renal venography shows complete occlusion of the proximal portion of the vein and no filling of the intrarenal venous system. Compare with normal venogram in Figure 2-10.

renal vein indicates clot. Amputation of the main renal vein is consistent with complete occlusion. An adjunctive advantage of venography is demonstration of the collateral venous network.

TREATMENT

In infants, correction of dehydration usually results in return to a normal renal status. The use of anticoagulation in this age group remains controversial. In adults, anticoagulation is the therapy of choice regardless of the underlying etiologic disease process. The purpose of this treatment is twofold: prevention of the intrarenal progression of thrombus and prevention of subsequent pulmonary emboli, which occur in as many as 50 percent of cases of renal vein thrombosis.

REFERENCES

1. Beckmann, C.F., and Abrams, H.L. Idiopathic renal vein varices: Incidence and significance. *Radiology* 143:649, 1982.
2. Blaufox, M.D., and Freeman, L.M. Renewed role of nuclear medicine in renovascular hypertension. *Urol. Radiol.* 10:35, 1988.
3. Braedel, H.-U.,and Schindler, E. Demonstration, importance, and origin of renal vacrices. *Urol. Radiol.* 2:241, 1981.
4. Clark, R.A., and Colley, D.P. Radiological evaluation of renal vein thrombosis. *CRC Crit. Rev. Diagn. Imag.* 13:337, 1980.
5. DuBrow, R.A., and Patel, S.K. Mycotic aneurysm of the renal artery. *Radiology* 138:577, 1981.
6. Easterbook, J.S. Renal and hepatic microaneurysms: Report of a new entirely simulating polyarteritis nodosa. *Radiology* 137:629, 1980.
7. Eknoyan, G., et al. Renal papillary necrosis: An update. *Medicine (Baltimore)* 61:55, 1982.
8. Erwin, B.C., et al. Renal infarction appearing as an echogenic mass. *A.J.R.* 138:759, 1982.
9. Fraley, E.E. Vascular obstruction of superior infundibulum causing nephralgia. *N. Engl. J. Med.* 275:1403, 1966.
10. Gatewood, O.M.B., et al. Renal vein thrombosis in patients with nephrotic syndrome: CT diagnosis. *Radiology* 159:117, 1986.
11. Glazer, G.M., et al. Computed tomography of renal infarction: Clinical and experimental observations. *A.J.R.* 140:721, 1983.
12. Glazer, G.M., et al. Computed tomography of renal vein thrombosis. *J. Comput. Assist. Tomogr.* 8:288, 1984.
13. Goldblatt, H., et al. Studies on experimental hypertension. I. The production of persistent elevation of systolic blood pressure by means of renal ischemia. *J. Exp. Med.* 59:347, 1934.
14. Grant, E.G., Tessler, F.N., and Perrella, R.R. Clinical Doppler imaging. *A.J.R.* 152:707, 1989.
15. Hann, L., and Pfister, R.C. Renal subcapsular rim sign: New etiologies and pathogenesis. *A.J.R.* 138:51, 1982.
16. Havey, R.J., et al. Screening for renovascular hypertension: Is renal digital-subtraction angiography the preferred noninvasive test? *J.A.M.A.* 254:388, 1985.
17. Hillman, B.J. Renal hypertension. *Urol. Radiol.* 10:31, 1988.
18. Hunt. J.C., et al. Renal and renovascular hypertension: A reasoned approach to diagnosis and management. *Arch. Intern. Med.* 133:988, 1974.
19. Keating M.A., and Althausen, A.F. The clinical spectrum of renal vein thrombosis. *J. Urol.* 133:938, 1985.
20. Klinge, J., et al. Percutaneous transluminal renal angioplasty: Initial and long-term results. *Radiology* 171:501, 1989.
21. Kopchick, J.H., et al. Congenital renal arteriovenous malformations. *Urology* 17:13, 1981.
22. Lalli, A.F. Renal papillary necrosis. *A.J.R.* 114:741, 1972.
23. Lindvall, N. Radiological changes of renal papillary necrosis. *Kidney Int.* 13:93, 1978.
24. Lisbona, R., Derbekyan, V., and Rosenthal, L. Observations on renal scanning and intravenous urography in acute segmental renal infarction. *Clin. Nucl. Med.* 6:253, 1981.
25. Mettler, F.A., Jr., and Christie, J.H. The scintigraphic pattern of acute renal vein thrombosis. *Clin. Nuc. Med.* 5:468, 1980.

26. Miller, G.A., et al. Percutaneous transluminal angioplasty vs. surgery for renovascular hypertension. *A.J.R.* 144:447, 1985.
27. Peterson, C., et al. Polyarteritis nodosa with bilateral renal artery aneurysms and perirenal haematomas: Angiographic and nephrotomographic features. *Br. J. Raaiol.* 43:62, 1970.
28. Poutasse, E.F. Renal artery aneurysms. *J. Urol* 113:443, 1975.
29. Re, R.N. The renin–angiotensin systems. *Med. Clin. North Am.* 71:877, 1987.
30. Regan, J.B., and Benson, R.C., Jr. Congenital renal arteriovenous malformations. *J. Urol.* 136:1184, 1986.
31. Rosenfield, A.T., et al. Ultrasound in experimental and clinical renal vein thrombosis. *Radiology* 137:735, 1980.
32. Schwartz, G.L., and Strong, C.G. Renal parenchymal involvement in essential hypertension. *Med. Clin. North. Am.* 71:843, 1987.
33. Subramanyam, B.R., Lefleur, R.S., and Bosniak, M.A. Renal arteriovenous fistulas and aneurysm: Sonographic findings. *Radiology* 149:261, 1983.
34. Sufrin, G. The Page kidney: A correctable form of arterial hypertension. *J. Urol.* 113:450, 1975.
35. Talner, L.B. Specific causes of obstruction. In H.M. Pollack (ed.), *Clinical Urography.* Philadelphia: Saunders, 1990.
36. Taylor, D.C., et al. Duplex ultrasound scanning in the diagnosis of renal artery stenosis: A prospective evaluation. *J. Vasc. Surg.* 7:363, 1988.
37. Tegtmeyer, C.J., Kellum, C.D., and Ayers, C. Percutaneous transluminal angioplasty of the renal artery: Results and long-term follow-up. *Radiology* 153:77, 1984.
38. Tegtmeyer, C.J., and Sos, T.A. Techniques of renal angioplasty. *Radiology* 161:577, 1986.
39. Wilms, G.E., et al. Renal artery stenosis: Evaluation with intravenous digital subtraction angiography. *Radiology* 160:713, 1986.
40. Wise, K.L., et al. Renovascular hypertension. *J. Urol.* 140:911, 1988.
41. Wong, W.S., et al. Renal infarction: CT diagnosis and correlation between CT findings and etiologies. *Radiology* 150:201, 1984.

The Kidney: Failure And Transplantation

Renal failure is defined as a decrease in renal function sufficient to cause retention of nitrogenous waste in the body. It can be either acute or chronic and in either instance can progress to end-stage renal disease. About a quarter of a million patients around the world are currently undergoing dialysis for end-stage renal disease, and tens of thousands of patients are living essentially normal lives with functioning renal transplants. This chapter will address the mechanisms and imaging of renal failure and the imaging evaluation of the failing renal transplant.

RENAL FAILURE

ACUTE RENAL FAILURE

Acute renal failure (ARF) can be due to prerenal, renal, or postrenal causes. In developed countries, ARF occurs most frequently in the hospital setting. Unfortunately, 5 percent of all patients in tertiary care hospitals develop this condition, and over half of these episodes are iatrogenic [14]. Common iatrogenic causes of ARF include dehydration, hypotension related to surgery, and the administration of nephrotoxic drugs and contrast agents. Twenty-five percent of these patients eventually die; the most common cause of death is infection.

Prerenal ARF is due to hypoperfusion of the kidney in the clinical setting of hypotension, resulting in decreased glomerular capillary filtration pressure. If prolonged, this ischemia results in acute renal failure which persists even if the hypotension is reversed. Renal causes of ARF include exacerbation of chronic renal failure, the acute onset of primary renal disease and the deposition of protein or various crystalline substances (e.g., uric acid) in the renal tubules. Postrenal ARF is due to obstruction of urine flow; this accounts for 2 to 5 percent of all cases of ARF [1].

Acute renal failure can be associated with either oliguria or anuria The prognosis is worse for the anuric patient. For patients with ARF who progress to the need for dialysis, survivors can be expected to recover renal function in about 12 days. Patients who die usually do so about 5 days after onset of dialysis. Of those who survive, up to 5 percent will progress to end-stage renal disease requiring chronic dialysis [14].

CHRONIC RENAL FAILURE AND END-STAGE RENAL DISEASE

Patients who suffer established chronic renal failure almost never regain normal renal function, even if the process that originally insulted the kidneys has been eradicated (e.g., obstructive uropathy). Most patients experience a constant, progressive loss of renal function, though there may be significant variability in the rate of this loss. This eventually results in end-stage renal disease requiring either dialysis or transplantation.

There are many causes of end-stage renal failure (Table 13-1). The most common is chronic glomerulonephritis, which accounts for about 40 percent of patients with failed kidneys [9]. Diabetic nephropathy is also an important disorder leading to renal failure in adults; in the United States, as many as 25 percent of patients entering renal support programs are diabetic [9]. Forty to forty-five percent of insulin-dependent patients will develop diabetic nephropathy.

Cystic disorders of the kidneys account for about 10 percent of end-stage renal failure. Of these disorders, autosomal dominant polycystic disease is by far the most common, followed by variants of medullary cystic disease [5]. Polycystic kidney disease was discussed in Chap. 8. As the kidneys fail, they tend to attain an enormous size, becoming as large as 40 cm in length and weighing up to 8 kg [8]. They usually retain

Table 13-1. Major causes of end-stage renal failure (approximate incidence)

Glomerulonephritis	40%
Diabetic nephropathy	25%
Chronic pyelonephritis	10%
Renal cystic disease	10%
Other	15%

their reniform shape, and in many instances the cysts can measure over 10 cm in diameter. This condition should not be confused with the acquired cystic disease seen in many patients undergoing chronic dialysis.

Medullary cystic disease is an inherited condition with a spectrum of presentations. If inherited recessively, it is known as juvenile nephronophthisis; the dominant variety has onset in adulthood. In the juvenile variety, clinical onset is seen after 3 to 5 years of age, usually progressing to renal insufficiency during the next 5 to 10 years. Patients afflicted with medullary cystic disease present with progressive renal failure associated with polyuria, thirst, renal salt-wasting, and severe anemia. The urine sediment is usually normal, and there is no edema or hypertension.

Reflux nephropathy, which will be discussed in Chap. 17, is responsible for about 10 percent of all cases of end-stage renal failure. Many other conditions are responsible for the remainder of end-stage kidneys; these include drug-induced or hypertensive nephropathy, congenital hypoplasia/dysplasia of the kidneys, hereditary chronic nephritis (Alport's syndrome), renal vascular disease, cortical necrosis, urinary stone disease, and chronic urinary tract obstruction.

RENAL OSTEODYSTROPHY

Renal osteodystrophy is a catch-all term for multiple skeletal responses to longstanding renal disease. Bone disease is typically a feature of slowly progressive renal failure; it usually develops insidiously but is only occasionally symptomatic. There is no bone lesion that is specific to renal failure; rather, osteomalacia, osteitis fibrosa, osteoporosis, and osteosclerosis occur singly or in combination. The most common abnormalities seen are those resulting from secondary hyperparathyroidism. Various forms of renal osteodystrophy are found in 80 to 90 percent of patients undergoing chronic dialysis.

The bone disease that occurs in renal failure results from two basic processes: retention of inorganic phosphates and altered vitamin D metabolism [11, 23]. Phosphate retention, due to diminished renal function, leads to hyperphosphatemia and concurrent hypocalcemia. This combination subsequently stimulates the parathyroids to secrete parathormone (secondary hyperparathyroidism). In order to be activated, vitamin D absorbed from the intestine or synthesized in the skin must first be hydroxylated in the liver to produce 25-hydroxycholecalciferol. A second hydroxylation occurs in the kidney to produce 1,25-dihydroxycholecalciferol, which aids absorption of calcium from the gut and has a direct effect on bone mineralization. In renal failure production of the active form of vitamin D is deficient.

The skeletal effects of secondary hyperparathyroidism are known as osteitis fibrosa. Eroded ungual tufts and subperiosteal cortical bone resorption at the radial margins of the middle phalanges of the second and third digits are typically seen. Brown tumors, which are well demarcated, single or multiple expansile lesions, are most commonly seen in the mandible and other facial bones. Other radiographic changes of osteitis fibrosa include pathologic fractures, more common in the ribs or vertebral bodies, and diminished skeletal density, particularly evident in the skull, where spotty deossification results in a "salt and pepper" pattern.

Vitamin D deficiency results in osteomalacia in adults after cessation of bone growth; this can be seen in a diffuse or localized form. In the diffuse form there is a diminution in the number of trabeculae and a compensatory thickening of the remaining "stress trabeculae." In the localized form, bilateral and symmetrical "milkman's fractures" are seen with little or no callus formation; these tend to involve the medial scapular borders, ribs, and ischial rami. In children with unfused epiphyses, altered vitamin D metabolism results in rickets. In this condition there is widening of the physes from a normal of 1 mm to 3.2 mm on the average, cupping and fraying of the metaphyses, swelling of the costochondral junctions (the rachitic rosary), and bowing of the long bones due to softness.

Osteoporosis is another cause of pain and fracture in chronic renal failure. Osteosclerosis, which may also be associated with secondary hyperparathyroidism, typically manifests as the "rugger jersey spine," best seen in the thoracolumbar area.

Several types of soft-tissue calcification may also complicate end-stage renal disease. These may involve the arteries of the distal extremities (medial sclerosis) or result in large, multinodular calcifications at the end of long bones adjacent to the joint (tumoral calcinosis).

Bone lesions tend to remain static or perhaps even to progress in patients on dialysis. With transplantation, skeletal lesions typically regress if the hypertrophied parathyroid glands involute.

IMAGING OF RENAL FAILURE

In many instances patients in renal failure do not require an imaging evaluation beyond that necessary for excluding extrarenal obstruction as the cause of the failure. This is particularly true in acute renal failure and in some instances of chronic disease in which the diagnosis can be made on the basis of the clinical history, physical examination, and appropriate laboratory studies. When radiologic workup of chronic failure is indicated, a systematized approach is recommended [10].

Plain-Film Radiography

The skeletal changes of renal osteodystrophy have already been described. Other skeletal changes that may suggest renal failure include diffuse metastatic disease or changes consistent with sickle-cell disease. Bilateral renal or ureteral calculi may suggest obstruction as the cause of renal failure. Cortical nephrocalcinosis, discussed more fully in Chap. 15, is indicative of a severe renal insult such as cortical necrosis, chronic glomerulonephritis, or oxalosis. Plain film tomography is occasionally used for determining renal size in patients with chronic renal failure.

Intravenous Urography

Though intravenous urography is rarely used in evaluating failing kidneys because of the occasional nephrotoxic effects of contrast media, it is important to be aware of the various urographic patterns that can occur; these patterns primarily involve the nephrogram. In acute renal failure, several nephrographic patterns can found, one of which is an almost immediate onset of a dense nephrogram, which can persist for hours or days and does not progress to the pyelogram phase. Even though there is severe tubular damage in these cases [usually secondary to acute tubular necrosis (ATN)], glomerular filtration is obviously occurring and tubular concentration may be due to leakage of fluid from the tubular lumen across the damaged wall [22]. In other cases, the nephrogram may have slow onset, but eventually becomes dense. The typical causes of this pattern include prerenal hypotension and intratubular obstruction by crystal or protein deposition. When the glomerulus has been severely compromised, as in acute glomerulonephritis, the nephrogram may be faint or not seen at all. Finally, with cortical necrosis, there is also no detectable nephrogram.

Urography in patients with chronic renal failure typically shows a poor nephrogram due to the reduced number of functioning nephrons. Perhaps more important than the density of the nephrogram is the morphology of the kidney revealed by the nephrogram. The large majority of patients with end-stage renal disease will have bilateral small, smooth kidneys. Most of the conditions previously discussed result in this finding (e.g., chronic glomerulonephritis, diabetic nephropathy, hypertensive nephropathy), with the exception of autosomal dominant polycystic kidney disease, in which the kidneys are bilaterally enlarged. With reflux nephropathy, the end-stage kidneys are usually small and irregular (scarred) bilaterally but on occasion may be relatively smooth.

Renal Ultrasonography

Because of its high sensitivity in detecting hydronephrosis, renal ultrasonography is an ideal screening examination for obstruction. However, hydronephrosis may be obstructive or nonobstructive in nature, and the false positive rate for obstruction can be as high as a fourth of cases. For example, renal sonograms showing bilateral hydronephrosis in a patient with renal failure should not automatically be construed as diagnostic of an obstructive cause for the failure. In some such cases, bilateral vesicoureteral reflux may be the actual cause of the dilation (Fig. 13-1). On the other hand, a false negative diagnosis is rare with sonography, making it an excellent screening examination.

Unfortunately, ureteral obstruction can occasionally lead to renal failure without causing a sonographically detectable dilation of the renal pelvis or calices [17, 21]. No dilation is found in about 5 percent of patients with urinary tract obstruction; this is often due to the failure of a small intrarenal pelvis to dilate significantly in the face of even considerable obstruction. In such cases, when obstruction is strongly suspected on a clinical basis, confirmation can only be obtained by direct opacification of the urinary tract in either antegrade or retrograde fashion for confirmation that obstruction is present. Conversely, if there is only mild splitting of the central renal echo complex (the sonographic criterion for hydronephrosis), one report indicates that vascular structures can account for this separation in 43 percent of patients diagnosed as having Grade I (mild) hydronephrosis [29]. A vessel in the renal sinus mimicking mild hydronephrosis can be diagnosed easily by the use of Doppler sonography.

The term *medical renal disease* is generally used to describe diffuse, bilateral renal parenchymal involvement by conditions such as glomerulonephritis or diabetic nephropathy. In the past, the standard teaching has been that there is a direct correlation between the echo intensity of the renal cortex and the presence of medical renal disease. The cortex of the kidneys in normal individuals is less echogenic than that of the liver. With an increase in renal cortical echoes to a level equal to or greater than that of the liver, medical renal disease could be inferred [28]. However, one study found that 63 percent of patients who had renal disease did not have echogenic kidneys [25]. Conversely, 72 percent of patients with renal cortical echogenicity equal to that of the liver had no evidence of renal disease. Therefore, one cannot confidently detect or exclude renal disease based on the echogenicity of the kidneys relative to the liver.

Sonographic findings in autosomal dominant

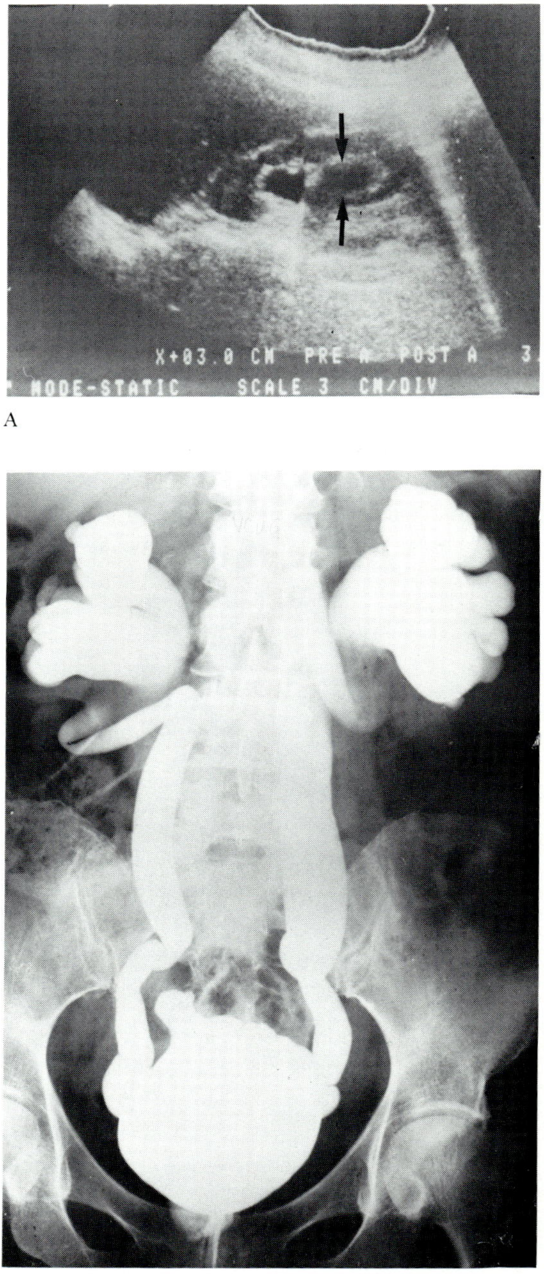

A

B

Figure 13-1. Renal failure secondary to bilateral reflux in an adult woman. A. Sonography of the right kidney shows splitting of the central echo complex (arrows) typical of moderate hydronephrosis. The left kidney showed a similar finding. B. Cystography demonstrates bilateral vesicoureteral reflux into the dilated collecting systems. (From E.S. Amis, Jr., and D.S. Hartman. Renal ultrasonography 1984: A practical overview. *Radiol. Clin. North Am.* 22(2): 315–332, 1984.)

polycystic kidney disease are typical and have been discussed in Chap. 8. Sonography may also be able to suggest the possibility of medullary cystic disease. In one report, the renal parenchyma was isoechoic or hyperechoic as compared with the adjacent liver in 15 cases of nephronophthisis, kidney size was slightly reduced, and a few small (5 mm or less) medullary cysts were seen in all patients who had progressed to end-stage disease [6]. However, the sonographic findings in medullary cystic disease are often nonspecific.

Another use of renal sonography is the determination of renal size. As discussed in Chap. 2, sonography tends to measure normal kidneys as slightly smaller than their actual size. However, significant reductions from normal suggest medical renal disease. Medical renal disease should be strongly suspected when small renal size is seen in conjunction with increased echogenicity of the renal cortex (Fig. 13-2).

Radionuclide Renal Scanning

While sonography is highly accurate in excluding hydronephrosis, renal scanning is occasionally used. ^{99m}Tc DTPA is the agent commonly employed for this purpose, and in the presence of obstruction, it shows delayed clearance of the tracer, eventual accumulation in a dilated collecting system, and decreased activity in the bladder. However, these findings are not specific for obstruction and may be seen in patients with a capacious collecting system (large extrarenal pelvis) or nonobstructive dilation of the collecting system and ureter such as might be found with severe vesicoureteral reflux. In such cases, administration of a diuretic (furosemide) results in rapid clearance of tracer, while with obstruction this does not occur.

Another cause of renal failure, severe bilateral renal artery stenosis, can be suggested when ^{99m}Tc-DTPA studies show diminished or no flow to the kidneys. In such cases, aortography may be indicated to image the renal arteries directly. When perfusion is normal (tracer seen in the kidneys within several seconds after injection) but there is a poor scintinephrogram, renal parenchymal disease can be suggested. More sophisticated computer-assisted studies using ^{131}I-labeled iodohippurate or other radionuclides are perhaps useful in differentiating various types of renal failure, but their discussion is beyond the scope of this book.

Computed Tomography

CT is capable of demonstrating significant renal obstruction and shows typical findings in autosomal dominant polycystic kidney disease as previously discussed. Even without the use of intravenous contrast medium, the renal size and shape can be determined, as can the presence of stone disease or nephrocalcinosis. In patients with end-stage renal disease, the kidneys are often quite small and the renal sinuses filled with replacement fibrolipomatosis (Fig. 13-3).

Figure 13-2. Medical renal disease demonstrated by sonography. The right kidney cortex is more echogenic than the liver, and the length of the kidney is 7.5 cm.

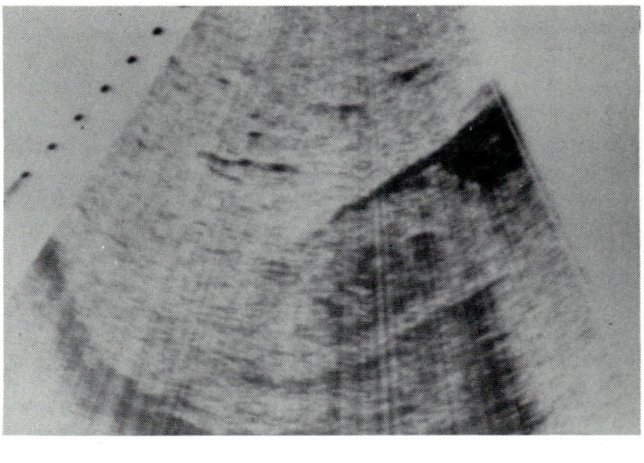

Figure 13-3. Medical renal disease demonstrated by CT. The kidneys are very small bilaterally, the parenchyma is thin, and fibrofatty tissue occupies the renal sinuses (replacement fibrolipomatosis).

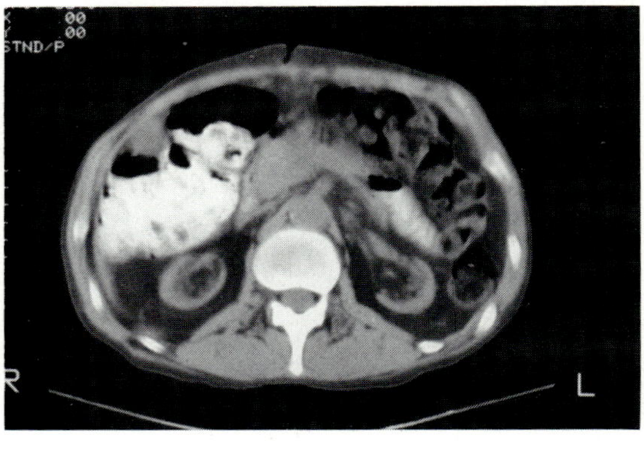

Further information can be obtained after the administration of an intravenous contrast agent, though the possibility of exacerbating renal failure exists, especially in patients with diabetic nephropathy. Studies done after the administration of contrast medium effectively demonstrate renal perfusion and permit evaluation of the renal vessels, aorta, and vena cava for thrombi. Furthermore, the CT nephrogram will exhibit changes similar to those described previously for intravenous urography in the various types of renal failure.

Magnetic Resonance Imaging

T1 weighted images, which in normal kidneys usually show good corticomedullary differentiation, often show loss of this distinction in renal failure (Fig. 13-4). While this finding almost always indicates renal disease, it is nonspecific in that it cannot differentiate among the various insults to the kidney. As with CT, obvious conditions such as well-developed autosomal dominant polycystic kidney disease, significant obstructive dilation of the collecting systems, or small renal size can be easily detected.

Recommended Imaging Sequence

Given the findings noted above for acute and chronic renal failure detected by various methods, how should imaging proceed for the patient recently discovered to be azotemic? Needless to say, the methods employed and their sequencing will vary from institution to institution based on the preferences of the referring physicians and demonstrated areas of expertise within the radiology department. Certainly, plain radiography of the abdomen is a logical first study for reasons previously described. After that, renal sonography is an excellent noninvasive study for excluding obstruction as a possible cause of failure, keeping in mind the instances that can result in erroneous conclusions. Sonography may also show polycystic kidneys or changes suggestive of medical renal disease. Aside from information provided by laboratory data regarding overall renal function, radionuclide scanning is also useful in this regard and may also be able to demonstrate obstruction or diminished perfusion suggesting renal artery stenosis. As we learn more about the capabilities of MRI and duplex or color flow Doppler techniques, these may provide more sophisticated analyses of the failing kidney. Once surgically correctable causes of renal failure are excluded, however, histologic examination of tissue obtained by renal core biopsy is usually necessary for determining the cause of failure.

Figure 13-4. Medical renal disease demonstrated by MRI. T1 weighted section in patient with diabetic nephropahty shows the kidneys to be small and there is loss of the corticomedullary distinction normally seen.

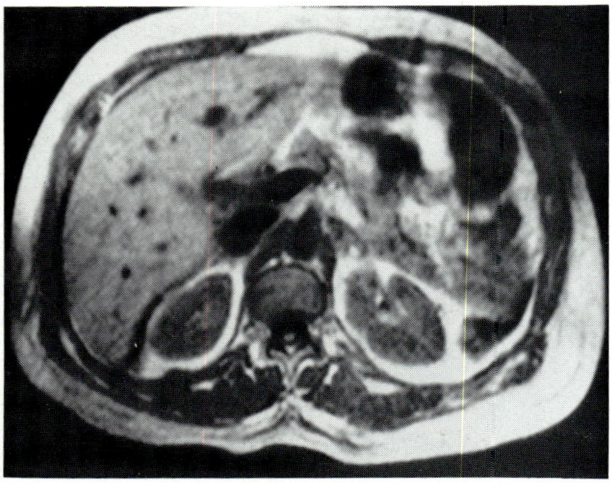

RENAL TRANSPLANTATION

Renal transplantation has become the treatment of choice for the majority of patients with end-stage renal disease. However, in some patients, medical or immunologic reasons require maintenance on hemodialysis. At any time, over 10,000 people are awaiting kidney transplants at one of the almost 200 kidney transplant centers in the United States.

PATIENT AND GRAFT SURVIVAL

Patient survival after renal transplantation is now about 90 percent at one year, and approximately 80 percent of all transplanted kidneys are functioning a year after the operation. However, the success rate 10 years after transplantation is only 30 percent. Of the patients whose transplanted kidneys continue functioning for 10 years, most received the organs from donors whose tissue closely matched their own. Survival of the graft is continuing to improve because of modified immunosuppression, rigid HLA matching, and the widespread use of cyclosporine. Survival after cadaver kidney transplantation is now approaching a level at which, given an adequate supply of cadaver kidneys, there may be little or no justification for continuing transplantation from living, related donors.

Multiple factors influence survival of transplant patients and their graft kidneys. With regard to age, maximum survival is seen in patients between the ages of 5 and 50 years. Patients undergoing bilateral removal of their failed native kidneys before transplantation experience better graft survival. Furthermore, as expected, the medical center at which the graft is performed has an effect on survival of patients and grafts; this is probably related to the number of patients undergoing operation and, undoubtedly, patient selection. In patients receiving sequential grafts, the regrafted kidney has a poorer chance of survival than does a first graft.

Recurrence of the recipient's original disease in the grafted kidney fortunately accounts for less than 2 percent of graft failures. However, the overall incidence of recurrent disease is probably 5 to 10 times more common [18].

PATIENT SELECTION FOR TRANSPLANTATION

At present, virtually all patients up to the age 65 who have end-stage renal disease are considered suitable for transplantation; this includes diabetics, though they are considered high-risk patients. Perhaps the only metabolic disorders that are contraindications to transplantation are oxalosis and Fabry's disease (progressive deposition of glycosphingolipids in most viscera) [20]. Other contraindications include severe ischemic heart disease, old age, persistent infections, and cancer. Certainly, neurogenic bladder dysfunction or an otherwise compromised lower urinary tract can adversely influence the outcome of transplantation and should be corrected preoperatively when possible. Evaluation of the lower urinary tract for neurogenic dysfunction is discussed in Chap. 21.

SURGICAL ASPECTS OF RENAL TRANSPLANTATION

Right or left graft kidneys can be placed in either iliac fossa. The vascular connection is typically an end-to-side anastomosis of the renal artery to the external iliac artery and a similar anastomosis of the renal vein to the external iliac vein. Occasionally, the internal iliac artery is divided distally and anastomosed end-to-end to the renal artery.

When the graft has multiple renal arteries, a patch of aorta containing all the openings can be removed (in cases of cadaver donors) and this patch anastomosed to the side of the common or external iliac arteries. Since this cannot be done when the graft is from a living donor, various types of anastomoses may be necessary when multiple renal arteries are present.

Urinary drainage is usually established by implantation of the ureter from the donor kidney into the bladder. A relatively long submucosal tunnel for the most distal portion of the ureter is employed to prevent vesicoureteral reflux.

MECHANISMS OF RENAL TRANSPLANT FAILURE

Both medical and surgical problems can affect the function of a transplanted kidney. Medical problems frequently encountered include graft rejection, acute tubular necrosis, and cyclosporine toxicity. Urologic complications occur in up to 10 percent of cases and include urinary obstruction, urine extravasation, perirenal fluid collections, and renal artery stenosis. Table 13-2 lists the common causes of complications that can affect graft survival and the temporal sequence of their occurrence.

When classified on a temporal basis, graft rejection includes hyperacute, accelerated acute, acute, and chronic varieties. The hyperacute and accelerated acute forms of rejection may be so overt as to be recognizable at the time of surgery; otherwise they present as graft malfunction immediately after surgery. These result in significant edema and may progress to kidney rupture and hemorrhage. Acute rejection usually occurs between 1 and 4 weeks postoperatively; this category of rejection may be either cellular (good prognosis) or vascular (poor prognosis). The cellular type of acute rejection

Table 13-2. Major causes and temporal sequence of graft failure

Medical Complications	
Acute tubular necrosis (ATN)	Can be found at time of surgery in cadaver kidney
Rejection	
Hyperacute	During surgery to a few hours afterward
Accelerated acute	First week after surgery
Acute	1–4 weeks after surgery
Chronic	Months to years after surgery
Cyclosporine toxicity	1 to 3 months after surgery (rare during first month)
Urologic Complications	
Leak, hematoma, anastomotic stricture	Few days to few weeks after surgery
Lymphocele with ureteral obstruction	1 to 4 months after surgery
Renal artery stenosis	1 month or more after surgery

Modified from Dubovsky, E.V., and Russell, C.D. Radionuclide evaluation of renal transplants. *Semin. Nucl. Med.* 18:181, 1988.

results in edema of the interstitium and cortical infiltration with mononuclear cells. The vascular type of acute rejection is typified by an endovasculitis that results in swelling of the endothelial cells and edema in the subendothelial space, both of which serve to increase vascular resistance in the kidney. Graft rejection is the most common cause of transplant dysfunction and loss; when cadaver kidneys are used, rejection episodes of some degree occur in as many as 93 percent of cases [13].

Up to half of cadaver kidney transplants exhibit poor function during the immediate postoperative period. This poor function is usually due to ischemia that has resulted in ATN. However, ATN can also present clinically during the first week or two after transplantation.

Cyclosporine, widely used for immunosuppression in transplant recipients, suppresses T lymphocytes, thereby preventing or delaying graft rejection. Unfortunately, in some patients it also has a nephrotoxic effect. This nephrotoxicity generally manifests itself between 1 and 3 months posttransplantation.

Urologic complications, particularly those causing ureteral obstruction or compromise of the blood supply to the graft, can occur independently or be found in association with the medical causes of decreased graft function.

The differential diagnosis of the failing transplant in the weeks after surgery poses a difficult clinical problem. The symptoms of graft enlargement and tenderness, fever, fluid retention, decreased renal function, oliguria, and increasing serum creatinine constitute a nonspecific symptom complex that can be seen with any of the medical or surgical causes of graft failure. However, it is extremely important to arrive at the correct diagnosis since the treatment is different for each of these conditions. While ATN will usually resolve spontaneously, graft rejection requires alteration of immunosuppressive treatment, cyclosporine toxicity requires a reduction in dosage of this drug, and urologic complications require rapid interventional or surgical treatment.

IMAGING THE FAILING RENAL TRANSPLANT

A normally functioning transplant kidney in either iliac fossa can easily be imaged by all current techniques and in general exhibits the same imaging characteristics as a normal native kidney (Fig. 13-5). However, when graft dysfunction occurs it is essential that urologic problems be excluded as the cause or, when they are found, be treated promptly. Delay in alleviating these complications may cause loss of the transplanted kidney; furthermore, mortality rates secondary to urologic complications exceed 20 percent in some series [2].

Fluid collections, especially hematomas or urinomas, are frequently seen in the early postoperative period. Lymphoceles, which are the most common fluid collections seen in association with renal transplants, typically occur from 3 weeks to several months after transplantation; these tend to be large and may contain septations. Commonly found medial or inferior

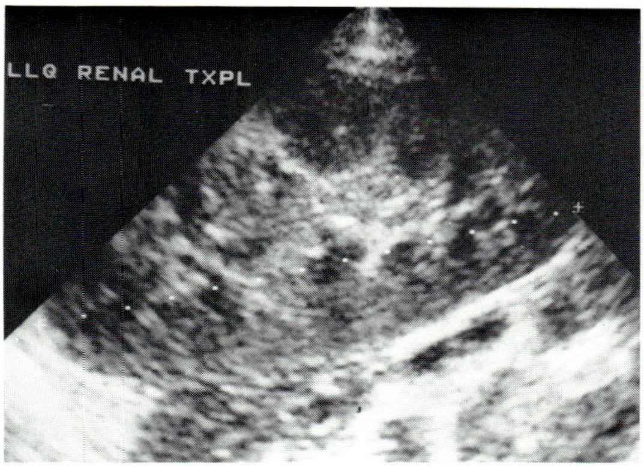

A

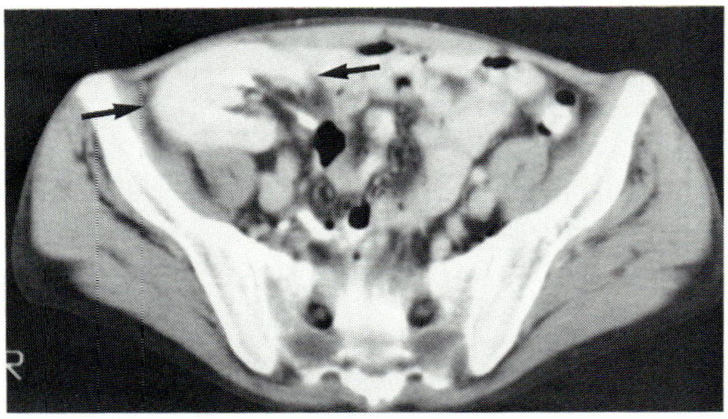

B

Figure 13-5. Normally functioning graft kidney. A. Transplant sonography shows normal parenchymal thickness and echogenicity. The pyramids are slightly prominent, which is not unusual. B. Contrast-enhanced CT of transplant (arrows) shows normal parenchymal enhancement and a nondilated collecting system.

to the transplant kidney, fluid collections are ideally situated to obstruct the ureter. Sonography is an excellent method for detecting these fluid collections (Fig. 13-6), though their characteristics are often nonspecific. CT can also easily detect fluid collections and, if an intravenous contrast agent is given, demonstrate urine leaks. Renal scintigraphy may suggest a fluid collection by showing mass effect between the kidney and bladder; it can also diagnose urine leakage and ureteral obstruction. MRI has the potential to further differentiate fluid collections; lymphoceles and urinomas, with or without infections, tend to exhibit low signal intensity on T1 weighted images and become bright on T2 images, while hematomas may have high signal intensities on both sets of images. Fluid

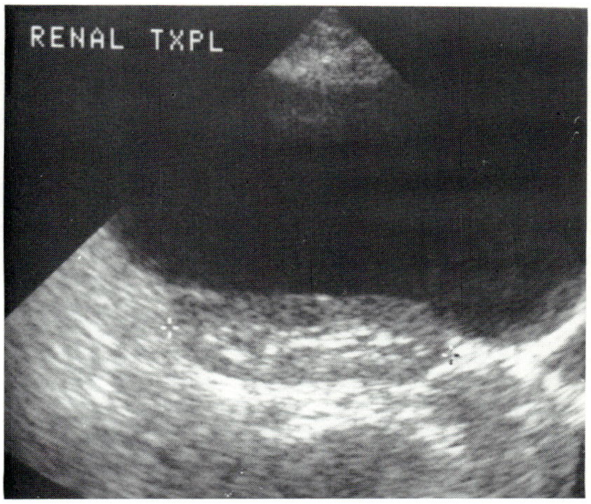

Figure 13-6. Lymphocele demonstrated by sonography. The transplanted kidney is compressed by a large fluid collection anteriorly and medially. There is nothing specific on this study to suggest the nature of the fluid, but aspiration confirmed a lymphocele and percutaneous drainage was performed.

collections can be further characterized by needle aspiration, and percutaneous drainage techniques have proven useful in their treatment.

Ureteral obstruction can be secondary to postoperative edema at the site of anastomosis of the ureter to the bladder. This will usually spontaneously resolve. As noted previously, fluid collections can compress the ureter and should be treated by percutaneous or surgical drainage. While sonography is excellent for detecting hydronephrosis (Fig. 13-7), in some cases, the exact point of obstruction can only be determined by antegrade pyelography. If necessary, percutaneous nephrostomy can then be performed for long-term drainage, or access to the collecting system established for ureteral stenting.

Stenosis or occlusion of the vascular supply to the transplant kidney may be manifested by hypertension, elevated serum creatinine, or both. Renal artery stenosis has been reported as developing in 1.6 to 16 percent of patients who have undergone transplantation [31]. This complication can be imaged with standard arteriography (Fig. 13-8), though digital subtraction angiography performed after intraarterial injections of very small doses of contrast medium has also been reported as effective in evaluating

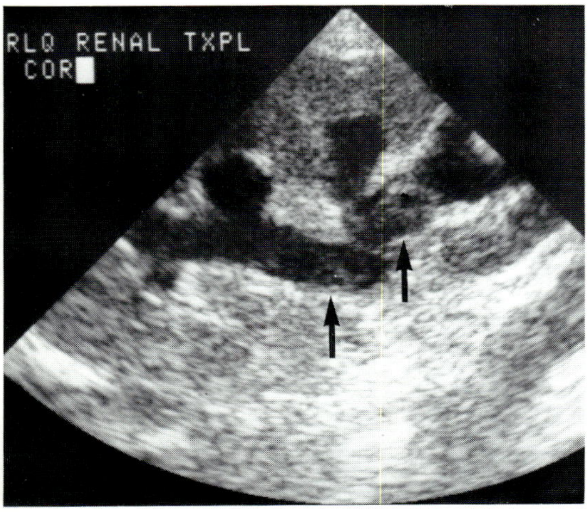

Figure 13-7. Transplant hydronephrosis demonstrated by sonography. Moderate dilation of the collecting system can be easily detected as can slightly echogenic material in the collecting system (arrows). The patient had obstruction due to passage of clots after a renal core biopsy.

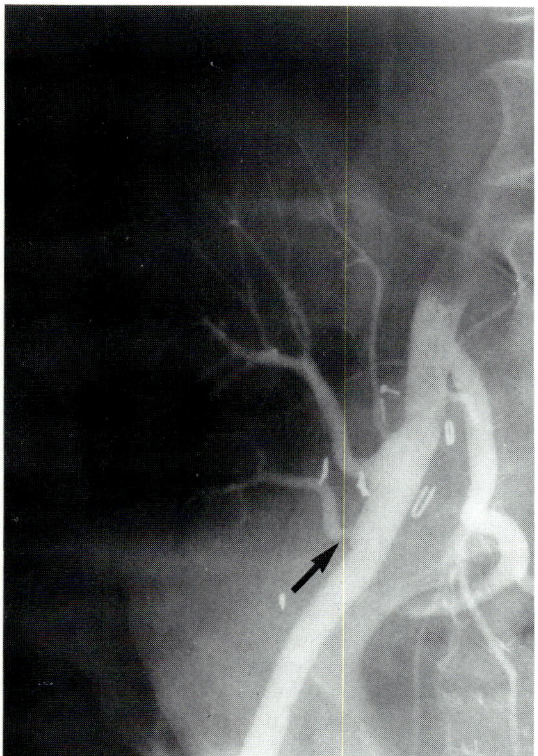

Figure 13-8. Graft renal artery stenosis. Right iliac arteriography shows three vessels to the graft, the most caudad of which has a severe stenosis near its origin from the external iliac artery (arrow).

vascular problems in renal transplant patients [24]. Doppler sonography has been reported to be useful in imaging the arterial flow to the transplanted kidney; an area of significant luminal narrowing (greater than 50%) in the renal artery should produce a segmental region of abnormal flow (high-velocity jet exceeding 7.5 kHz and distal turbulence) [30]. However, the tortuosity and small size of this vessel create some problems in identification of stenoses.

While urologic complications involving the transplanted kidney can be readily diagnosed by various imaging methods and often treated by interventional techniques, the differentiation of the various medical complications is less well defined. Perhaps the most critical determination in the evaluation of the failing transplant is the differentiation of graft rejection from acute tubular necrosis or cyclosporine toxicity. At the time of this writing, no single imaging method has permitted accurate differentiation of these processes with sufficient sensitivity and specificity to obviate the need for graft biopsy [15].

Multiple sonographic findings have been associated with graft rejection; these include enlargement of the medullary pyramids, increased cortical echogenicity, thickening of the collecting system wall, decreased renal sinus fat, and swelling of the transplanted kidney. However, these findings are nonspecific and cannot routinely differentiate the causes of graft failure [16]. Recently, duplex scanning techniques have been used for measuring the resistive index of blood flow within the transplanted kidney. The mean resistive index can be calculated from Doppler measurements within main, segmental, or interlobar renal arteries:

$$\text{Resistive Index} = \frac{\text{Peak systolic blood flow velocity} - \text{Minimum end diastolic blood flow velocity}}{\text{Peak systolic blood flow velocity}}$$

The usefulness of this measurement is based on the fact that the resistive index is increased in cases of acute vascular rejection and is more likely to remain normal in other conditions [26]. Generally speaking, a resistive index greater than 0.90 is highly suspicious for vascular rejection, while an index of less than 0.70 indicates normal vascular impedance (Fig. 13-9). How-

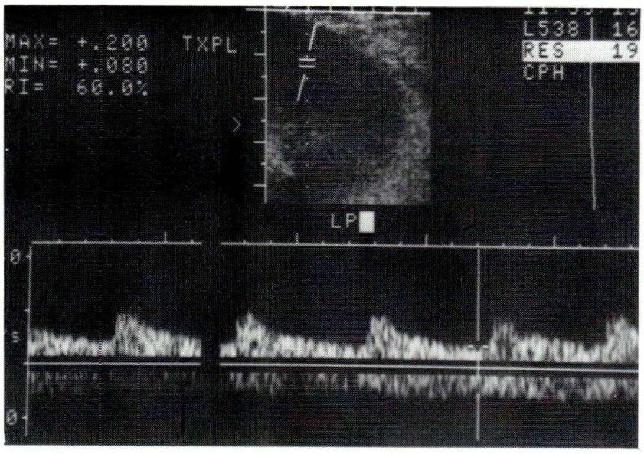

A

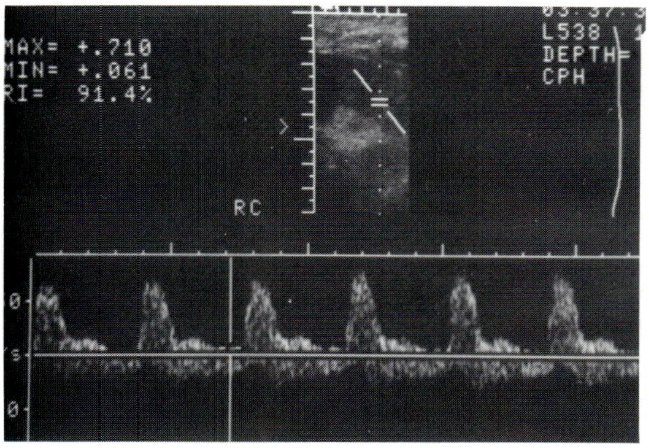

B

Figure 13-9. Duplex Doppler determination of resistive index. A. Normal resistive index (0.60) measured over interlobar artery (marker) in normally functioning graft. B. Significantly elevated resistive index (0.91) measured over interlobar artery (marker) in graft undergoing acute vascular rejection. Note the rapid drop-off of systolic flow to almost zero on the wave form at the bottom of the illustration, indicating a severe impedance to normal flow.

ever, stenosis of the main transplant renal artery, renal vein thrombosis or obstruction, severe ATN, pyelonephritis, extrarenal compression of the graft, and ureteral obstruction have all been shown to increase vascular impedance within the transplanted kidney [3, 7, 33].

Radionuclide studies using both ^{99m}Tc-DTPA (perfusion) and sometimes ^{131}I iodohippurate (tubular function) are often employed in a serial fashion to evaluate failing grafts. Though none of the radionuclide agents is specific enough to diagnose a particular cause of failure, improvement or deterioration in perfusion of the graft and its parenchymal function can be documented by quantitative radionuclide studies performed over a period of time [27]. When correlated with the clinical status of the patient and other imaging findings, this technique is of significant clinical value. Since all medical causes of graft dysfunction exhibit deteriorating tubular function, diminished renal perfusion is the key in distinguishing rejection from cyclosporine toxicity or ATN. Using ^{99m}Tc-DTPA, a normally functioning graft demonstrates rapid uptake of the radionuclide and maximum activity is seen at about 5 minutes. Poor graft function is seen as a decreased uptake of the radionuclide; this may occur in conjunction with good perfusion, as would be expected with ATN or cyclosporine toxicity, or poor perfusion, which suggests rejection [4] (Fig. 13-10).

At this point it must be emphasized that, while the vascular resistive index determined by duplex Doppler studies and renal "perfusion" determined by radionuclide scanning are undoubtedly of clinical significance, so-called normal values do not necessarily correlate with normal blood flow to the kidney. For example, a normal resistive index and normal radionuclide perfusion in the face of graft dysfunction suggest that vascular rejection can be excluded as the cause of the dysfunction, leaving ATN or cyclosporine toxicity as the possible causes. However, with either of these last conditions, it is well known that renal blood flow in the graft is lower than that found in a normally functioning graft.

MRI was initially thought to be a promising method in evaluating the failing transplant kidney. While decrease or loss of corticomedullary distinction on T1 weighted images was initially reported to be relatively specific for graft rejection [12], a more recent report indicates that, when applying this finding, there is significant overlap between rejection, ATN, cyclosporine toxicity, and pyelonephritis [34].

Given the nonspecific nature of the findings in the failing transplant kidney when imaged by the above methods, it is no surprise that percutaneous core needle biopsy remains the gold standard in differentiating rejection from other causes of graft dysfunction. In one series of 64 biopsies, the results differed from the prebiopsy

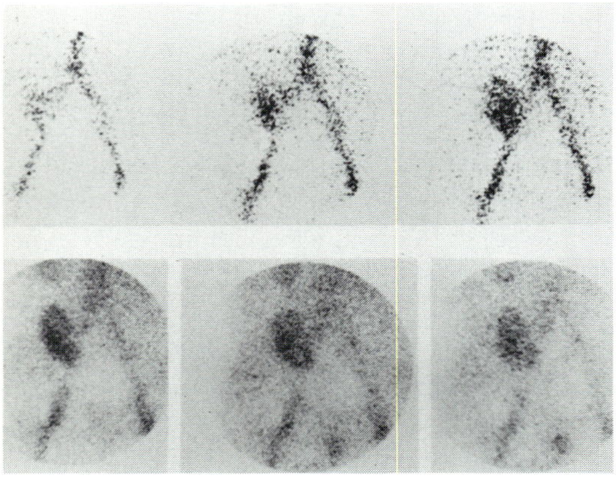

A

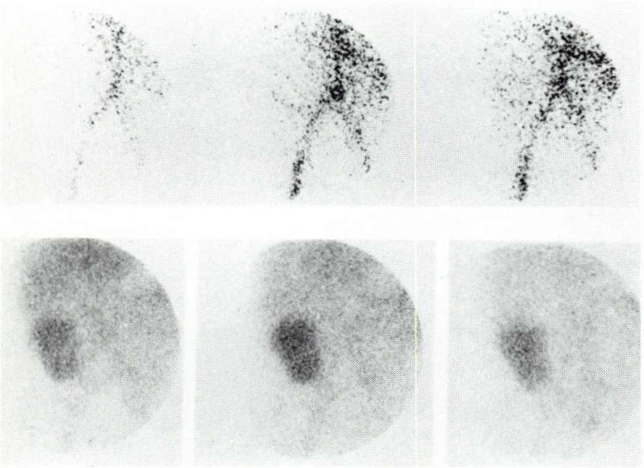

B

Figure 13-10. ^{99m}Tc-DTPA radionuclide renal scanning for determining the cause of a failing graft kidney. A. ATN—Selected images show good perfusion to the graft (top row). Later images (bottom row) demonstrate a poor scintinephrogram (poor function). B. Acute vascular rejection—Perfusion images (top row) show poor perfusion of the graft. Later images also demonstrate poor function. (From J.M. Rosen. Scintigraphic examination of the urinary tract. In *Radiology: Diagnosis-Imaging-Intervention,* ed. J.M. Taveras and J.T. Ferrucci. Philadelphia: J.B. Lippincott, 1989.)

diagnosis in 42 percent of cases and directly affected treatment of patients [32]. Perhaps as more experience is gained with duplex sonographic techniques and with MRI, the sensitivity and specificity of these examinations will be improved to a point at which needle biopsy, with its attendant complications, will no longer be needed.

Generally speaking, in patients with transplant dysfunction sonography is an excellent initial examination for excluding urologic complications such as fluid collections or obstruction, while at the same time a duplex Doppler study can evaluate the renal artery and determine intrarenal vascular impedance. Serial radionuclide renal scans also provide useful information regarding graft perfusion and function. These studies, combined with laboratory data, the clinical course of the patient, and the time frame of graft dysfunction, often allow noninvasive diagnosis and proper treatment of the condition responsible for the failing transplant kidney.

REFERENCES

1. Anderson, R.J., and Schrier, R.W. Acute tubular necrosis. In R.W. Schrier and C.W. Gottschalk (eds.), *Diseases of the Kidney* (4th ed.) Boston: Little, Brown, 1988. Pp. 1413–1446.
2. Bennet, L.N., et al. Urologic complications following renal transplantation: Role of interventional radiologic procedures. *Radiology* 160:531, 1986.
3. Don, S., et al. Duplex doppler US of renal allografts: Causes of elevated resistive index. *Radiology* 171:709, 1989.
4. Dubovsky, E.V., and Russell, C.D. Radionuclide evaluation of renal transplants. *Semin. Nucl. Med.* 18:181, 198.
5. Gardner, K.D., Jr. Medullary and miscellaneous renal cystic disorders. In R.W. Schrier and C.W. Gottschalk (eds.). *Diseases of the Kidney* (4th ed.). Boston: Little, Brown, 1988. Pp. 559–571.
6. Garel, L.A., et al. Juvenile nephronophthisis: Sonographic appearance in chidren with severe uremia. *Radiology* 151:93, 1984.
7. Genkins, S.M., Sanfilippo, F.P., and Carroll, B.A. Duplex Doppler sonography of renal transplants: Lack of sensitivity and specificity in establishing pathologic diagnosis. *A.J.R.* 152:535, 1989.
8. Grantham, J.J., and Gabow, P.A. Polycystic kidney disease. In R.W. Schrier and C.W. Gottschalk (eds.). *Diseases of the Kidney* (4th ed.). Boston: Little, Brown, 1988. Pp. 583–615.
9. Halasz, N.A., et al., Kidney transplantation in the cyclosporine era. *Arch. Surg.* 122:1001, 1987.
10. Hennessy, W.T., et al. Radiologic evaluation of anuric patient: Systematized approach. *Urology* 18:435, 1981.
11. Hosking, D.J. Renal osteodystrophy. *Br. Med. J.* 2:110, 1977.
12. Hricak, H., Terrier, F., and Demas, B.E. Renal allografts: Evaluation by MR imaging. *Radiology* 159:435, 1986.

13. Kim, E.E., et al. Cyclosporine-A nephrotoxicity and acute cellular rejection in renal transplant recipients: Correlation between radionuclide and histologic findings. *Radiology* 159:443, 1986.
14. Kjellstrand, C.M., Ebben, J., and Davin, T. Time of death, recovery of renal function, development of chronic renal failure and need for chronic hemodialysis in patients with acute tubular necrosis. *Trans. Am. Soc. Artif. Intern. Organs* 27:45, 1981.
15. Letourneau, J.G., et al. Imaging of renal transplants. *A.J.R.* 150:833, 1988.
16. Linkowski, G.D., et al. Sonography in the diagnosis of acute renal allograft rejection and cyclosporine nephrotoxicity. *A.J.R.* 148:291, 1987.
17. Maillet, P.J., et al. Nondilated obstructive acute renal failure: Diagnostic procedures and therapeutic management. *Radiology* 160:659, 1986.
18. Mathew, T.H. Recurrence of disease following renal transplantation. *Am. J. Kidney Dis.* 12:85, 1988.
19. Mogensen, C.E., Mauer, S.M., and Kjellstrand, C.M. Diabetic Nephropathy. In R.W. Schrier and C.W. Gottschalk (eds.). *Diseases of the Kidney* (4th ed.). Boston: Little, Brown, 1988. Pp. 2395–2437.
20. Morris, P.J. Renal transplantation: Indications, outcome, complications, and results. In R.W. Schrier and C.W. Gottschalk (eds.). *Diseases of the Kidney* (4th ed.). Boston: Little, Brown, 1988. Pp. 3211–3234.
21. Naidich, J.B., et al. Nondilated obstructive uropathy: Percutaneous nephrostomy performed to reverse renal failure. *Radiology* 160:653, 1986.
22. Newhouse, J.H., Pfister, R.C. The nephrogram. *Radiol. Clin. North Am.* 17:213, 1979.
23. Nortman, D.F., and Coburn, J.W. Renal osteodystrophy in end-stage renal failure. *Postgrad. Med.* 64:123, 1978.
24. Picus, D., et al. Intraarterial digital subtraction angiography of renal transplants. *A.J.R.* 145:93, 1985.
25. Platt, J.F., et al. The inability to detect kidney disease on the basis of echogenicity. *A.J.R.* 151:317, 1988.
26. Rifkin, M.D., et al. Evaluation of renal transplant rejection by duplex Dopper examination: Value of the resistive index. *A.J.R.* 148:759, 1987.
27. Rosen, J.M, Scintigraphic Examination of the Urinary Tract. In J.M., Taveras, and J.T. Ferrucci (eds.). *Radiology: Diagnosis-Imaging-Intervention.* Philadelphia: Lippincott, 1989. Chap. 105, Pp.1–7.
28. Rosenfield, A.T., and Siegel, N.J. Renal parenchymal disease: Histopathologic-sonographic correlation. *A.J.R.* 137:793, 1981.
29. Scola, F.H., Cronan, J.J., and Schepps, B. Grade I hydronephrosis: Pulsed Doppler US evaluation. *Radiology* 171:519, 1989.
30. Snider, J.F., et al. Transplant renal artery stenosis: Evaluation with duplex sonography. *Radiology* 172:1027, 1989.
31. Taylor, K.J.W., et al. Vascular complications in renal allografts: Detection with duplex Doppler U.S. *Radiology* 162:31, 1987.
32. Waltzer, W.C., et al. Value of percutaneous core needle biopsy in the differential diagnosis of renal transplant dysfunction. *J. Urol.* 137:1117, 1987.
33. Warshauer, D.M., et al. Unusual causes of increased vascular impedance in renal transplants: Duplex Doppler evaluation. *Radiology* 169:367, 1988.
34. Winsett, M.Z., et al. Renal transplant dysfunction: MR evaluation. *A.J.R.* 150:319, 1988.

The Renal Sinus

The renal sinus is a true anatomical entity, and many lesions can occur within it (Table 14-1). When imaged, many of these lesions may present similar appearances and result in confusing radiographic patterns; errors in diagnosis can therefore occur. This chapter will define the sinus, enumerate the diseases that can occur there and their imaging appearances, and discuss the differential diagnoses of various radiographic patterns.

The renal sinus is a well-defined anatomical compartment that surrounds and contains the intrarenal collecting system and communicates medially with the perinephric space through the renal hilus. It is otherwise bounded by the renal medulla and cortical columns. Normal contents of the sinus are renovascular structures, lymphatics, and nerves, all of which are invested by fatty tissue (Fig. 14-1). While the intrarenal collecting system is obviously contained within the sinus, only lesions that can be confused with sinus lesions will discussed in this chapter, the remainder being covered in the chapters on diseases of the renal pelvis and ureter.

The portal to the renal sinus is the hilus of the kidney. This may have several anatomical appearances based on the depth of the anterior and posterior medial parenchymal notches of the kidney. These may be of equal depth, though in the majority of cases the posterior notch is deeper than the anterior. Volumetric studies have shown that the cortex and medulla of the kidney constitute about 90 percent of the total kidney volume in the neonate. This decreases to slightly over 80 percent in the adult. The remainder of the renal volume is occupied by the sinus, whose increase in size with age is due to the deposition of renal sinus fatty tissue, often in response to renal parenchymal atrophy. This adipose tissue is virtually absent at birth, as can be seen on sonographic studies in infants, which show absent or minimal central echoes. The normal adult pattern is found almost invariably after the age of 10.

FAT DEPOSITION IN THE RENAL SINUS

After the development of normal amounts of sinus fat, there is a spectrum of excess fat deposition that can be seen in the renal sinus. In the normal young adult there is a rather thin layer of loose adipose tissue enveloping the collecting system and other sinus structures. With aging, there is a mild normal increase in this fat, constituting one end of the spectrum (Fig. 14-2). These fatty deposits can proliferate to the point at which mass effect in the sinus results in pyelocaliceal deformity, yielding the classic pattern on urography of stretched and bowed infundibula associated with an enlarged, radiolucent sinus. This is referred to as *renal sinus lipomatosis* (RSL) [10]. Causes other than aging include obesity and loss of renal parenchyma due to chronic pyelonephritis or ischemia. Increased sinus fat is also seen in patients undergoing steroid therapy and in association with Cushing's disease and pelvic lipomatosis. In the early days of urography, the incidence of renal sinus lipomatosis was thought to be less than 1 percent. However, with the advent of high-quality nephrotomography, the incidence is now reported at around 10 percent. There is no sex predilection, and the typical age at which RSL is seen is in the sixth decade and beyond.

The extreme of the spectrum of fat deposition is termed *replacement lipomatosis*, or perhaps more appropriately, *replacement fibrolipomatosis*. In these patients there is a reactive deposition of dense fibrofatty tissue in the renal sinus in response to severe loss of renal parenchyma [17]. This parenchymal wasting is usually due to atrophy or destruction, the latter often being associated with stone disease; renal calculi have

Table 14-1. Pathologic lesions presenting within the renal sinus

Excessive deposition of fat in the renal sinus
Renal sinus lipomatosis (RSL)
Replacement fibrolipomatosis
Cysts in the renal sinus
Peripelvic cysts (probably from renal lymphatics)
Parapelvic cyst (from adjacent renal parenchyma)
Other nonneoplastic lesions in renal sinus
Originating from adjacent parenchyma
Column of Bertin
Originating within renal sinus
Vascular lesions (aneurysm, varix, tortuous vessel)
Spontaneous hemorrhage
Urine extravasation (uriniferous pseudocyst)
Originating from perinephric space
Pancreatic pseudocyst
Neoplastic lesions in renal sinus
Originating from adjacent parenchyma
Renal cell carcinoma, oncocytoma, angiomyolipoma, etc.
Originating from sinus structures
Teratoma, sarcoma, myxoma, neural tumors, etc.
Originating from perinephric space
Lymphoma, metastatic disease
Originating from collecting system
Transitional cell carcinoma

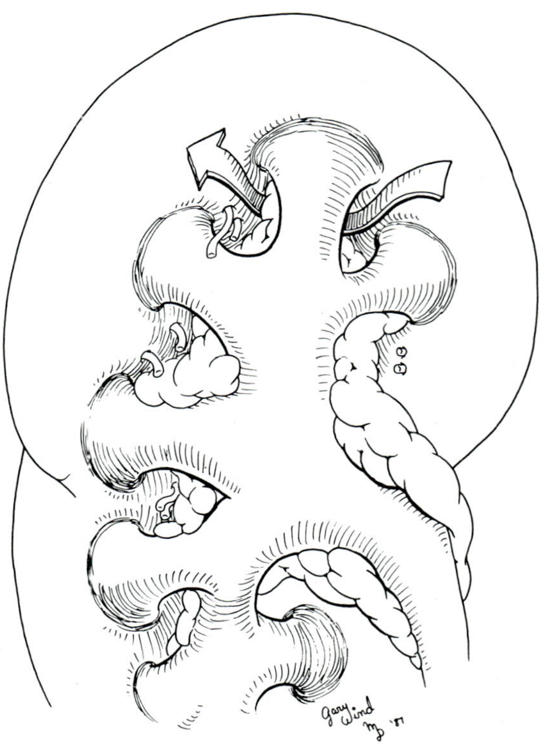

Figure 14-1. Diagram of the renal sinus demonstrating its three-dimensional nature surrounding the collecting system (arrow) and normal small amount of fat. (From E.S. Amis, Jr., and J.J. Cronan. The renal sinus: An imaging review and proposed nomenclature for sinus cysts. *J. Urol.* 139:1151–1159, © by Williams & Wilkins, 1988.)

been reported in 75 percent of such cases. Radiographically, the atrophic kidney is seen to be small, the parenchyma thin, and the sinus relatively enlarged and filled with radiolucent tissue. The radiologic finding of a large lucent renal sinus surrounding a staghorn calculus in a nonfunctioning kidney is another presentation of this process. The differential diagnosis of replacement fibrolipomatosis includes lipoma, liposarcoma, or angiomyolipoma, any of which can originate in the sinus or from adjacent parenchyma and protrude into the sinus. However, these lesions are usually more tumefactive.

On nephrotomography the radiolucent renal sinus seen with RSL is often indistinguishable from the similar finding occurring with cysts in the renal sinus. However, renal sonography will easily differentiate between these two entities. In cases of RSL, the central echo complex of the kidney is prominent and quite echodense (Fig. 14-2B). In the past, several investigators have reported sonolucent fat in the renal sinus. Review of these cases, however, indicates that when nephrotomography showed a lucent renal sinus and subsequent renal ultrasonography showed echolucency in the central complex, the assumption was made that sonolucent fat was the cause of the findings. In fact, these cases were undoubtedly misinterpretations of peripelvic cysts. It is currently accepted that all fat occurring in the renal sinus is echodense, and this has been proved by studying such cases with CT, cyst puncture, or MRI [9]. CT or MRI findings for fat are specific, as they are for cystic structures. Table 14-2 compares the findings for RSL and sinus cysts by the methods useful in imaging these entities. In the past, puncture of sinus cysts, though no longer indicated for diagnosis, was used to confirm the cystic cause of a radiolucent sinus.

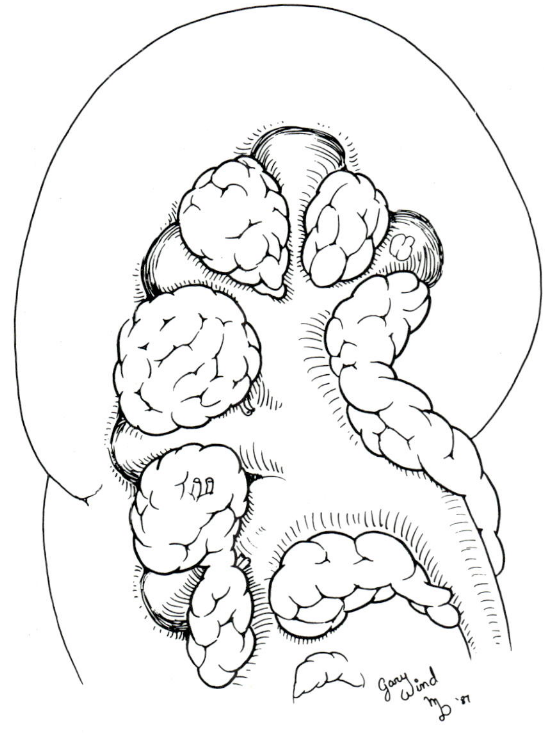

A

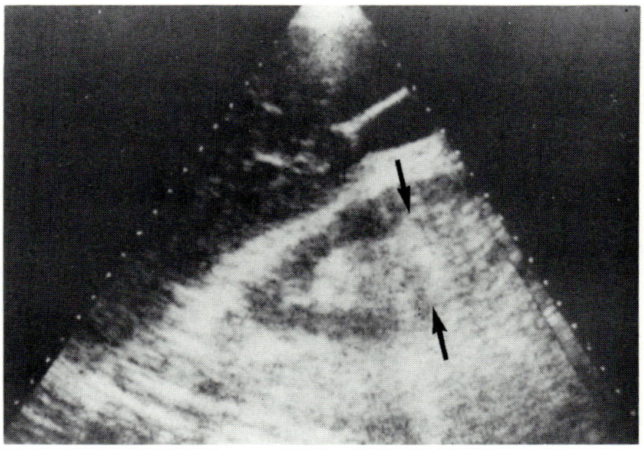

B

Figure 14-2. Renal sinus lipomatosis. A. Diagram showing excess fat deposition in renal sinus. (From E.S. Amis, Jr., and J.J. Cronan. The renal sinus: An imaging review and proposed nomenclature for sinus cysts. *J. Urol.* 139:1151–1159, © by Williams & Wilkins, 1988.) B. Renal sonography shows prominent, highly echogenic renal sinus (arrows).

Table 14-2. Imaging results in renal sinus lipomatosis and sinus cysts

	Renal sinus lipomatosis	Sinus cysts
Nephrotomography	Lucent sinus	Lucent sinus
Sonography	Echodense	Echolucent
Computerized tomography	−15 Hounsfield units or less	−10 to +10 Hounsfield units
Magnetic resonance imaging	T1 weighted: high signal T2 weighted: intermediate signal	T1 weighted: low signal T2 weighted: high signal

RENAL SINUS CYSTS

Over the years many names have been applied to cysts in the renal sinus. More recently the terms *peripelvic* and *parapelvic* have come into common use, though they are often used interchangeably. To prevent this ambiguity, the term *peripelvic cysts* should be reserved for the pattern of small, multiple, confluent, irregularly shaped cysts that appear to arise within the sinus itself [1] (Fig. 14-3). On the other hand, a *parapelvic cyst* is a single, larger cyst most likely arising from renal parenchyma adjacent to the renal sinus and projecting into the sinus (Fig. 14-4). Cystic lesions in the renal sinus can almost invariably be placed into one of these two categories, though some overlap may occasionally occur. The term *sinus cysts* encompasses both parapelvic and peripelvic cysts.

Historically, all cysts in the renal sinus have been considered to have a common cause. However, there is evidence to suggest that

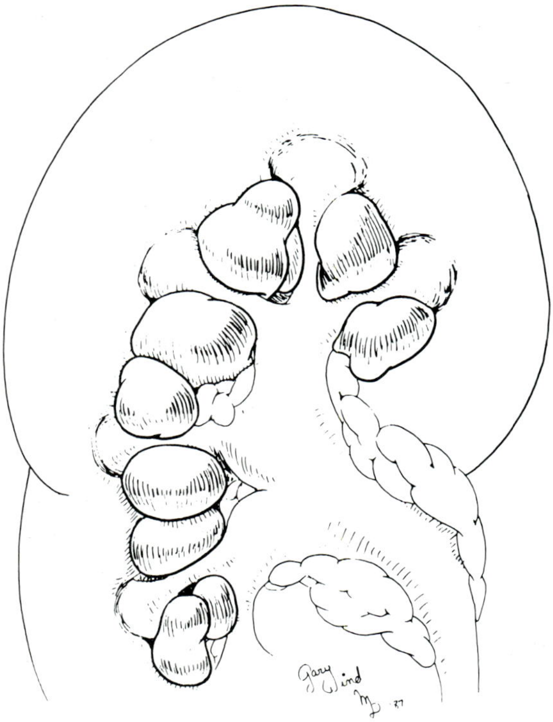

A

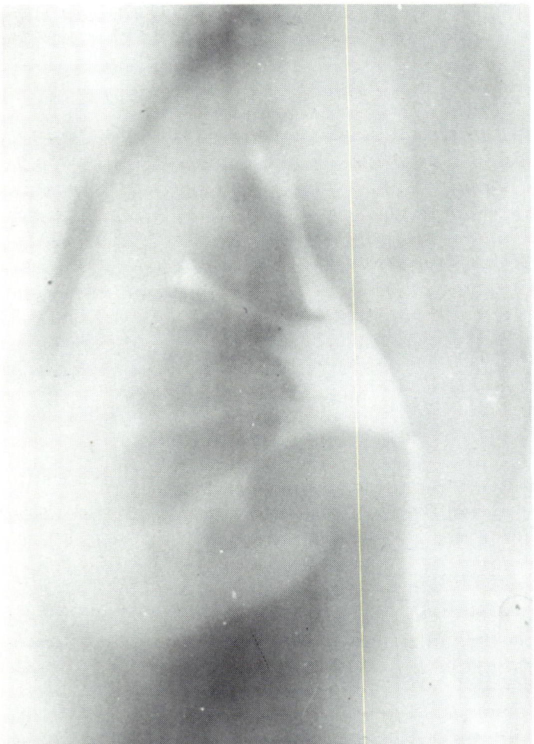

B

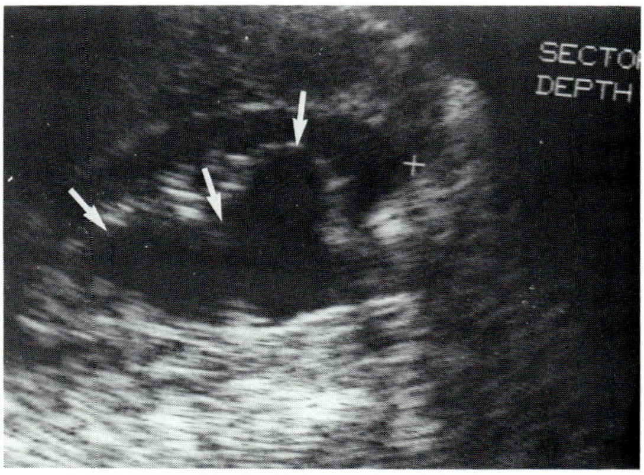

C

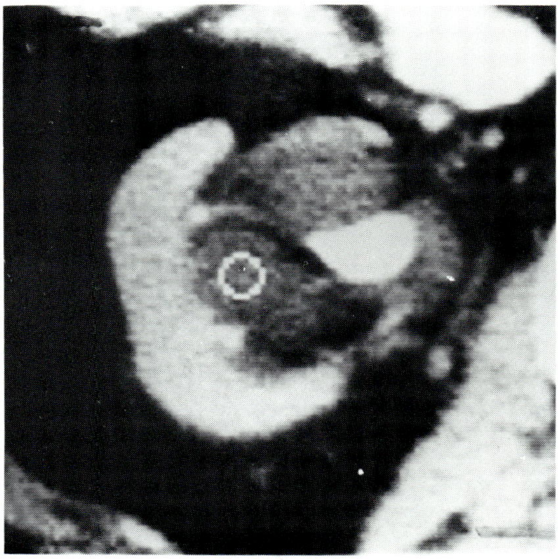

D

Figure 14-3. Peripelvic renal sinus cysts. A. Diagram showing multiple, small, confluent cyst in renal sinus. (From E.S. Amis, Jr., and J.J. Cronan. The renal sinus: An imaging review and proposed nomenclature for sinus cysts. *J. Urol.* 139:1151–1159, © by Williams & Wilkins, 1988.) B. Nephrotomography shows a lucent renal sinus and thinning/stretching of the infundibula. This nephrotomographic pattern is indistinguishable from that seen with renal sinus lipomatosis. C. Renal sonography (coronal view) shows the appearance of a dilated, fluid-filled (echo-free) collecting system (arrows). This is a false positive study for hydronephrosis. D. Contrast-enhanced CT showing the opacified collecting system surrounded by peripelvic cysts. (RO1 = 3 Hounsfield units)

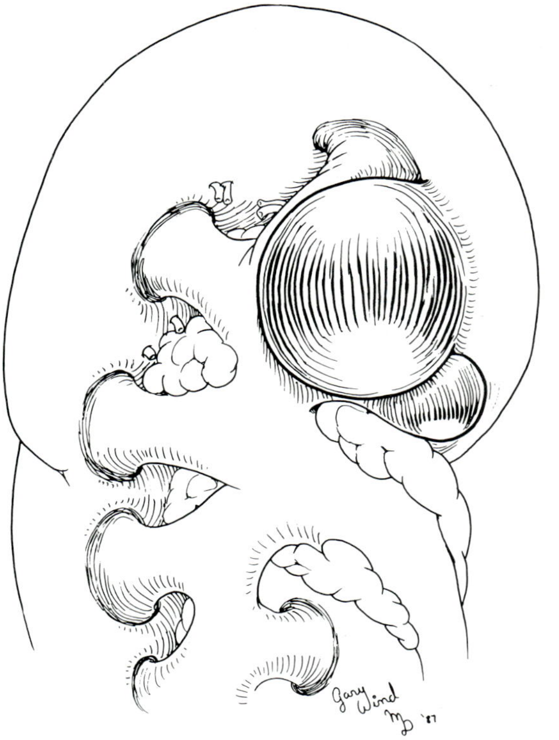

A

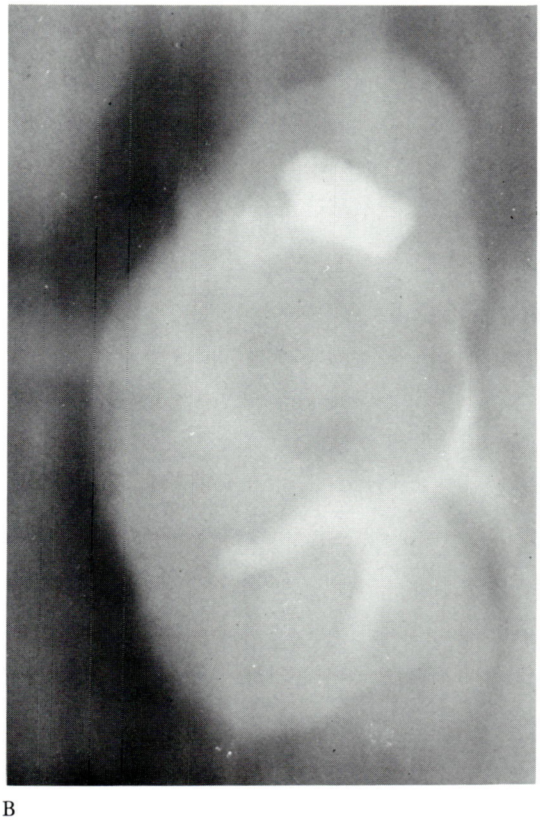

B

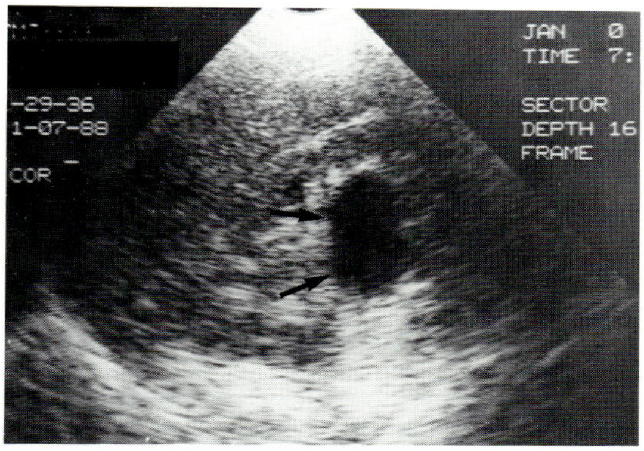

C

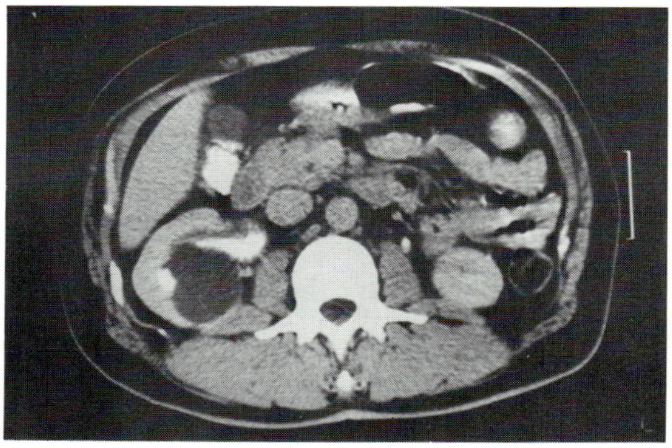

D

Figure 14-4. Parapelvic renal sinus cyst. A. Diagram showing a single, large cyst encroaching on the renal sinus from its origin in the renal parenchyma. (From E.S. Amis, Jr., and J.J. Cronan. The renal sinus: An imaging review and proposed nomenclature for sinus cysts. *J. Urol.* 139:1151–1159, © by Williams & Wilkins, 1988.) B. Nephrotomography shows the parapelvic cyst compressing the upper-pole infundibulum, resulting in a hydrocalix. C. Sonography shows the cyst extending into the renal sinus echoes (arrows). D. Contrast-enhanced CT shows the cyst compressing the collecting system.

peripelvic cysts arise from dilated lymphatics in the sinus itself, probably on the basis of blockage of the renal hilar lymphatics. On the other hand, a parapelvic cyst, which simply has its major presentation in the sinus, probably has the same parenchymal cause as simple renal cysts found elsewhere in the kidney.

The incidence of cysts in the renal sinus is about 1 to 3 percent in the older population. Symptoms secondary to sinus cysts are rare and, when they occur, are due to pressure effects of parapelvic cysts as they enlarge in the sinus. If the pressure within a parapelvic cyst is high enough, there can be compression of renal vasculature with resultant hypertension, though this is extremely rare. More commonly, compression of an adjacent infundibula can result in localized hydronephrosis. The size of an obstructive parapelvic cyst does not correlate directly with the degree of obstruction caused. Rather, the position of the cyst in relation to the renal pelvis and infundibulum, coupled with its ability to expand within the sinus, determines the degree of obstruction.

Treatment is necessary only when parapelvic cysts cause symptoms such as hypertension or flank pain or when localized hydronephrosis is resulting in loss of functioning renal parenchyma. Simple percutaneous aspiration of the cyst in such cases may not be adequate treatment, as the dynamic nature of the cyst wall can result in rapid reaccumulation of fluid [13]. If this occurs, percutaneous cyst ablation may be indicated [3]. Currently, 95 percent ethanol is the most effective agent for sclerosing the cyst wall and preventing reaccumulation of fluid [6]. The technique for cyst ablation involves placing a small-bore pigtail catheter into the cyst cavity percutaneously. The cyst fluid is then aspirated in toto and the volume measured. After opacifying the cyst with contrast medium and obtaining views in multiple obliquities to evaluate the wall, the contrast is also removed. Then an amount of ethanol equal to 25 percent of the aspirated cyst volume is instilled into the cyst cavity and left for 10 minutes, at which time the ethanol is aspirated and the catheter removed. If a leak is identified at the time of cyst opacification, ablation should not be performed. Another caveat is that calculi that might have formed in obstructed calices tend to migrate distally after ablation of the obstructing cyst and subsequently may obstruct the ureter [8].

Parapelvic and peripelvic cysts often cause confusion on imaging studies. As mentioned previously, on nephrotomography they are often indistinguishable from fat because of the resultant radiolucent sinus (see Fig. 14-3B). Sonography is then helpful in differentiating cysts from fat. However, both processes are benign, barring hypertension or infundibular obstruction in the cases of some parapelvic cysts. It is therefore adequate to report such excretory urograms as being consistent with either RSL or sinus cysts. Further confusion may result when renal sonography is performed as a screening examination for hydronephrosis, since an anechoic area within the central echo complex of kidney is the criterion for dilation of the collecting system. While this anechoic area may be due to urine in a hydronephrotic collecting system, peripelvic or parapelvic cysts may have a similar appearance, resulting in a false positive diagnosis of hydronephrosis [7]. The false positive rate for sonographic screening for hydronephrosis has been reported as varying from 11 to 26 percent, and sinus cysts are by far the most common culprit in false positive cases [4]. Coronal views of the kidney on sonography usually allow the identification of dilated infundibula connecting to a dilated renal pelvis in hydronephrosis, while an intact collecting system cannot be identified in cases of sinus cysts [16]. However, in rare instances a sinus cyst may lie adjacent to the renal pelvis and, while effacing it, be mistakenly imaged as the dilated pelvis (see Fig. 14-3C). Furthermore, sinus cysts can also, on very rare occasion, extend through the renal hilus and parallel the proximal ureter, giving the sonographic impression of a dilated ureter. If sonography is not absolutely clear in diagnosing a dilated collecting system, given the somewhat high false positive rate, other imaging studies may be necessary to delineate the cause of echolucency in the renal sinus.

CT without a contrast agent may yield transaxial images of the kidney that resemble hydronephrosis even though none is present [2]. A large parapelvic cyst or a cluster of smaller peripelvic cysts in the renal sinus may closely resemble a dilated renal pelvis (Fig. 14-5A). However, a contrast study will clearly demonstrate the attenuated collecting system winding its way around the sinus cyst (or cysts) (Fig. 14-5B). Similarly, absence of radiopharmaceutical in the region of the renal sinus during the perfusion phase of a ^{99m}Tc-DTPA dynamic renal study is usually ascribed to hydronephrosis. If the kidney is hydronephrotic, the photon-deficient area will eventually fill in as

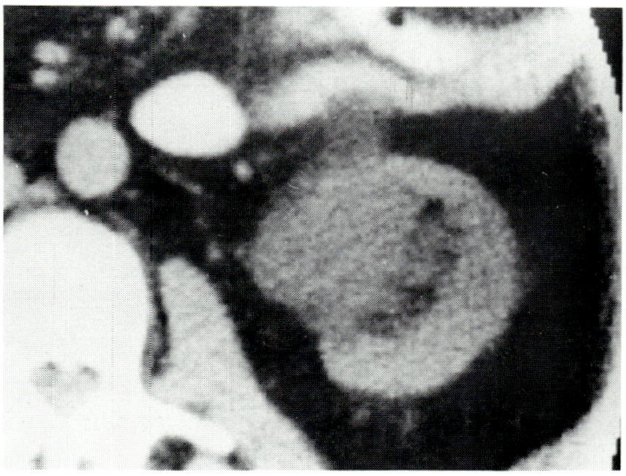

A

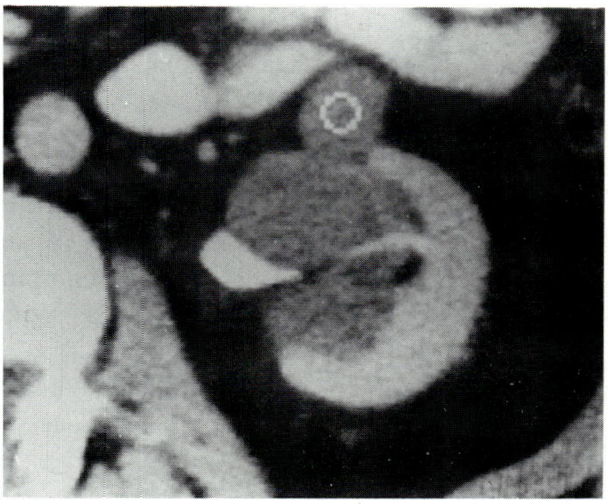

B

Figure 14-5. Pseudohydronephrosis on nonenhanced CT scan. A. Nonenhanced CT shows what appears to be dilated, fluid-filled left renal pelvis. B. After administration of an intravenous contrast agent, the collecting system is seen to be attenuated by peripelvic cysts. A small cyst also extends anteriorly.

radioactivity is slowly excreted into the dilated collecting system. However, when this filling does not occur on delayed scans, sinus cysts or other sinus masses should be considered, especially if the ureter becomes visible.

OTHER NONNEOPLASTIC LESIONS IN THE RENAL SINUS

While RSL and peripelvic cysts are the most common entities found arising from normal sinus structures, other nonneoplastic lesions may also occur in the sinus, encroach on the sinus from the adjacent renal parenchyma, or extend through the hilus from the perinephric space. While uncommon, vascular lesions may involve the renal vessels in the sinus and present as masses in the sinus. Such lesions include aneurysm of an intrarenal arterial branch, a varix of the renal vein, and a tortuous renal vein seen en face. Doppler ultrasonography or contrast-enhanced dynamic CT can be used to diagnose these conditions.

Rarely, pancreatic pseudocysts have been known to invade the renal sinus via the hilus, resulting in a thick-walled, debris-containing cystic lesion in the sinus.

Spontaneous processes can also occur in the renal sinus, resulting in mass lesions. Patients on anticoagulants have been reported to hemorrhage into the sinus [11]. This is a self-limiting process, and the pattern may be tumefactive or resemble peripelvic cysts. Extrinsic compression of the collecting system is a common accompanying finding, though this is reversed with resolution of the clot over a period of 2 or 3 weeks. Another self-limiting condition is the peripelvic renal pseudocyst, or uriniferous pseudocyst [5]. This process is seen as a radiolucent sinus mass in an obstructed kidney and is due to pyelosinus urine leakage caused by increased pressure in an obstructed collecting system. This also resolves over a period of a few weeks after relief of the obstruction.

Hypertrophy of a normal cortical column of Bertin may present as a pseudotumor encroaching on the renal sinus. One sonographic study of normal kidneys found that 16 percent had enlarged columns of Bertin that projected into the lateral portion of the sinus on coronal views [14]. In these cases the renal outline remained smooth. This same study also reported that renal cell carcinoma, while it could protrude from the renal parenchyma into the sinus, always distorted the renal outline. The investigators concluded that the characteristics of a hypertrophied column, namely a mass protruding into the sinus but not distorting the renal outline, and with an echotexture the same as adjacent renal parenchyma, readily differentiated it from renal cancer and obviated the need for further investigation. Another study reached a similar conclusion, stating further that renal cell carcinoma has a different echotexture from kidney parenchyma, allowing it to be differentiated from a column even more readily [15]. While these guidelines are generally valid, renal cell carcinoma or other renal parenchymal tumors can mimic a benign hypertrophied column on sonography. The resemblance can be striking (Fig. 14-6), thus compromising the use of sonography alone to establish the diagnosis of this type of pseudotumor.

Figure 14-6. Nonspecificity of renal sonography for differentiating prominent column of Bertin from parenchymal neoplasm. A. Sonogram of prominent column of Bertin extending into renal sinus echo complex (arrows). The renal outline is not distorted. B. Sonogram of renal cell carcinoma extending into renal sinus echo complex (arrows). The echotexture of the tumor is the same as that of normal renal parenchyma, and there is no distortion of the renal contour. (From E.S. Amis, Jr., and J.J. Cronan. The renal sinus: An imaging review and proposed nomenclature for sinus cysts. *J. Urol.* 139:1151–1159, © by Williams & Wilkins, 1988.)

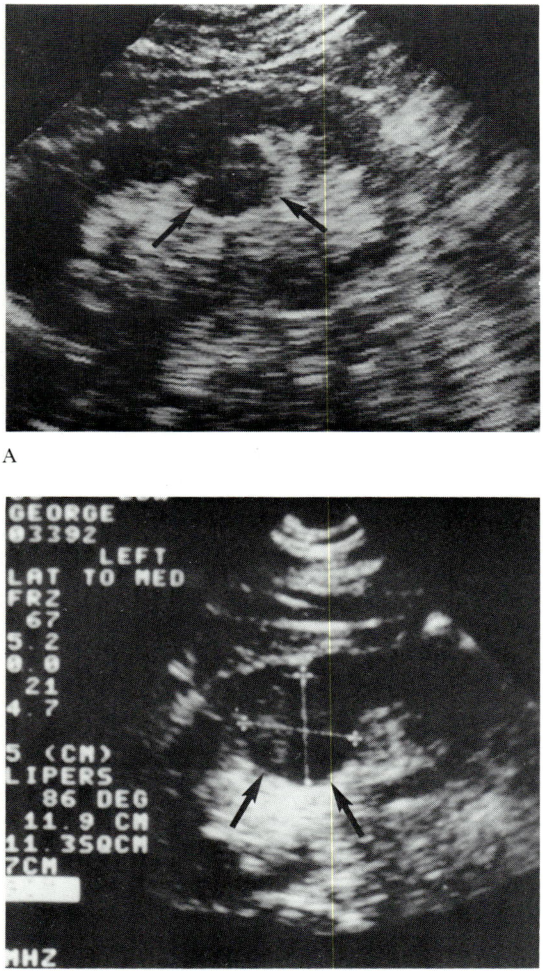

A

B

NEOPLASTIC LESIONS PRESENTING IN THE RENAL SINUS

Benign and malignant neoplastic lesions can arise from sinus structures or project into the sinus from adjacent renal parenchyma; the latter group includes renal cell carcinoma, oncocytoma, angiomyolipoma, multilocular cystic nephroma, and Wilms' tumor. Reported tumors arising from sinus structures include teratoma, sarcoma, myxoma, paraganglionoma, and angiomyolipoma. Diagnostic imaging of these lesions is the same as for other renal neoplasms. On urography, a noncystic mass will be seen in the sinus area, often displacing or obstructing (or both) infundibula. While ultrasonography can determine the solid nature of the mass, it can suggest the diagnosis only when certain characteristics are found, e.g., the dense echotexture of an angiomyolipoma. CT is useful in determining vascularity of a lesion but also is specific only when fat is found within an angiomyolipoma.

A soft-tissue mass surrounding the collecting system in the sinus should lead to the suspicion of lymphoma. This is true even in the absence of renal parenchymal abnormality or retroperitoneal adenopathy. On sonography the homogeneous nature of lymphoma, which replaces renal sinus fat, can result in a relative paucity of echoes and thus resemble the appearance of hydronephrosis. However, CT shows the soft-tissue nature of the sinus lesion. Though sinus hemorrhage may have a similar appearance, it should resolve in a few weeks. With complete replacement of the kidneys by lymphoma, the central echo complex may also be absent because of destruction and replacement of renal sinus fat.

Invasive transitional cell carcinoma arising from the intrarenal collecting system can present as a mass in the renal sinus (Fig. 14-7A). While some may be enhanced significantly

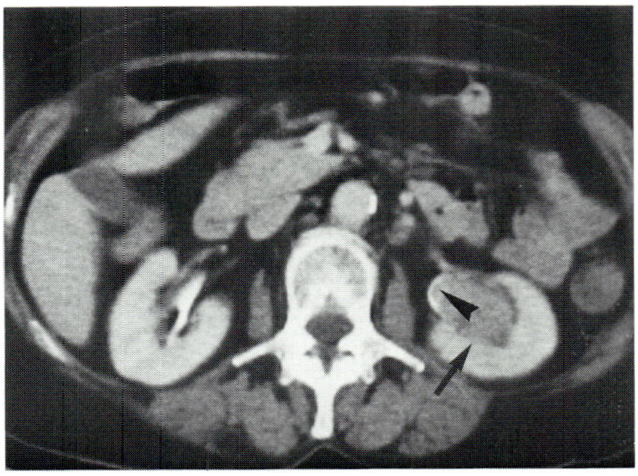

A

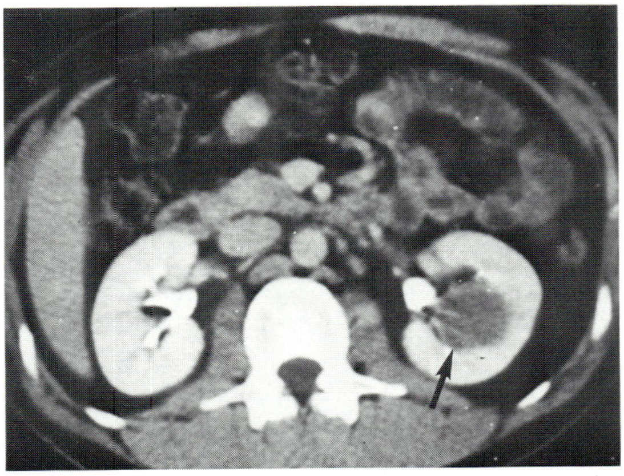

B

Figure 14-7. Similar appearance of invasive transitional cell carcinoma and renal cell carcinoma presenting predominantly in the renal sinus. A. CT shows transitional cell carcinoma in the renal sinus (arrow), which appears to have at least some intrapelvic component (arrowhead). B. CT shows renal cell carcinoma (arrow) encroaching on the renal sinus from its parenchymal origin.

with contrast medium, the majority are enhanced only minimally. It may be difficult to differentiate this tumor from those protruding into the sinus from adjacent parenchyma, notably a poorly enhancing renal cell carcinoma (Fig. 14-7B).

REFERENCES

1. Amis, E.S., Jr., and Cronan, J.J. The renal sinus: An imaging review and proposed nomenclature for sinus cysts. *J. Urol.* 139:1151, 1988.
2. Amis, E.S., Jr., Cronan, J.J., and Pfister, R.C. Pseudohydronephrosis on noncontrast computed tomography. *J. Comput. Assist. Tomogr.* 6:511, 1982.
3. Amis, E.S., Jr., Cronan, J.J., and Pfister, R.C. Needle puncture of cystic renal masses: A survey of the Society of Uroradiology. *A.J.R.* 148:297, 1987.
4. Amis, E.S., Jr., et al. Ultrasonic inaccuracies in diagnosing renal obstruction. *Urology* 19:101, 1982.
5. Barbaric, Z.L., and Frank, I.N. Peripelvic renal pseudocyst due to obstruction. *A.J.R.* 129:1097, 1977.
6. Bean, W.J. Renal cysts: Treatment with alcohol. *Radiology* 138:329, 1981.
7. Cronan, J.J., et al. Peripelvic cysts: An impostor of sonographic hydronephrosis. *J. Ultrasound Med.* 1:229, 1982.
8. Cronan, J.J., et al. Obstructive migration of renal calculi following cyst aspiration. *Radiology* 152:317, 1984.
9. Cronan, J.J., et al. The myth of anechoic renal sinus fat. *Radiology* 144:149, 1982.
10. Faegenburg, D., Bosniak, M., and Evans, J.A. Renal sinus lipomatosis: Its demonstration by nephrotomography. *Radiology* 83:987, 1964.
11. Fishman, M.C., et al. Radiographic manifestations of spontaneous renal sinus hemorrhage. *A.J.R.* 142:1161, 1984.
12. Han, B.K., and Babcock, D.S. Sonographic measurements and appearance of normal kidneys in children. *A.J.R.* 145:611, 1985.
13. Jacobsson, L., et al. Fluid turnover in renal cysts. *Acta Med. Scand.* 202:327, 1977.
14. Lafortune, M., et al. Sonography of the hypertrophied column of Bertin. *A.J.R.* 146:53, 1986.
15. Prando, A., Pereira, R.M., and Marins, J.L. Sonographic evaluation of hypertrophy of septum of Bertin. *Urology* 24:505, 1984.
16. Ralls, P.W., et al. Severe hydronephrosis and severe renal cystic disease: Ultrasonic differentiation. *A.J.R.* 134:473, 1980.
17. Subramanyam, B.R., et al. Replacement lipomatosis of the kidney: Diagnosis by computed tomography and sonography. *Radiology* 148:791, 1983.

Urinary Stone Disease

Stones in the urinary tract are an age-old problem, as evidenced by the finding of a large bladder stone in the pelvis of an Egyptian skeleton estimated to be more than 7,000 years old. Stone disease was also recognized by Hippocrates in his oath for the physician when he wrote "I will not cut, even for stone, but leave such procedure to the practitioners of the craft." In fact, for many centuries, cutting for stone was the exclusive purview of numbers of itinerant lithotomists.

Until the past century, urinary stone disease appears to have occurred almost exclusively in the bladder. Bladder stones are still common in some underdeveloped nations, primarily as a disease of children. However, in the past century, the incidence of bladder stones has markedly decreased in the industrialized nations. This has been paralleled by a significant increase in the formation of calcium-containing stones in the upper urinary tract. This dramatic change can probably be attributed to dietary factors as well as altered lifestyles in these countries.

There are two major types of involvement of the urinary tract by calculus disease: nephrocalcinosis and urolithiasis. Nephrocalcinosis is the formation of concretions within the renal parenchyma, while urolithiasis denotes stones within the lumina of the urinary tract. There is actually a significant overlap between these two categories, since calculi formed within the renal medulla (medullary nephrocalcinosis) may erode into the collecting system (urolithiasis).

The large majority of all stones forming in the urinary tract, whether in the renal parenchyma or in the collecting system, contain calcium. The large majority of these calcium-containing stones are idiopathic. The remaining stones have diverse compositions. Furthermore, in addition to the idiopathic stones there are multiple disease processes that can result in urinary calculi.

INCIDENCE OF URINARY TRACT STONES

Autopsy studies have revealed renal calcifications in more than 1 percent of the general population [12]. This high incidence is reflected in the lifetime risk for suffering stone disease in the urinary tract, which approaches 20 percent for males and 5 to 10 percent for females. The recurrence rate for stone disease is high—about 50 percent of patients experience another stone within 5 to 10 years from the onset of the disease. Stone disease occurs primarily in adults, with the peak incidence in the fourth and fifth decades. Urinary stones in children are rare, comprising less than 1 percent of all urinary stone disease. Males are affected more than females by a ratio of 2 or 3 : 1, and blacks are affected far less frequently than whites [18].

FACTORS CONTRIBUTING TO STONE DISEASE

The existence of "stone belts," or geographic areas in which cases of urinary calculi occur with unusual frequency, has long been recognized. The highest incidence has been reported in the Southeastern United States, with the second highest incidence occurring in New England. These areas are followed by the Midwest and the far Western states. Factors in this geographic distribution probably include the climate and the hardness of the drinking water. The risk of forming renal stones also appears to be increased in individuals with a family history of urinary stone disease. Although genetic factors may play a role in such cases, it should be recognized that family members tend to adopt similar habits of living.

Other contributing factors in stone formation are the affluence and dietary habits prevalent in the Western world. Patients with stones tend to be more overweight, to have higher serum cholesterol levels, and to have impaired glucose tolerance. There is also a generally accepted relation between hypertension and urinary stones. Finally, a sedentary lifestyle is also associated with a higher incidence of urinary stones.

SYMPTOMATOLOGY OF URINARY STONE DISEASE

Nephrocalcinosis is essentially asymptomatic unless, in the medullary variety, a stone erodes into the collecting system. Moreover, it is not until an upper tract stone moves into the ureter and produces obstruction that it causes renal colic. Renal colic produces pain that is excruciating and may be continuous or, more typically, intermittent. It is often associated with diaphoresis, nausea, and vomiting. The pain is due to distention of the proximal collecting system and of the renal capsule as well as hyperperistalsis and is usually referred to the ipsilateral costovertebral angle, flank, or both. Patients with stone colic are unable to find a comfortable position and are extremely restless.

As the stone continues its path down the ureter, the pain may radiate around the flank into the ipsilateral lower abdominal quadrant or groin. As the stone reaches the ureterovesical junction, bladder irritative systems or atony with urinary retention may result. If the urine is infected, the clinical picture may be complicated by chills and fever.

On the other hand, ureteral calculi may be totally asymptomatic or heralded only by gross or microscopic hematuria. The classic combination of flank pain accompanied by hematuria is seen in only about 50 percent of cases. Staghorn calculi remain confined to the intrarenal collecting system and may be asymptomatic or associated with aching ipsilateral back pain, gastrointestinal symptoms, or both.

Calculi in the urinary bladder may be asymptomatic or associated only with recurrent urinary tract infections. Forty to fifty percent of patients will complain of frequency and urgency of urination. Only 30 to 40 percent of patients complain of interruption of the urinary stream due to a temporary lodging of the stone in the region of the bladder neck. Certainly, however, pain and hematuria can accompany bladder calculi. Stones small enough to enter the posterior urethra willl usually pass without difficulty. On occasion, however, stones can be retained within the urethra, resulting in dysuria and weak or intermittent urinary stream.

THEORIES OF STONE FORMATION

Urinary stones are composed of about 97.5 percent polycrystalline aggregate and 2.5 percent glycoprotein or mucoprotein matrix. Virtually any crystalline substance excreted in the urine in sufficient concentrations can form a stone. There are several theories regarding the formation of stones. The first, crystallization, presumes that the urine must be supersaturated, at least from time to time, with the substance in question. As supersaturation continues, the solution becomes unstable, and spontaneous nucleation can occur. Another theory, which explains the composition of most urinary stones, is that of a matrix nidus on which crystallization can occur, again in a supersaturated urine. Other investigators have defined modifiers of stone formation that include both promoters and inhibitors of crystallization. Matrix and, in some situations, Tamm-Horsfall protein may be considered promoters [23]. Multiple inhibitors of stone formation have been identified, including pyrophospates and mucopolysaccharides. Perhaps it is the lack of these inhibitors in urine that contributes to the formation of some stones. In all likelihood, the formation of urinary stones may involve all of the above processes.

Urinary pH is also a significant factor in the solubility of certain crystalline components of the urine, most notably uric acid and struvite. Struvite precipitation begins at a pH of approximately 7.5 and increases with increasing alkalinity of the urine. Since this is above the upper limits of normal urine alkalinization, the presence of bacteria that alkalinize urine by splitting urea is required for the precipitation of struvite crystals. Furthermore, uric acid has very limited solubility in acidic urine, predisposing to the formation of uric acid stones when urine pH is low. When the pH is increased to 6.5, the compound is present in the form of a urate which has a significantly increased solubility.

Another factor in the formation of stones is

the concept of fixation. Formation of tiny concretions, as discussed in the previous paragraphs, does not adequately explain the retention and growth of a stone within the urinary tract, as it is assumed that any concretion less than 1 mm in diameter can freely pass down the ureter and be voided from the bladder. Therefore, at least during early stone growth, anatomic fixation to some portion of the urinary tract has most likely occurred. The physiochemical basis for stone formation and growth is still under active investigation.

COMPOSITION AND RADIOGRAPHIC APPEARANCE OF URINARY STONES

The large majority of stones seen in clinical practice are composed of calcium oxalate, calcium phosphate, magnesium ammonium phosphate, uric acid, and cystine. Table 15-1 gives the incidence of the various types of stones found within the urinary tract. Almost three-fourths of all urinary stones are composed of calcium oxalate, calcium phosphate, or a combination of these. Furthermore, while struvite stones, which are almost always associated with infected urine, comprise 15 percent of all urinary stones, the large majority of these are combined with calcium phosphate to form the so-called triple phosphate calculus (magnesium ammonium calcium phosphate). Therefore, approximately 87 percent of urinary stones contain calcium. These calcium-containing stones plus cystine stones constitute the 90 percent of stones that are radiopaque. The remaining 10 percent of urinary stones are radiolucent on plain-film radiography, though they can be detected by CT or ultrasonography.

Calcium-containing stones are easily detected on plain radiographs if they are of sufficient size. While pure struvite stones are radiolucent, it has been previously noted that the large majority of these stones are admixed with calcium phosphate, resulting in easily seen radiopacity. Less opaque, though usually easily visualized, are the cystine stones. Stones that are truly radiolucent include uric acid, xanthine, and pure matrix stones.

CAUSES OF NEPHROCALCINOSIS

There are two different types of nephrocalcinosis, which differ etiologically and radiologically: cortical and medullary. Both forms of nephrocalcinosis involve the deposition of calcium concretions within the renal parenchyma. The common causes of nephrocalcinosis are listed in Table 15-2.

CORTICAL NEPHROCALCINOSIS

Cortical nephrocalcinosis is characterized by diffuse foci of calcific densities in the renal cortex that have a tendency to coalesce. The kidneys are often smaller than normal, and the calcification occurs in the thin rim of remaining cortex. The mechanism of calcification in cortical nephrocalcinosis is frequently dystrophic, indicating the deposition of calcium salts in previously damaged tissue. This is particularly true in cases of cortical necrosis and chronic glomerulonephritis. Cortical necrosis is often the result of renal ischemia secondary to shock or may occur secondary to the ingestion of toxins

Table 15-1. Chemical composition and incidence of stones

Chemical name	*Crystal name*	*Incidence (%)*
Calcium oxalate monohydrate	Whewellite	33
Calcium oxalate dihydrate	Weddellite	
Calcium phosphate	Apatite	6
Calcium hydrogen phosphate	Brushite	
Calcium oxalate/phosphate (mixed)		34
Magnesium ammonium phosphate	Struvite	15
"Triple" phosphate	Struvite + apatite	
Uric acid/urate	Uric acid/urate	8
Cystine	Cystine	3
Other (xanthine, matrix)		1

Table 15-2. Common causes of nephrocalcinosis

Cortical Nephrocalcinosis
Cortical necrosis
Chronic glomerulonephritis
Hyperoxaluria
Medullary Nephrocalcinosis
Hypercalcemic states (see Table 15-3)
Renal tubular acidosis (Type I)
Medullary sponge kidney

such as ethylene glycol (antifreeze) or exposure to the anesthetic agent methoxyflurane (Penthrane). On the other hand, metastatic deposition of calcium oxalate in normal cortex occurs in secondary hyperoxaluria. This is usually due to any one of multiple factors, including increased ingestion of food rich in oxalates, increased formation of oxalates in cases of ethylene glycol poisoning or methoxyflurane anesthesia, and increased absorption of oxalates in small-bowel inflammatory disease.

MEDULLARY NEPHROCALCINOSIS

In medullary nephrocalcinosis, calcium salts are deposited in the distal tubules in the region of the pyramids. These calcium concretions may be small and poorly defined or larger, coarse granulations. On occasion, as in the case of hyperparathyroidism, some of these calcific deposits are within the basement membrane of the tubule or actually in the medullary interstitium. Small stones forming within the distal tubules can erode into the collecting system, thus resulting in a significant overlap of this condition with urolithiasis.

Approximately 40 percent of cases of medullary nephrocalcinosis are secondary to hyperparathyroidism, 20 percent to renal tubular acidosis, 20 percent to medullary sponge kidney, and the remainder divided among a variety of causes, including other hypercalcemic states.

Papillary necrosis can also result in the dystrophic deposition of calcium in the necrotic papilla before sloughing occurs. If a sloughed necrotic papilla is retained within its adjacent calix, rimlike calcification of the retained papilla is not uncommon.

The only anatomic cause of medullary nephrocalcinosis is medullary sponge kidney. In this condition there is a fusiform or cystic dilation of the collecting ducts in the renal pyramid. This dilation results in stasis of urine, which can lead to the precipitation of calcium salts. While the other causes of medullary nephrocalcinosis almost invariably lead to bilateral renal involvement, medullary sponge kidney may affect both kidneys, one kidney, or even only one papilla. Therefore, unilateral or segmental medullary nephrocalcinosis should lead to the suspicion of this condition as opposed to the other causes of medullary nephrocalcinosis.

On occasion, diffuse coalescent calcification can occur throughout the cortex and medulla of the kidney. This is usually due to primary hyperoxaluria and is a bilateral condition. This should be differentiated from the autonephrectomized tuberculous kidney, which can result in a diffusely calcified kidney, though it is almost always unilateral.

CAUSES OF UROLITHIASIS

The majority of all stones formed in the urinary tract are composed of calcium oxalate or calcium phosphate or both. Of this large group of patients, 70 to 80 percent of stones form idiopathically, and half of these are found to have idiopathic hypercalciuria without associated hypercalcemia [10]. The remainder of urinary stones have varied compositions and causes (Table 15-3). These are discussed in the following sections.

CYSTINURIA

Cystinuria is a tubular syndrome inherited as a autosomal recessive trait. Clinically, the formation of cystine urinary stones is the only recognizable abnormality. Cystine stones are quite hard and, radiographically, are faintly to moderately opaque and homogeneous. They may occur as a single stone, multiple large stones, or even as a staghorn calculus. Cystinuria commonly begins in childhood and should be considered when opaque calculi are seen in younger patients.

RENAL TUBULAR ACIDOSIS

Renal tubular acidosis may be an autosomal dominant familial process, but more commonly it occurs spontaneously. It is divided into prox-

Table 15-3. Etiologic classification of urolithiasis

Idiopathic stone disease
Idiopathic hypercalcuria
Tubular syndromes
Cystinuria
Renal tubular acidosis (distal, Type I)
Enzyme disorders
Xanthinuria
Primary hyperoxaluria
Secondary hyperoxaluria
Hypercalcemic states
Hyperparathyroidism
Sarcoidosis
Immobilization
Hypervitaminosis D
Milk-alkali syndrome
Neoplastic disorders
Cushing's disease
ACTH therapy
Hyperthyroidism
Hyperuricosuria
Idiopathic
Gout
Myeloproliferative disorders
Gastrointestinal disorders/surgery
Ileostomy (uric acid stones)
Small bowel disease/resection/bypass (calcium oxalate stones)
Urinary infection
Urinary obstruction/stasis
Medullary sponge kidney
Caliceal diverticulum
Ureteropelvic junction obstruction
Ureterocele
Bladder outlet obstruction
Urinary diversion

imal and distal varieties. The proximal form (Type II) almost never results in nephrocalcinosis or renal calculi. Distal renal tubular acidosis (Type I), frequently associated with urinary stones, can be either primary or secondary to some systemic diseases [3]. The distal renal tubule in this condition cannot effectively secrete hydrogen ions to lower the urinary pH. This results in a metabolic acidosis and a urine with a pH consistently greater than 5.5. Urinary wasting of calcium occurs, and medullary nephrocalcinosis and calcium urolithiasis are found in up to 73 percent of the primary cases. Renal tubular acidosis is usually the underlying cause when massive medullary nephrocalcinosis is seen.

XANTHINURIA

Xanthinuria results from a deficiency of xanthine oxidase. It is very rare familial disorder. These patients have an increased urinary excretion of xanthine, which can result in the formation of lucent stones in the urinary tract. Probably a more common cause of xanthine stones is the use of allopurinol (a xanthine oxidase inhibitor) for the treatment of gout. Xanthine stones of either cause are rare.

HYPEROXALURIA

Hyperoxaluria may be the result of overproduction or excessive intestinal absorption of oxalates. Humans cannot metabolize oxalate, and it can be eliminated from the body only by renal excretion. Hyperoxaluria may be primary or secondary. Primary hyperoxaluria is a rare autosomal inherited disease in which there is an enzyme deficiency resulting in an accelerated conversion of hydroxypyruvate to L-glyceric acid. This leads to oxidation of glycoxalate to oxalate [9]. The excess endogenous oxalate so produced results in diffuse nephrocalcinosis and urolithiasis. The majority of the patients suffer progressive renal failure and an early death. Secondary hyperoxaluria, as previously noted, also produces calcium oxalate urolithasis as well as cortical nephrocalcinosis.

HYPERCALCEMIC STATES

Calcium urolithiasis may be a complication of virtually any systemic disease associated with hypercalcemia, whether from increased bone resorption or enhanced intestinal absorption of calcium. The most common disorder in this group of diseases is primary hyperparathyroidism, which accounts for 1 to 5 percent of all calcium stones [2]. In fact, clinical stone disease may be the first evidence of excessive secretion of parathyroid hormone. Approximately 10 percent of all patients with this disease will eventually form stones. Urolithiasis may also be the first clinical manifestation of other hypercalcemic states such as vitamin D intoxication, sarcoidosis, and the milk-alkali syndrome. In these conditions there is enhanced gastrointestinal absorption of calcium, as opposed to the increased bone resorption seen with hyperparathyroidism.

Forced immobilization of the body, usually occurring during recuperation from major trauma, may also result in hypercalcemia and subsequent rapid stone formation. This problem is prevalent in children and young adults. In most of the other hypercalcemic conditions, urinary stones present as a late complication. This is especially true in the hypercalcemia associated with various neoplastic conditions, the patient usually being in the terminal phase of the disease. The urinary stones seen in patients with Cushing's disease or undergoing adrenocorticotropic hormone (ACTH) therapy are probably due to the effect of steroids on bone.

HYPERURICOSURIA

The formation of uric acid is the end point of purine metabolism in humans, apes, and the Dalmatian dog. The hyperuricosuria associated with gout causes 20 to 40 percent of uric acid stones. Another source of excess uric acid excretion is a diet high in purines such as fish, meat, and poultry. In many instances, however, uric acid stones are formed idiopathically.

It is advisable to evaluate patients with uric acid stones for myeloproliferative disorders, since the formation of stones may be the presenting complaint in these patients. Rapid cell destruction, especially in lymphomas being treated, may result in uric acid stones in up to 40 percent of cases.

GASTROINTESTINAL DISORDERS/SURGERY

There are several gastrointestinal diseases that may be associated with increased absorption of oxalate and subsequent hyperoxaluria. These include Crohn's disease, celiac sprue, and pancreatic insufficiency. Calcium oxalate stone disease has been reported in approximately 7 percent of patients with inflammatory intestinal disease. Another condition that can result in hyperoxaluria is either a resection or bypass of the small intestine. In these cases there is increased absorption of oxalate in the colon. This is likely due to abnormalities of fatty acid metabolism within the gut [26].

Uric acid stones are not uncommon in patients who have undergone an ileostomy for diversion of the fecal stream. In these patients there are large losses of water and bicarbonate, resulting in low-volume, acidic urine. Uric acid is poorly soluble in this environment.

URINARY INFECTION

Urinary tract infection may lead to magnesium ammonium phosphate (struvite) stones. These stones are rarely pure and are usually mixed with calcium phosphate (apatite) to form the "triple" phosphate stones (magnesium ammonium calcium phosphate) frequently described in association with infected urine. *Proteus mirabilis* is the most common organism associated with struvite stones, though on occasion infection with pseudomonas, klebsiella, or staphyloccus species has been reported [11]. These bacteria have the capability of producing urease, an enzyme that facilitates the formation of ammonia from urea. Ammonia (NH_3) then buffers H^+ and forms ammonium (NH_4^+). The abundance of ammonia buffer causes a highly alkaline urine that promotes the precipitation of magnesium ammonium phosphate [13]. The high urinary pH in these patients is also conducive to the crystallization of calcium phosphate, which becomes mixed with the struvite stone in the large majority of cases.

Because of the mixture of struvite and calcium phosphate, infection stones are readily apparent on plain films. These stones tend to grow rapidly and can often assume a staghorn configuration that conforms to part or all of the intrarenal collecting system. Approximately 70 percent of all staghorn calculi are composed of triple phosphate. Other stones that can assume a staghorn configuration include cystine and uric acid.

The chronic urinary infection associated with triple phosphate stones can frequently be traced to stasis of urine from anatomic defects, neurogenic bladder dysfunction, or urinary diversion procedures.

URINARY STONES IN CHILDREN

As previously noted, urinary stones are distinctly uncommon in children; this group comprises only about 1 percent of all patients with stones. There are four general etiologic categories usually found in children: metabolic disorders, developmental anomalies with urinary stasis (with or without infection), immobilization, and idiopathic. In a child who has not been immobilized and in whom infected urine is not found, there should be a complete and thorough evaluation for metabolic problems. These may include hyperparathyroidism, renal tubular acidosis, cystinuria, or hyperoxaluria. Furthermore, the child may have diseases that produce excessive uric acid such as Lesch–Nyhan syndrome (juvenile gout) or leukemia. The presence of infected urine may indicate an anatomic abnormality of the urinary tract such as vesicoureteral reflux or obstruction.

Immobilization, often necessary after skeletal fracture, is accompanied by bone demineralization and subsequent stone formation. Idiopathic stone formation accounts for 25 to 45 percent of urinary stones in children. These stones are usually composed of calcium oxalate, although the urine does not typically show evidence of excessive excretions of any crystalloid. The condition may be genetic in origin and result from a primary renal defect in the handling of calcium.

In the past, urolithiasis occurring below the age of 1 year was virtually unknown. In the neonatal period, urinary stones are now usually found in premature infants after long-term furosemide therapy for respiratory distress syndrome complicated by bronchopulmonary dysplasia [6]. Furosemide therapy can cause alkalosis and hypercalciuria, which, coupled with the relative high rates of urinary excretion of calcium from immature kidneys, predisposes these premature neonates to the development of medullary nephrocalcinosis and urolithiasis. The incidence of renal calcifications after furosemide treatment is inversely related to the gestational age and to birth weight. Renal sonography to screen for stone disease is recommended for all such premature infants. Other causes of intrarenal calcifications in the neonatal period include renal cortical necrosis and renal vein thrombosis. Renal cortical necrosis results in linear calcification in the periphery of the kidney, while renal vein thrombosis results in reticular intravascular calcifications.

IMAGING OF URINARY STONE DISEASE

RENAL STONE DISEASE

Stone disease constitutes one of the major indications for radiologic evaluation of the urinary system. Although approximately 90 percent of all urinary calculi are radiopaque, the degree of opacity depends on the chemical composition of the stone. Calcium oxalate and phosphate stones are the most radiodense, followed by triple phosphate stones and cystine stones. Plain films of the abdomen will usually identify with ease calcium-containing stones at least 2 mm in diameter. Less opaque stones, such as cystine, may not be appreciated unless they are 3 to 4 mm in size. When calcifications are seen overlying the renal shadows on plain films, the ipsilateral posterior oblique view should be obtained to confirm that the calcification remains in constant relation to the renal shadow before diagnosing an intrarenal calcific process.

Nephrocalcinosis, if significant, can also be easily detected by plain films. Cortical nephrocalcinosis presents as a peripheral increased density in kidneys that are often smaller than normal. This decrease in size is due to the etiologic factors of the nephrocalcinosis, such as cortical necrosis or chronic glomerulonephritis. Dense cortical nephrocalcinosis may result in the appearance of diffuse renal density on plain films because the x-ray beam must penetrate both the anterior and posterior cortex (Fig. 15-1A).

Medullary nephrocalcinosis presents as scattered discrete calcifications or clusters of small calculi in the region of the renal pyramids. The metabolic causes of this entity, such as a hypercalcemic state or renal tubular acidosis, usually result in a bilateral and often somewhat symmetric distribution of the calculi. Renal tubular acidosis (Type I) is responsible for the most dense aggregates of calculi in the renal pyramids (Fig. 15-2A). Segmental or unilateral medullary nephrocalcinosis should suggest the diagnosis of medullary sponge kidney as opposed to metabolic disease.

Precontrast tomography of the kidney can result in increased sensitivity in the detection of renal calculi. Reports indicate that calculi not

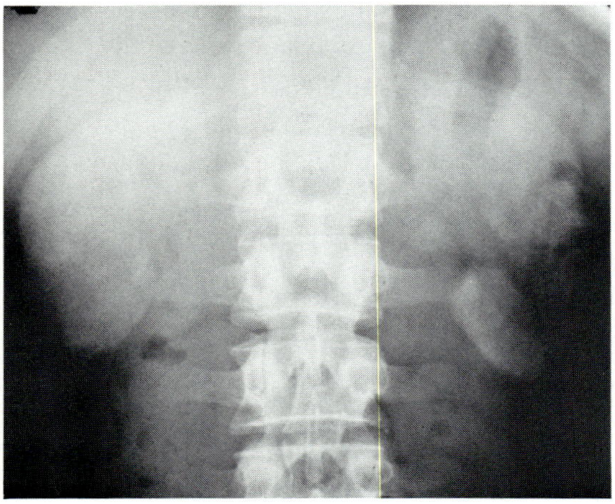

A

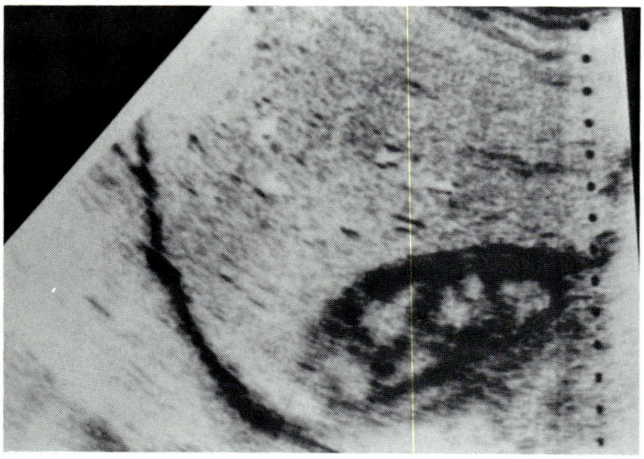

B

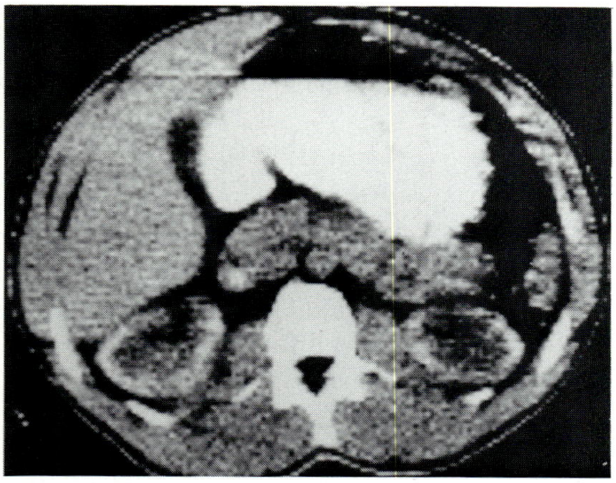

C

Figure 15-1. Imaging of cortical nephrocalcinosis (chronic glomerulonephritis). A. Plain radiograph shows dense renal shadows. B. Right renal sonography demonstrates highly echogenic cortex, while the medullary pyramids are of normal echogenicity. C. CT without a contrast agent reveals the renal cortices to be quite dense.

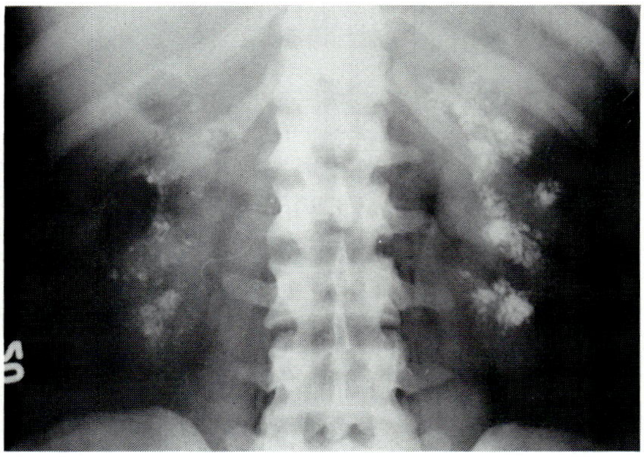

A

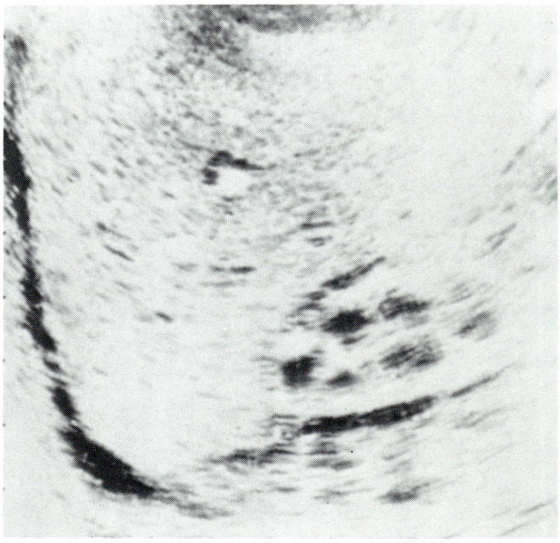

B

Figure 15-2. Imaging of medullary nephrocalcinosis (renal tubular acidosis). A. Plain radiograph demonstrates dense clusters of calculi in the renal papillae. B. Right renal sonography shows highly echodense pyramids without significant acoustic shadowing.

seen on plain film can be detected on tomograms in 13 to 39 percent of patients with known or suspected stone disease [21]. However, even precontrast tomography will not detect lucent stones.

"Milk of calcium" stones are a special condition that require mention. Milk of calcium is a liquid suspension of calcium carbonate usually found within a renal cyst or an obstructed caliceal diverticulum. On rare occasions, it has been reported to occur in the ureter secondary to a ureterocele or other form of obstruction.

Usually occurring in renal cysts, milk of calcium is seen as a vague rounded radiodensity on plain supine films of the abdomen. If this condition is suspected, upright or decubitus radiography should be performed. In these positions, because the specific gravity of the calcium carbonate is greater than that of its suspending fluid, it will form a layer with a horizontal upper border. In caliceal diverticula, 50 percent of which contain calculi, it is more common to see a single calculus or multiple microcalculi rather than milk of calcium. The presence of a caliceal diverticulum can often be suspected on the plain film of the abdomen if a stone or cluster of tiny stones is seen outside the normal location of the calices (Fig. 15-3).

Staghorn calculi, usually composed of triple phosphate, are seen on plain films adapting to all or part of the configuration of the intrarenal collecting system. Staghorn calculi may also be composed of cystine, which should be apparent with high-quality films, and uric acid, which is radiolucent and will not be appreciated until urography is performed.

After the plain films, urography is usually the next evaluative step in patients with stones. In some patients, calculi seen in the region of the renal medulla on plain film may subsequently be found to lie within the intrarenal collecting system. Thus, after administration of an intravenous contrast agent the stones will no longer be seen, since they are contained within the opacified collecting system. In patients with medullary sponge kidney, the major diagnostic finding is contrast medium surrounding the medullary stones in the cystically dilated distal collecting ducts (Fig. 15-4). Other causes of medullary nephrocalcinosis will result in the calculi remaining visible in the tips of the pyramids adjacent to the opacified calices.

Figure 15-3. Stones in caliceal diverticulum. A. Plain radiograph shows cluster of tiny stones outside the normal location of the calices. B. Intravenous urography demonstrates these stones to be in a caliceal diverticulum (arrow).

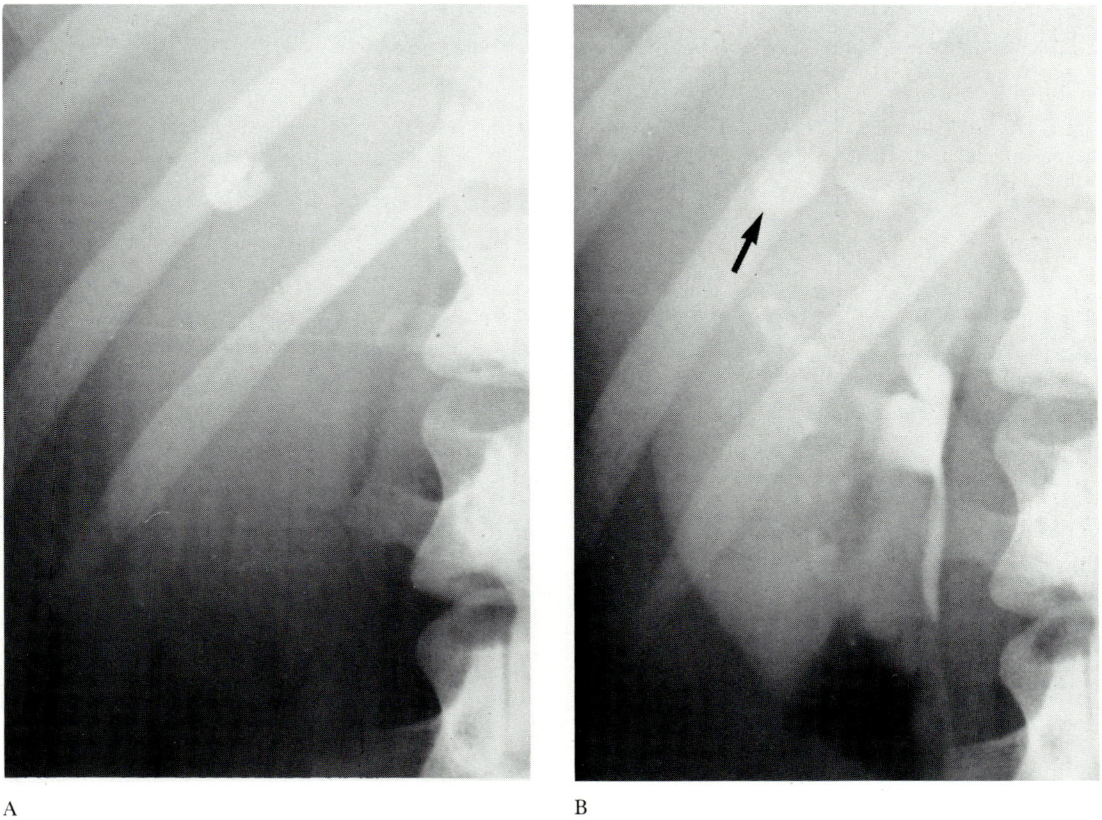

A B

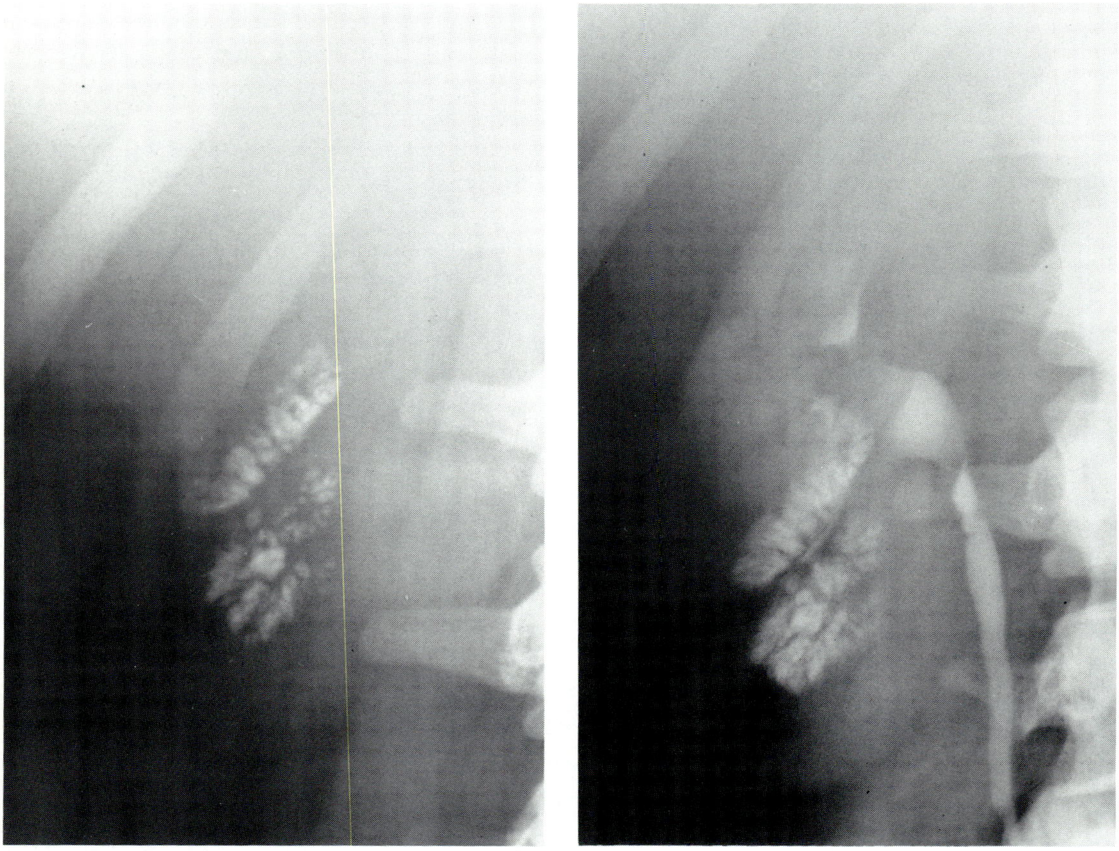

A B

Figure 15-4. Medullary sponge kidney. A. Plain radiograph reveals multiple linear calcifications located in the lower pole of the right kidney in the region of the medulla. B. Intravenous urography shows these stones to be in dilated collecting ducts surrounded by contrast.

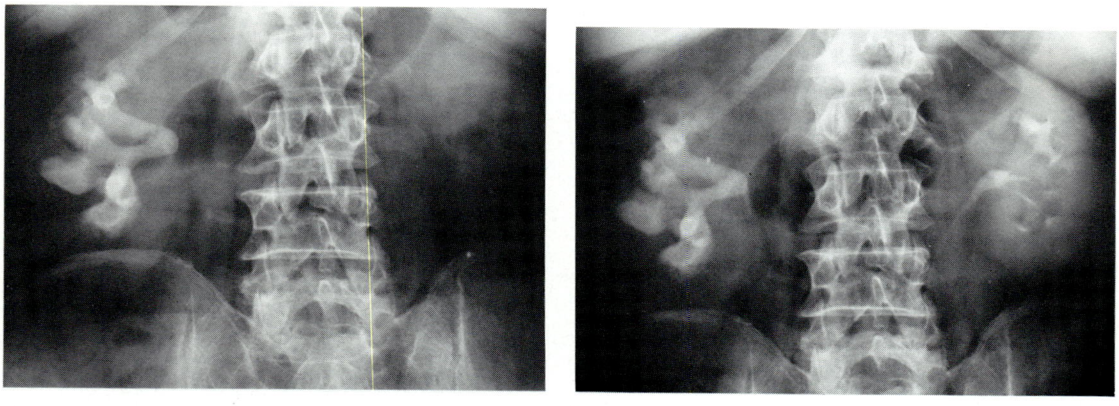

A B

Figure 15-5. Staghorn calculus. A. Plain film of kidneys shows a complete staghorn calculus on the right. B. Five-minute urography shows normal function on the left, but on the right no change is seen from the preliminary film. (Courtesy of Dr. John J. Cronan, Rhode Island Hospital, Providence, RI.)

On urography staghorn calculi are frequently seen to be nonobstructive. On occasion, they can be lost to view in the opacified intrarenal collecting system (Fig.15-5), though commonly they are seen as a filling defect in the contrast column.

Renal sonography is obviously superior to plain abdominal radiography for the detection of radiolucent renal calculi [14]. However, it is slightly less sensitive than the combination of abdominal radiography and precontrast renal tomography for imaging opaque stones. Calculi in the intrarenal collecting system typically appear as dense echogenic foci with acoustic shadowing (Fig. 15-6). Of particular concern are the false positive results resulting in a specificity of only 89 percent for sonographic detection of stones. These false positive results can be caused by catheters or renal arterial calcifications, but in some cases there is no radiographic explanation for the sonographic findings. To reduce the number of false positive findings, a definite acoustic shadow should be identified before a diagnosis of renal stones can be made. It has been reported that diagnostic accuracy for renal stones is high if an acoustic shadow is produced, though gas in the collecting system and calcified transitional cell carcinomas can also produce shadowing. Unfortunately, not all renal stones show discernible acoustic shadows since shadowing varies directly with stone size [8].

Sonography is highly sensitive for the detection of mild degrees of medullary nephrocalcinosis, even when abdominal radiographs are negative. This is seen as increased echogenicity of the renal pyramids, usually without shadowing (see Fig. 15-2B). This suggests that macroscopic aggregates of calcifications are necessary to produce acoustic shadowing [7]. Ultrasonography is also highly sensitive for detecting microcalcifications in the renal cortex, showing

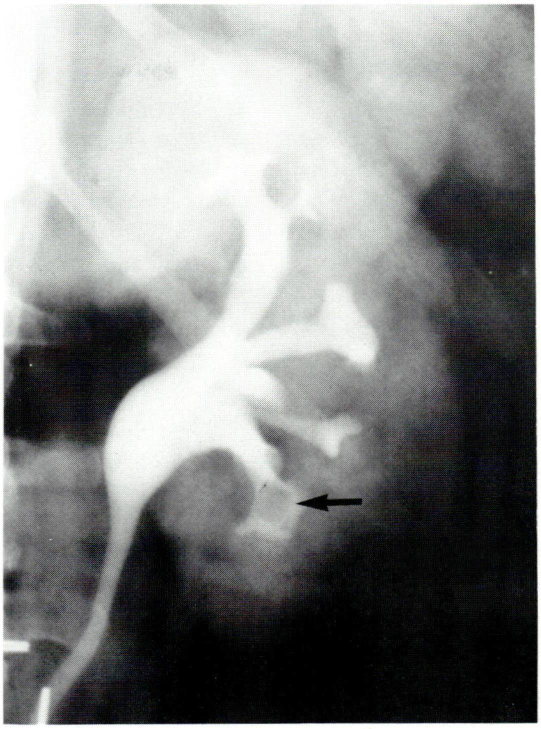

A

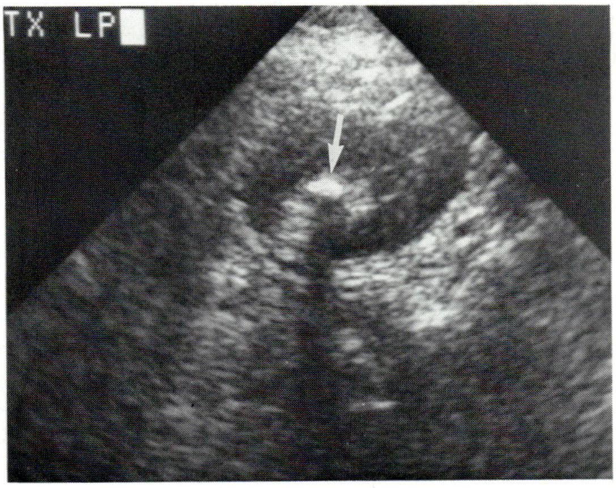

B

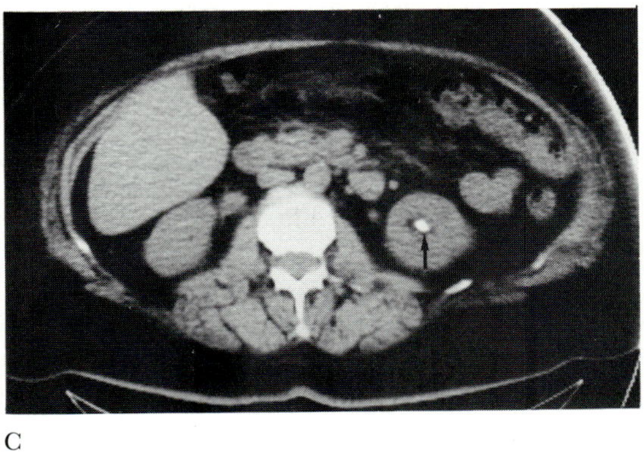

C

Figure 15-6. Evaluation of uric acid stone in calix (plain film showed no calcifications). A. Urography shows 1-cm filling defect in left lower calix (arrow). B. Left renal sonography demonstrates echogenic focus in region of collecting system (arrow) with acoustic shadowing. C. CT without a contrast agent shows the high-attenuation uric acid stone in the left-lower-pole collecting system (arrow).

increased echogenicity in the cortical region of the kidney (see Fig. 15-1B).

All urinary tract stones, with the exception of matrix, have a high-attenuation appearance on CT. This applies even in the case of stones that are radiolucent on plain films. For example, uric acid stones usually have attenuation values of 300 to 400 Hounsfield units, while calcium-containing stones are even higher. Studies have been performed in an attempt to determine whether CT attenuation values would allow accurate analysis of stone composition. Although uric acid and cystine calculi can often be identified by their discrete attenuation, calcium-containing stones of various compositions, including triple phosphate, cannot be reliably distinguished from one another. Therefore, CT analysis of stone density is not likely to be more accurate than standard radiography in characterizing stone composition [17]. The main benefit of CT appears to be in determining whether filling defects in the intrarenal collecting system are lucent stones rather than neoplasms, blood clots, fungus balls, or other soft tissue lesions (see Fig. 15-6C). In this regard, CT is highly accurate. CT is also highly sensitive in detecting mild degrees of cortical (see Fig. 15-1C) or medullary nephrocalcinosis on precontrast scans.

URETERAL CALCULI

Stones that are passed into the ureter may be totally nonobstructive, though more commonly they result in proximal hydronephrosis, accompanied by a prolonged dense nephrogram and late opacification of the collecting system on urography. In some instances delayed films must be obtained up to 24 hours after injection of contrast medium to allow opacification of the ureter down to the suspected stone and thus to confirm the stone as the cause of the obstruction (Fig. 15-7). There is poor correlation between the size of a ureteral stone and the degree of obstruction it can cause. The physiology and radiography of obstruction will be discussed more fully in Chap. 16.

Stones passing into the ureter tend to hang up at the ureteropelvic junction, at the point where the ureter crosses the iliac vessels, or at the ureterovesical junction. Overall, however, 75 percent of stones passing into the ureter are found at initial evaluation to be lodged within the pelvic ureter. The large majority of these are less than 1 cm in size. Virtually all stones seen within the ureter were originally formed within the renal medulla or intrarenal collecting system. Stones forming primarily in the ureter are distinctly uncommon and usually are found proximal to a point of anatomic obstruction such as a ureterocele.

Retrograde pyelography is frequently used for evaluation of ureteral obstruction when the cause is unclear. This is especially true in cases of lucent stones. A stone can usually be seen as a discrete rounded or oval defect in the ureteral lumen at the point of obstruction. If tumor remains part of the differential diagnosis, brushing can then be performed for cytologic study. Usually, however, the ureter immediately below a transitional cell carcinoma is more dilated than that found with a stone; this is due to expansile growth of the tumor. This finding on retrograde studies should raise the suspicion of malignancy. On the other hand, the ureteral edema secondary to a small stone may be indistinguishable from a mural tumor. Thin-section CT through the area of concern may detect the small stone responsible for the obstruction. Often a drainage stent is placed in the ureter at the time of retrograde study for relief of obstruction.

BLADDER CALCULI

Stones within the bladder may be difficult to appreciate on plain films because the overlying sigmoid is filled with gas and feces. Bladder stones are multiple in 25 to 30 percent of cases, and these are often faceted (Fig. 15-8A); solitary calcium oxalate stones may have an irregular border, in which case they are referred to as "mulberry stones" (Fig. 15-8B), or may be spiculated and look like the jacks children play with ("jack stones") (Fig. 15-8C). In the United States, the most common cause of bladder stones is bladder outlet obstruction in the male secondary to benign prostatic hypertrophy. Thus, it is not unusual to detect an enlarged prostate protruding into the bladder base and an associated trabeculated bladder. Calculi in these cases are usually seen as lucent rounded defects in the contrast-filled bladder (Fig. 15-9). Bladder stones may also form on a foreign-body

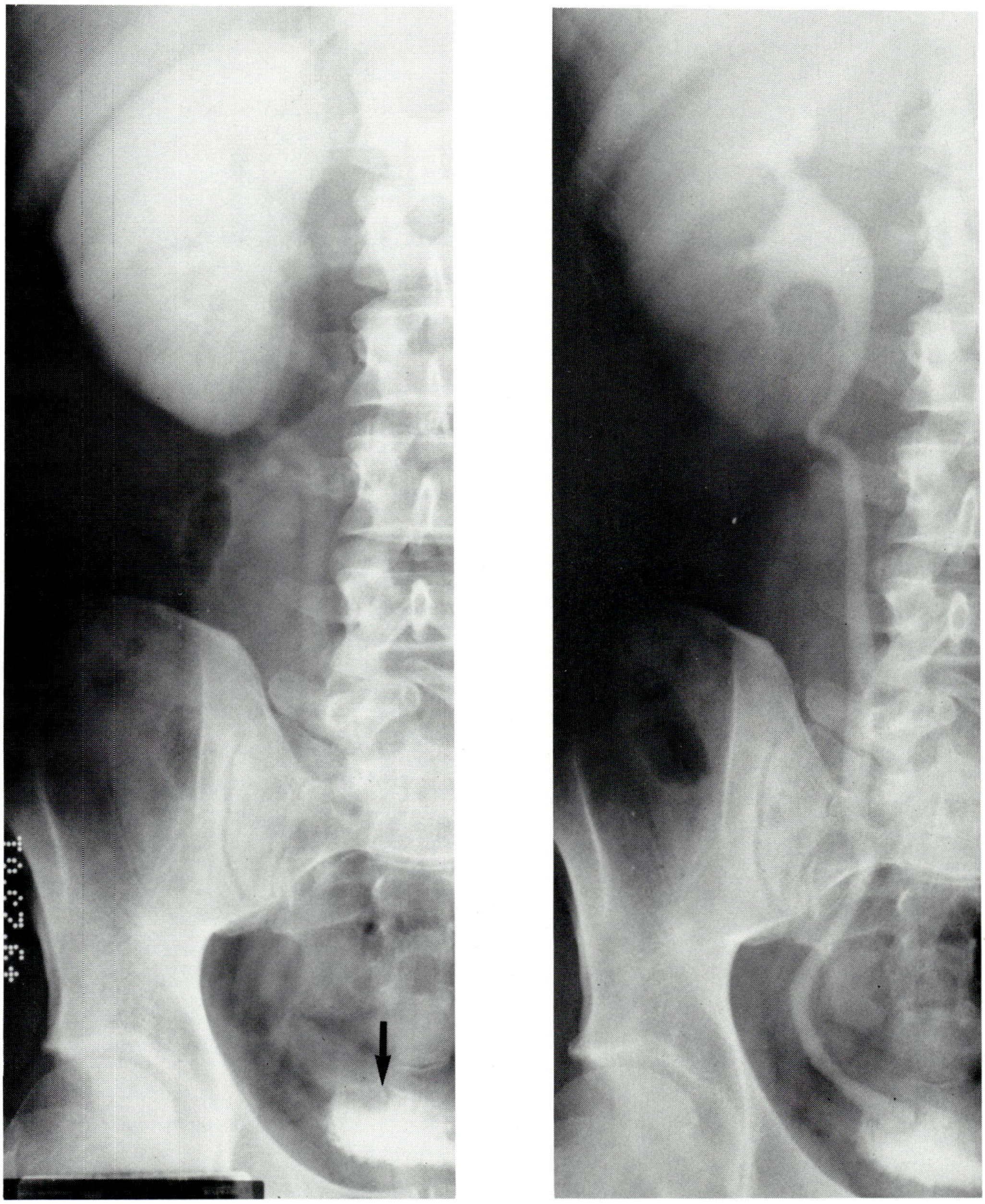

A B

Figure 15-7. Obstructive distal ureteral calculus. A. Two-hour postvoiding urography shows dense nephrogram and contrast medium in a mildly dilated collecting system and proximal ureter. There is a 2-mm calcification at the expected location of the ureterovesical junction (arrow) with surrounding trigonal edema. B. Four-hour delay film demonstrates contrast medium columning in the ureter to previously mentioned calcification, confirming it as the cause of the obstruction.

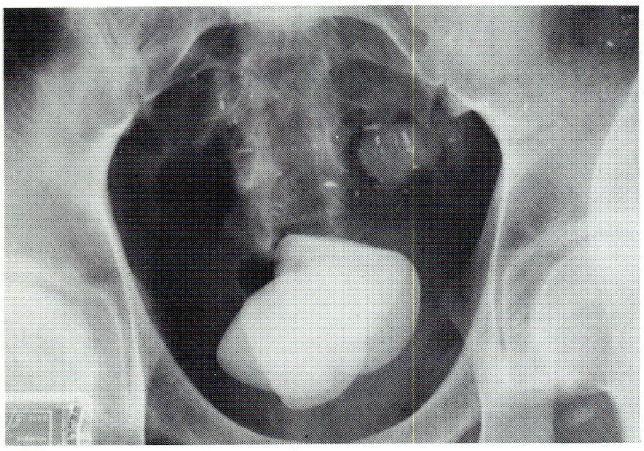

A

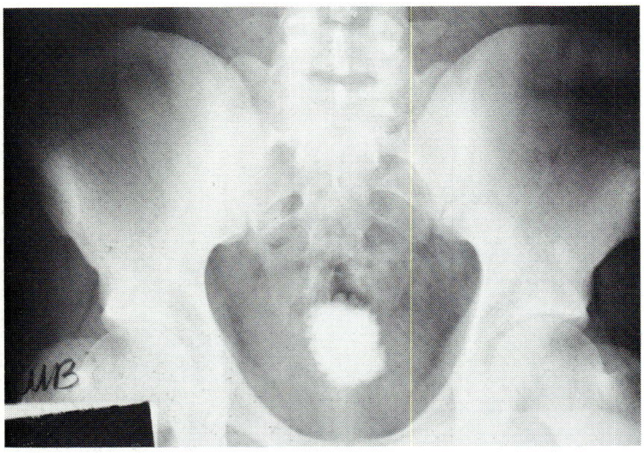

B

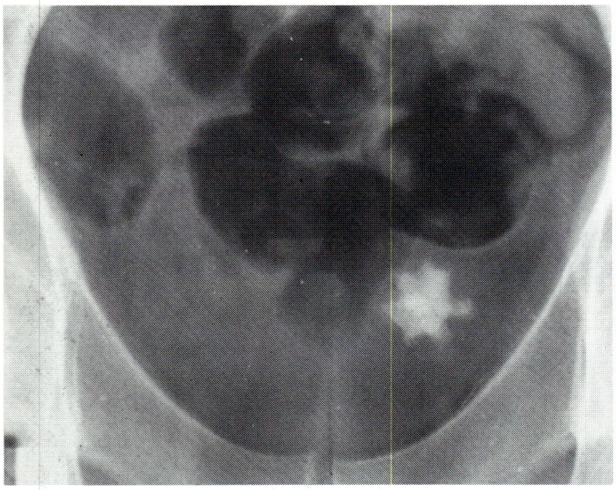

C

Figure 15-8. Radiopaque bladder calculi. A. Plain radiograph shows multifaceted bladder stones. B. Plain radiograph shows single "mulberry stone." C. Plain radiograph shows single "jack stone."

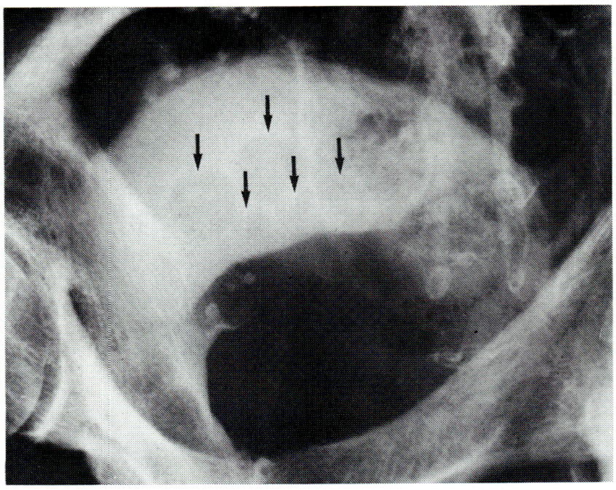

Figure 15-9. Radiolucent bladder calculi (plain radiograph showed no abnormal calcifications). Coned view of the bladder on urography shows round filling defects (arrows) above the significantly enlarged prostate, which is causing outlet obstruction.

nidus, such as a surgical clip that has eroded into the bladder or a retained catheter fragment [1].

URETHRAL CALCULI

Migrant calculi originate in the bladder or kidney and descend into the urethra. These are 10 times more frequent than primary calculi, which are actually formed within the urethra. Most primary urethral stones form in association with chronic urinary stasis and urinary infection, either within a congenital anterior urethral diverticulum or proximal to a urethral obstruction. Usually, only a single stone is found, though several calculi may be found within a large diverticulum.

The majority of urethral calculi are missed during urography. This is probably because of exclusion of the external genitalia from most routine urograms and inattention to the areas below the symphysis pubis that are included. Certainly, the entire pubic symphysis should be included in preliminary films during urography, as opaque calculi will occasionally be noted on these films as the cause of voiding symptoms or hematuria (Fig. 15-10A). When a stone is suspected, confirmation of the diagnosis requires either retrograde or antegrade urethrography (Fig. 15-10B). Not only does this localize a suspicious calcification to the urethral lumen, it

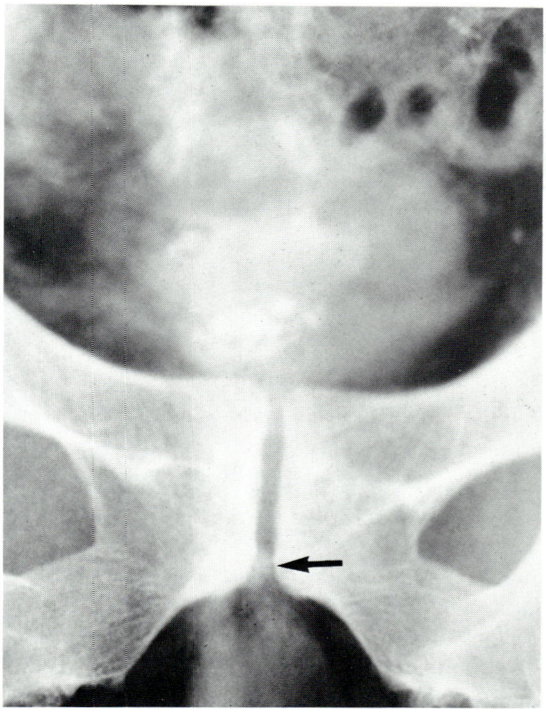

A

also reveals any associated urethral pathology that may require correction. The differential diagnosis of urethral calculi includes phleboliths in the pampiniform plexus of the spermatic cord and calcification of fibrous plaques involving the corpora cavernosa in Peyronie's disease [1].

COMPLICATIONS OF URINARY TRACT STONES

The large majority of complications ascribed to urinary calculus disease occur as a result of infection or obstruction. Also, there is an increased incidence of leukoplakia, a premalignant condition, and squamous cell carcinoma of the collecting system with calculus disease. In patients afflicted with these processes, stones are reported to be present in 25 to 50 percent of cases.

With acute obstruction from ureteral calculi, it is not unusual to note pyelosinus extravasation of contrast material during urography (Fig. 15-11). This can occur with even mild

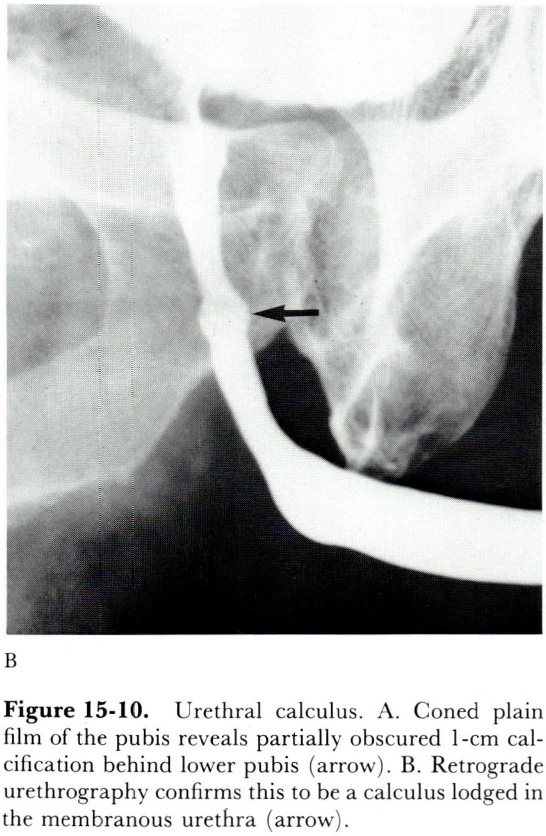

B

Figure 15-10. Urethral calculus. A. Coned plain film of the pubis reveals partially obscured 1-cm calcification behind lower pubis (arrow). B. Retrograde urethrography confirms this to be a calculus lodged in the membranous urethra (arrow).

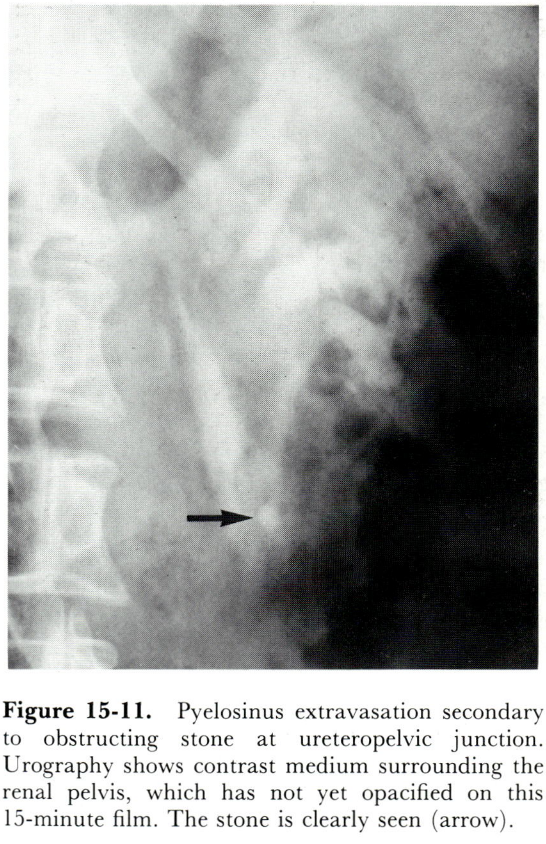

Figure 15-11. Pyelosinus extravasation secondary to obstructing stone at ureteropelvic junction. Urography shows contrast medium surrounding the renal pelvis, which has not yet opacified on this 15-minute film. The stone is clearly seen (arrow).

degrees of obstruction and is secondary to leakage of contrast material at the fornix of a calix. This contrast containing urine can then be seen tracking through the renal sinus, exiting through the renal hilus, and even enveloping the proximal ureter. This resolves spontaneously and is of no clinical consequence if the urine is uninfected.

With long-term uninfected obstruction, hydronephrotic atrophy of the kidney may result, with subsequent inability to resume normal function once the obstruction is relieved. These kidneys exhibit thinned parenchyma in response to the chronically elevated pressure in the dilated collecting system, and their overall size may be decreased. If infection supervenes, pyonephrosis can occur, with rapid progression of significant renal damage. Extensive perirenal inflammatory disease is not unusual in these cases and can best be evaluated with CT, which shows soft-tissue stranding or frank abscess formation in the perirenal space. Renal and ureteral calculi associated with secondarily infected kidneys are a major cause of perirenal abscess. Approximately 83 percent of perirenal abscesses are of renal origin, with about 34 percent being associated with renal calculus disease [20]. An unusual inflammatory response of the kidney is xanthogranulomatous pyelonephritis. About 70 percent of these cases are associated with an obstructing calculus in the intrarenal collecting system. This entity is discussed further in Chap. 11.

The urographic findings of focal clubbing of the renal calices and adjacent parenchymal scarring usually prompt a diagnosis of chronic pyelonephritis, which is frequently thought to be due to ongoing or previous vesicoureteral reflux. However, recent work indicates that upper tract stone disease appears to be the condition that most often precedes or accompanies caliceal clubbing and parenchymal scarring in adults. In one group of adults with clubbing and scarring, 67 percent had stone disease but only 8 percent had a history of reflux [16]. Caliceal or staghorn calculi that cause episodes of obstruction at the infundibular level can produce focal parenchymal thinning and caliceal flattening with the same pattern that is seen in reflux nephropathy.

TREATMENT OF URINARY STONE DISEASE

There are currently five methods available for treatment of urinary stones. These include medical management, open surgical removal, retrograde transurethral techniques, percutaneous nephrolithotomy, and extracorporeal shock-wave lithotripsy (ESWL). Treatment must be individualized for each case, and there may be a need for a combined approach.

MEDICAL MANAGEMENT

Uric acid calculi can often be dissolved by systemic alkalinization using oral therapy. Cystine calculi have also been successfully treated using oral therapy including alkalinization and penicillamine. Chemical dissolution of certain stones can be accomplished via a percutaneously placed nephrostomy tube or ureteral catheter; for cystine calculi, tromethamine-E has proven effective, as has hemiacidrin for struvite calculi [24].

SURGERY

Surgical removal of urinary calculi has been largely replaced by less-invasive techniques. It is currently necessary in less than 1 percent of cases. A major indication for surgical intervention is an associated anatomic obstruction that would require open correction. Another indication for surgery is extreme obesity, which contraindicates ESWL or percutaneous techniques.

RETROGRADE TECHNIQUES

Retrograde techniques, including ureteroscopy with associated stone basketing or fragmentation, are highly effective in the treatment of distal ureteral stones. ESWL is limited in its capabilities in this area because of the underlying bony pelvis. Retrograde techniques are successful in removing distal ureteral stones in over 90 percent of cases, with very few complications. Bladder stones can also be successfully fragmented and extracted by way of the urethra.

PERCUTANEOUS TECHNIQUES

Percutaneous nephrolithotomy (PNL) involves creation of a large-caliber percutaneous access to the involved portion of the intrarenal collecting system followed by direct extraction (Fig. 15-12) or ultrasonic fragmentation of the calculus. Stone fragments produced by fragmentation are either passed down the ureter or extracted via the percutaneous tract. There is a relatively steep learning curve for this technique, but once mastered it is highly successful.

PNL is currently appropriate therapy for a variety of renal and ureteral stones. General indications for PNL include large renal pelvic stones or staghorn calculi, cystine stones, obstructive uropathy, young age (children), and ESWL failures. Large renal pelvic stones or staghorn calculi occupying virtually the entire intrarenal collecting system often require debulking by PNL prior to ESWL therapy. Cystine stones, because of their hardness, are difficult to fragment with ESWL.

PNL is an invasive procedure and complications may occur. Probably the most significant of these is arteriovenous fistula formation resulting from trauma to a peripheral artery [22]. Other complications include hemorrhage,

Figure 15-12. Percutaneous nephrolithotomy. A. A large-caliber sheath has been placed percutaneously into the collecting system after dilation of the track over the guide wire that was initially placed down the ureter. A faintly opaque 1-cm calculus is seen at the end of the sheath (arrow). B. After extraction of the stone, opacification of the collecting system shows typical spasm and edema where the stone had been lodged at the ureteropelvic junction (arrow) and minimal extravasation around the renal pelvis.

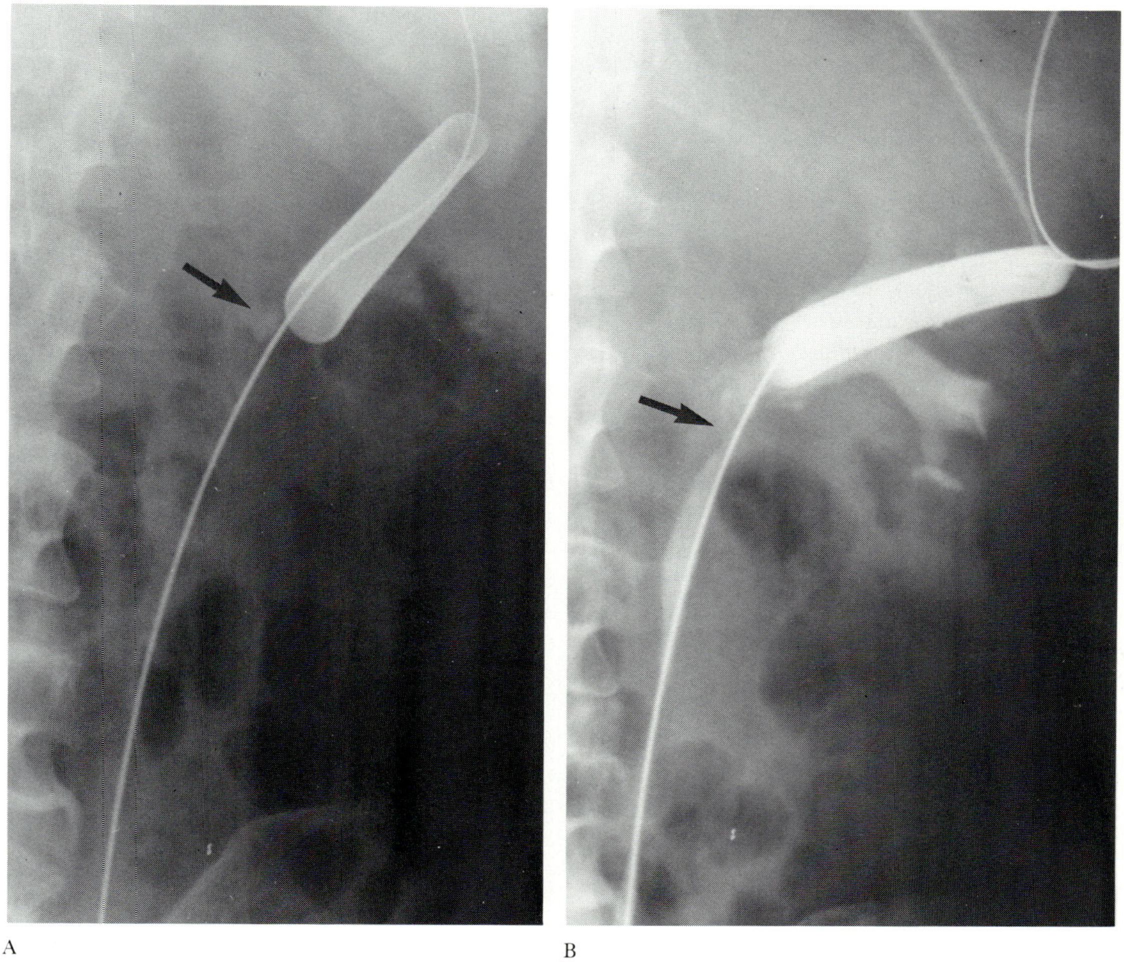

A B

catheter dislodgement, urine extravasation, infection, pneumothorax, and prolonged ileus [5].

EXTRACORPOREAL SHOCK-WAVE LITHOTRIPSY

ESWL has now been in clinical use for almost a decade and has largely replaced other treatment techniques for the majority of calculi occurring in the upper urinary tract. The current range of its indications includes approximately 70 percent of patients with upper urinary tract stones [4]. An additional 25 percent of patients with more complex stone problems in the upper urinary tract can be treated with ESWL combined with endourologic procedures.

This technique is noninvasive and uses focused shock waves generated outside the body for disintegration of stones. Focusing of the shock wave is accomplished by fluoroscopic or sonographic triangulation after localization of the stone. Refinement of this technique has resulted in equipment that has the capability of fragmenting stones with less requirement for anesthesia. While the original lithotriptors required submerging of the patient in a water bath, the machines now require only a localized coupling of the shock-wave generator to the patient's back in the renal area.

For solitary kidney stones of 1.0 cm or less, ESWL is 90 percent effective in complete eradication. On the other extreme, when complete staghorn stones are treated with ESWL, it is reported that only 31 to 50 percent of patients become stone-free. Overall, the incidence of totally stone-free kidneys after ESWL therapy ranges from 50 to 90 percent. The annual recurrence rate of stones after removal of the primary calculus by ESWL is only 4 to 8 percent, which compares favorably to other treatment methods [15].

ESWL appears to be associated with a low frequency of serious renal trauma. However, when studied with CT after ESWL treatments, the kidney may demonstrate subcapsular hematomas of varying size, intrarenal hematomas, subcapsular collections of urine, and an overall increase in size [19]. The majority of patients show perinephric soft-tissue stranding and fascial thickening. It has been shown that the renal trauma associated with ESWL can result in mildly decreased renal function of the treated kidney and that this decrease may be permanent [25]. ESWL is also associated with the onset of hypertension in about 8 percent of patients. This may occur immediately or be delayed by several weeks or months. The pathogenesis of this hypertension remains unknown.

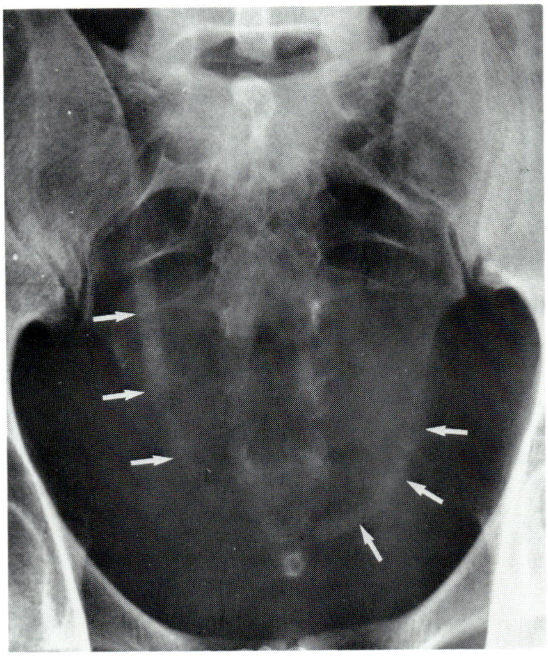

Figure 15-13. Steinstrasse in patient who has undergone ESWL therapy for bilateral renal stones. Plain radiograph reveals stone fragments impacted in both distal ureters (arrows).

After either PNL or ESWL (or a combination of the two), small stone fragments are usually passed through the ureter with ease. However, on occasion, multiple fragments may cluster in the distal ureter and produce obstruction (Fig. 15-13). Radiographically this finding is known as steinstrasse, or street of stones. If the obstruction is significant, antegrade or retrograde stenting or extraction of these distal ureteral stones becomes necessary.

REFERENCES

1. Banner, M.P., and Pollack, H.M. Urolithiasis in the lower urinary tract. *Semin. Roentgenol.* 17:140, 1982.

2. Broadus, A.E. Primary hyperparathyroidism. *J. Urol.* 141:723, 1989.
3. Buckalew, V.M., Jr. Nephrolithiasis in renal tubular acidosis. *J. Urol.* 141:731, 1989.
4. Chaussy, C.G., and Fuchs, G.J. Current state and future developments of noninvasive treatment of human urinary stones with extracorporeal shock wave lithotripsy. *J. Urol.* 141:782, 1989.
5. Dunnick, N.R., et al. Complications of percutaneous nephrostolithotomy. *Radiology* 157:51, 1985.
6. Gilsanz, V., et al. Nephrolithiasis in premature infants. *Radiology* 154:107, 1985.
7. Glazer, G.M., Callen, P.W., and Filly, R.A. Medullary nephrocalcinosis: Sonographic evaluation. *A.J.R.* 138:55, 1982.
8. King, W., III, Kimme-Smith, C., and Winter, J. Renal stone shadowing: An investigation of contributing factors. *Radiology* 154:191, 1985.
9. Lalli, A.F. Renal parenchymal calcifications. *Semin. Reontgenol.* 17:101, 1982.
10. Lemann, J., Jr., and Gray, R.W. Iodiopathic hypercalciuria. *J. Urol.* 141:715, 1989.
11. Lerner, S.P., Gleeson, M.J., and Griffith, D.P. Infection stones. *J. Urol.* 141:753, 1989.
12. Ljunghall, S. Incidence of upper urinary tract stones. *Mineral Electrolyte Metab.* 13:220, 1987.
13. Margolin, E.G., and Cohen, L.H. Genitourinary calcification: An overview. *Semin. Roentgenol.* 17:95, 1982.
14. Middleton, W.D., et al. Renal calculi: Sensitivity for detection with US. *Radiology* 167:239, 1988.
15. Miles, S.G., et al. Extracorporeal shock-wave lithotripsy: Prevalence of renal stones 3-21 months after treatment. *A.J.R.* 150:307, 1988.
16. Newhouse, J.H., and Amis, E.S., Jr. The relationship between renal scarring and stone disease. *A.J.R.* 151:1153, 1988.
17. Newhouse, J.H., et al. Computed tomographic analysis of urinary calculi. *A.J.R.* 142:545, 1984.
18. Rous, S.N. A review of 171 consecutive patients with urinary lithiasis. *J. Urol.* 126:376, 1981.
19. Rubin, J.I., et al. Kidney changes after extracorporeal shock wave lithotripsy: CT evaluation. *Radiology* 162:21, 1987.
20. Saksouk, F.A., et al. Computed tomography of perirenal and pararenal inflammatory disease complicating renal calculi. *Urology* 24:200, 1984.
21. Scwartz, G., Lipschitz, S., and Becker, J.A. Detection of renal calculi: The value of tomography. *A.J.R.* 143:143, 1984.
22. Segura, J.W. The role of percutaneous surgery in renal and ureteral stone removal. *J. Urol.* 141:780, 1989.
23. Smith, L.H. The medical aspects of urolithiasis: An overview. *J. Urol.* 141:707, 1989.
24. Smith, T.P., et al. Current trends in the management of urinary stones. *Acta Radiol.* 29:145, 1988.
25. Williams, C.M., et al. Extracorporeal shock-wave lithotripsy: Long-term complications. *A.J.R.* 150:311, 1988.
26. Williams, H.E., and Wandzilak, T.R. Oxalate synthesis, transport and the hyperoxaluric syndromes. *J. Urol.* 141:742, 1989.

16

Urinary Tract Obstruction

In urologic imaging and clinical practice, obstructive phenomena may be the most frequently encountered manifestations of urinary tract diseases. An extremely wide variety of conditions produce obstruction, obstruction itself is extremely common, and clinical findings suggesting obstruction virtually always require confirmatory diagnosis by imaging. For all of these reasons, a thorough familiarity with the imaging manifestations of obstruction is essential for uroradiologic practice [14, 26].

Since the causes of urinary tract obstruction are so numerous and varied, they will not be described in detail in this chapter but will instead be found in other sections of this book that deal with specific disease entities. A few general comments are in order, however. First of all, obstruction may be due to processes that occur entirely within the lumina of the hollow urinary viscera; stones, urothelial tumors, and blood clots are common causes of such obstruction. Functional and anatomic abnormalities of the mural portions of the urinary tract constitute another group; congenital and acquired urethral and ureteral stenoses, intramural tumors, and disorders of the bladder detrusor and sphincter muscles are examples of this group of diseases. Finally, processes extrinsic to the hollow urinary viscera may impinge on these structures and occlude them; retroperitoneal tumors and fibrosis and prostatic hypertrophy are examples of this category.

In addition, cases of urinary tract obstruction exhibit extreme variety with regard to severity, rapidity of onset, duration, and, when relieved, persistence of residual abnormalities. It should be clear, therefore, that the manifestations of obstruction are quite varied and that it is necessary to be familiar with all of them.

PATHOPHYSIOLOGY

Acute obstruction of the ureter produces a rise in urine pressure proximal to the obstruction [22]; if the affected kidney is healthy, the amount of pressure rise depends on the degree of obstruction. If the obstruction is anything but very mild, the pressure rise is transmitted retrograde to the calices, since peristalsis becomes ineffective [40], and the ureter and collecting system become one continuous column of urine [6]. Elevated caliceal pressure causes a well-known chain of events within the kidney. The pressure in the tubular lumina also rises [12] as glomerular filtration continues; ultimately, pressure in Bowman's capsule rises, and glomerular filtration rate begins to decrease [7]. If the pressure in Bowman's space remains elevated, ultimately the blood flow in the affected kidney begins to drop [8–10, 42]. The flow rate of tubular fluid decreases, and the ability of the kidney to concentrate many solutes—including radiographic contrast material—also decreases.

The elevated urine pressure in the calices and collecting system impairs normal peristalsis. These structures become distended (although acute obstruction, even if severe, does not produce a great increase in diameter), and peristaltic waves no longer completely close the lumen or may cease altogether. In some patients markedly elevated caliceal pressure may cause a rupture at the caliceal fornix [13], so that urine escapes into the renal sinus and ultimately into the perinephric space. Extravasated urine has been known to enter the peritoneal space to form ascites [5] if the patient is very young and the obstruction is severe.

If obstruction is complete and if it persists, the renal changes progress: Renal blood flow continues to drop and glomerular filtration may diminish and, for all practical purposes, disappear; the volume of the renal parenchyma (which increases slightly with acute obstruction) begins to diminish as tubular cells atrophy.

If persistent obstruction is partial, so that the kidney continues to produce urine, the renal changes are different. Some tubular atrophy occurs, but glomeruli remain unless renal damage becomes very severe [36]. Concentrating capacity remains low; the relative urine output from the affected kidney is variable but, with persistent moderate or severe obstruction, tends to diminish. Tubular-cell atrophy produces loss of renal parenchymal mass; this is at the expense, at first, of medullary tissue. Although the parenchyma thins, the overall outer dimensions of the kidney may increase, so that a hydronephrotic kidney may become considerably longer and wider than normal; this is in contradistinction to acute persistent complete obstruction, in which case the outer dimensions of the kidney, as well as renal parenchymal mass, tends to diminish. Parenchymal loss from obstruction is called hydronephrotic atrophy.

With persistent ureteral obstruction, the changes undergone by the collecting system and ureter depend on the degree and severity of the obstruction. In general, there is a tendency for the collecting system and ureter to dilate and for peristalsis to become ineffective or absent. Very mild obstruction produces relatively little dilation; at the other extreme, complete persistent obstruction usually does not cause massive dilation either. The most severe dilation occurs at an intermediate state, which appears when there is ureteral obstruction sufficiently severe to raise the urine pressure in the lumen but not so severe as to produce severe oliguria or anuria in the affected kidney. As might be expected, the degree of dilation in cases of partial obstruction tends to increase as the duration of obstruction increases.

If the actual obstruction is removed, there is a tendency for the system superior to it to revert toward normal. If the obstruction has been short-lived—that is, some days or less—the kidney, collecting system, and ureter often return entirely to normal, or at least to their preobstructive base-line state. If the obstruction is complete and persists for a number of weeks or longer before being relieved, mild degrees of ureterocaliectasis may remain after relief, and the overall renal size and parenchymal mass may be irrevocably diminished; at the extreme, a kidney whose ureter has been completely obstructed for months or more may become quite small and never regain significant function.

If the obstruction has been partial, abnormalities may or may not persist after relief. Mild short-lived obstruction may, of course, permit a complete return to normal. If, however, the caliceal and ureteral dilation has become moderate or severe, some degree of dilation of these structures persists even after the obstruction has been relieved and decompression permits some reduction in their volume. The effects on the kidney depend primarily on the degree of tubular-cell atrophy that has occurred: Atrophic parenchyma does not regenerate, so that parenchymal thinning persists after relief of obstruction. If the kidney has been distended into a thin shell of parenchyma by longstanding partial obstruction, its morphology usually changes very little after relief of the obstruction; there may be minimal diminution in the overall dimensions of the organ.

Bladder-outlet obstruction and its effects on the bladder itself are described in detail elsewhere in this book, but this phenomenon may affect the upper tracts as well [27]. If the mean pressure of urine in the bladder is elevated by severe urethral obstruction of any kind, the ureteral peristaltic mechanism may not be sufficiently strong to force each ureteral urine bolus entirely into the bladder. When this occurs, a continuous column of urine in the ureteral lumen appears, pressure throughout the ureters and collecting systems rises, and these structures begin to distend. Peristaltic contraction waves no longer completely coapt the walls of the ureter and may disappear entirely. The collecting system and ureteral changes are bilaterally symmetrical or nearly so, since both ureters empty into the same bladder lumen and thus are exposed to the same urine pressure. Prolonged elevated upper tract pressure may produce hydronephrotic atrophy of the medullary parenchyma; although bladder-outlet obstruction may progress to complete urinary retention and thus to clinical anuria, upper tract pressure rarely, if ever, is elevated to the point at which the kidneys completely stop making urine. Their concentrating capacity may be significantly compromised, however.

IMAGING OF ACUTE OBSTRUCTION

PLAIN FILMS

Abdominal radiography may occasionally reveal urinary tract stones as the cause of acute obstruction. Acute urinary retention usually distends the bladder to the point at which it can be seen as a pelvic mass.

UROGRAPHY

In cases of very mild acute obstruction, the nephrogram [23] and the timing of caliceal opacification may be normal; only the mildest of caliceal and ureteral dilation may indicate that an obstruction exists (Fig. 16-1). With moderate or severe obstruction, the nephrogram shows a delayed onset; its eventual peak density may be very great, however, so that the renal parenchyma becomes much more opaque than the densest normal nephrogram (Fig. 16-2), and the obstructive nephrogram may persist for many minutes to many hours. The obstructive nephrogram may demonstrate faint radial striations [3]. Not all cases of severe acute obstruction produce an obstructive nephrogram, however; the nephrogram may sometimes be very faint or even absent. The kidney may become slightly enlarged [7].

If the obstructed kidney is oliguric, the calices may be opacified later than those on the contralateral normal side. Opacified urine may be seen to proceed down the collecting system and ureter at a slower rate than on the normal side, due both to the increased volume of the collecting system and ureter and to the slower production of urine. The contrast agent is usually less concentrated on the obstructed side [17]. Obviously, a completely obstructed kidney that is anuric may not opacify the collecting system at all. If the upper tract begins to opacify, it is good practice to obtain serial delayed films until

Figure 16-1. Minimal right ureteral obstruction. Intravenous urography shows the caliceal fornices on the right to be minimally but unquestionably blunted. The fornices on the left are normal and appear sharp.

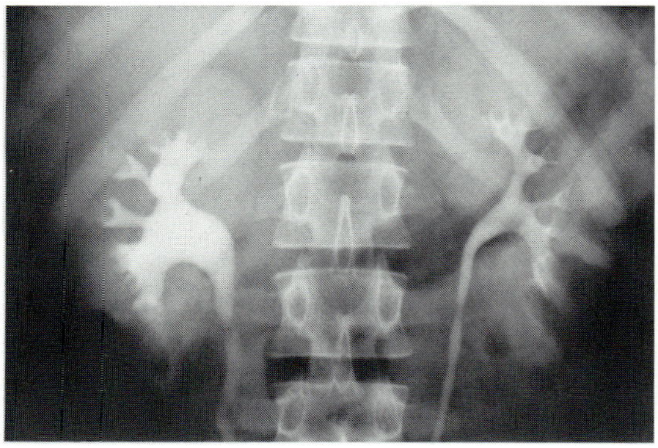

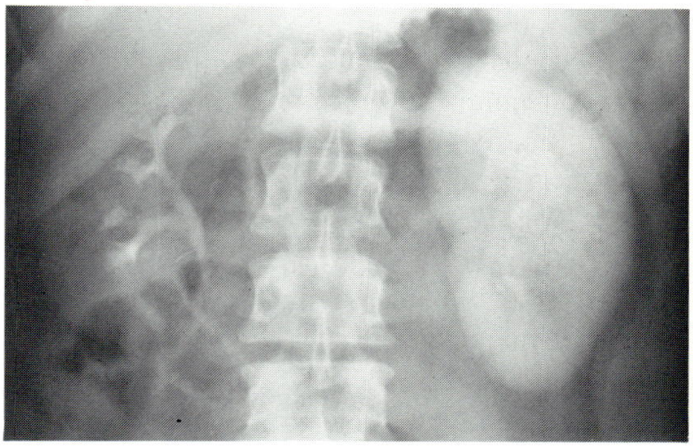

Figure 16-2. Acute left ureteral obstruction; 30-minute urographic film. The nephrogram on the left is very dense, and there is very little contrast in the collecting system. This film was obtained 30 minutes after contrast agent administration; the nephrogram on the right has already faded to a density considerably less that its peak.

Figure 16-3. Recently relieved left-sided obstruction; 15-minute urographic film. Note that the left collecting system is poorly opacified and the contrast material is faint. The right collecting system appears normal; there is dense papillary blush on the right, which is normal.

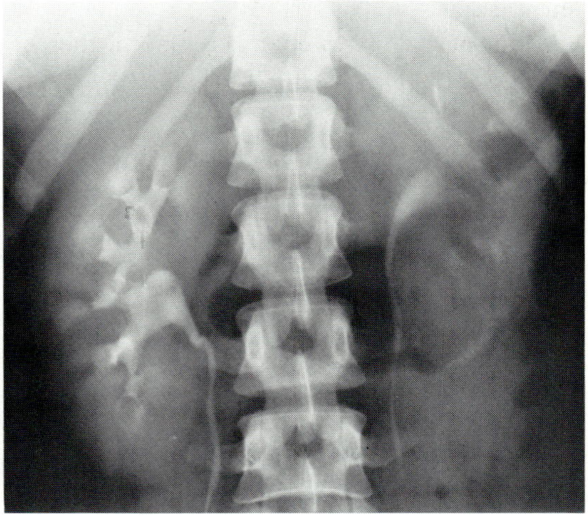

the obstructed level of the ureter becomes apparent; this may require many hours. An acutely obstructed kidney may remain relatively oliguric and concentrate contrast material poorly for several hours to days after the obstruction has been relieved (Fig. 16-3).

The elevated pressure of acute ureteral obstruction produces dilation of the collecting system proximal to the point of obstruction (Fig. 16-4). Even with severe obstruction, the degree of enlargement is mild, unless the ureter or collecting system musculature has been stretched by prior episodes of obstruction. The caliceal fornices will become blunted by the elevated pressure.

If the elevated caliceal pressure has ruptured a fornix, opacified urine will be seen to dissect throughout the soft tissues of the renal sinus [28] ("pyelosinus backflow"); this opacified urine may find its way through the renal hilus and spread throughout the perinephric space (Fig. 16-5).

RETROGRADE URETEROPYELOGRAPHY

If the obstructing ureteral lesion permits contrast medium to be injected past it to the more proximal collecting system, that collecting system will be seen to be distended, just as it would be with intravenous pyelography. The combination of distention and relative oliguria may cause the contrast material proximal to the obstruction to persist if delayed films are obtained; however, since oliguria or caliceal distention caused by conditions other than ongoing obstruction may also cause contrast material to be washed out relatively slowly, this sign is not entirely reliable as an independent indicator of obstruction. The pressure produced by injection of a contrast agent during retrograde pyelography may distend the calices even in the absence of obstruction; therefore, caliectasis should be diagnosed only if it persists after the catheter has been removed from the ureter.

CT

The abnormalities in contrast opacification of the renal parenchyma, collecting system, and ureter that have been described for urography may be equally well demonstrated by CT, as may pyelosinus backflow and extravasation into

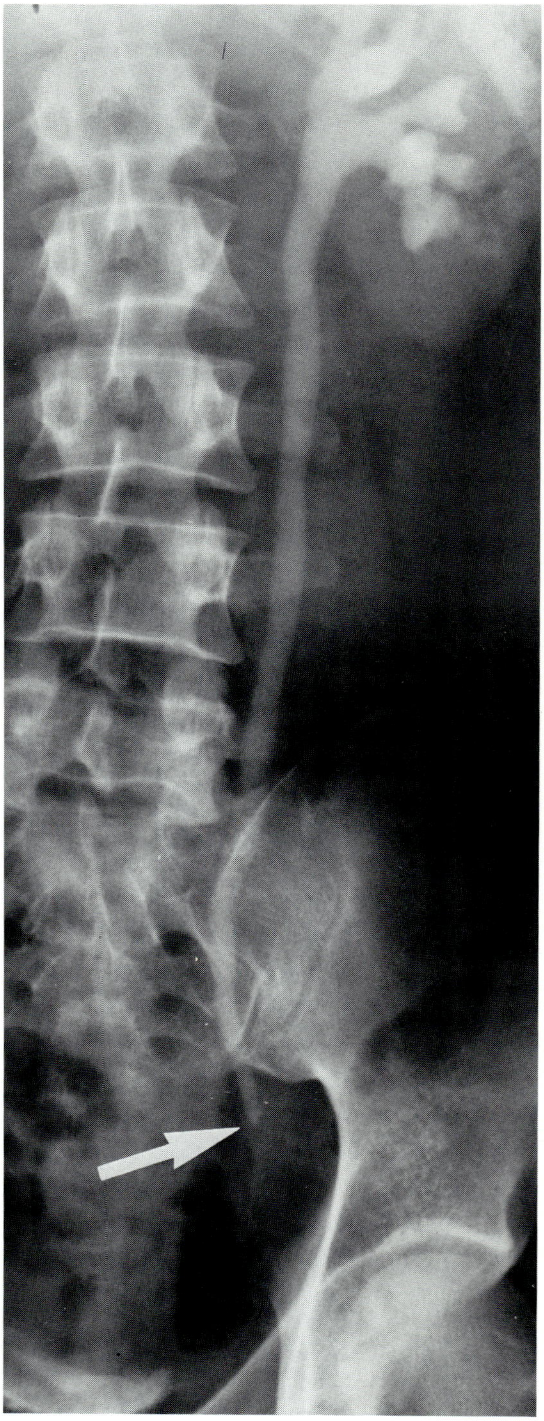

Figure 16-4. Partial left ureteral obstruction. Intravenous urography shows a stone that has lodged in the left distal ureter just inside the pelvic brim (arrow). The ureter is distended and columned down to the point of the obstruction; the collecting system is slightly dilated.

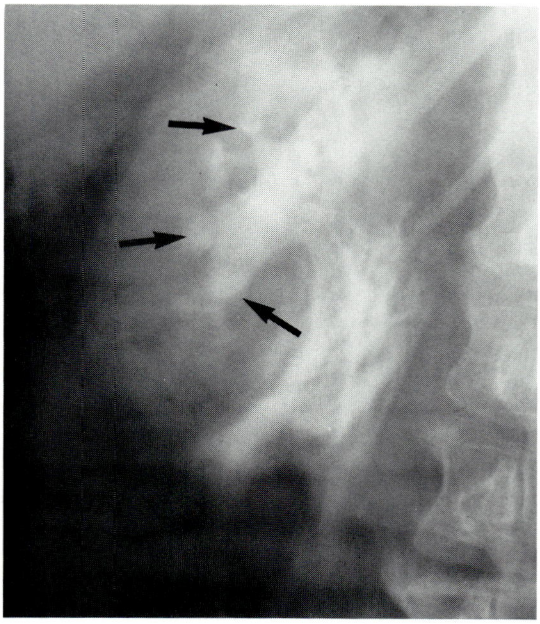

Figure 16-5. Urinary extravasation from acute ureteral obstruction. The collecting system (arrows) is only minimally distended with contrast medium in this intravenous urogram. All of the rest of the contrast agent has escaped through a forniceal rupture and is dissecting through the renal hilus into the perinephric space.

the perinephric space. Dilation of the collecting system and ureter may also be seen, of course; details of forniceal dilation—which may be the only reliable imaging finding in cases of mild obstruction—are difficult to evaluate with CT, however.

RADIONUCLIDE STUDIES

If a compound is used for imaging whose pharmacodynamics are the same as radiographic contrast agents—such as technetium DTPA—the changes in distribution of contrast material demonstrated at urography and CT may also be seen with urinary tract scintigraphy: Activity in the parenchyma may rise at a slower rate [20, 30] than in the normal side and may reach a peak that is lower than, about the same as, or considerably greater than normal; the peak concentration of isotope in the parenchyma persists as the scintigraphic equivalent of the obstructive nephrogram. Isotope concentrates in the collecting system more slowly than in the normal side; the ultimate amount seen in the collecting system may be less than, about the same as, or greater than normal, depending on the degree of distention of the system and amount of concentration of isotope. The leading edge of collecting-system activity will proceed down the ureter at a slower rate than on the normal side and will require a longer time to wash out than normal [34]. Any significant degree of urine leakage from the fornix will be demonstrated by isotope activity seen in the perinephric space.

ULTRASONOGRAPHY

The hallmark of acute ureteral obstruction seen on ultrasonography is dilation of the collecting system (Fig. 16-6). As we have seen, the collecting system usually does not undergo massive distention with acute obstruction—at least if the kidneys were previously normal—so that the size of echo-free regions [39] that split the normal echogenic renal sinus complex may not be great. Indeed, there may be overlap between the degree of pyelocaliceal distention seen in some perfectly normal patients and that seen in some patients with unquestionable obstruction whose collecting systems were originally diminutive [9].When mild distention of the intrarenal collecting system is seen on ultrasonography in patients who are not thought to be at risk for ureteral obstruction, the finding is usually an anatomic variant; when the same degree of collecting-system distention is seen in patients whose clinical picture suggests obstruction, it usually means that obstruction is indeed present

Figure 16-6. Mild ureteral obstruction. Sonography shows the dilated calices as round, echo-poor regions (arrows) in the renal sinus.

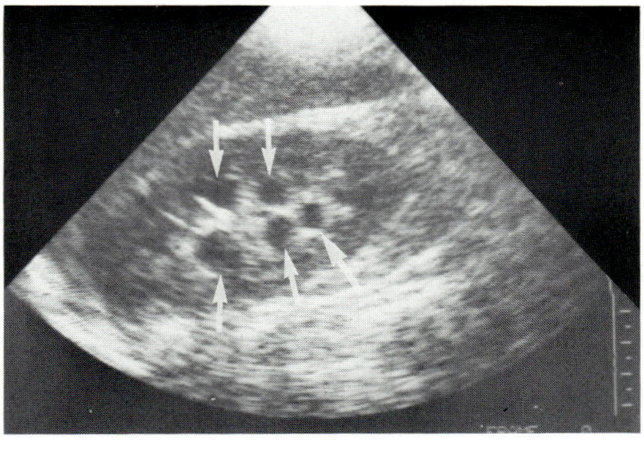

[16]. Doppler ultrasonography may reveal elevated renal vascular resistance in obstructed kidneys [32].

MRI

Acute ureteral obstruction has not been shown to produce unequivocal abnormalities in MRI of the renal parenchyma. Mild pyelocaliceal and ureteral distention may be visualized [18].

IMAGING OF CHRONIC OBSTRUCTION

PLAIN FILMS

If chronic obstruction has produced severe hydronephrotic enlargement of a kidney, the organ may be visible on plain film as a soft-tissue mass in the renal fossa [11]. As in cases of acute obstruction, the plain film may visualize stone disease.

UROGRAPHY

The obstructive nephrogram is not seen in cases of chronic obstruction (although it may appear if acute severe obstruction is superimposed upon a chronic milder obstruction). The dynamics of the nephrogram are either normal or show a diminished peak density [38]. The nephrogram defines the morphology of the parenchyma: As hydronephrotic atrophy destroys the medulla, this portion of the parenchyma disappears. As mentioned previously, the outer dimensions of the kidney may increase as the parenchymal thickness diminishes; severe hydronephrosis may leave the kidney's only remaining parenchyma as a layer a few millimeters thick, which then appears as a faintly opacified rim on urography (Fig. 16-7).

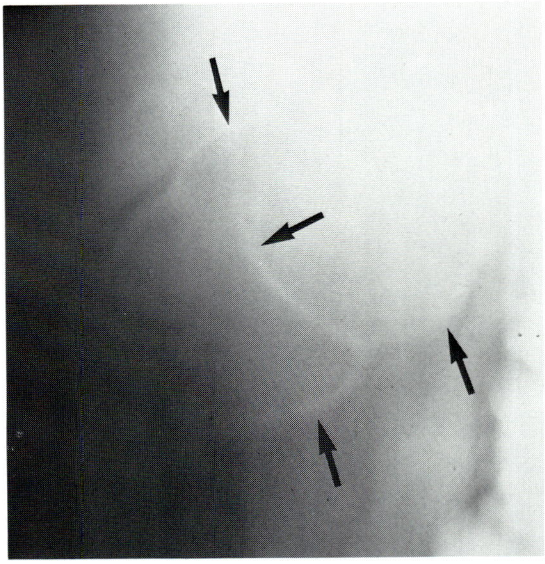

Figure 16-7. Severe hydronephrosis. The collecting system has been so expanded by chronic obstruction that the kidney has only a thin shell of parenchyma, which appears in this nephrotomogram as a series of faintly opacified rims (arrows).

Chronic obstruction produces various degrees of pyelocaliceal dilation [8, 10], which may be severe. During the nephrographic phase, no contrast material may have entered caliceal urine [37], so that the dilated calices are outlined by the opacified remaining parenchyma and form a "negative pyelogram" [4] (Fig. 16-8). The large volume of these calices, combined with oliguria, causes opacification of the calices to take a long time. Occasionally, contrast material forms thin rings or crescents [19] at the interface of the calix and parenchyma (Fig. 16-9); these are called Dunbar's Crescents. Further opacification of the collecting system is slow, and contrast material progresses down the dilated ureter much more slowly than on the normal side. In long-term stable obstruction, pyelosinus extravasation of contrast agent is not seen, but severe obstruction that persists may begin with urine extravasation, which if voluminous may persist as an encapsulated

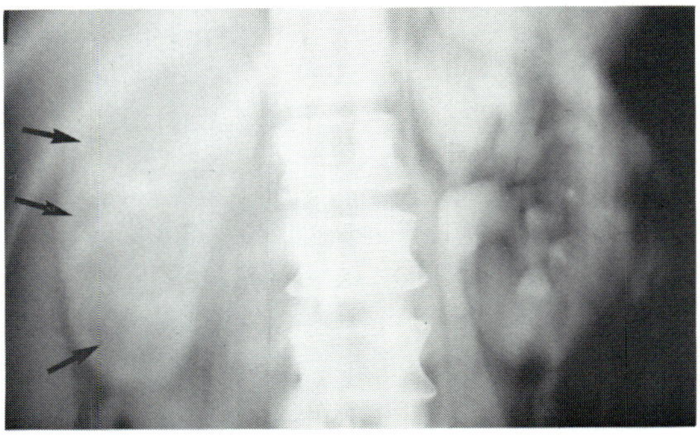

Figure 16-8. Bilateral chronic ureteral obstruction; intravenous urogram. The right kidney is severely oliguric; although the nephrogram has appeared, the dilated calices appear as a "negative pyelogram" (arrows). There is mild hydronephrosis on the left with diminished concentration of contrast in the calices.

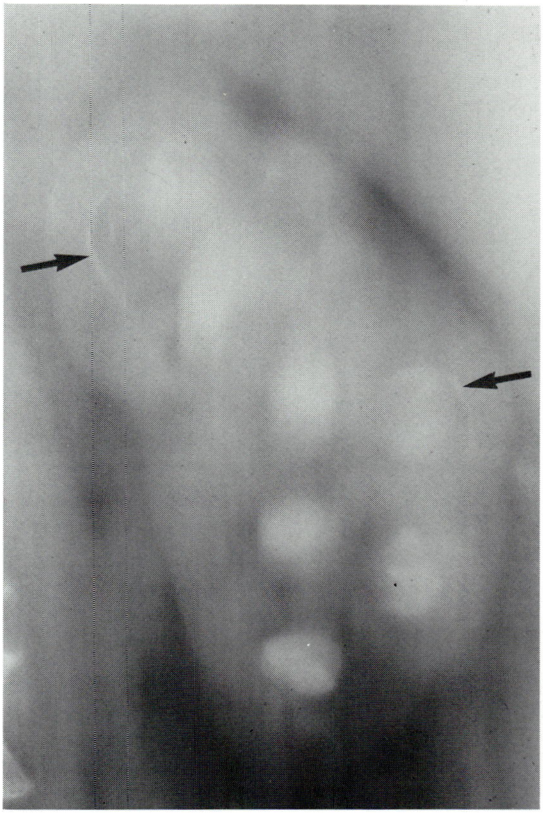

Figure 16-9. Chronic left ureteral obstruction. In addition to the dilated calices, this nephrotomogram shows caliceal crescents (arrows); these will disappear when the collecting system fills entirely with contrast material.

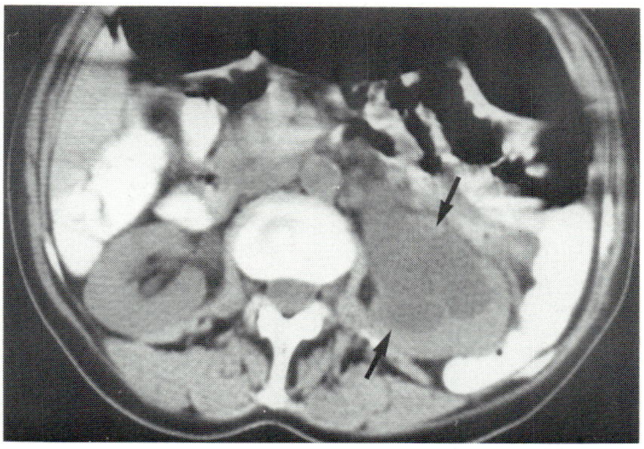

Figure 16-10. Left hydronephrosis. In this CT without contrast medium the left renal pelvis and calices are seen to be dilated (arrows). The parenchyma of the left kidney is mildly thinned when compared to the normal right kidney.

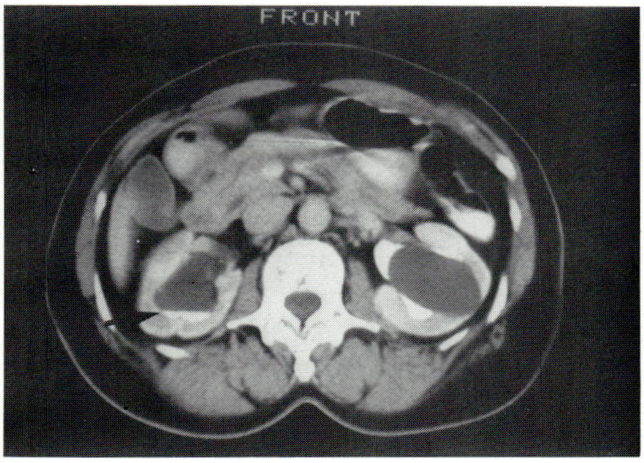

Figure 16-11. Right hydronephrosis; CT with contrast. Contrast medium is layering in the dependent portions of the right collecting system (arrow); most of the urine in the right kidney is not yet opacified. The lucency in the center of the left kidney is a parapelvic cyst; the calices are distorted but well opacified.

urinoma [21] adjacent to the kidney. Kidneys whose collecting systems fill very slowly because of chronic obstruction also display prolonged washout of contrast material from the collecting system.

RETROGRADE URETEROPYELOGRAPHY

Retrograde pyelography demonstrates the morphology of the dilated collecting system and ureter; as with acute obstruction, increased volume and oliguria may produce delayed washout of contrast material introduced by retrograde injection [25].

CT

CT reflects the same findings visualized at urography. The overall renal dimensions may be abnormal; varying degrees of renal parenchymal thinning and caliceal and pelvic dilation may be seen (Fig. 16-10). As with urography, the obstructive nephrogram seen with acute ureteral occlusion is not demonstrated with chronic obstruction. Since most CT is done in transverse planes with the patient lying supine, the calices may be shown by CT to opacify from posterior to anterior (Fig. 16-11), because urine laden with contrast material is heavier than urine without contrast material and there is no active mixing.

RADIONUCLIDE STUDIES

As in cases of acute obstruction, radionuclide examinations in chronic obstruction [15] display findings similar to those seen on urography or CT as long as a compound is used that is handled via the kidneys in the same way as contrast material (i.e., DTPA). The uptake of activity in the renal parenchyma may be slowed; its peak may be somewhat delayed as compared with the normal kidney, but the intensity of isotope in the parenchyma never reaches the intensity seen with an acute obstructive nephrogram. Activity appears within the collecting system more slowly than on the normal side; by virtue of its increased size, however, the total amount of activity in the collecting system may, at its peak, be considerably greater than that ever seen on the normal side (Fig. 16-12A). Washout of isotope from the collecting system is prolonged, and progress of the leading edge of isotope down the ureter may be slow.

In hydronephrotic kidneys, the rise and fall of activity levels in the collecting system may both be prolonged, and the peak activity may be prolonged as well; these findings may be encountered whether the hydronephrosis is either produced by ongoing obstruction or by a previous episode of obstruction not accompanied by current obstruction. In order to distinguish these two conditions, a diuretic may be administered (usually furosemide, 40 mg intravenously) when a large amount of isotope has accumulated within the affected collecting system [29]. If the isotope washes out very rapidly after a diuretic is administered, the system is said not to be obstructed (Fig. 16-12B); if the isotope in the collecting system remains at a high level or even increases in amount, ureteral obstruction is presumed to be present.

There are, of course, intermediate cases, in which very slow washout of contrast material after diuretic administration produces an intermediate pattern of the time–activity curve, so that the presence or absence of obstruction cannot be determined.

Diuretic-assisted scintigraphy rests on the proposition that nonobstructed kidneys respond to the drug with diuresis, whereas partially-obstructed kidneys cannot. Clearly, this is not always the case; a severely damaged but nonobstructed kidney may not be able to increase

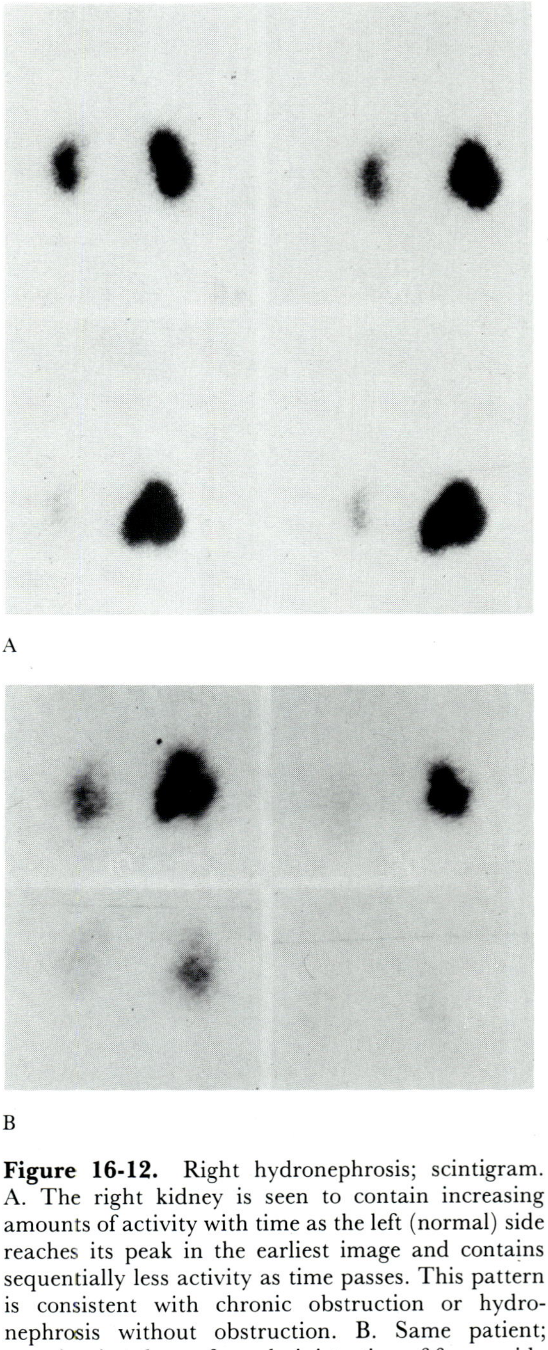

A

B

Figure 16-12. Right hydronephrosis; scintigram. A. The right kidney is seen to contain increasing amounts of activity with time as the left (normal) side reaches its peak in the earliest image and contains sequentially less activity as time passes. This pattern is consistent with chronic obstruction or hydronephrosis without obstruction. B. Same patient; examination done after administration of furosemide (Lasix). Note that the abnormal kidney contains less and less isotope after the diuretic is administered. This finding is consistent with nonobstructive hydronephrosis.

its urine flow even when a strong diuretic is administered, and some mildly obstructed kidneys may respond with considerable diuresis. The test is therefore not always accurate in distinguishing obstructed from nonobstructed dilated systems [33], but it remains in common use, primarily because of its noninvasiveness.

Nuclear medicine studies are also useful in obstructive disease in conditions in which a severely hydronephrotic kidney may be resected or may have its obstructing lesion repaired. Measures of the accumulation of isotope within the two kidneys provides an estimate of the fraction of total renal function contributed by each one. When such surgical decisions need to be made, a better, if more time-consuming, procedure is to treat the obstruction temporarily with a percutaneous nephrostomy tube; after a week or more of relief, the obstructed kidney may have regained most of the function it could hope to acquire after surgical relief of obstruction, so that radioisotope estimates of fractional renal function may be more accurate. CT, ultrasonography, and nephrotomography may all contribute to this decision as well. Each of these studies is able to provide an estimate of the volume of remaining parenchyma, which provides at least a qualitative estimate of the maximum amount of function the affected kidney can be hoped to have.

ULTRASONOGRAPHY

The ultrasound manifestations of chronic ureteral obstruction consist of demonstration of the dilated renal pelvis and calices as echo-free fluid-containing regions within the renal sinus (Fig. 16-13). A reasonable estimate of remaining parenchymal thickness can usually be made; if the hydronephrosis is moderate or severe, medullary destruction usually makes it impossible to demonstrate separate medullary pyramids by ultrasonography. Occasionally, chronically obstructed renal parenchyma may be more echogenic than normal cortex. There are limitations in the ultrasonographic evaluation of hydronephrosis: Peripelvic cysts [1] may not be distinguishable from dilated calices and obstructed calices may not be distinguishable from residual hydronephrosis in patients whose obstruction has been relieved.

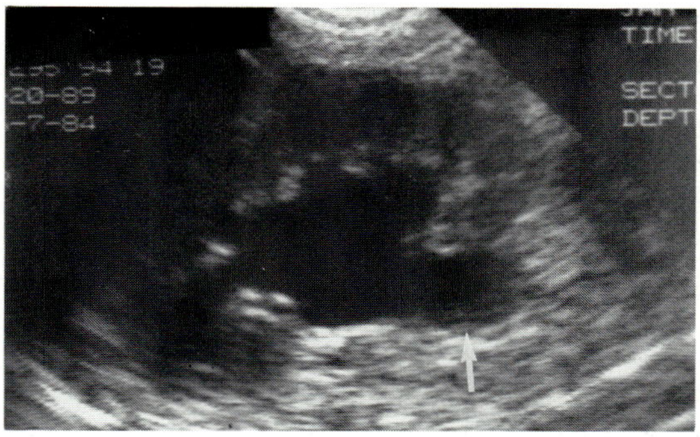

Figure 16-13. Moderate chronic obstruction. Sonography shows the dilated collecting system as an echo-free region in the center of the kidney; part of the dilated left ureter (arrow) can also be seen.

MRI

Chronically obstructed kidneys may be demonstrated by MRI so that their morphologic characteristics become clear. The corticomedullary distinction usually demonstrable on T1 weighted images may disappear, since the medulla is often destroyed. The dilated calices are seen as low-signal-intensity regions on T1 weighted images and bright regions on T2 weighted images.

WHITAKER TEST

The technique for performing the Whitaker test has been described in Chap. 3; it is useful in patients with dilated upper tracts in whom it is not clear whether ureteral obstruction is present [41]. In brief, the test permits exact measurement of the resistance to flow of fluid along a ureter. The study calculates resistance by measuring the pressure in the renal pelvis and the pressure in the bladder as the ureter is being perfused with fluid in an antegrade fashion at a rate of 10 ml per minute (Fig. 16-14). Experience with normal and abnormal ureters shows that with perfusion pressures (renal pelvis pressure minus bladder pressure) of 13 cm of water or below, no significant ureteral obstruction exists [24]; perfusion pressures above this level indicate degrees of ureteral obstruction commensurate with the pressure. The examination has the advantage of directly assessing ureteral obstruction but is limited in that it provides no information about current or recoverable renal function, and it is invasive.

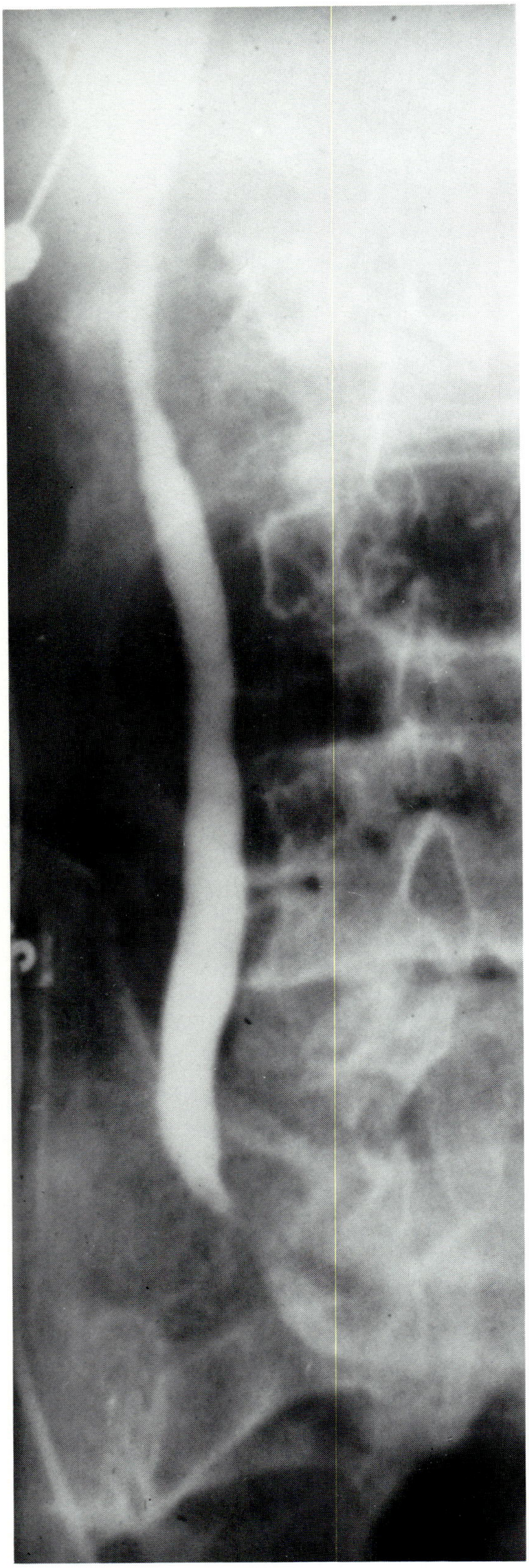

Figure 16-14. Right distal ureteral obstruction. Antegrade pyelography is being performed via the needle seen in the collecting system. A Whitaker test is being performed; as contrast medium is perfused through the needle and ureter, the pressure in the right collecting system becomes abnormally elevated, confirming obstruction.

INTERVENTIONAL THERAPY OF OBSTRUCTION

Since the development of percutaneous nephrostomy, image-guided techniques have been used for therapeutic maneuvers aimed at relieving upper urinary tract obstruction. Patients with ureteral obstruction may, of course, be treated by a variety of surgical techniques and by the placement of retrograde ureteral stents via a cystoscopic approach, but percutaneous nephrostomy drainage and its variants are useful in a large number of conditions [31].

The technique of placing a percutaneous nephrostomy catheter has been briefly outlined in Chap. 3. The establishment of a route for a percutaneous catheter permits a number of therapeutic maneuvers; although the details of percutaneous interventional techniques in the kidney are beyond the scope of this textbook, some general principles are worth reviewing.

The simple relief of obstruction by placing a percutaneous catheter and allowing the urine to drain through it may provide effective therapy in a number of situations. In patients in whom total renal function is compromised by obstruction to the point at which they become uremic, percutaneous drainage is valuable. If the obstructing lesion is a transient one or if subsequent surgery removes it, the percutaneous drainage may be relatively brief; alternatively, patients have lived for many months or longer with indwelling percutaneous nephrostomy tubes as primary therapy. Sometimes percutaneous drainage is crucial even when surgery is available; for example, when patients have obstructive pyonephrosis [43] and are severely septic, percutaneous drainage combined with antibiotic therapy may buy sufficient time so that the patient may undergo definitive surgery after uremia and generalized sepsis have been treated. Patients with infravesical obstruction usually are treated by use of transurethral catheter; however, in patients in whom the urethra cannot be catheterized, or in whom a lengthy period of urethral catheterization is not desirable, a percutaneous cystostomy tube may be placed. Although this maneuver is usually performed by urologists occasionally imaging guidance is used, and the catheter is inserted using radiologic techniques.

The percutaneous nephrostomy catheter route may be used for a number of other maneuvers as well. Although since the introduction of extracorporeal shock wave lithotripsy (ESWL) percutaneous direct stone therapy (by extraction, ultrasound disintegration, or primary dissolution) has diminished in importance, these maneuvers may continue to form a part of therapy in patients whose stones are not entirely successfully treated by ESWL. Percutaneous nephrostomy drainage that overcomes obstruction when multiple stone fragments obstruct the ureter after ESWL may also be useful.

A percutaneous nephrostomy catheter track may be used for antegrade ureteral stenting [35] or dilating as well. Under fluoroscopic guidance, the obstructed ureteral segment is traversed by a guide wire, over which a stent with multiple side holes is then passed. The final stent may be entirely indwelling (the most commonly used is a double-pigtail catheter whose ends rest in the renal pelvis and bladder), or may be one that is capped at the skin but continues to traverse the renal parenchyma and end in the bladder, or may even be one that is placed by a combined radiologic–urologic technique so that it traverses the renal parenchyma and the ureter and exits through the urethra. Such stents may be used to treat obstruction simply by keeping the ureter open, or may be used as primary therapy to dilate benign ureteral strictures (long-term results of this therapy are mixed) [2], or may be used to provide a mold around which an injured ureter may heal. Some ureteral strictures are also amenable to balloon dilation.

REFERENCES

1. Amis, E.S., et al. Ultrasonic inaccuracies in diagnosing renal obstruction. *Urology* 19:101, 1982.
2. Banner, M.P., et al. Catheter dilatation of benign ureteral strictures. *Radiology* 144:753, 1982.
3. Bigongiari, L.R., et al. Visualization of the medullary rays in excretory urography in experimental ureteric obstruction. *A.J.R.* 129:89, 1977.
4. Brown, C.B., et al. High-dose excretion urography in oliguric renal failure. *Lacet* 2:952, 1970.
5. Cremin, B.J. Urinary ascites and obstructive uropathy. *Br. J. Radiol.* 48:113, 1975.
6. Djurhuus, J.C., et al. Experimental hydronephrosis. *Acta Chir. Scand.* (Suppl. 472), 1976.
7. Elkin, M. Radiological observations in acute ureteral obstruction. *Radiology* 81:484, 1963.
8. Elkin, M. Obstructive uropathy and uremia. *Radiol. Clin. North Am.* 10:421, 1972.
9. Ellenbogen, P.H., et al. Sensitivity of gray scale ultrasound in detecting urinary tract obstruction. *A.J.R.* 130:731, 1978.
10. Emmett, J.L., Witten, D.M. Urinary stasis: The obstructive uropathies, atony, vesicoureteral reflux and neuromuscular dysfunction of the urinary tract. In J.L. Emmet and D.M. Witten (eds.), *Clinical Urography*, Philadelphia: Saunders, 1971. Pp. 369–605.
11. Griscom, N.T. The roentgenology of neonatal abdominal masses. *A.J.R.* 93:447, 1965.
12. Harris, R.H., Gill, J.M. Changes in glomerular filtration rate during complete ureteral obstruction in rats. *Kidney Int.* 19:603, 1981.
13. Hinman, F. Peripelvic extravasation during intravenous urography: Evidence for an additional route for backflow after ureteral obstruction. *Trans. Am. Assoc. Genitourin. Surg.* 52:45, 1960.
14. Hydronephrosis. *Br. Med. J.* 2:1736, 1978.
15. Joekes, A.M. Obstructive uropathy. *Semin. Nucl. Med.* 4:187, 1974.
16. Kamholtz, R.G., Cronan, J.J., and Dorfman, G.S. Obstruction and the minimally dilated renal collecting system: US evaluation. *Radiology* 170:51, 1989.
17. Korobkin, M., et al. Diminished radiopacity of contrast material: A urographic sign of ureteral calculus. *A.J.R.* 131:847, 1978.
18. Kressel, H.Y., et al. NMR imaging of the abdomen at 0.12T: Initial clinical experience with a resistive magnet. *A.J.R.* 141:1179, 1983.
19. Levine, M., et al. The crescent sign. *Radiology* 81:971, 1963.
20. Lundstam, S., et al. Acute radiorenography during attacks of renal colic. *J. Urol.* 130:855, 1983.
21. McInerny, D., Jones, A., Roylance, J. Urinoma. *Clin. Radiol.* 28:345, 1977.
22. Michaelson, G. Percutaneous puncture of the renal pelvis, intrapelvic pressure and the concentrating capacity of the kidney in hydronephrosis. *Acta Med. Scand.* (Suppl 559), 1974.
23. Newhouse, J.H., Pfister, R.C. The nephrogram. *Radiol. Clin. North Am.* 17:213, 1979.
24. Newhouse, J.H., et al. The Whitaker test following successful pyelopasty: Establishment of normal ureteral perfusion values *A.J.R.* 137:223, 1981.

25. Newhouse, J.H., Amis, E.S., Pfister, R.C. Urinary obstruction: Pitfalls in the use of delayed contrast material washout for diagnosis. *Radiology* 152:319, 1984.
26. Newhouse, J.H. Acute and chronic upper urinary tract obstruction. In J. Taveras and J. Ferrucci (eds.), *Radiology: Diagnosis-Imaging-Intervention.* Philadelphia: Lippincott, 1989, Pp. 1–11.
27. Olbrich, O., et al. Renal function in prostatism. *Lancet* 1:1322, 1957.
28. Olsson, O. Frequency of backflow in acute renal colic. *Acta Radiol. Diag.* 12:469, 1972.
29. O'Reilly, P.H., et al. Diuresis renography in equivocal urinary tract obstruction *Br. J. Urol.* 50:76, 1980.
30. O'Reilly, P.H. Obstructive uropathy. In A.M. Joekes et al. (Eds.), *Radionuclides in Nephrology.* New York: Grune & Stratton, 1982.
31. Pfister, R.C., and Newhouse, J.H. Interventional percutaneous pyeloureteral techniques. II. Percutaneous nephrostomy and other procedures. *Radiol. Clin. North Am.* 17:351, 1979.
32. Platt, J.F., et al. Duplex Doppler US of the kidney: Differentiation of obstructive from nonobstructive dilatation. *Radiology* 171:515, 1989.
33. Poulsen, E.U., et al. Diuresis renography and simultaneous renal pelvic pressure in hydronephrosis. *J. Urol.* 138:272, 1987.
34. Powers, T.A., et al. Detection of obstructive uropathy using 99m technetium DTPA. *J. Urol.* 124:588, 1980.
35. Reznek, R.H., Talner, L.B. Percutaneous nephrostomy. *Radiol. Clin. North Am.* 22:393, 1984.
36. Robbins, S.L. *Textbook of Pathology with Clinical Application.* Philadelphia: Saunders, 1962, P. 819.
37. Siegel, N.J., et al. Renal cortical blood flow distribution in obstructive nephropathy in rats. *Circ. Res.* 40:379, 1977.
38. Talner, L.B. Urographic contrast media in uremia. *Radiol. Clin. North Am.* 10:421, 1972.
39. Taylor, K.J.W., Kraus, V. Grey-scale ultrasound imaging: Assessment of acute hydronephrosis. *Br. J. Urol.* 47:593, 1975.
40. Tscholl, R., Keller, U., and Spreng, P. Investigation of urine transport in the ureter of the pig by x-ray video densitometry. *Invest. Urol.* 13:410, 1976.
41. Whitaker, R.H. Methods of assessing obstruction in dilated ureters. *Br. J. Urol.* 45:15, 1973.
42. Yarger, W.E., and Griffith, W. Intrarenal hemodynamics following chronic unilateral ureteral obstruction in the dog. *Am. J. Physiol.* 227:816, 1974.
43. Yoder, I.C., Lindfors, K.K., and Pfister, R.C. Diagnosis and treatment of pyonephrosis. *Radiol. Clin. North Am.* 22:407, 1984.

Vesicoureteral Reflux

PATHOPHYSIOLOGY OF REFLUX

The normal ureterovesical junction acts as a one-way valve that prevents the flow of urine from the bladder into the ureter. This valve mechanism depends on the structure of the ureterovesical junction. As the distal ureter courses inferiorly it traverses the muscular bladder wall at an oblique angle; the musculatures of the ureter and the bladder wall are not separated by any discrete plane. The ureter then continues to travel medially and anteriorly in the space just deep to the transitional epithelium of the bladder and finally opens into the bladder lumen at the end of this subepithelial tunnel (Fig. 17-1A). The valve mechanism is effective because the pressure of urine in the bladder lumen compresses the epithelium overlying the most distal ureter, thus occluding the ureteral orifice, and also because the portion of the ureter that traverses the bladder-wall musculature is kept occluded except when a bolus of urine is being actively propelled through it.

In infants, the bladder wall is thinner than it is in adults, and the subepithelial course of the ureter is shorter. In infancy, therefore, less deviation from the normal anatomy is required for the valve mechanism to become faulty and for reflux to occur (Fig. 17-1B). As the infant grows, the maturing ureterovesical junction comes closer to its normal adult anatomic configuration [43], so that there is a tendency for vesicoureteral reflux to resolve spontaneously with increasing age [34].

Vesicoureteral reflux may be primary or secondary. Primary reflux is that resulting from an isolated abnormality of the ureterovesical junction that is neither acquired nor due to a predisposing condition. It is both congenital and familial [5, 50]. As mentioned above, it has a tendency to resolve with increasing age and is seen much more frequently in parents, offspring, and siblings of patients with reflux than in the general population. Although reflux is more commonly unilateral than bilateral, it occurs bilaterally more frequently than would be accounted for by chance alone.

The prevalence of vesicoureteral reflux in a general pediatric population is not known; since the tests for diagnosing it are all invasive to some degree, they have not been applied to an unselected group. Urinary tract infection is the most common reason for screening for reflux. A number of studies of infected children have been done; these have found reflux of some degree in up to half of the tested patients [4, 35].

Vesicoureteral reflux may also be associated with a number of diseases that, directly or indirectly, affect the anatomy of the ureterovesical junction. A bladder diverticulum [1] near the ureterovesical junction (a periureteral diverticulum) may cause reflux (Fig. 17-2). Male infants with bladder outlet obstruction from posterior uretheral valves have a higher incidence of reflux than do otherwise normal children (although the bladder outlet obstruction seen in men with prostatism does not seem to be associated with a particularly high incidence of reflux). Inflammatory processes such as schistosomiasis or tuberculosis, which may markedly alter the pliability and anatomy of the bladder wall, may be associated with acquired reflux. Bladders with a variety of neurogenic dysfunctional states may ultimately be associated with reflux. Ureteral duplication anomalies are often associated with reflux, as are other congenital urinary tract abnormalities, especially imperforate anus [39]. Apparently, the continuous peristalsis of normal amount of urine through the ureterovesical junction is required to maintain the effectiveness of the valve; reflux may develop in ureters whose kidneys have been resected or are chronically anuric. Finally, surgery that involves the ureterovesical junction may produce reflux. Renal transplantation using a transplanted ureter and resection of periureteral bladder tumors [15] are examples of techniques that may produce reflux. In both primary and acquired reflux, partial obstruction at the

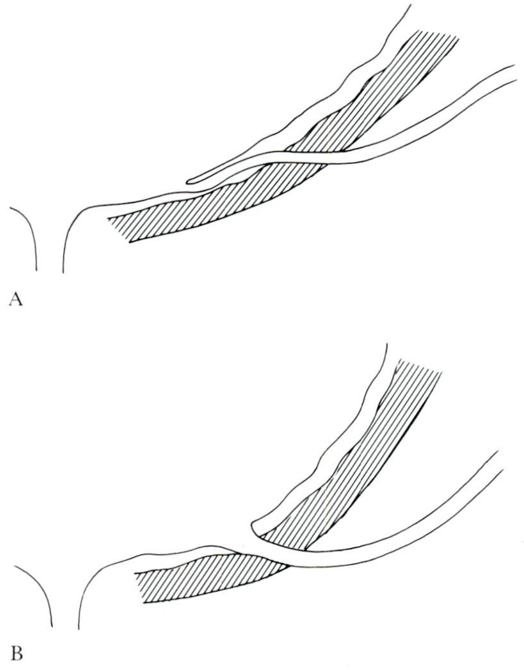

Figure 17-1. Diagram of ureterovesical junction. A. Normal—The ureter traverses the muscle wall (shaded) at an angle and courses submucosally before emerging at the orifice. This anatomy functions as a competent valve. B. Refluxing—There is no submucosal ureteral course; vesicoureteral reflux occurs.

ureterovesical junction may coexist with the reflux but is unusual.

Vesicoureteral reflux may produce secondary changes in the urinary tract anywhere from the peripheral renal cortex to the urethra. If the reflux is intermittent and very mild (when, for example, only a milliliter or two of urine transiently passes into the distal ureter) these changes may be negligible. But if the reflux is severe, the anatomic, physiologic, and pathologic changes may be considerable.

With high-volume reflux, the bladder may become enlarged. The detrusor contraction occurring with each voiding causes most of the bladder urine to reflux into the ureter rather than traverse the urethra. Within a minute or so after voiding, the dilated ureter refills the bladder with urine, and the additional urine produced by the kidneys prior to the next voiding distends the bladder even more.

The ureter may undergo various degrees of dilation when chronic reflux occurs. When the

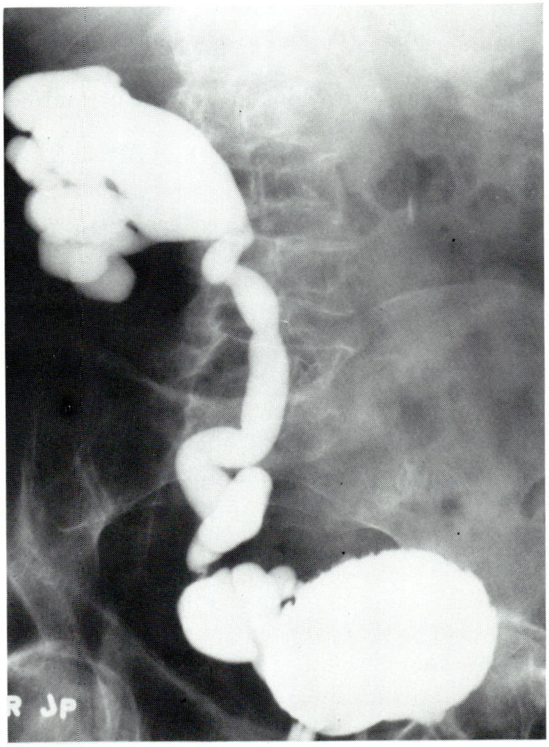

Figure 17-2. Bladder diverticulum with reflux. Cystography reveals a right-sided bladder diverticulum into which the right ureter empties. Contrast agent flows from the bladder through the diverticulum into the ureter and collecting system. This is not a periureteral diverticulum, which would exist adjacent to, but would not include, the ureterovesical junction.

bladder contracts, a retrograde wave of urine travels up the ureteral lumen; the considerable pressure and volume of this urine wave stretches the relaxed ureteral musculature well beyond any state that occurs in the normal ureter. Its muscular wall thins and stretches; this increases both the diameter and the length of the ureter so that the ureter ultimately becomes flaccid, dilated, and tortuous; its peristaltic contraction waves may no longer coapt the ureteral walls. Between bladder contractions the ureteral lumen is constantly exposed to urine whose pressure is equal to that within the bladder, and although the resting pressure of the bladder is usually low, as the bladder reaches maximum distention, pressure within it begins to rise, as does that within the ureter. Finally, as previously mentioned, reflux may coexist with bladder outlet obstruction, and in some patients the partially obstructed bladder wall becomes thickened and noncompliant, so that the resting pressure within it begins to rise, the pressure to which the ureter is subjected rises concomitantly, and the ureteral dilation becomes worse. In the most severe cases of vesicoureteral reflux, the ureteral dilation may be massive. In patients with severe reflux, there may be considerable dilation of both the ureters and the bladder by the mechanisms outlined above. In pediatric patients this is sometimes called the megaureter–megacystis syndrome; in the past it was ascribed to bladder outlet obstruction, and although it certainly may be associated with posterior urethral valves in some patients, severe vesicoureteral reflux may produce it without any bladder outlet obstruction at all.

Before discussing the effect of vesicoureteral reflux on the kidney, the relationship between reflux and urinary tract infection should be reviewed. Although reflux does not cause urinary infection per se [18], and although patients with reflux probably do not have episodes of bacterial inoculation of the urinary tract any more often than people without reflux, there is certainly a correlation between reflux and urinary infection.

Patients with significant reflux have their bladders partially filled with urine draining from the ureters immediately after voiding; for all practical purposes, they have a nearly immediate postvoid residual. Under normal circumstances, the urothelium of the bladder is bactericidal. However, since the bladder does not secrete any bacteriostatic or bacteriotoxic materials into the urine, the bactericidal capacities of the bladder wall can sterilize the bladder only if the bladder is completely emptied at each voiding so that the tiny amount of urine remaining in it comes into close contact with the urothelium; the bladder is then filled by sterile urine from normal ureters. Clearly, this mechanism cannot operate if large amounts of infected urine are propelled from the bladder into the ureter with every bladder contraction.

Another normal mechanism for clearing the urinary tract of bacteria, which is interfered with by reflux, is ureteral peristalsis. Normally, a ureteral contraction wave propels urine inferiorly much faster than bacteria can move superiorly, and the contraction wave completely removes urine from the contracted portion of the ureter. As sterile urine is formed in the kidneys, bacteria in the upper tract are simply washed away faster than they can reproduce. But with moderate or high-grade reflux, retrograde flow of boluses of infected urine from the bladder into the ureter clearly interfere with this mechanism. Finally, it has been suggested that when infected urine is forced into the renal parenchyma by high-pressure reflux, bacteria may reproduce within the renal parenchyma, thus converting a case of simple pyelitis to one of pyelonephritis, which may be harder for natural mechanisms to eradicate.

The association of urinary infection with vesicoureteral reflux produces the symptoms that cause patients to be subjected to radiologic workup. In adults, and in children who are old enough to describe symptoms accurately, the urinary infection may be easy to suspect: Flank pain, fever, and dysuria may all appear. But in infants, urinary infection may produce much more protean effects: Fever or failure to thrive may be nonspecific indicators of urinary infection; occasionally, foul-smelling urine may be noted.

The clinical diagnosis of vesicoureteral reflux is complicated by the fact that urinary infection may be asymptomatic or transient. Patients may have no clinical sequelae of vesicoureteral reflux at all until reflux nephropathy makes itself known by producing renal failure or hypertension.

REFLUX NEPHROPATHY

Mild reflux may have no effect at all on the morphology and function of the kidney; at the other extreme, reflux may produce severe renal parenchymal damage, chronic renal failure, proteinuria, loss of concentrating capacity, and hypertension [7, 22, 29, 41, 42, 46–48, 52].

If the renal pelvis and calices are subjected to transient or sustained high urine pressure due to severe reflux, these structures may dilate. The morphology of this pyelocaliectasis may be indistinguishable from that seen in cases of ureteral obstruction. Persistent or recurrent elevated pressure in the upper urinary tract may lead at first to medullary tissue loss and then to cortical thinning, so that the kidney adopts the morphology of chronic obstruction. The functional changes of obstructive hydronephrosis also appear: Concentrating capacity is lost, and ultimately, glomerular filtration rate diminishes. If the reflux resolves spontaneously or is surgically corrected, the pyelocaliectasis usually diminishes; the degree of recovery of renal parenchyma depends on the amount of initial loss, the functional state of the contralateral kidney, and the age of the patient.

A more characteristic form of reflux nephropathy is that of focal renal parenchymal scarring with associated caliectasis. These lesions are thought to be due to intrarenal reflux [40]. It has been observed when performing voiding cystourethrography in patients with severe reflux that opacified urine may travel not only from the bladder to the calices but retrograde from the calices into the renal tubules as far peripherally as the renal capsule. This intrarenal reflux does not occur uniformly throughout the renal parenchyma; it tends to occur in the polar regions [16], where multiple fused papillae [19] are frequently found supplying one calix (compound calix); in these papillae, the orifices of the ends of the renal collecting ducts are shaped differently from the orifices in simple papillae and are more likely to allow intrarenal reflux. When repeated bouts of intrarenal reflux occur, they tend to affect the same segments of the kidney. Intrarenal reflux has been shown to produce a local diminution in renal blood flow [49]; this, together with an inflammatory response caused by intrarenal reflux with infected urine, ultimately causes the affected renal segment to form a scar. Documentation of the serial histopathologic changes that occur during scar formation is lacking, but the mature lesion is well characterized [2, 10]. In it, there is complete or nearly complete destruction of the tubules and most of the glomeruli; the affected tissue shrinks and develops primarily fibrous and collagenous tissue that, by the time of ultimate pathologic examination, contains little or no evidence of inflammation. Retraction of the scarred tissue produces an indentation in the external surface of the kidney and an eversion of the normal papillary contour, so each scar is associated with a dilated or blunted calix. These calices are often described as "clubbed" in appearance. The parenchymal scars may be single or multiple and may appear unilaterally or bilaterally. If there has been sufficient loss of renal substance, the remaining renal parenchyma undergoes compensatory hypertrophy [8]. This hypertrophy simply enlarges the entirety of the kidney if the scars are all in the contralateral organ; if compensatory hypertrophy occurs in the scarred kidney, the unscarred enlarging portions may mimic masses.

If the reflux that has caused the scars resolves or is corrected, dilation of the ureter, pelvis, and calices may resolve as well. The degree of caliceal dilation caused by papillary destruction does not revert to normal, however, so that the calices affected remain permanently clubbed.

The natural history of reflux nephropathy depends, of course, on that of the reflux itself [14]. As we have seen, primary reflux is most prevalent and tends to be most severe in the newborn; it tends to diminish in severity and prevalence with increasing age. Experimental evidence also suggests that immature kidneys are more prone to intrarenal reflux at a given caliceal pressure than are mature kidneys; the combination of these factors causes most renal damage in cases of intrarenal reflux to take place during infancy. Cases of new scars, or progression of preexisting scars, in late childhood or adulthood are very unusual in cases of primary reflux. If severe secondary reflux is acquired later in life, of course, reflux nephropathy may appear after the onset of reflux.

The natural history of reflux nephropathy [23, 28, 45, 51] is not simple, however, even in cases of congenital primary reflux. A baby may acquire renal scars and undergo compensatory hypertrophy of the remaining renal parenchyma and remain healthy for a number of years, but the compensatory hypertrophy may have exhausted the patient's renal growth reserve; when the child approaches adulthood, the total renal volume may not be sufficient to prevent some degree of renal failure, even though the scarring took place many years earlier. Also, in cases of severe renal scarring, the remaining functional parenchyma may undergo the sort of functional impairment that is seen in virtually all diseases in which there is moderate to severe persistent chronic renal failure: Proteinuria and glomerulosclerosis [11] may appear and progress, with inexorable slow progression of the renal failure many years after the scars have stabilized. In a few cases, systemic hypertension appears; in some of the hypertensive patients the renin–angiotensin system has been implicated both by renal vein renin measurements and by noting the effect of resection of the severely scarred kidney. Finally, upper tract stones may form in a small number of patients with reflux nephropathy.

In most patients, it appears necessary for moderate to severe vesicoureteral reflux and urinary infection to coexist if scars are to form [14, 17]. It is much less clear whether reflux can produce renal scarring in patients who have had no infections, if for no other reason than that it is very difficult to prove that a patient with reflux and scarred kidneys never had urinary infection, even though he or she may not be infected at the time of workup.

It is beyond the scope of this book to discuss in detail the therapy of vesicoureteral reflux. Certainly, all practitioners would concur that careful monitoring of the urine for infection is appropriate, with prompt treatment of any infection or continuous antibiotic suppression of urinary infection or both. The role of surgery is less clear [12]. There are practitioners who claim that sterilizing the urine is sufficient and that surgery neither halts the progression of scars [13, 53] nor improves renal function. Most clinicians agree that surgical correction of vesicoureteral reflux by any of the commonly used methods of ureteroneocystostomy at least prevents cases of bacterial cystitis from progressing to upper tract infection [13]; in addition, some studies suggest that certain patients who undergo ureteral implantation may also display a consequent improvement in function of the treated kidney [20]. Other studies [26] do not confirm this, however, and the exact role of surgery remains controversial.

RADIOLOGY OF VESICOURETERAL REFLUX AND REFLUX NEPHROPATHY

Prior to discussing the actual findings on specific examinations, the issue of whom to screen with any imaging method needs to be decided [31, 32]. In children, urinary infection usually prompt radiologic screening, and a large literature discusses the issue of how many urinary infections a given child should be allowed to have before screening is instituted [44]. In very young infants, most authors agree that the first urinary infection should prompt screening, especially in males, in whom posterior ureteral valves are sufficiently frequent and dangerous that their diagnosis should not be postponed. In young girls past their second birthday, urinary infections occur sufficiently often that some authors have suggested that two or even three infections should be permitted before instituting screening; however, many suggest that in this group a single urinary infection should prompt screening, and we concur. Many studies have shown that as many as half of all children so screened will display abnormalities. Screening in young women with urinary tract infection has yielded many fewer positive examinations, and most of the abnormal patients do not have reflux or reflux nephropathy.

Screening examinations such as radiographic, fluoroscopic, or radionuclide cystography [21] are necessary to demonstrate reflux. Radionuclide cystography has the advantages of a lower radiation dose and a higher sensitivity [6, 9] for reflux than fluoroscopic or radiographic cystography; however, the radiographic and fluoroscopic studies have a greater capacity to reveal urethral abnormalities and subtle abnormalities elsewhere in the urinary tract than do the radionuclide examinations. Reflux nephropathy is best shown by high-quality intravenous urography, although radionuclide renal scintigraphy, ultrasonography, and CT have all been reported to show the abnormalities of reflux nephropathy.

Some authors suggest that urography should be done first, on the grounds that if the examination is normal reflux is unimportant, and to miss it by omitting cystography [30] is permissible. Others suggest that certain patients with reflux who have infection and initially normal urograms may subsequently develop renal scars, so both tests should be performed. Still others [3] suggest that cystography should be performed first, claiming that normal results render it unimportant to determine whether there are renal scars; others, pointing out that patients with renal scarring may need closer follow-up and that reflux may be intermittent, suggest that urography should follow even if cystography is normal. Our own view is that patients screened for possible reflux disease should undergo both cystography and urography.

Although the techniques of performing the various examinations have been described elsewhere, there are additional worthwhile points to be made regarding screening examinations. The technique of cystography is important. First of all, cystography alone is not sufficient; all patients should have voiding cystourethrography in order to examine the urethra and because reflux may not occur during standard cystography but may be present during voiding. The patient should be awake and should void as normally as possible; an examination performed by instilling contrast medium into the bladder in a patient anesthetized for cystoscopy is not sufficient to exclude reflux. The patient should be catheterized with a catheter small enough to permit voiding around it so that the bladder may be filled several times if necessary; 5 French and 8 French pediatric feeding catheters are good choices. The examination should be performed under fluoroscopic control; not only should the presence and degree of any reflux be recorded, but the appearance of the bladder mucosa, the anatomy and functioning of the urethra, and the mechanics of micturition should be observed as well.

Radionuclide cystography should also be performed with a small catheter and on conscious patients. We feel that the examination is not sufficiently accurate in evaluation of bladder wall abnormalities or of abnormal urethras to be used as an initial test, but it may be quite useful for follow-up studies. We feel that there is insufficient evidence to date that intravenous radionuclide scintigraphy is accurate enough in the depiction of small renal scars and in the differential diagnosis of renal parenchymal loss to be used as an initial examination for reflux nephropathy.

Renal scars have been described in ultrasonographic examinations [27], but there is no evidence that ultrasonography is particularly sensitive in discovering them. The added expense of CT prohibits substituting it for urography in the investigation of patients for reflux-induced renal scarring.

Urography in children ought to be performed in such a way that the entirety of the renal outlines can be well seen. This may require multiple oblique views and maneuvers such as filling the stomach with gas in order to displace smaller intestinal air bubbles from the kidney. In adults, nephrotomography is frequently required.

FINDINGS

During fluoroscopy, vesicoureteral reflux is diagnosed by observing contrast material in either ureter after it has been instilled into the bladder. Contrast material may fill only the distal ureter or the entire ureter and collecting system. The ureter and collecting system may be normal or dilated. These findings have been codified in grading systems; unfortunately, more than one such system exists. In a common one, Grade I indicates reflux into only part of the ureter, without dilation; Grade II (Fig. 17-3) indicates reflux filling the entire ureter and collecting system, without dilation; Grade III indicates reflux filling the entire ureter and collecting system, with mild dilation (Fig. 17-4); and Grades IV and V connote complete filling of the ureter and collecting system, with moderate and severe dilation, respectively (Fig. 17-5) (Table 17-1). A practical approach for radiologists is to describe carefully the level of the upper tract to which the refluxed contrast medium flows and the degree of dilation, irrespective of the grading system. The reflux grading systems do not attempt to quantify the degree of renal scarring.

In patients with severe reflux, cystography may occasionally demonstrate intrarenal reflux. When this occurs, contrast material is seen extending from the dilated calices into the collecting tubules of the renal parenchyma (Fig. 17-6). This reflux of contrast material may appear relatively homogeneous or faintly striated, may extend to the periphery of the kidney, and is virtually always focal—that is, it involves certain parts of the parenchyma and spares others, with a predilection for the polar regions. Care must be taken, especially in infants, to distinguish intrarenal reflux from other kinds of pyelorenal backflow.

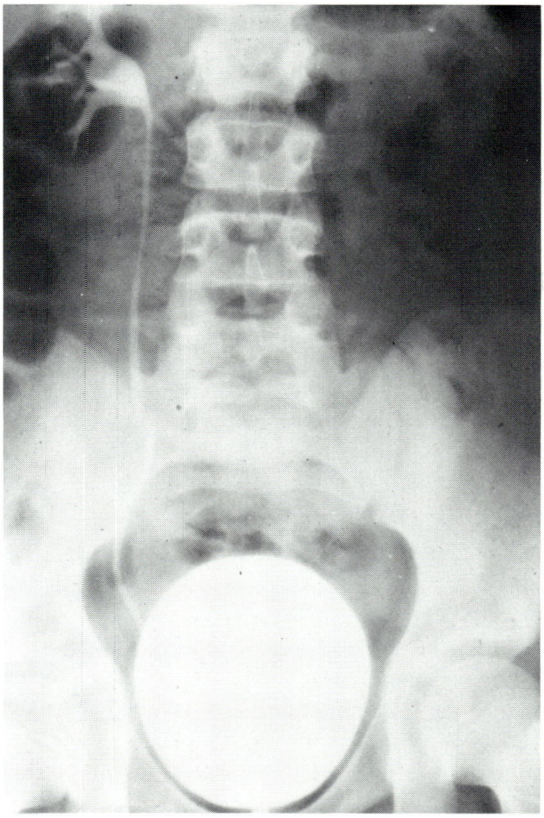

Figure 17-3. Grade II vesicoureteral reflux. In this cystogram contrast medium has flowed from the bladder into the entire ureter and collecting system but has not caused dilation. (Courtesy of Robert Cleveland, M.D., Massachusetts General Hospital, Boston, MA.)

Radionuclide scintigraphy demonstrates reflux by revealing linear streaks of radioactivity extending cephalad from the bladder in the course of the ureters and collecting systems. Specific grading systems are not commonly agreed on, but the percentage of the total radioactivity that appears in the upper tracts can be quantitated; this may be useful if serial examinations are performed in order to monitor a patient's progress.

It is important, both for radionuclide cystography and for standard contrast cystography, not to perform the examination immediately after an intravenous examination. This could lead to a misdiagnosis of reflux in patients in whom the isotope or contrast material is still being excreted by the kidneys at the time of cystography.

Table 17-1. International classification of vesicoureteral reflux

Grade I	Reflux only into ureter
Grade II	Reflux into collecting system, without dilation
Grade III	Reflux into collecting system, with mild dilation
Grade IV	Reflux into collecting system, with moderate dilation
Grade V	Reflux into collecting system, with severe dilation

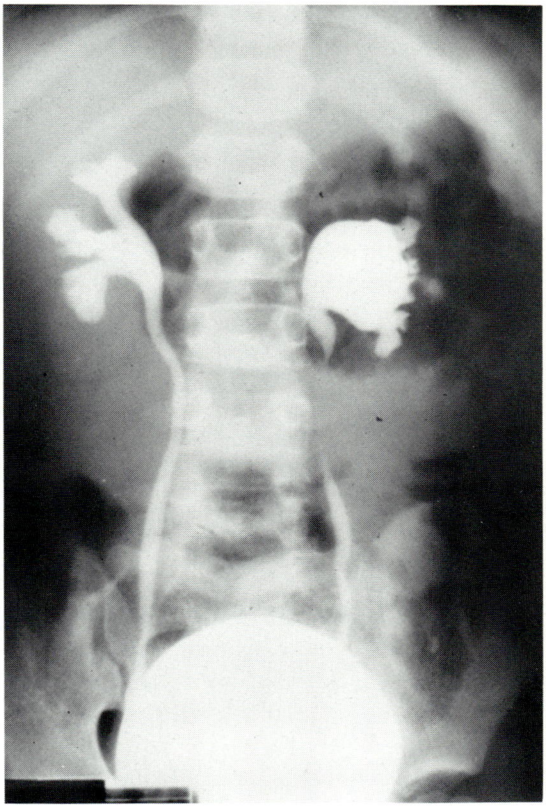

Figure 17-4. Grade III vesicoureteral reflux (bilateral). Cystography reveals bilateral opacification of the ureters and collecting systems with mild pyelocaliectasis. (Courtesy of Robert Cleveland, M.D., Massachusetts General Hospital, Boston, M.A.)

The radiographic hallmark of reflux nephropathy is the focal renal parenchymal scar associated with a blunted calix (Fig. 17-7). The scars may be unilateral or bilateral and may be mild (that is, causing only a small indentation in the renal outline) or severe (so that the caliceal lumen and the renal outline virtually meet with

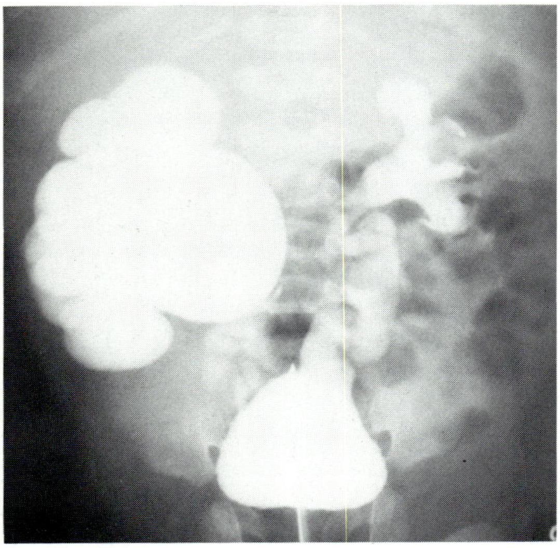

Figure 17-5. Grade V vesicoureteral reflux on right; Grade III–IV on left. Cystography demonstrates reflux with severe upper tract dilatation, especially on the right.

no intervening visible renal parenchyma). The scars do not form adjacent to calices whose papillae are normal. If the scars have destroyed a great deal of the patient's renal parenchyma, the remaining parenchyma may have undergone compensatory hypertrophy. If only one kidney is scarred, the entirety of the other kidney may appear enlarged. If the compensatory hypertrophy occcurs in parenchyma between scars, the enlarged portions may distend the renal outline and bow or stretch the adjacent calices and thus mimic a mass (Fig. 17-8). If reflux nephropathy has destroyed enough of the parenchyma to cause moderate or severe renal failure, there are usually few, if any, remaining normal calices, and the affected kidneys may be quite small.

The scars may be subtle and difficult to find. They have a predilection for the polar regions, especially the upper poles, and may be visible only by causing a thinning of the parenchyma just medial to the upper-pole calix. Once present, the scars never regress; they may remain stable or become more severe on subsequent examinations. The scars may be aassociated with ipsilateral reflux, or the reflux may have resolved or been cured by the time the scars are demonstrated. Conversely, patients known to have reflux may not have associated renal scars. In

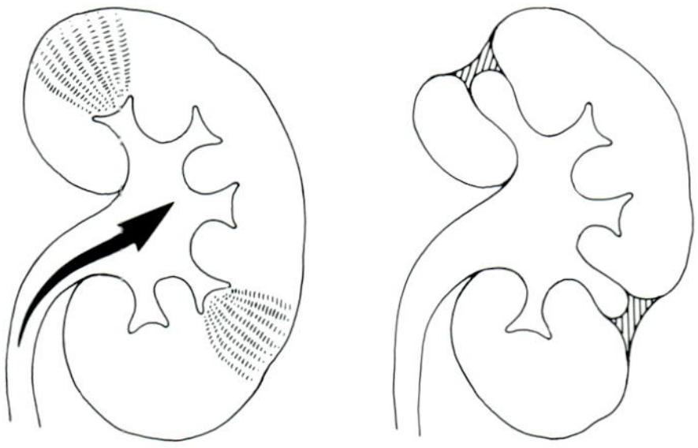

A

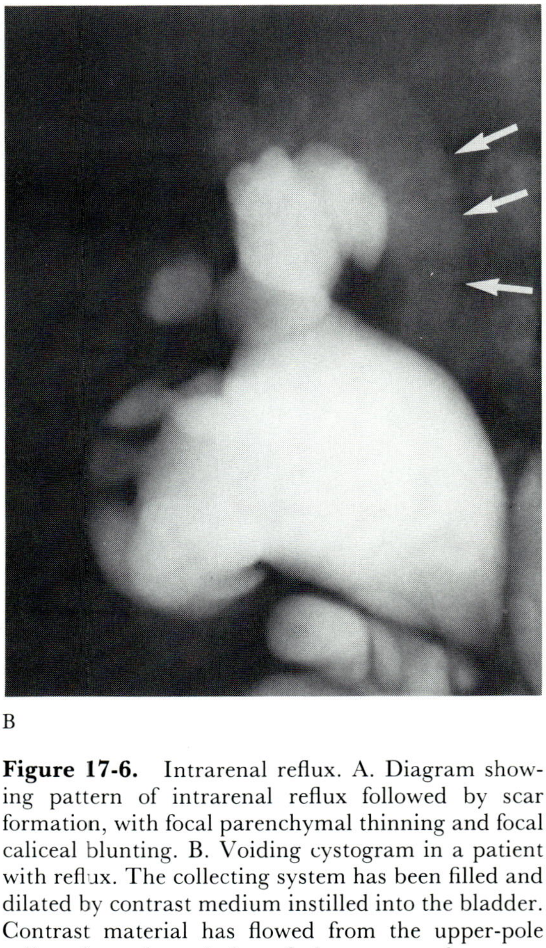

B

Figure 17-6. Intrarenal reflux. A. Diagram showing pattern of intrarenal reflux followed by scar formation, with focal parenchymal thinning and focal caliceal blunting. B. Voiding cystogram in a patient with reflux. The collecting system has been filled and dilated by contrast medium instilled into the bladder. Contrast material has flowed from the upper-pole calices into the tubules of the upper-pole parenchyma, causing faint opacification (arrows). (Courtesy of Walter Berdon, M.D., Columbia–Presbyterian Medical Center, New York, NY.)

patients with complete ureteral duplication and reflux into the lower-pole moiety, the scars invariably appear adjacent to the portion of the collecting system into which the reflux occurs. CT may show the scars equally well (Fig. 17-9);

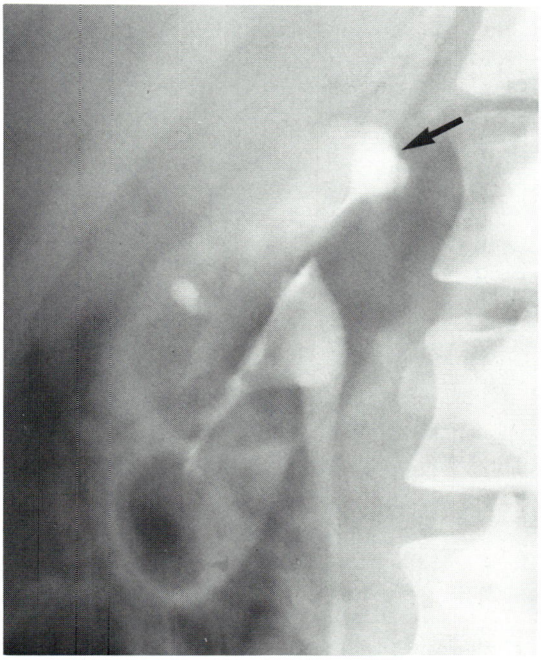

Figure 17-7. Chronic atrophic pyelonephritis (reflux nephropathy). Urography reveals a blunted upper-pole calix with a parenchymal scar that has virtually destroyed the upper-pole parenchyma (arrow). The lower pole appears normal; the lateral calix in the middle of the kidney is mildly blunted and is associated with moderate parenchymal thinning.

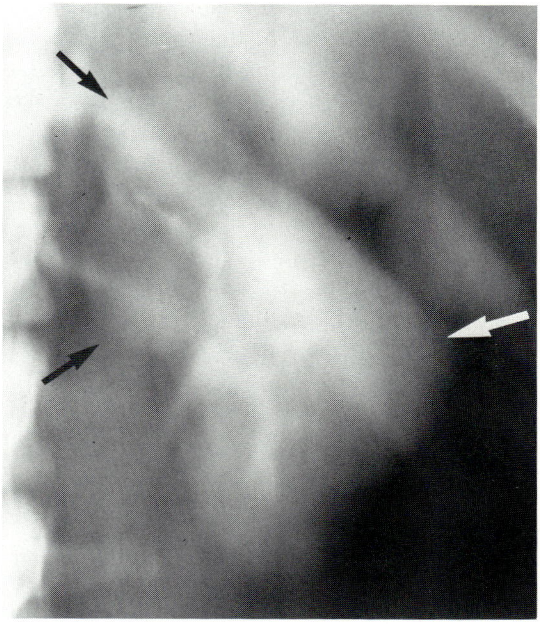

Figure 17-8. Chronic atrophic pyelonephritis (reflux nephropathy) with pseudotumors. The parenchyma immediately medial to the upper pole calix has been thinned; the adjacent parenchyma is not diminished in volume and mimics masses (black arrows). There is a dromedary hump in the lateral aspect of the kidney (white arrow).

it probably reveals anterior and posterior scarring better than urography, but urography may reveal polar scars and subtle caliceal changes better than CT.

Ultrasonography [24, 33] may reveal the scars to be regions of focal parenchymal thinning; the scarred portions may be more echogenic than the remaining kidney. Radionuclide scintigraphy may reveal reflux nephropathy [25, 36, 38] by virtue of diminished activity over the affected kidney and, possibly, by focal regions of diminished activity within the kidney itself.

Reflux nephropathy, or chronic atrophic pyelonephritis, may sometimes pose a serious exercise in differential diagnosis. Focal scars with associated caliceal blunting may be caused by caliceal stones [37]; the differentiation may be easy for patients in whom the stones remain or in whom the history is clear, but for adults who are poor historians and have no current stones, differentiation may be difficult. Focal scars caused by lesions of the major branches of the renal arteries may look similar but are not classically associated with caliceal blunting. The peripheral indentations of the renal outline that constitute fetal lobation are usually smaller than chronic pyelonephritic scars, exist between major caliceal groups, and are not associated with

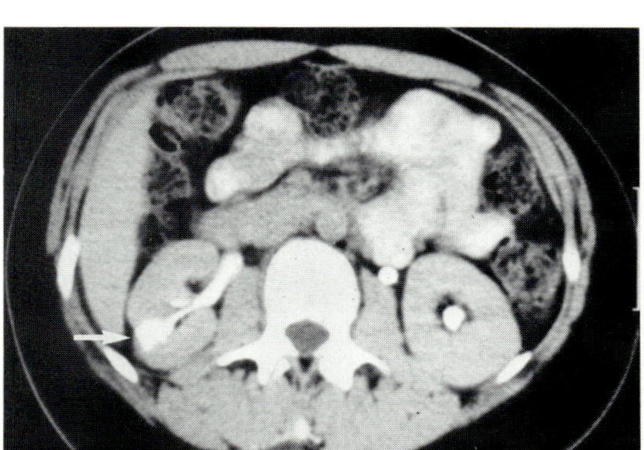

Figure 17-9. Chronic atrophic pyelonephritis (reflux nephropathy). CT reveals a dilated calix with focal parenchymal scarring (arrow).

caliceal abnormalities. Parenchymal loss can be safely assumed not to be due to reflux nephropathy if the loss is uniform around the kidney and is bilaterally symmetrical. Papillary necrosis may produce blunted calices but rarely produces deep parenchymal scars. Renal tuberculosis may produce dilated calices and focal scars, but the parenchymal calcifications and ureteral and caliceal strictures often encountered in tuberculosis are not seen in reflux nephropathy. Hydronephrotic atrophy can usually be distinguished from reflux nephropathy, since the former does not produce focal scars; nevertheless, as we have seen, severe vesicoureteral reflux may cause uniform caliceal distention and parenchymal loss, so only voiding cystography can be used to distinguish between cases of obstruction and reflux. Finally, the pseudotumors of focal compensatory hypertrophy may be distinguished from renal tumors, since only the pseudotumors excrete isotopes or show a normal nephrogram on CT.

REFERENCES

1. Armar, A.D., Das, S. Vesicoureteral reflux in women with primary bladder diverticulum. *J. Urol.* 134:33, 1985.
2. Bernstein. J., and Arant, B.S., Jr. Renal scars and vesicoureteral reflux: pathology and pathogenesis of segmental atrophy. In *Proceedings of The Ninth International Congress of Nephrology* (Los Angeles, June 1984). Berlin: Springer-Verlag, 1984, P. 948.
3. Blickman, J.G., Taylor, G.A., and Lebowitz, R.L. Voiding cystourethrography: The initial radiologic study in children with urinary tract infection. *Radiology* 156:659, 1985.
4. Bourchier, D., Abbott, G.D. and Maling, T.M.J. Radiological abnormalities in infants with urinary tract infections. *Arch. Dis. Child.* 59:620, 1984.
5. Bredin, H.C., et al. Family study of vesicoureteral reflux. *J. Urol.* 113:623, 1975.
6. Brendstrup, L., et al. Micturition cystourethrography using x-ray or scintigraphy in children with reflux. *Acta. Pediatr. Scand.* 72:559, 1983.
7. Cardiff-Oxford Bacteriuria Study Group. Long-term effects of bacteriuria on the urinary tract in schoolgirls. *Radiology* 132:343, 1979.
8. Claesson, I., et al. Compensatory kidney growth in children with urinary tract infection and unilateral renal scarring: An epidemiologic study. *Kidney Int.* 20:759, 1981.
9. Conway, J.J., and Kruglik, G.D. Effectiveness of direct and indirect radionuclide cystography in detecting vesicoureteral reflux. *J. Nucl. Med.* 17:81, 1976.
10. Cotran, R.S. Glomerulosclerosis in reflux nephropathy. *Kidney Int.* 24:528, 1982.
11. Conway, J.J., et al. Detection of vesicoureteral reflux with radionuclide cystrography: A comparison study with roentgenographic cystography. *A.J.R.* 115:720, 1972.
12. Elo, J., et al. The role of vesicoureteral reflux in paediatric urinary-tract infection. *Scand. J. Urol. Nephrol.* 15:243, 1981.
13. Elo, J., et al. Character of urinary tract infections and pyelonephritic renal scarring after antireflux surgery. *J. Urol.* 129:343, 1983.
14. Filly, R., et al. Development and progression of clubbing and scarring in children with recurrent urinary tract infections. *Radiology* 113:145, 1974.
15. Freed, S.Z. Vesicoureteral reflux following transurethral resection of bladder tumors. *J. Urol.* 116:184, 1976.
16. Funston, M.R., and Cremin, B.J. Intrarenal reflux, papillary morphology and pressure relationships in children's necropsy kidneys. *Br. J. Radiol.* 51:665, 1978.
17. Gillenwater, J.Y., Harrison, R.B., and Kunin, C.M. Natural history of bacteriuria in schoolgirls: A long-term case control study. *N. Engl. J. Med.* 301:396, 1979.
18. Gross, G.W., and Lebowitz, R.L. Infection does not cause reflux. *A.J.R.* 137:929, 1981.
19. Hannerz, L., et al. Distribution of renal scars and intrarenal reflux in children with a past history of urinary tract infection. *Acta Radiol.* 28:443, 1987
20. Hawtrey, C.E., et al. Ureterovesical reflux in an adolescent and adult population. *J. Urol.* 130:1067, 1983.
21. Hedman, J.K., Kempi, V., and Voss, H. Measurement of vesicoureteral reflux with intravenous 99mTc-DTPA compared to radiographic cystography. *Radiology* 126:205, 1978.
22. Hodson, C.J., et al. The pathogenesis of reflux nephropathy (chronic atrophic pyelonephritis). *Br. J. Radiol.* 13:1, 1975.
23. Ibsen, K.K., Uldall, P., and Frokjer, O. The growth of the kidneys in children with vesicoureteric reflux. *Acta Paediatr. Scand.* 66:741, 1977.
24. Kay, C.J., et al. Ultrasonic characteristics of chronic atrophic pyelonephritis. *A.J.R.* 132:47, 1979.
25. Kullendorf, C.M., Laurin, S., and White, T. Evaluation of renal parenchyma in children by DMSA scintigraphy, x-ray computed tomography and intravenous urography. *Acta Paediatr. Scand.* 76:284, 1987.
26. Huland, H., and Busch, R. Pyelonephritic scarring in 213 patients with upper and lower urinary tract infections: Long-term followup. *J. Urol.* 132:936, 1984.

27. Kangarloo, H., et al. Urinary tract infection in infants and children evaluated by ultrasound. *Radiology* 154:367, 1985.
28. Kincaid-Smith, P.S. Natural history and treatment of reflux nephropathy. In *Proceedings of the Ninth International Congress of Nephrology* (Los Angeles, June 1984). Berlin: Springer-Verlag, 1984. Pp. 959–979.
29. Kincaid-Smith, P., and Fairley, K.F. (eds). *Renal Infection and Renal Scarring*. Melbourne, Australia: Mercedes Publishing, 1970.
30. Lanning, P., et al. Prediction of vesico-ureteral reflux in children from intravenous urography films. *Clin. Radiol.* 30:67, 1979.
31. Lebowitz, R.L. Urography in children. *Postgrad. Med.* 64:63, 1978.
32. Lebowitz, R.L., and Mandell, J. Urinary tract infection in children: Putting radiology in its place. *Radiology* 165:1, 1987.
33. Leonidas, J.C., et al. Sonography as a substitute for excretory urography in children with urinary tract infection. *A.J.R.* 144:815, 1985.
34. Manley, C.B., Neuman, N., and McAlister, W.H. Prognosis for resolution of moderate, primary reflux in girls. *J. Urol.* 115:307, 1976.
35. McLachlan, M.S.F., et al. Urinary tract in schoolgirls with covert bacteriuria. *Arch. Dis. Child.* 50:253, 1975.
36. Merrick, M.V., Uttley, W.S., and Wild, S.R. The detection of pyelonephritic scarring in children by radioisotope imaging. *Br. Jr. Radiol.* 53:544, 1980.
37. Newhouse, J.H., and Amis, E.S., Jr. The relationship between renal scarring and stone disease. *A.J.R.* 151:1153, 1988.
38. Nielsen, J.B., et al. Renal parenchymal appearance on 123 iodine-hippurate renoscintigrams and excretory urograms. *J. Urol.* 133:179, 1985.
39. Parrott, T.S., and Woodard, J.R. Importance of cystourethrography in neonates with imperforate anus. *Urology* 13:607, 1979.
40. Rose, J.S., Glassberg, K.I., and Waterhouse, K. Intrarenal reflux and its relationship to renal scarring. *J. Urol.* 113:400, 1975.
41. Salvatierra, O., Jr., and Tanagho, E.A. Reflux as a cause of end stage kidney disease: Report of 32 cases. *J. Urol.* 117:441, 1977.
42. Savage, J.M., et al. Renin and blood-pressure in children with renal scarring and vesicoureteral reflux. *Lancet.* 2:441, 1978 Vol. 441, 1978.
43. Schulman, C.C., and Gregoir, W. Die physiopathologie des primaren vesikoureteralen refluxes. *Urologe [A]* 16:118, 1977.
44. Shah, K.J., Robins, D.G., and White, R.H.R. Renal scarring and vesicoureteric reflux. *Arch. Dis. Child.* 53:210, 1978.
45. Smellie, J.M., et al. Development of new renal scars: A collaborative study. *Br. Med. J.* 290:1957, 1985.
46. Stecker, J.F., Jr., Read, B.P., and Poutasse, E.F. Pediatric hypertension as a delayed sequela of reflux-induced chronic pyelonephritis. *J. Urol.* 118:644, 1977.
47. Steinhardt, G.F. Reflux nephropathy. *J. Urol.* 134:855, 1985.
48. Thomsen, H.S. Vesicoureteral reflux and reflux nephropathy. *Acta Radiol. Diagn.* 26:3, 1985.
49. Thomsen, H.S., et al. Intrarenal backflow and renal perfusion during increased intrapelvic pressure in excised porcine kidneys. *Acta Radiol. Diagn.* 24:327, 1983.
50. Van den Abbeele, A.D., et al. Vesicoureteral reflux in asymptomatic siblings of patients with known reflux: Radionuclide cystography. *Pediatrics* 79:147, 1987.
51. Wikstad, I., et al. Vesicoureteric reflux and pyelonephritis. *Acta Radiol. Diagn.* 20:252, 1979.
52. Wikstad, I., et al. Long-time effect of large vesicoureteral reflux with or without urinary tract infection. *Acta Radiol. Diagn.* 22:325, 1981.
53. Winter, A.L., et al. Acquired renal scars in children. *J. Urol.* 129:1190, 1983.

18

Duplex Collecting Systems

Duplication of the collecting system is the most frequently occurring congenital anomaly in the urinary tract. The duplex collecting system and its related abnormalities are responsible for some of the most complicated patterns detected on imaging studies in both children and adults and affect virtually all levels of the urinary tract.

The autopsy incidence of partial duplication is about 1 in 150 cases, while complete duplication is found once in every 500 cases. However, the incidence in clinical series is up to six times higher, probably reflecting the propensity of this anomaly to produce symptoms. Complete duplications of the collecting system are bilateral in 10 to 20 percent of cases. Females are affected two to five times more frequently than males. The typical clinical presentation of a complicated duplication is urinary infection or continual dribbling incontinence of urine in a young girl.

EMBRYOLOGY OF DUPLICATIONS

Embryologically, the ureter forms as a bud from the mesonephric duct. The normal kidney is formed when this bud invaginates the metanephric blastema and through multiple branchings forms the collecting system and distal collecting ducts. Figure 18-1 diagrammatically depicts the development of single and duplicated collecting systems. Partial duplication results from a branching of the ureteral bud before it connects with the metanephric blastema; the point at which the ureteral bud branches will determine the level at which the two ureters join; this may be anywhere from the bladder wall immediately proximal to a single ureteral orifice to the renal pelvis. The latter will result in a bifid renal pelvis. On rare occasions, the single ureteral bud may trifurcate or even branch into four or five segments before meeting the metanephric blastema; these multiple branchings are almost always quite high and result in multiplication of the renal pelvis.

Complete duplication of the ureter occurs when two separate buds arise from the mesonephric duct. These invaginate the metanephric blastema separately, resulting in formation of upper and lower intrarenal collecting systems. Each of these collecting systems is known as a moiety, and each is drained by a separate ureter. As the mesonephric duct migrates caudally, the ureter from the lower moiety is deposited near its expected normal location in the bladder, and its ureterovesical junction is therefore usually in its normal position on the trigone or slightly laterally and superiorly placed. The ureter from the upper moiety remains attached to the mesonephric duct longer during its caudal migration and eventually connects with the bladder inferiorly and medially as compared with the lower-moiety ureter. The Meyer–Weigert law states that the ureter from the upper moiety will enter the bladder inferiorly and medially in relation to the ureter draining the lower moiety [2].

DUPLICATIONS AND RELATED ABNORMALITIES

The majority of both complete and incomplete duplications are associated with normal function and are thus incidental findings on urography. In most cases, the upper moiety is the smaller of the two (usually only two or three calices) and drains about a fourth of the overall kidney (Fig. 18-2A). On rare occasions, however, this configuration can be reversed (Fig. 18-2B). As previously noted, with incomplete duplication, the point at which the two proximal ureters join can be anywhere from the renal pelvis (bifid collecting system) to the level of the bladder wall. In this latter instance it may be impossible to differentiate partial from complete duplication without cystoscopic evaluation of the bladder to determine whether there are one or two orifices on the side in question. With complete duplications of the uncomplicated

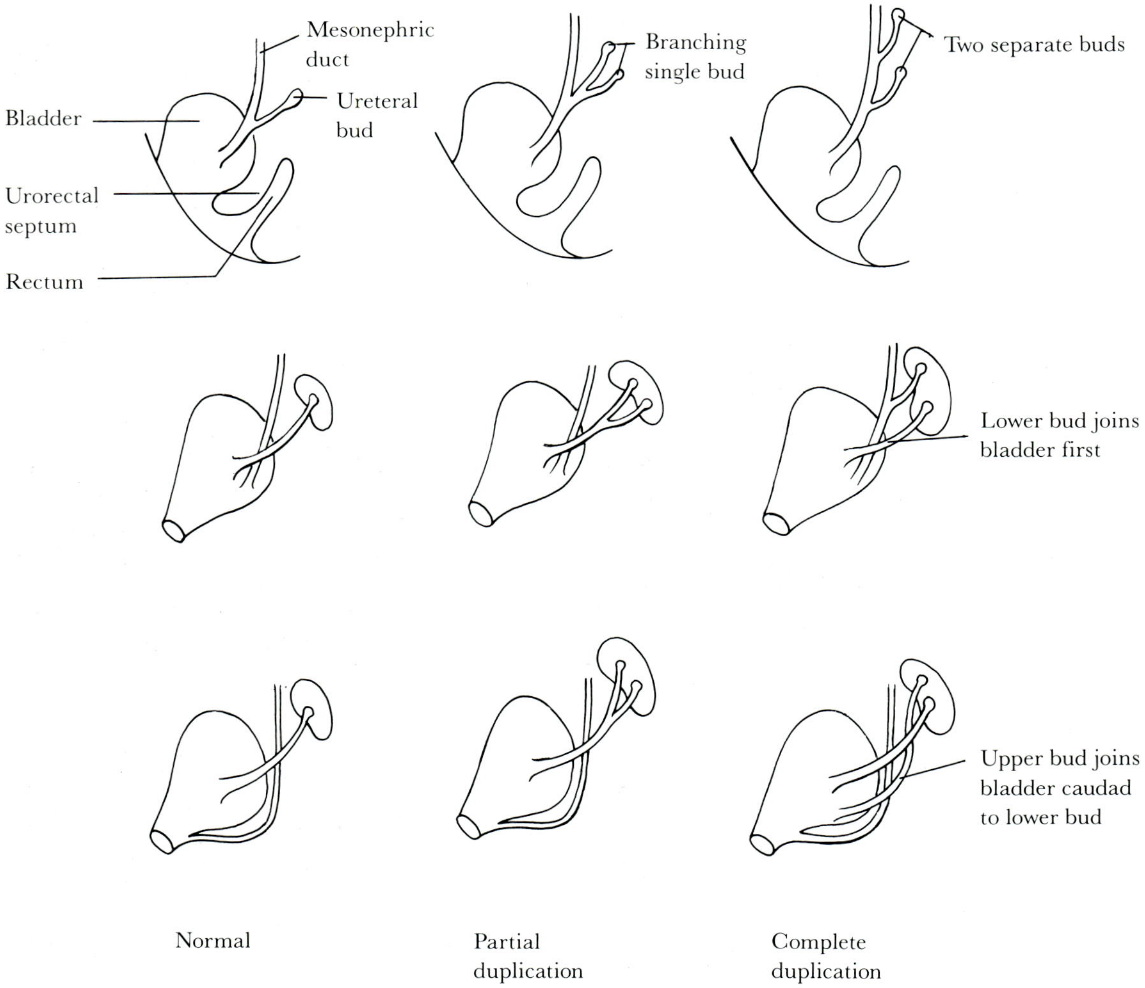

Figure 18-1. Embryology of duplex collecting systems.

variety, the orifices usually enter the bladder adjacent to each other in a relatively normal position on the trigone.

There are three discrete abnormalities of the termination of the ureters in complete duplications that can result in significant pathologic changes in the duplicated kidney. These include maldevelopment of the valve mechanism at the ureterovesical junction of the lower-moiety ureter, ectopic insertion of the ureter draining the upper moiety, and ectopic ureterocele involving the ureter draining the upper moiety [6]. Generally speaking, these abnormalities result in either obstruction of the upper moiety, reflux into the lower moiety, or both. However, in many instances the findings are not so straightforward. These abnormalities and their resultant changes in the kidney will be individually discussed below.

MALDEVELOPMENT OF THE VALVE MECHANISM OF THE LOWER-MOIETY URETER

Maldevelopment of the valve mechanism at the ureterovesical junction involves the orifice of the ureter draining the lower moiety. As previously noted, this orifice may be slightly above and lateral to its normal position on the trigone. Because of this abnormal location, there is a shorter submucosal tunnel for the distal ureter and thus a more direct course through the bladder wall—a condition that facilitates reflux. This mechanism has been discussed in more detail in Chap. 17. In complete duplications,

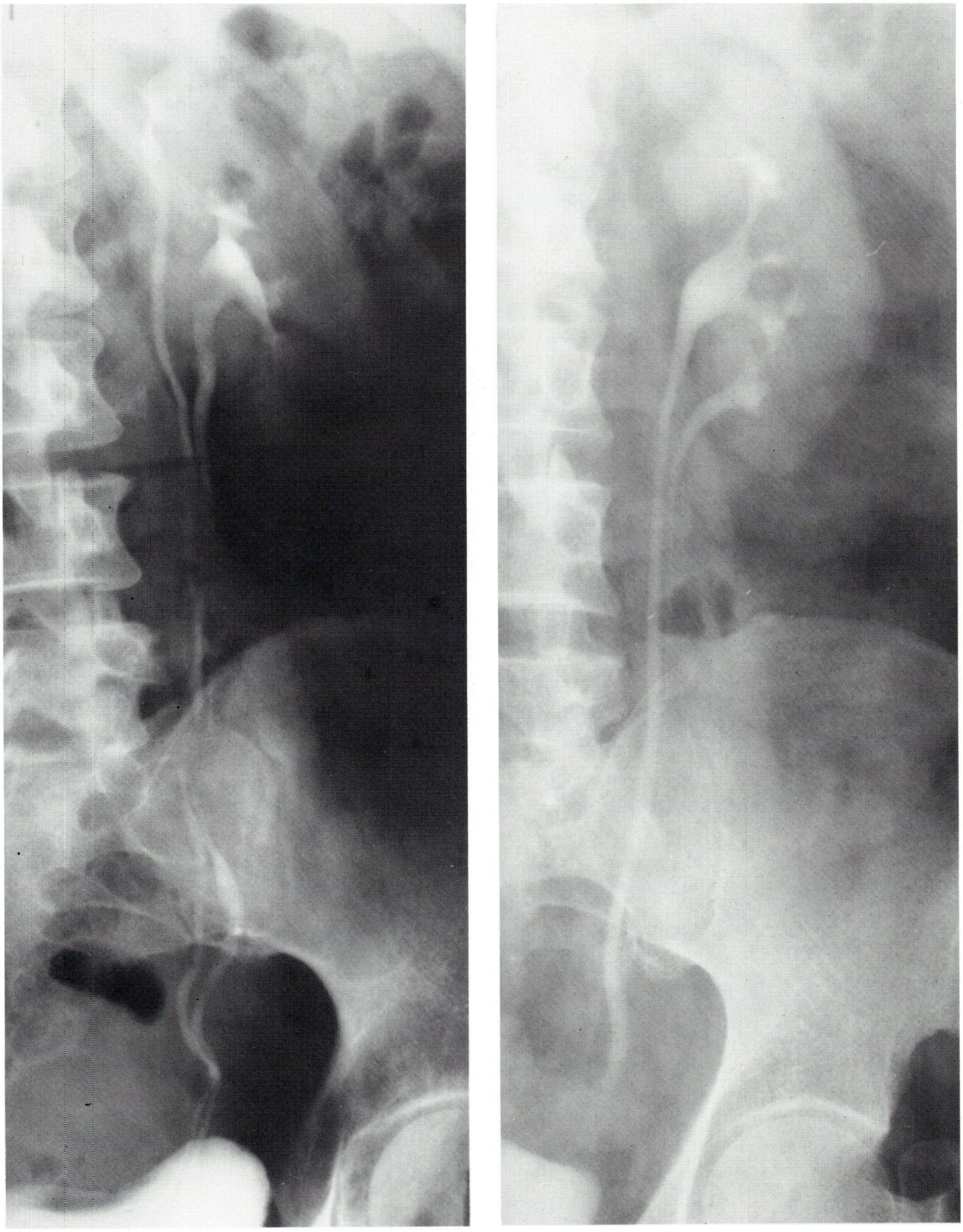

A B

Figure 18-2. Variations in configuration of moieties in nonpathologic duplications. A. Urography shows common pattern of diminutive upper moiety. B. Urography shows rare pattern of diminutive lower moiety.

the incidence of reflux into the lower moiety is approximately 6 percent. If there is further distortion of this valve mechanism by a ureterocele of the ureter from the upper moiety, reflux occurs in about a third of cases. Vesicoureteral reflux is the most common abnormality associated with completely duplicated systems.

In girls with urinary tract infection, complete duplication is found in 5 percent, and in over two-thirds of these duplex systems reflux is seen, usually into the lower-moiety ureter [3]. In girls with incomplete duplications, the incidence of reflux when urinary infection is present is no higher than if they had a single collecting system. This is not surprising, as in both cases there is a single normal ureteral orifice.

Radiographically, reflux can be demonstrated by voiding cystourethrography. There is a significant spectrum of radiographic appearances that can be seen with reflux. These range from filling of a nondilated normal lower collecting system to massive dilation of the lower moiety with associated parenchymal thinning. In addition, the typical findings of reflux nephropathy are often seen, including focal or diffuse renal scarring with clubbing of the underlying calices. On execretory urography, these changes may also be demonstrated (Fig. 18-3). Furthermore, reflux can rarely produce enough damage to result in minimal or no function in the lower moiety on urography.

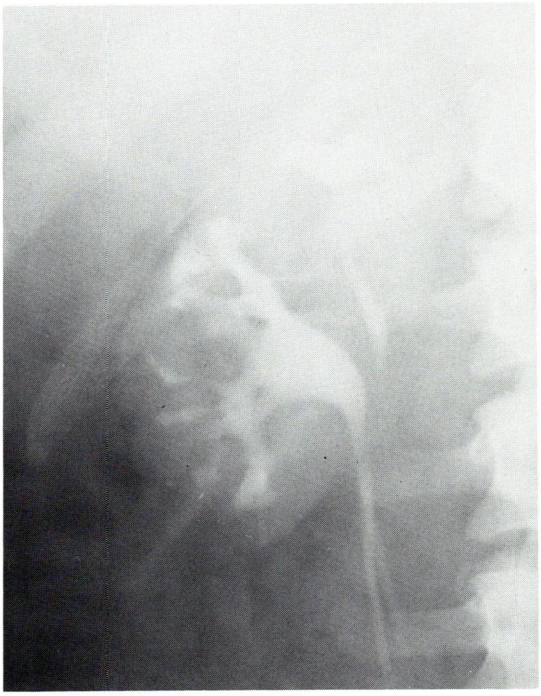

Figure 18-3. Reflux nephropathy (chronic atrophic pyelonephritis) of lower-pole moiety in complete duplication. Urography demonstrates clubbing of the lower-moiety calices and significant associated lower-pole parenchymal thinning.

ECTOPIC INSERTION OF THE URETER

Ectopic insertion of the ureter means that a ureteral orifice is removed from its normal position on the trigone. Ectopic insertions can occur near or at the bladder neck, in the posterior urethra, or in extravesical locations. The ectopic ureter invariably drains the upper moiety in duplicated systems; furthermore, more than two-thirds of all extravesical ectopic insertions of the ureter are associated with complete duplications. Figure 18-4 demonstrates the sites of extravesical ectopic insertion and their frequencies of occurrence in both males and females. Remnants of the embryonic mesonephric duct can be found in the walls of the vagina, uterus, and broad ligaments in 25 percent of all adult females. These vestigial structures establish the relationship of the mesonephric duct to the vagina and uterus and explain ectopic insertion of the ureter into these female organs. In the male, ectopic insertion into the vas deferens and seminal vesicles is explained by the fact that these organs are derived from the mesonephric duct, which also gives rise to the ureter.

Ectopic orifices located at the bladder neck or in the posterior urethra may demonstrate reflux during voiding; otherwise, they are usually obstructed because of the fact that they empty into a predominantly closed space. Ectopic ureters terminating outside the urinary tract are usually obstructed. Reflux or obstruction may therefore result in dilation and poor or no function of the upper moiety on imaging studies. Generally speaking, the more distally situated the ectopic orifice (posterior urethra, other extravesical locations), the more dysplastic, and hence bizarre appearing, will be the upper moiety it drains [8].

Clinically, extravesical ectopic ureteral insertions in girls, aside from those entering into the

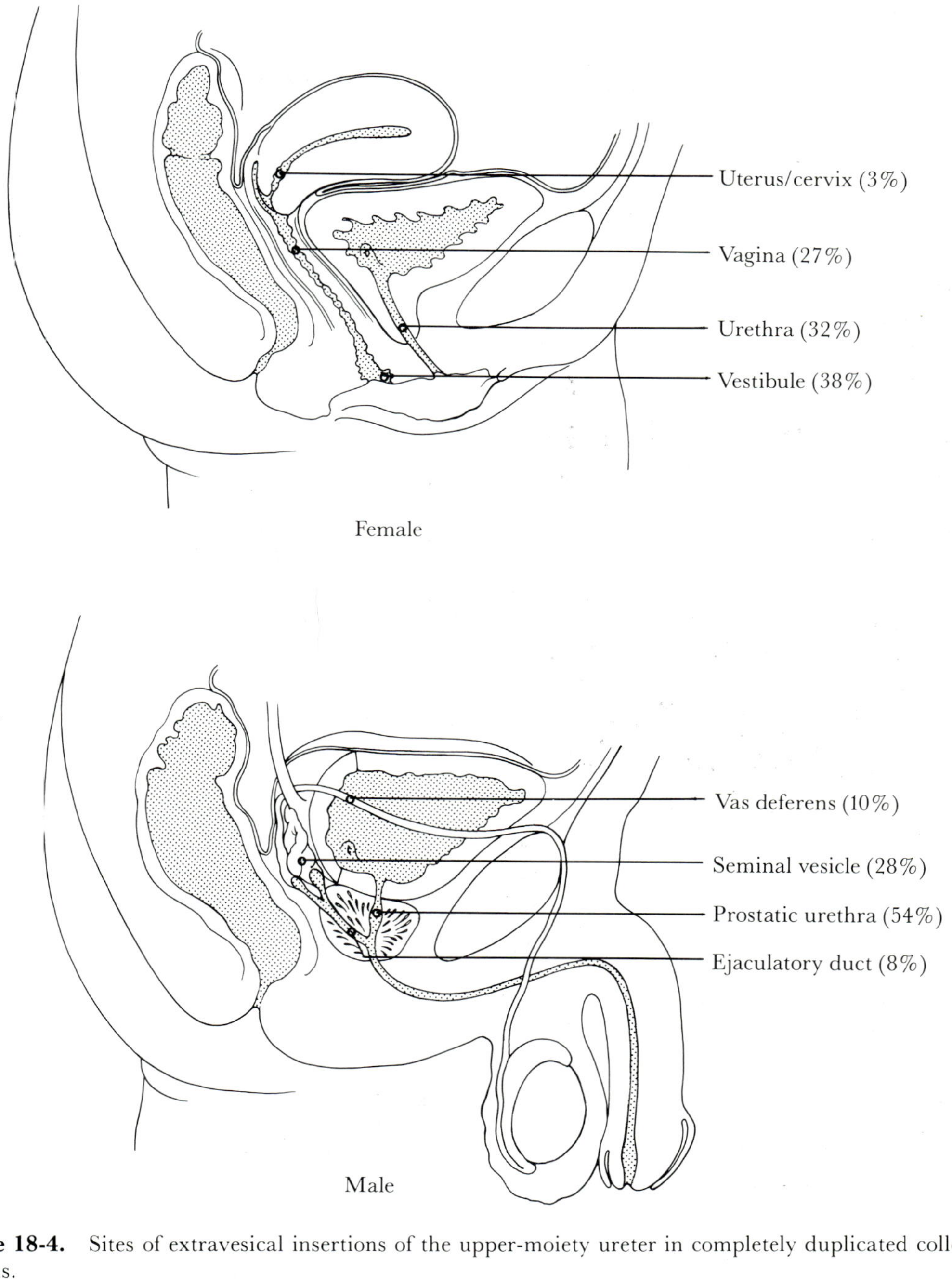

Figure 18-4. Sites of extravesical insertions of the upper-moiety ureter in completely duplicated collecting systems.

posterior urethra, are beyond sphincter control; assuming even a minimally functional upper moiety, this results in a continual dribbling incontinence of urine. This is not the case in males, since all ectopic orifices occur above the level of the external urethral sphincter. However, males may present with chronic or recurrent epididymitis due to ectopic insertion of the ureter into the ipsilateral vas deferens or seminal vesicle. In both sexes, recurrent or chronic urinary tract infection can be found with refluxing ectopic ureteral orifices located in the posterior urethra or at the bladder neck.

Urographic findings may range from a readily visualized dilated or dysplastic upper-pole collecting system to complete nonvisualization of

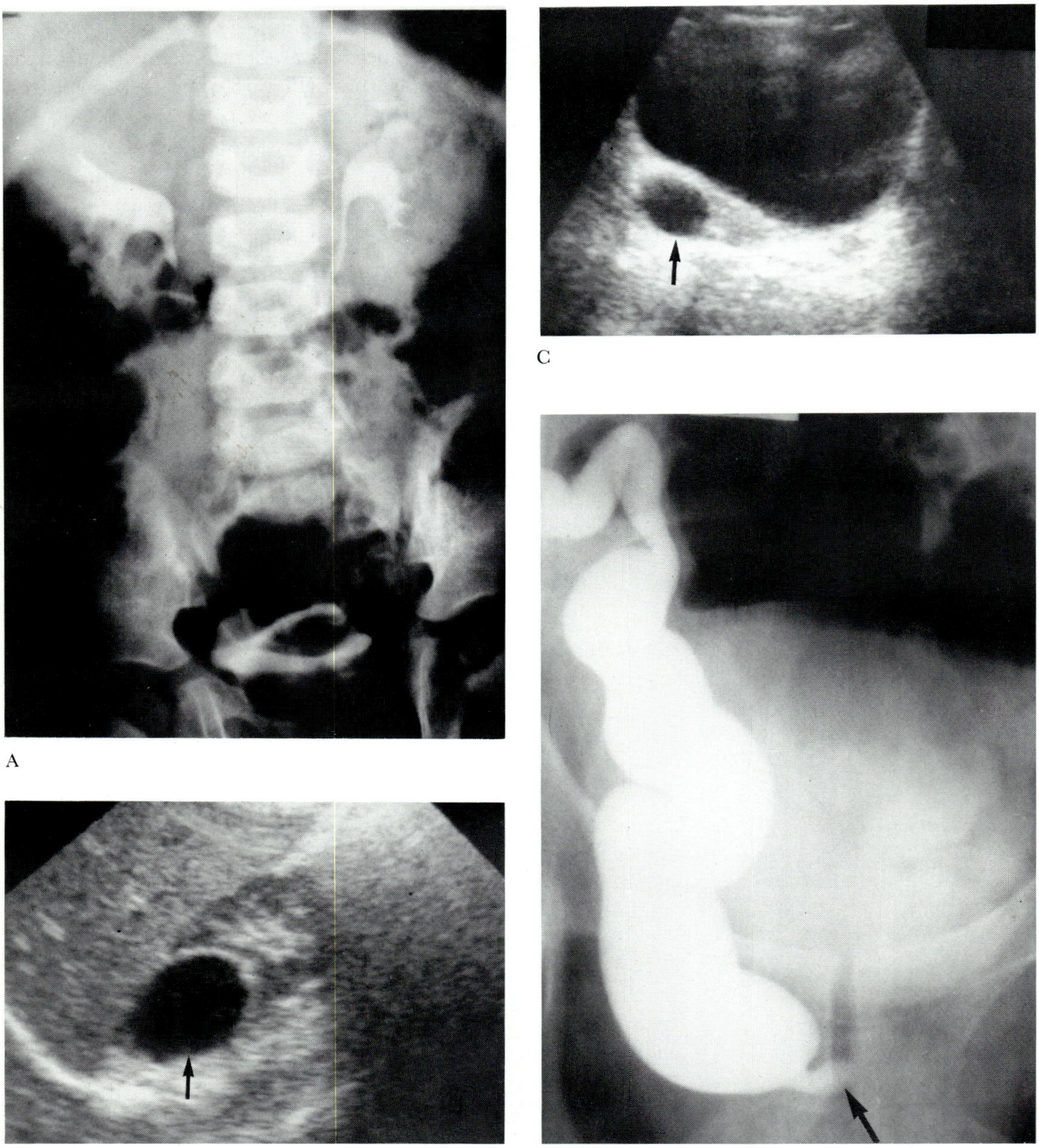

A B C D

Figure 18-5. Ectopic insertion of upper-moiety ureter into urethra. A. Urography shows tilted axis of right collecting system, fewer than normal number of calices, and cystic-appearing upper pole. B. Right renal sonography shows cystic area in upper pole (arrow). C. Transverse sonography of pelvis shows a dilated ureter coursing behind bladder on right (arrow). D. Coned view of antegrade pyelogram performed via upper moiety shows dilated, tortuous ureter from upper moiety inserting into urethra below bladder base (arrow).

the upper moiety. The presence of a nonfunctioning upper moiety can often be inferred based on the appearance of the visualized lower moiety. In these cases, the lower moiety will usually exhibit deviation from its normal axis, fewer than the normal number of calices expected for a nonduplicated kidney, and mild lateral deviation of the proximal ureter (due to the medial location of the dilated ureter from the nonfunctioning upper pole). Most importantly, the altered axis (upper pole tilted laterally) of the functioning lower moiety should strongly indicate mass effect in the upper pole of the kidney (Fig. 18-5A). The appearance of the lower collecting system has been called the "drooping lily" sign. The dilated ureter from the upper moiety, as it courses toward its ectopic location, may spiral around the lower-moiety ureter in its distal half, resulting in tortuosity of both ureters, and may cause mass effect on the ipsilateral bladder wall.

In cases in which a nonfunctioning, obstructed upper moiety is suspected, sonography typically shows an echo-free cystic area in the upper pole of the kidney (the dilated upper collecting system) (Fig. 18-5B) and can often trace the dilated ureter from the upper moiety as it courses behind or beside the bladder to its ectopic insertion (Fig. 18-5C). CT can also demonstrate the hydronephrotic upper-pole moiety and trace its dilated ureter distally in serial transverse sections. If necessary, antegrade pyelography permits anatomic delineation of the ectopic insertion (Fig. 18-5D). In some cases, careful physical inspection of the vestibule, vagina, and cervix or cystoscopic examination of the posterior urethra will result in identification of a small draining dimple representing the ectopic orifice. In these cases, the nonvisualized system can be opacified in retrograde fashion via the ectopic orifice. Voiding cystourethrography should be performed in all cases of duplication in which pathology is suspected, since it may demonstrate reflux into either moiety.

ECTOPIC URETEROCELE

Ninety-nine percent of ectopic ureteroceles are associated with ipsilateral complete duplication; the ectopic ureteroceles in these cases are always associated with the ureter from the upper moiety. An ectopic ureterocele is closely related to ectopic insertion of the ureter in that it is formed by a focal dilation of the lower submucosal portion of an ectopic ureter opening near the bladder neck or in the posterior urethra [5]. About half of all ectopic ureteroceles terminate within the bladder, and the large majority of these have stenotic orifices that usually do not reflux (Fig. 18-6A). However, a small number will have patulous orifices, which can reflux.

Figure 18-6. Configurations of ectopic ureteroceles. A. Terminating within bladder. Opening usually stenotic. B. Terminating in urethra. Opening usually wide enough to reflux during voiding.

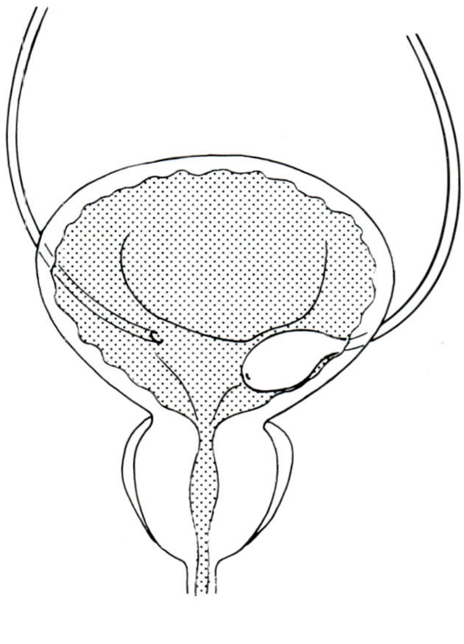
A

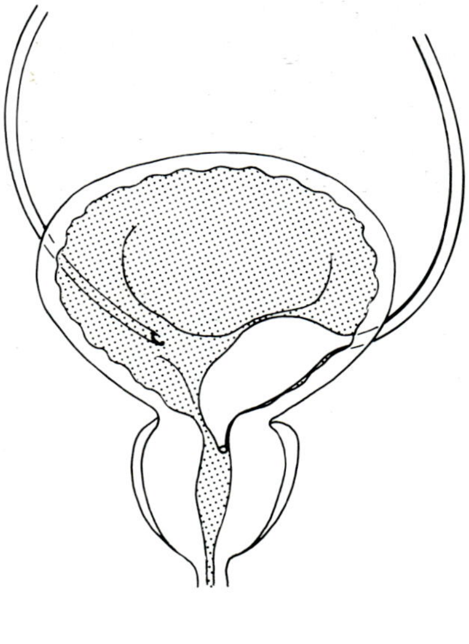
B

The other half of ureteroceles course submucosally through the bladder neck and terminate in the posterior urethra, where a widely patent orifice is the rule rather than the exception (Fig. 18-6B). This latter system often refluxes on voiding, but as in the case with ectopic ureteral insertion in the posterior urethra, when the patient is not voiding the ureterocele is obstructed, since it empties into a closed space. Overall, about 45 percent of ureteroceles demonstrate reflux during cystourethrography, at least during voiding.

Ectopic ureteroceles are often associated with little or no function of their associated ipsilateral upper-pole moieties. Furthermore, because of their size and location, large ectopic ureteroceles can also distort the ipsilateral lower-pole orifice and significantly increase the incidence of reflux into the lower moiety as previously noted. They may even directly compress, and thus obstruct, the ipsilateral lower-pole orifice. They may also be large enough to obstruct the contralateral ureteral orifice or prolapse into the bladder neck, resulting in bladder outlet obstruction.

An ectopic ureterocele is typically seen during urography or cystography as a smooth round or ovoid filling defect in the bladder (Fig. 18-7A). Although they are usually somewhat laterally oriented, their location can be midline. They may range in size from one to several centimeters in diameter. A ureterocele may have a low internal pressure, which can result in its efface-

Figure 18-7. Ectopic ureterocele obstructing upper moiety. A. Urography shows tilted axis of mildly dilated right collecting system and large oval filling defect (ectopic ureterocele) in bladder. Dilation of right lower moiety is due to partial obstruction of its ureteral orifice by the ureterocele. Left collecting system, obscured by bowel gas, is normal. B. Right renal sonography shows cystic area in upper pole (arrow) representing the obstructed upper moiety. C. Sonography of bladder depicts the thin-walled ureterocele (arrows).

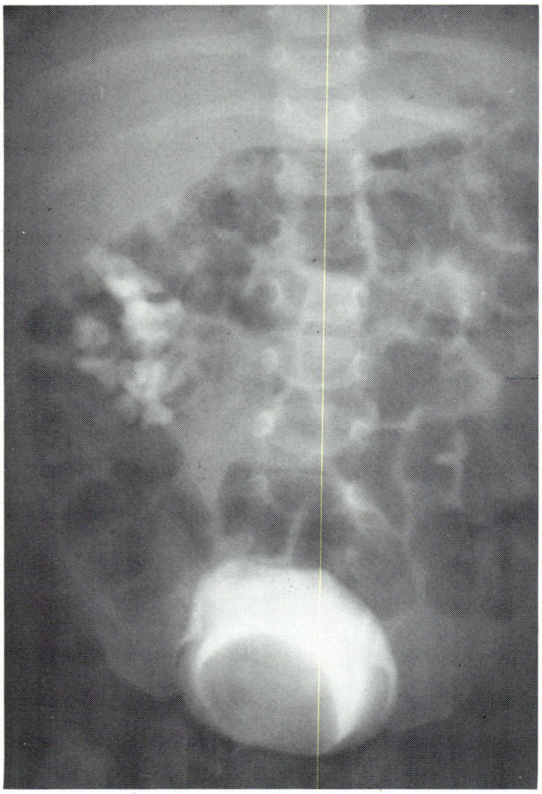

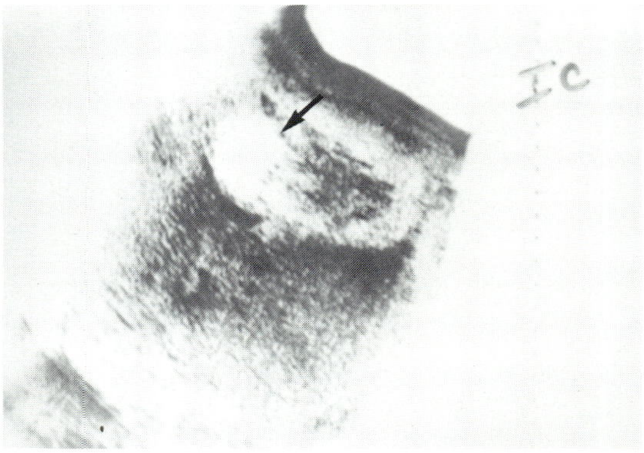

B

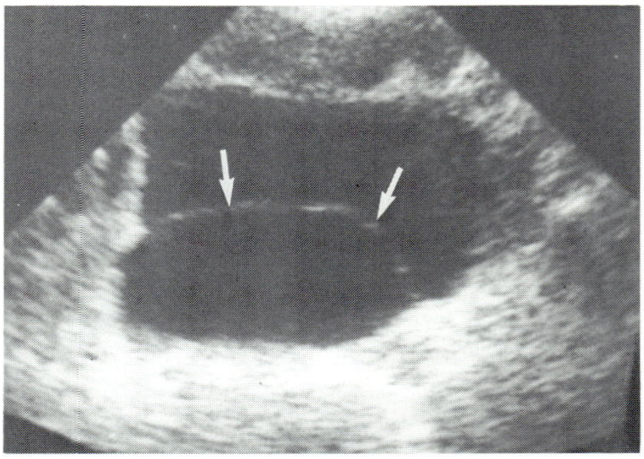

C

ment as the bladder fills, particularly during cystography. Therefore, it is important during cystography to evaluate the bladder fluoroscopically as it fills to prevent missing the diagnosis of ureterocele. In some cases, as intravesical pressure increases, the ureterocele may even evert into the extravesical portion of the ureter feeding it; this is usually seen during the voiding phase, when pressure within the bladder is at its maximum [7].

Urographic upper tract findings in completely duplicated systems complicated by either ectopic ureteral insertion or ureterocele are identical, as both affect the upper moiety, often causing dilation, nonfunction, and tilting of the renal axis as previously described (Fig. 18-8). As in the cases of ectopic insertion of the ureter from a duplicated upper-pole moiety, the further evaluation of an upper moiety suspected to be obstructed because of ectopic ureterocele should include sonography of the involved kidney. This typically shows an anechoic, fluid-filled structure in the region of the upper pole (see Fig. 18-7B). If a bladder defect consistent with ectopic ureterocele is not easily appreciated, antegrade pyelography via the nonfunctioning dilated upper-pole system will allow opacification of the entire pathologic drainage system. However, only rarely is it necessary to proceed to antegrade pyelography, since the ectopic ureterocele can usually be demonstrated in views of the partially filled bladder during urography or cystography. Unlike the case of ectopic insertion of the ureter, in which the dilated distal ureter is seen coursing posteriorly or laterally to the bladder, pelvic sonography in the case of ectopic ureterocele will demonstrate a thin septation in the bladder representing the distended ureterocele (see Fig. 18-7C).

Figure 18-8. Diagram showing the similar upper tract changes caused by extravesical ectopic ureteral insertion (A) and ectopic ureterocele (B).

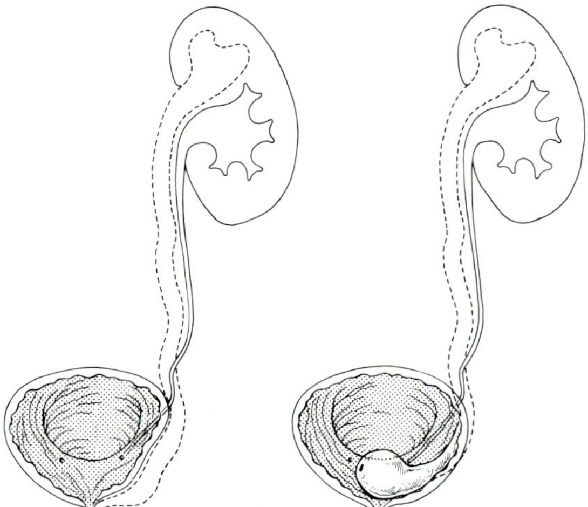

UNUSUAL RADIOGRAPHIC PATTERNS WITH DUPLEX COLLECTING SYSTEMS

The typical abnormalities seen with duplex collecting systems as described in the above sections usually result in radiographic findings that cause suspicion of a duplication and subsequent rapid diagnosis. However, not all duplications result in these easily recognizable patterns.

In some patients with complete duplications and ectopic ureteral insertions, the upper moiety may be very small and dysplastic and its ureter diminutive also, unlike the more common case, in which significant dilation of the entire upper-pole system is seen. Furthermore, the remainder of the kidney (the lower moiety) in such cases can have a normal axis and look essentially like a normal nonduplicated kidney (Fig. 18-9A). Because even the small dysplastic upper moiety can produce small amounts of urine, suspicion for this condition should be prompted by the clinical history of continual urine leakage in females or of recurrent or chronic epididymitis in men. On urography, the only evidence of a small nonvisualized upper moiety may be a slight flattening of the upper pole of the kidney or a small radiolucent bulge in this area. Sonography may demonstrate a small cystic lesion contiguous with the upper pole. As previously noted, careful physical examination of the vestibule, vagina, and cervix may reveal the ectopic orifice, allowing retrograde study of the covert system. In men CT or sonography can be used to evaluate the seminal vesicles for cystic dilation, a finding that would suggest ectopic insertion of the upper ureter into those organs. Rarely, a large typical ureterocele can be seen in the bladder in association with this tiny dysplastic upper-pole moiety; this is known as ureterocele disproportion [10] (Fig. 18-9B).

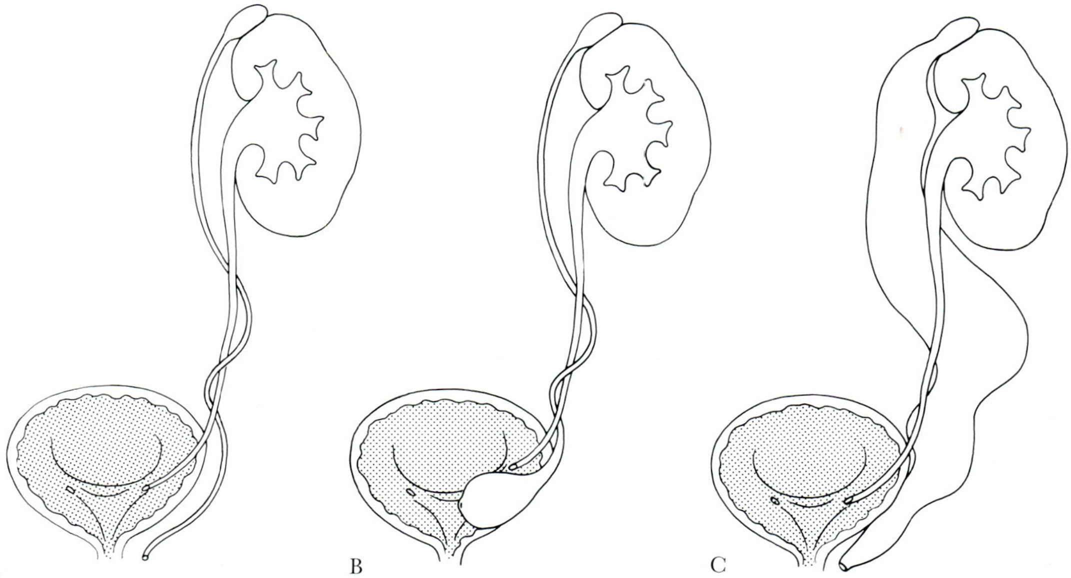

Figure 18-9. Unusual configurations of completely duplicated collecting systems. A. Diminutive upper moiety and ureter with ectopic insertion outside the bladder. B. Ureterocele disproportion—Large ureterocele but diminutive upper moiety and ureter. C. Diminutive upper moiety with grossly dilated ureter inserting ectopically outside the bladder.

Conversely, the ureter draining a small, dysplastic upper moiety (as well as a dilated upper moiety) may be grossly dilated and virtually fill the abdomen as it meanders on its tortuous course to either an ectopic insertion (Fig. 18-9C). or termination in an ectopic ureterocele. In these cases of extreme dilation and tortuosity, the ectopic ureter may sonographically mimic a multiseptated, cystic abdominal mass. Furthermore, large tortuous ureters with ectopic insertions can sometimes indent the lower vesical wall in a manner simulating a ureterocele [9]. Even with this significant degree of ureteral dilation, the upper moiety may be difficult to detect because it may be tiny.

Because of the high incidence of reflux into the lower moiety of a completely duplicated system, decreased, delayed, or absent opacification of a hydronephrotic lower-pole moiety is usually initially attributed to reflux nephropathy (Fig. 18-10A). Obstruction in completely duplicated systems is typically found to involve the upper moiety, as previously noted, because of an ectopic ureteral orifice or ureterocele. However, obstruction of the lower moiety is not uncommon. As previously noted, obstruction of the lower moiety can occur at the level of the ureterovesical junction if a ureterocele from the upper moiety is large enough to block the lower orifice. Aside from this, virtually any pathologic entity that can obstruct a nonduplicated ureter can involve the ureters in a duplicated system [1]. These include congenital ureteropelvic-junction obstruction, ureteral calculi, ureteral tumors, and retroperitoneal processes that can extrinsically constrict the ureters (Fig. 18-10B).

In the typical duplicated collecting system, only the lower moiety has a true renal pelvis and ureteropelvic junction. Therefore, it is almost always the lower moiety that is involved with congenital ureteropelvic-junction obstruction when this occurs (Fig. 18-10C). Also, the lower moiety, by virtue of its normally larger volume, runs the greater risk of urine stasis and hence stone formation. In cases of partial duplication, ureteropelvic-junction obstruction involving the lower moiety typically occurs at the point where the ureter bifurcates at the level of the renal pelvis of the lower moiety (Fig. 18-10D).

In imaging patients with duplication and lower-moiety obstruction, the urographic findings are rather typical. A diminutive, normally opacified upper-pole collecting system is seen, and with acute obstruction of the lower

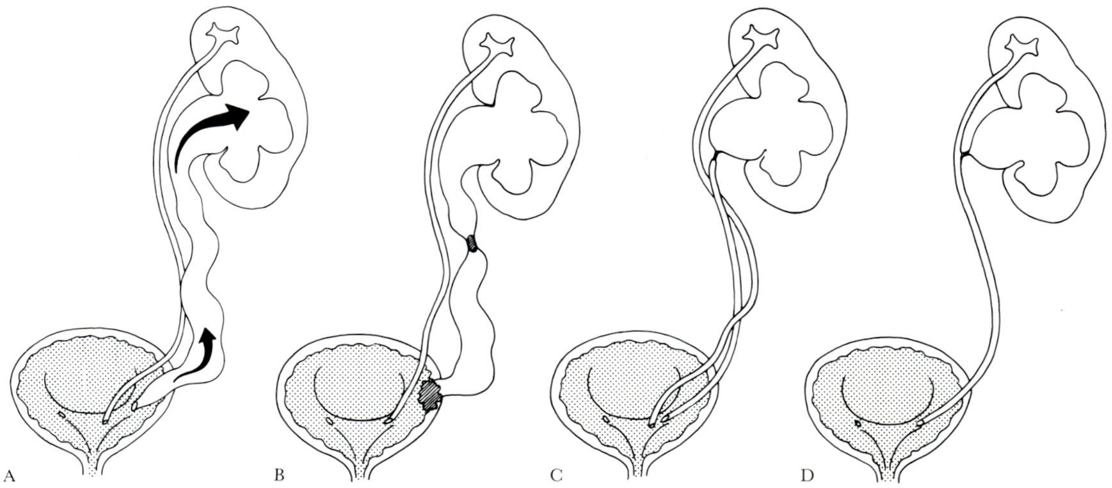

Figure 18-10. Lower-moiety hydronephrosis. A. Complete duplication with refluxing lower collecting system (most common cause). B. Ureteral stone or bladder tumor selectively obstructing lower collecting system. C. Complete duplication with ureteropelvic-junction obstruction of lower moiety. D. Partial duplication with ureteropelvic-junction obstruction of lower moiety at point where ureter bifurcates.

moiety there is usually a prolonged, dense, segmental nephrogram involving approximately the lower two-thirds to three-fourths of the kidney. Delayed films will usually show subsequent opacification of the dilated lower-moiety collecting system. With longstanding, severe lower-moiety obstruction, dilation may be massive, and no function or only a thin, opacified rim of parenchyma is seen. Voiding cystourethrography should be performed to rule out reflux into the lower moiety as a cause of nonfunction or poor function when there is no evidence of an obstructive nephrogram. If delayed films during urography do not delineate the point of lower-moiety obstruction, retrograde ureteropyelography may be necessary for this purpose. CT has also been reported to be useful in evaluating patients with obstructed, duplicated systems [4].

REFERENCES

1. Amis, E.S., Jr., Cronan, J.J., and Pfister, R.C. Lower moiety hydronephrosis in duplicated kidneys. *Urology* 26:82, 1985.
2. Berdon, W.E., et al. Ectopic ureterocele. *Radiol. Clin. North Am.* 6:205, 1968.
3. Bisset, G.S., III, and Strife, J.L. The duplex collecting system in girls with urinary tract infection: Prevalence and significance. *A.J.R.* 148:497, 1987.
4. Cronan, J.J., et al. Obstruction of the upper-pole moiety in renal duplication in adults: CT evaluation. Radiology 161:17, 1986.
5. Friedland, G.W., and Cunningham, J. The elusive ectopic ureteroceles. *A.J.R.* 116:792, 1972.
6. Hartman, G.W., and Hodson, C.J. The duplex kidney and related abnormalities. *Clin. Radiol.* 20:387, 1969.
7. Lebowitz, R.L., and Avni, F.E., Misleading appearances in pediatric uroradiology. *Pediatr. Radiol.* 10:15, 1980.
8. Mackie, G.G., and Stephens, F.D. Duplex kidneys: A correlation of renal dysplasia with position of the ureteric orifice. *Birth Defects* 13:313, 1977.
9. Nussbaum, A.R., et al. Ectopic ureter and ureterocele: Their varied sonographic manifestations. *Radiology* 159:227, 1986.
10. Share, J.C., and Lebowitz, R.L. Ectopic ureterocele without ureteral and calyceal dilatation (ureterocele disproportion): Findings on urography and sonography. *A.J.R.* 152:567, 1989.

The Ureter

The ureters are muscular tubes whose function is to conduct urine from the renal pelves to the bladder. They undergo active peristalsis; the functional combination of descending contraction waves that completely occlude the ureteral lumen with the one-way valve mechanism at the ureterovesical junction serves also to keep the pressure of urine within the renal calices low, even during periods of relatively high bladder pressure. This function is at least as important as that of urine transport since it protects the renal medulla from elevations in caliceal urine pressure, which would be detrimental to renal function.

The ureter is subject to a number of innate diseases [28] and, by virtue of its considerable length and the great number of structures that are anatomically close to it, is affected by a number of periureteral conditions. Not all of these are described in this chapter. Most congenital abnormalities are discussed in Chaps. 5 and 18. Certain retroperitoneal conditions, such as retroperitoneal fibrosis, primary and secondary retoperitoneal tumors, and pelvic lipomatosis are discussed in Chaps. 6 and 20. Upper urinary tract stone disease is discussed in Chap. 15, trauma of the ureter in Chap. 25, vesicoureteral reflux in Chap. 17, and tuberculosis and schistosomiasis in Chap. 11. The generic effects on the ureter of ureteral obstruction are found in Chaps. 16 and 20. Finally, ureteral alterations caused by surgery are treated in Chap. 26.

URETERAL COURSE

The normal ureter begins at its junction with the renal pelvis, which is either at or just inferior to the renal hilus. The most proximal part of the ureter courses inferiorly, usually immediately adjacent to the anteromedial surface of the inferior half of the kidney. It runs through retroperitoneal fat, initially at the lateral border of the superior portion of the psoas muscle. Farther inferiorly, the ureter climbs to the anterior portion of the psoas muscle. Urography in an anteroposterior projection usually reveals the midureter to be superimposed on the lateral portions of the transverse processes of the vertebral bodies; however, the side-to-side position of the ureter is normally quite variable, and it may run as far medially as the vertebral pedicles or be lateral to the transverse processes.

More inferiorly, the ureter courses anteriorly to the common iliac vessels. Within the true pelvis, the ureter courses posterolaterally and then anteromedially to reach the ureterovesical junctions. Anteroposterior views at urography show the distal third of the ureter to parallel the medial margin of the iliac bone.

The course of the ureter may display a variety of anatomic variations. These are, for the most part, clinically insignificant, but it is important to be aware of them so they are not mistaken for manifestations of disease. In patients with ptotic kidneys (which may be idiopathic or produced by severe lumbar spine compression from osteoporosis and fractures or caused by flattened diaphragms caused in turn by chronic obstructive pulmonary disease), the ureter may be seen to be tortuous in its proximal course. Tortuous ureters may undergo relatively sharp bends, and at points of maximum curvature they may seem to have webs or kinks traversing them. These kinks, although they appear at urography as though they ought to obstruct the ureter, do not do so and are merely a normal variant. Unusually large psoas muscles, which are sometimes present in athletic or heavily muscled men, may deviate the course of the ureter [4]; in this case, the proximal ureter lies at the lateral margin of the muscle but then jogs medially to a position anterior to the middle portion of the psoas muscle; the proximal ureters are thus seen to be laterally deviated while their middle portions are medially deviated.

A number of pathologic conditions may alter the course of the ureter. Space-occupying lesions that arise from the medial aspect of the lower renal poles may deflect the ureters medially. Retroperitoneal lymphadenopathy may deflect the ureters either focally and subtly or markedly and over a long portion of their course. Lymphadenopathy usually deflects the proximal ureter laterally (Fig. 19-1) and the pelvic portions of the ureter medially; the midureters may be displaced anteriorly by massive retroperitoneal lymphadenopathy.

Abdominal aortic aneurysms may alter the course of the ureter [32]. Usually, the left ureter is involved; the aneurysm (or, in the case of a leaking aneurysm, its attendant hematoma) may push the left ureter laterally. As the ureter crosses the iliac arteries, it may be displaced anteriorly if the arteries are markedly tortuous (Fig. 19-2). If they are sufficiently large, aneurysms of the common, internal, or external iliac arteries may displace the ureters as well.

Figure 19-1. Carcinoma of the prostate with malignant lymphadenopathy deviating the left ureter. Urography shows the left proximal ureter to be deviated laterally (arrows) but not obstructed. The prostate is enlarged and irregular and has directly invaded and partially obstructed the right vesicoureteral junction.

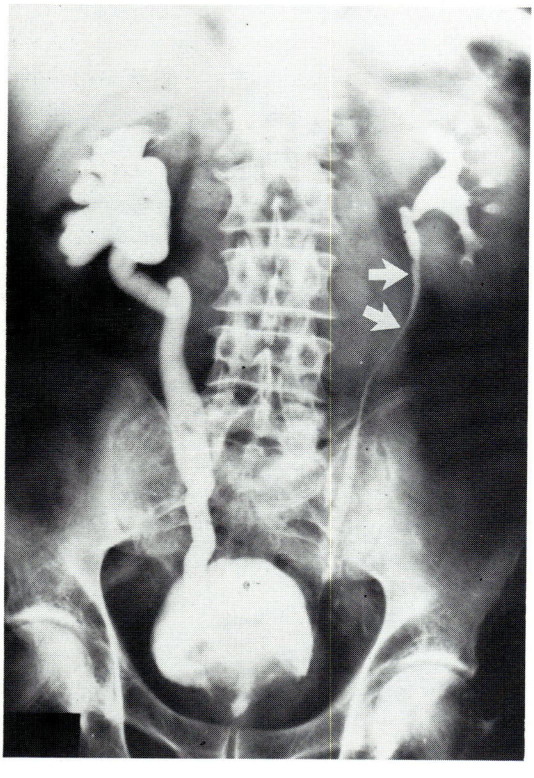

Deviations of the ureter caused by other retroperitoneal masses, by retroperitoneal fibrosis, by surgery, and by certain congenital anomalies are discussed elsewhere.

VARIATIONS IN URETERAL DIAMETER

Ureteral peristalsis often produces variations in luminal diameter seen on intravenous urography. The normal contraction wave of peristalsis completely coapts the ureteral wall so that no contrast material can be seen in the portion of the ureter that is contracting. The relaxed ureter proximal and distal to a contraction wave contains contrast material and may be as wide as 8 mm in normal diameter. In some patients, a segment of the middle third of the ureter superior to the crossing of the iliac vessels may be slightly dilated normally (Fig. 19-3); this appearance is called the "midureteral spindle." The most distal portion of the ureter—that is, the last centimeter or so, which traverses the bladder wall—is usually less distensible than the remainder of the ureter and may dilate to a maximum of 2 to 3 mm in diameter. When a bolus of urine is pushed across the distal ureter by a peristaltic wave, it may form a narrow jet as it squirts into the bladder lumen; if this jet contains more contrast material than the urine in the lumen, it may be visualized either on urography or CT; the ureteral jet has been seen on ultrasonography as well.

PRIMARY MEGAURETER

The term *primary megaureter* refers to a condition in which part or all of the ureter is dilated because of a particular abnormality that involves only the most distal portion of the ureter [27]. The condition does not include megaureters caused by reflux, by most acquired lesions that obstruct the ureter, or by intrinsic abnormalities of the dilated portion of the ureteral wall (such as that seen in the prune-belly syndrome). A bewildering array of names has been attached to this condition, including megaloureter, aperistaltic megaloureter, ureteral achalasia, and a host of others.

The abnormality that appears to be common to all cases of primary megaureter involves the

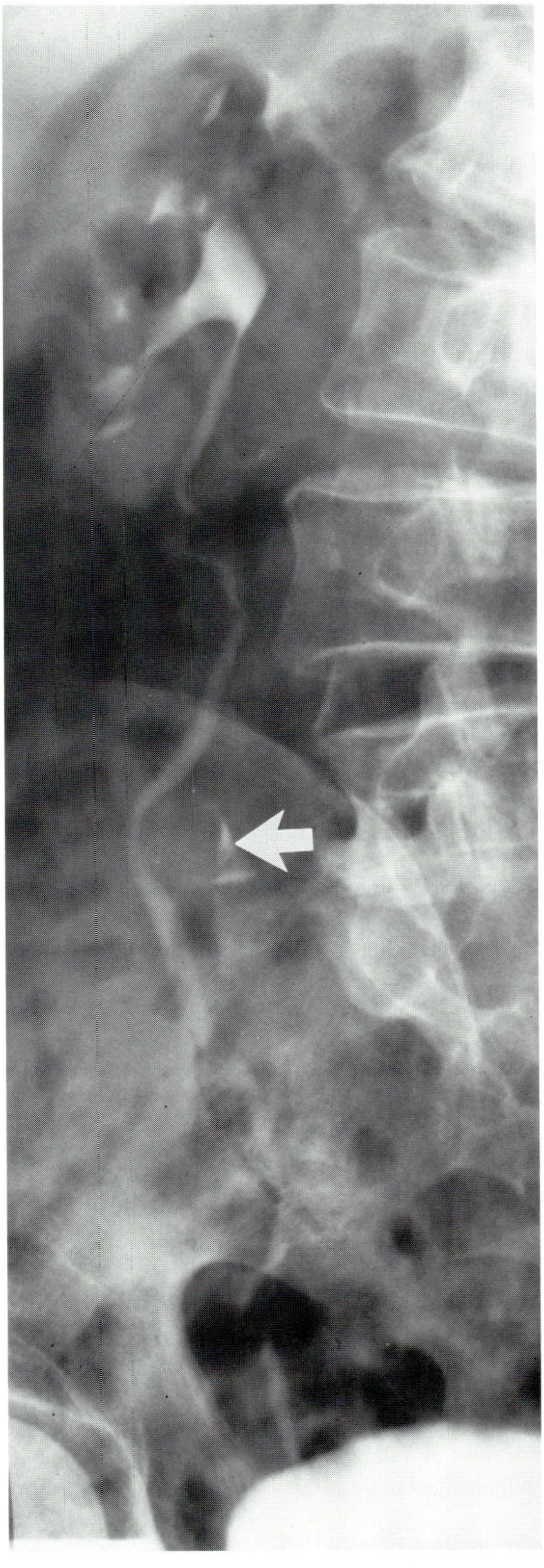

Figure 19-2. Right ureter deviated by tortuous common iliac artery. Urography shows the calcification (arrow) in the posterior part of the artery. The right ureter is deviated anteriorly as it crosses the vessel.

Figure 19-3. Midureteral spindle. Intravenous urography reveals mild fusiform dilation of the right midureter.

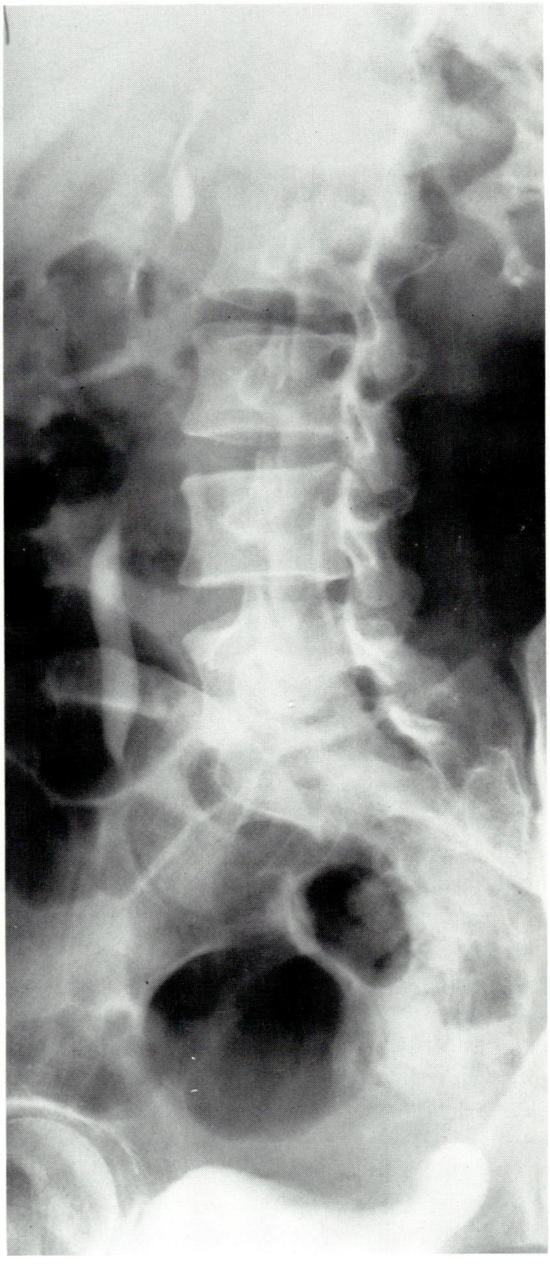

musculature of the most distal ureter; the involved segment ranges from a few millimeters to several centimeters in length. This segment does not appear to be able to dilate to accept the full width of a bolus of urine as it is propelled from above; neither does it appear to conduct the phase of the peristaltic wave in which the muscle contracts to coapt the ureteral walls. Abnormalities in the ureteral wall [38] are noted in all cases, but they vary in type. The total amount of ureteral musculature may be normal or diminished, the orientation of the individual muscle cells may be abnormal, and there may be an abnormally large amount of fibrous tissue or collagen present [16]. The ureter immediately proximal to this segment is dilated, and the dilated segment tapers smoothly into the aperistaltic portion. The dilated portion may extend a variable length proximally along the ureter. It may involve only a distal segment of the ureter or may involve most of the ureter but leave the proximal portion and collecting system looking normal or may even extend as far proximally as the calices. Usually, the more distal dilated segment is wider than the more proximal portions. Occasionally, caliectasis may be seen without dilation of the proximal ureter and renal pelvis but with dilation of the more distal segment of the ureter.

If the ureters are observed fluoroscopically in cases in which the proximal ureter is not dilated at all, the proximal segment displays normal peristalsis. As the contraction wave proceeds down the ureter, it becomes progressively weaker. Within the dilated segment of the ureter the contraction wave becomes harder to see and fails to bring the walls of the ureter together. The contraction wave does not pass through the aperistaltic distal segment at all, so that the bolus of urine propelled distally from the proximal ureter does not get swept entirely into the bladder but merely adds to the urine in the dilated distal segment, from which a disorganized trickle presumably passes through the aperistaltic distal segment into the bladder.

Many cases of primary megaureter were noted by early investigators to have an aperistaltic distal segment that could be catheterized by a standard catheter; the distal segment was therefore presumed not to be obstructed. These tended to be the cases in which caliectasis and dilation of the proximal ureter were less severe. Subsequent examination with ureteral perfusion confirmed that these ureters were not obstructed. This group of patients is said to have primary nonobstructive megaureter. But in other cases, ureteral catheterization suggests that the aperistaltic segment is indeed narrower than normal; ureteral perfusion suggests that this group has a distal aperistaltic segment that is sufficiently stenotic to produce a partial obstruction. These patients tend to have more severe dilation of the ureter proximal to the aperistaltic segment, and the dilation tends to extend as far proximally as the calices. The kidneys themselves may show evidence of obstructive atrophy or dysplasia.

Patients with this condition may be asymptomatic or present with clinical evidence of infection, ureteral stones, or pain. In addition to the stones and infection, clinical complications include obstructive damage to the ipsilateral kidney.

Urography (intravenous, antegrade, or retrograde) reveals a characteristic ureteral morphology (Fig. 19-4). There is a distal aperistaltic relatively nondistensible segment, ranging from slightly less than a centimeter to several centimeters in length; this segment usually involves the intramural segment of the ureter and the segment immediately proximal to it. The condition may be bilateral; when it is unilateral, it more frequently appears on the left. The condition may be suggested by ultrasonographic findings of a dilated distal ureter [43] that tapers to an aperistaltic distal segment and that is associated with either no caliectasis in the ipsilateral kidney or caliectasis that is less severe than the degree of distal ureterectasis would suggest. CT findings have not been described, but it is reasonable to assume that when the ureter is opacified it will be demonstrated on CT to have dilation that progresses in severity as the CT images progress from the proximal to the distal ureter, with the possible demonstration of a relatively narrow short terminal segment.

URETERECTASIS OF PREGNANCY

Pyelocaliectasis and ureterectasis commonly accompany normal pregnancy [39]. The condition may appear at any time during pregnancy but is commonly seen at about 20 weeks of

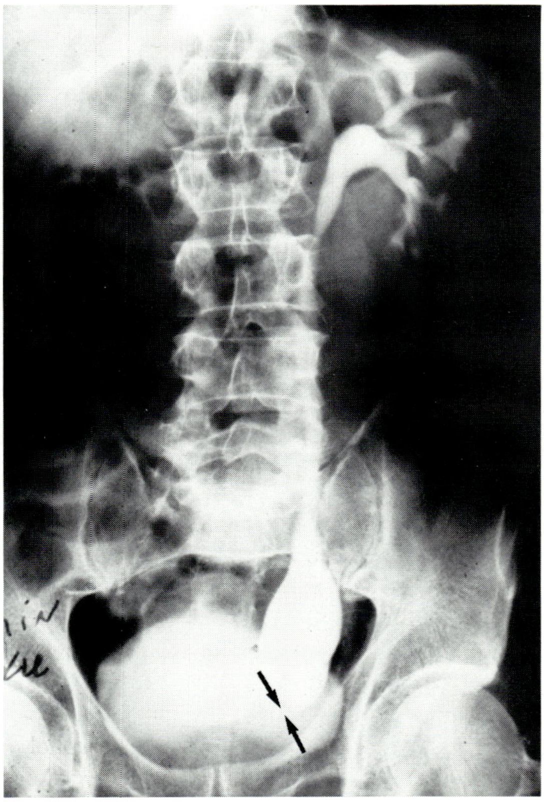

Figure 19-4. Primary megaureter. There is narrowing of the most distal centimeter of the left ureter (arrows); the ureter immediately superior to this segment is dilated, and it tapers smoothly into a nondilated proximal ureter. The right kidney is congenitally absent.

gestation. Dilation is seen more commonly and is usually more severe on the right; by the end of pregnancy, the right side is dilated in almost all patients and the left side in a majority of patients. It has been postulated that changing levels of circulating hormones are at least in part responsible for the ureterectasis, but since the ureters are not dilated distal to the pelvic inlet, this theory does not seem entirely plausible. More likely is compression of the ureters against the bony pelvis by the enlarged uterus. Probably, mild differences in the relationship between the uterus and the right and left common iliac arteries are responsible for the bilateral asymmetry of dilation. The degree of dilation is usually mild and almost never produces lasting morphologic change or renal damage; the upper urinary tract of most patients returns to normal within a couple of months after childbirth. Both intravenous and retrograde urography have been used to demonstrate this condition; ultrasonography may demonstrate progressive caliectasis during pregnancy as well [26].

BENIGN EPITHELIAL DISEASE OF THE URETER

URETERITIS CYSTICA

Ureteritis cystica consists of multiple small cysts in the epithelial or subepithelial portions of the ureter [23]. The lesions are thought to be the result of inflammation, and a prior or current urinary tract infection can usually be documented in patients who have the condition. It is usually seen in middle-aged adults, it has a predilection for the proximal ureter, and it may also be associated with stone disease. When the condition involves the renal pelvis as well (as it not infrequently does), it is called pyeloureteritis cystica.

Although the discovery of the lesion should prompt a workup for urinary infection, the condition itself has little intrinsic significance. The lesions do not obstruct the ureter, and they are not premalignant; they may, however, cause microscopic hematuria. They may or may not resolve when any associated infection is treated.

The lesions consist of small cysts lined with epithelial cells. They are most commonly a few millimeters in diameter. They may rest primarily within the wall of the ureter, existing within the lamina propria, or may protrude into the ureteral lumen and appear nearly pedunculated in configuration. The nature of the fluid within the cyst varies: It may be clear or not, may be thin or viscous, and may contain evidence of hemorrhage. It is usually not infected, however.

Ureterography—either intravenous or retrograde—is the primary method of establishing the diagnosis of ureteritis cystica. The condition appears as multiple small filling defects within the ureteral lumen (Fig. 19-5). The number may vary from a very few to many dozens; individual lesions may be isolated or clustered. As mentioned above, there is a tendency for the proximal ureter and pelvis to be affected. Although a group of lesions may produce a ragged appearance of the ureteral wall, each individual cyst has a smooth surface.

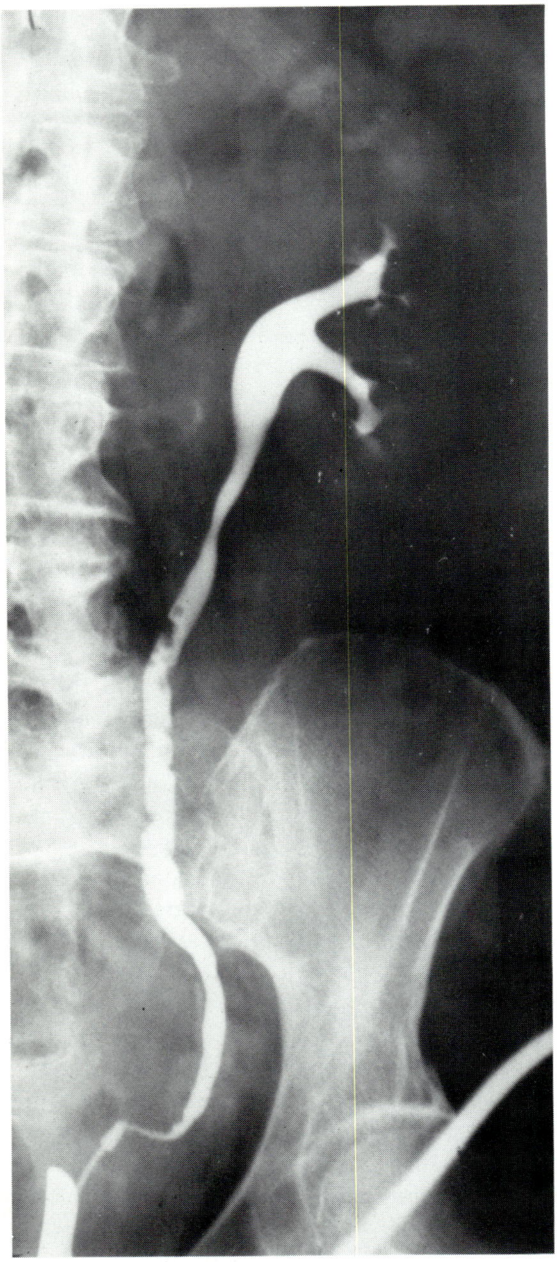

Figure 19-5. Ureteritis cystica. Retrograde ureteropyelography reveals multiple hemispherical filling defects in the midureter. This patient also has a left-upper-pole renal mass, which has deviated the superior calices laterally.

Multiple ureteral filling defects may require differential diagnosis, but ultimately the diagnosis of ureteritis cystica can usually be made with certainty. Air bubbles, introduced at retrograde pyelography may mimic pyeloureteritis cystica, but they usually can be shown to move, and unlike the cysts of ureteritis cystica, they cannot be shown to elevate the ureteral epithelium when viewed in tangent. Primary urothelial tumors are usually more irregular in surface outline and not as numerous as the cysts of ureteritis cystica, even when multiple. Crossing vessels that indent the ureter do not produce spherical or ovoid filling defects and are usually not as numerous as the cysts of ureteritis cystica. Although hemorrhage into the ureteral wall may produce multiple filling defects, accompanying evidence of trauma, venous occlusion, or bleeding diathesis usually exists, and unlike ureteritis cystica, the small ureteral hematomas usually resolve fairly quickly.

MALACOPLAKIA

Malacoplakia is a relatively rare condition, inflammatory in nature, which may appear in a number of sites but most frequently affects the urinary tract [13, 36]. The bladder is most frequently involved, with the kidney and ureter being affected next most frequently. There is a decided female predominance, and although the disease can be found at nearly any age, most patients are middle-aged.

The exact cause of the disease is not known, but it is thought to be a response to infection. Both the biochemistry and the pathology of the condition suggest that the inflammatory response is not one that usually follows urinary tract infection, however. Many patients who have malacoplakia have not only infection but an accompanying condition that causes compromise of the immune system.

In the ureter, malacoplakia produces yellow-brown plaques, which initially appear in the subepithelial region. The plaques are relatively soft, demonstrate peripheral hyperemia, and may ultimately form small central ulcerations. The lesions are usually multiple and tend to involve the distal ureter. They may cause strictures and ureteral obstruction but usually do not. The lesions consist of clusters of large mononuclear histiocytes, which have characteristic inclusions called Michaelis–Gutmann bodies; these small calcified bodies may also be found outside the histiocytes and have a lamellated appearance. Other kinds of inflammatory cells are also found. There are no clinical signs specific for malacoplakia. Patients have a lengthy history of urinary infection, usually with coliform bacteria. In cases in which malacoplakia has obstructed the ureter and caused renal obstruction, or in which the condition has destroyed all or part of the kidney directly, there may be only nonspecific symptoms referring to the renal disease.

Like ureteritis cystica, malacoplakia of the ureter is clinically diagnosed by intravenous or retrograde ureterography (Fig. 19-6). The lesions appear as ureteral filling defects whose surface may appear either convex or relatively flat. They are usually multiple and may coalesce, resulting in a cobblestone appearance

Figure 19-6. Ureteral malacoplakia; retrograde ureteropyelogram. The ureter is slightly dilated, and its margins are scalloped throughout its length. (Courtesy of Richard C. Pfister, M.D., Massachusetts General Hospital, Boston.)

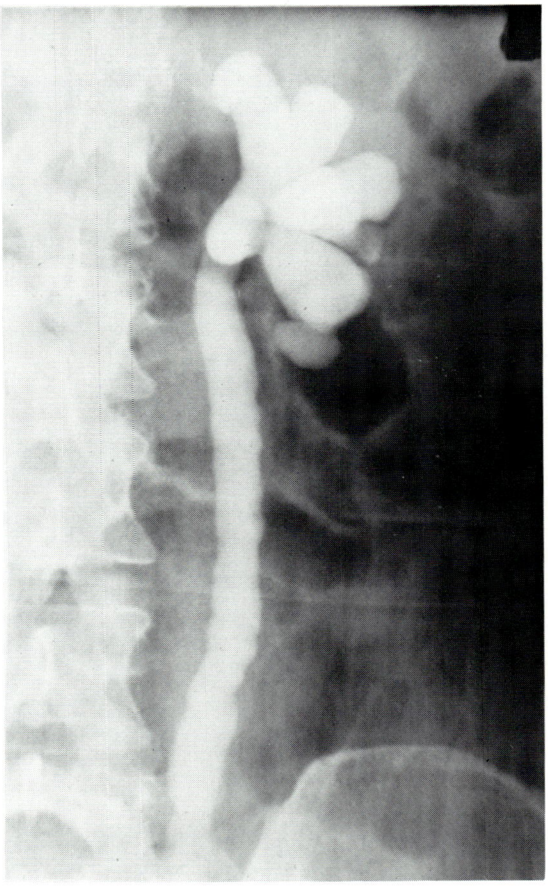

of the ureter. The ureter may be slightly dilated, even in the absence of a specific obstructing lesion; occasionally, malacoplakia may produce sufficient stenosis to cause more severe hydronephrosis or hydroureter and to interfere with or completely destroy the function of the associated kidney. The lesions may regress if treatment of the associated infection is successful, but there is an unfortunate tendency for the condition to reappear after therapy, sometimes in another part of the urinary tract.

The differential diagnosis of ureteral malacoplakia includes a number of conditions. Ureteritis cystica may look similar, but the lesions of ureteritis cystica are usually rounder and the ureter is rarely dilated. Tuberculosis may produce a thickening of the ureteral wall with focal stenoses. Malignant lesions of the ureter are rarely as widespread as malacoplakia.

LEUKOPLAKIA

Leukoplakia is a condition that may appear anywhere in the epithelium of the urinary tract; it is more common in the bladder than in the upper tracts and more common in the renal collecting system than in the ureter. It is a rare lesion, with no well-established sex or side predilection. It usually occurs in adults.

The abnormality consists of a squamous metaplasia of the urothelium with keratinization and a desquamation of the affected membrane [18]. Some investigators feel that it is the same lesion as that denoted by the term *cholesteatoma* [34]; others feel that there are subtle differences between the two. Disagreement also exists with regard to whether the lesion is a response of originally normal transitional epithelium to chronic irritation or whether it possibly consists of an embryonic rest of ectodermal tissues. The condition is almost always associated with chronic infection, irritation (as by a stone), or both. There is probably an association of leukoplakia with carcinoma of the upper tract [3].

Clinically, patients often have a history of longstanding stone disease, urinary infections, or symptoms of these conditions. They may have mild hematuria. Desquamated tissue may cause colic and may be recovered in the urine.

Radiographic manifestations vary. In the ureter and the remaining urinary tract the disease may present as an irregular filling defect. The defect may be small, or there may be irregular thickening of large areas of the collecting system, ureter, or both. The size and extent of the abnormality may progress slowly over a long period. The lesion itself or desquamated tissue arising from it may obstruct the ureter, producing various degrees of hydronephrosis and diminished function in the ipsilateral kidney. Descriptions of the abnormal findings exist only for intravenous or retrograde urography.

When a lesion is localized and appears as a filling defect, the major differential diagnosis is primary transitional cell carcinoma. Cases in which the lesion is more widespread may mimic malacoplakia or nonspecific ureteritis.

MURAL DISEASES

URETERAL DIVERTICULA

Radiographically demonstrable diverticula of the ureter are unusual and appear to fall into two distinct groups. One group consists of patients who demonstrate a single unilateral diverticulum. These abnormalities may appear at any level and probably constitute incomplete ureteral duplications. The diverticulum contains all layers of the normal ureteral wall, usually extends cephalad alongside the ureter from the point of connection, and contains a lumen that may be approximately the size of the normal ureter or considerably dilated. Diverticula are not associated with a dysplastic portion of the kidney, and when they are very long, they are usually called blind-ending duplications rather than diverticula. Complications such as stones or tumors forming within diverticula may occur but are exceedingly rare. Urographic manifestations are those that would be expected: The ureter demonstrates a Y-shaped branching with the blind-ending superior limb being either of equivalent diameter to the normal ureter or dilated.

The other kind of ureteral diverticula are called pseudodiverticula by some authors [40]; these are also rare. In this condition, hyperplastic buds of ureteral epithelium project outward from the ureteral lumen into—but usually not entirely through—the muscular layers of the ureteral wall [7]. The small diverticula that these epithelial buds form are usually multiple and often bilateral; commonly, they are no larger than approximately 2 mm in diameter. They may be associated with hematuria and a history of urinary infection but have no specific signs or symptoms. They are not thought to be premalignant, but in cases that have been reported, there is an unusually high association with transitional cell carcinoma, usually arising within the bladder. These diverticula are usually demonstrated by intravenous or retrograde urography. They consist of multiple small outpouchings extending from the ureteral lumen (Fig. 19-7); the ureter may be otherwise normal or may appear to be narrowed within

Figure 19-7. Ureteral diverticulosis. Retrograde ureterography reveals small diverticula (arrows) protruding from the ureteral lumen. The fusiform configuration of the ureter immediately distal to the diverticula is a midureteral spindle.

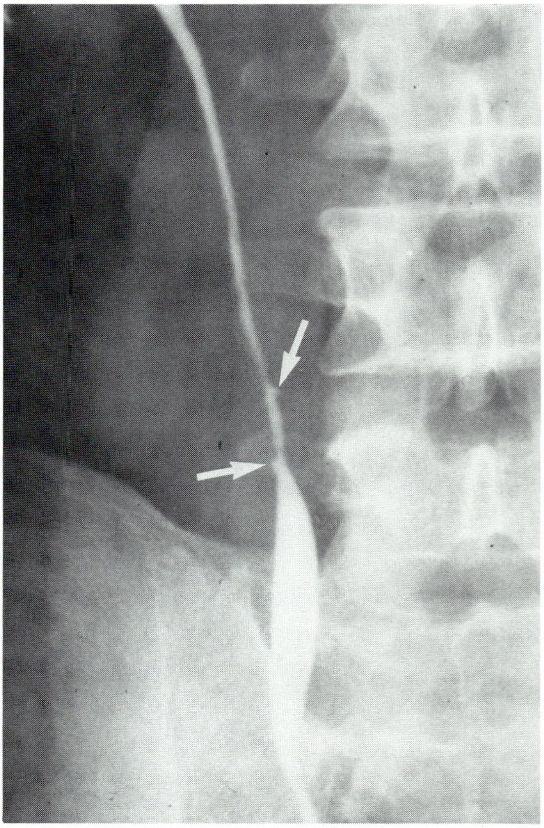

the segments that contain the diverticula. The diverticula are not associated with ureteral obstruction.

SUBUROTHELIAL HEMORRHAGE

Suburothelial hemorrhage is exceedingly rare; only a few cases have been reported [5]. It is distinct from the condition of ureteral displacement caused by retroperitoneal hematomas, and it apparently consists of hemorrhage within the wall of the ureter, usually associated with coagulopathies. The patients usually present with various degrees of hematuria. Urography reveals multiple filling defects projecting into the ureteral (or pyelocaliceal) lumen that are less discrete than those seen in pyeloureteritis cystica and that resolve spontaneously when the coagulopathy is corrected. CT [21] may reveal the focal urothelial thickening to be of relatively high attenuation, similar to that seen with hemorrhage elsewhere.

AMYLOIDOSIS

Ureteral amyloidosis is extremely rare [24, 42]. There are no specific findings; the patients usually have signs and symptoms of longstanding ureteral obstruction. Ureterography usually reveals an irregular, relatively lengthy ureteral narrowing; the images have no features that permit specific diagnosis.

URETEROPELVIC-JUNCTION OBSTRUCTION

Any pathologic process (such as tumor, postinflammatory stricture, stones, and so forth) that obstructs the ureter may occur at the proximal end of the ureter and cause ureteropelvic-junction obstruction. But there is a specific condition that is usually, if not always, congenital, that is due to an abnormality in the muscular ureteral wall, and that produces obstruction at the ureteropelvic junction [37]. This condition is the one usually referred to when a patient is said to have ureteropelvic-junction (UPJ) obstruction without mention of a specific cause; the condition is often called congenital hydronephrosis in Europe.

The primary abnormality involves the muscular wall [16]. At the UPJ, the muscle cells are diminished in number and overall volume and are often maloriented. There is an abnormally increased amount of interstitial collagen, which renders the UPJ relatively nondistensible. There may be histologic evidence of inflammatory change, but this is unusual. Proximal to the UPJ, the dilated renal pelvis is abnormal; the muscle cell layers may be either thinned or hypertrophic, and there may be an increased amount of collagen. Obstructive atrophy of the ipsilateral kidney ranges in degree from minimal to severe; the kidney may be markedly enlarged, and its function may range from nearly normal to virtually absent.

Inferior to the UPJ obstruction, the ureter is usually normal. Not infrequently, the main renal artery, an aberrant artery, or a renal artery branch may press against the UPJ. Whether the crossing vessel is responsible for the original narrowing or whether the distention of the renal pelvis causes its structure to drape over the artery (so that the artery appears to contribute secondarily to the obstruction) is not always clear. With or without a crossing vessel, the gross configuration of the UPJ is such that the ureter often emerges from the midportion of the spherical pelvis (a so-called high take-off) rather than appearing as the inferior continuation of the normally tapering renal pelvis.

Although the histologic changes at the UPJ suggest that the degree of stenosis should be observed to change very slowly, if at all, there are a few patients in whom the degree of obstruction appears to change quite rapidly. In some patients, a transient diuresis may distend the abnormal renal pelvis in such a way that the configuration of the UPJ is changed and obstruction becomes suddenly severe. In others, changes in body position may accomplish the same effect. In any case, both the symptoms and radiographic manifestations of congenital UPJ obstruction may acutely worsen and be just as quickly relieved.

In some patients who have dilated ureters and pelves due to vesicoureteral reflux or distal ureteral obstruction, the proximal ureter may become elongated, tortuous, and kinked. Often, a kink appears at the UPJ, so that it appears as if a UPJ obstruction exists in conjunction with a more distal ureteral abnormality. In these cases, it is often difficult to determine whether a UPJ obstruction really exists at all or is simply mimicked by the combination of a proximal ureteral kink and a dilated renal pelvis.

In addition to usually being congenital, this sort of UPJ obstruction may be familial. There is a definite increased incidence of the abnormality in siblings and parents of children with the disease. The condition is also associated with other urinary tract abnormalities; in particular, there is an increased incidence of multicystic dysplastic kidney as an abnormality involving the opposite side, which suggests that ureteral obstruction in utero, occurring in various degrees, constitutes a common cause of the two conditions.

The clinical presentation of congenital UPJ obstruction varies. It may be asymptomatic for many years; clearly, the less severe the condition, the more likely it is to be silent. It is one of the most common causes of palpable abdominal masses in infants. If UPJ obstruction is bilateral or associated with multicystic dysplastic kidney, it may present with uremia. Severely hydronephrotic kidneys are said to be more susceptible to injury when traumatized; congenital UPJ obstruction may become apparent when blunt abdominal or flank trauma produces hematuria or pain. Severely hydronephrotic kidneys are susceptible to forming stones; stones, in turn, may produce hematuria or acute exacerbations of the UPJ obstruction and so come to clinical attention. The affected kidneys are also more likely to become infected, and pyelonephritis or obstructive pyonephrosis may be the episode that brings the underlying condition to attention.

Even in the absence of complications, chronic abdominal or flank pain may be the presenting sign of congenital UPJ obstruction. In the small fraction of patients in whom the obstruction is transient, acute pain associated either with diuresis or particular body positions may prompt the workup that reveals the lesion.

The manifestations of congenital UPJ obstruction on imaging examinations depend in part on the severity of the obstruction. The affected kidney may be normal in size or enlarged. The parenchyma is reduced in volume; this may range in severity from mild papillary flattening to obstructive atrophy so severe that only a shell of parenchyma a few millimeters thick remains. If contrast medium is administered intravenously, the renal findings at urography or CT are those of chronic obstruction (these are reviewed in greater detail in Chap. 16). In the small group of patients in whom the obstruction changes rapidly in degree, findings of acute obstruction may be superimposed.

The calices are uniformly dilated, and the renal pelvis is distended (Fig. 19-8); in some patients the pelvic dilation may seem disproportionately severe as compared with the degree of caliectasis. The UPJ itself may appear narrowed, and the junction is often placed near the equator of the renal pelvis rather than at its inferior margin. The ureter is not dilated; the

Figure 19-8. Congenital UPJ obstruction. Antegrade pyelography reveals dilated renal pelvis and calices. There is transient complete obstruction: no contrast medium is flowing into the ureter.

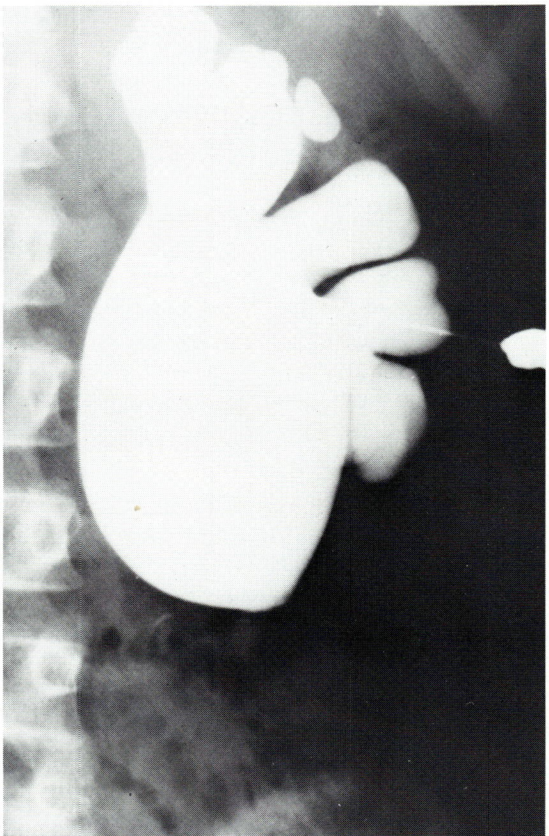

proximal ureter may be displaced medially by the enlarged pelvis. Sonography and radionuclide scintigraphy reveal the findings of chronic hydronephrosis without hydroureter; these findings often fail to distinguish congenital UPJ obstruction from other conditions causing obstruction at the UPJ or proximal ureter. Ureteral perfusion reveals an elevated ureteral resistance; in the occasional patient in whom diuresis or particular body positions cause transient increases in the degree of obstruction, antegrade pyelography with ureteral perfusion may demonstrate complete occlusion at the UPJ.

TUMORS OF THE URETER

PRIMARY CARCINOMA

Primary carcinomas of the ureter are usually transitional cell carcinomas [15]; squamous cell carcinomas are much less common, and adenocarcinomas are vanishingly rare [2]. Primary carcinoma appears less frequently in the ureter than in the renal collecting system, and all primary carcinomas of the upper tract are much less frequent than primary carcinomas of the bladder.

The important concepts regarding the biology of primary ureteral tumors are similar to those of primary carcinomas of the intrarenal collecting system and bladder, and they will not be entirely represented here. Some features are worthy of review, however. Ureteral carcinomas are more frequently found in the distal than in the proximal ureter, although they can appear at any level. At least half of patients with squamous cell carcinoma have had a lengthy history of stone disease, and many have had leukoplakia or squamous metaplasia. Patients with chronic schistosomiasis, which has a predilection for involving the distal ureters, are at risk for squamous cell carcinomas developing in this region.

A variety of signs and symptoms may herald a ureteral carcinoma; most frequently, hematuria is present. If the carcinoma obstructs the ureter, the hydronephrotic kidney may produce pain and, if sufficiently large, may be palpable. Obviously, distant metastases produce symptoms determined primarily by their location; metastases appear in the lung, mediastinum, liver, skeleton, and other sites.

Both the stage and grade of ureteral tumors are important in determining therapy and in prognosis. Some investigators feel that the lowest grade of tumors, when polypoid, represent benign papillomas; others regard these as true malignancies, albeit of low metastatic potential. The staging of ureteral carcinomas is given in Table 19-1 [41].

Patients who have been treated for transitional cell carcinoma of the ureter have a 20-fold increase in the likelihood of acquiring a subsequent transitional cell carcinoma of the bladder and a smaller increase in the likelihood of acquiring a tumor in the contralateral or (if the patient has been treated by segmental ureteral resection) ipsilateral upper tract [17].

Urography, either intravenous or retrograde, is the primary method of detecting ureteral carcinoma. The appearance depends on the size and extent of the tumor. When the tumors are quite small, they may appear as intraluminal filling defects and may be round, lobulated, or irregular. An intraluminal tumor may grow, and the resulting mass effect may distend the ureter surrounding it (Fig. 19-9A), when tumors like this are outlined by retrograde ureterography, the opacified normal–caliber ureter distal to the tumor and the distended but centrally tumor-filled ureter around the inferior margin of the tumor may produce a classic appearance known as a goblet sign or Bergman's sign (Fig. 19-9B). Alternatively, the tumor may appear primarily mural and initially look like a thickened irregularity of the ureteral wall. Tumors may encircle the ureter and produce a napkin-ring or apple-core appearance similar to that produced by some carcinomas in the alimentary tract. The tumors may obstruct the

Table 19-1. Staging of transitional cell carcinoma in the ureter

Stage A	Tumor restricted to mucosa or lamina propria
Stage B	Tumor invades, but does not extend through, ureteral muscle
Stage C	Tumor invades periureteral fat
Stage D	Tumor invades periureteral structures, or distant metastases have occurred

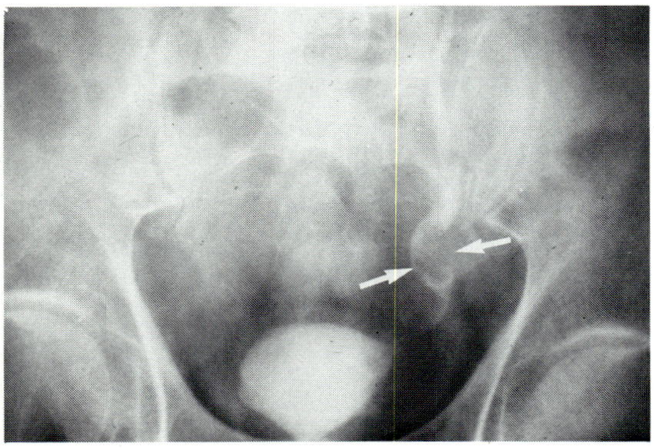

A

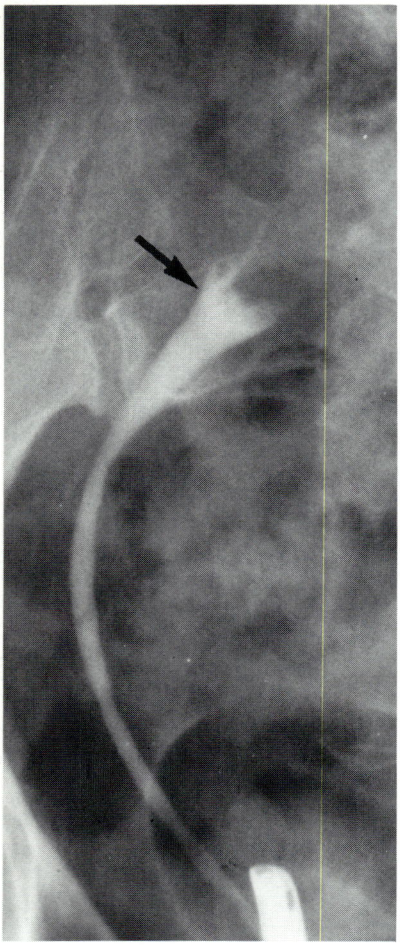

B

Figure 19-9. Polypoid transitional cell carcinoma of the ureter. A. Urography shows this tumor to be a lucent filling defect (arrows) that has distended the ureter around it but has not produced obstruction. B. In another patient, retrograde ureterography shows the classic goblet sign (arrow) below a ureteral tumor.

ureter so that intravenous urography reveals the ipsilateral kidney to be hydronephrotic to various degrees and to have diminished or absent function.

The differential diagnosis of the polypoid intraluminal variety of tumor includes a number of conditions [6, 14]. Uric acid stones may look like intraluminal filling defects; demonstrating that these can be dislodged or that they cast ultrasonic shadows or that they are denser than soft tissue when imaged by CT may permit the differential diagnosis. Clots within the ureter may mimic tumors; they may be distinguished by demonstrating that they resolve spontaneously within a few days or a few weeks. Sloughed papillae are usually associated with evidence in the kidney of papillary necrosis (although the coexistence of papillary necrosis and urothelial tumors in patients with analgesic abuse or Balkan nephropathy may be confusing); there may also be pieces of sloughed papillae in the urine. Intramural hemorrhage may be diagnosed by clinical means and by demonstrating spontaneous resolution. Fibroepithelial polyps usually have a smoother surface than carcinoma. Squamous cell carcinoma has no features to distinguish it from transitional cell carcinoma radiographically, but squamous cell carcinoma is less likely to form a polypoid tumor.

Ultrasonography very rarely directly demonstrates a ureteral tumor, although it may display the hydronephrosis that such a tumor produces. CT is primarily useful in evaluating the tumor once urography has revealed its location [20]. It shows the tumor to be a tissue-density mass that may represent an intraluminal filling defect (Fig. 19-10) or an irregular mass involving the wall of the ureter. The rare very large ureteral tumor will produce a CT appearance of an irregular retroperitoneal mass involving the ureter, and may be difficult to distinguish from other retroperitoneal malignancies. CT cannot distinguish Stage A from Stage B ureteral tumors, but it can distinguish Stage A and Stage B tumors from tumors of more advanced stage with reasonable accuracy. Sources of error include periureteral edema, which mimics tumor invasion, and microscopic periureteral fat invasion, which is altogether invisible to CT. CT of

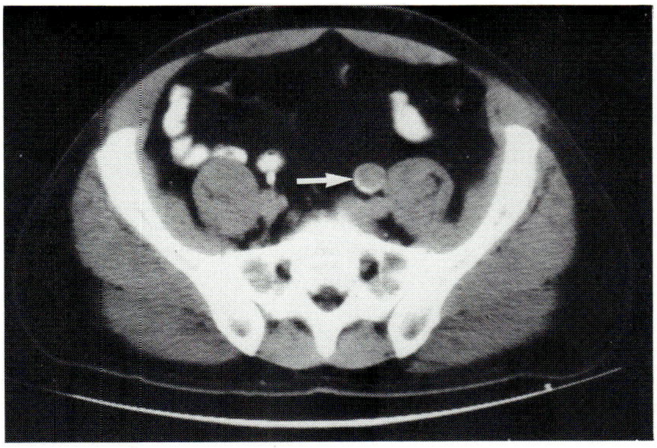

Figure 19-10. Polypoid left ureteral transitional cell carcinoma. CT reveals the tumor as a tissue-density lesion that has distended the left ureter; a rim of contrast material (arrow) surrounds the lesion.

patients who have ureteral tumors should include the entire retroperitoneum, in order to demonstrate any retroperitoneal lymphadenopathy, and should also include the liver and adrenals. At the least, workup for patients with ureteral carcinoma ought to include chest roentgenography; chest CT is probably more sensitive in detecting pulmonary and mediastinal metastases. Radionuclide skeletal imaging should be routinely obtained to search for bony metastases.

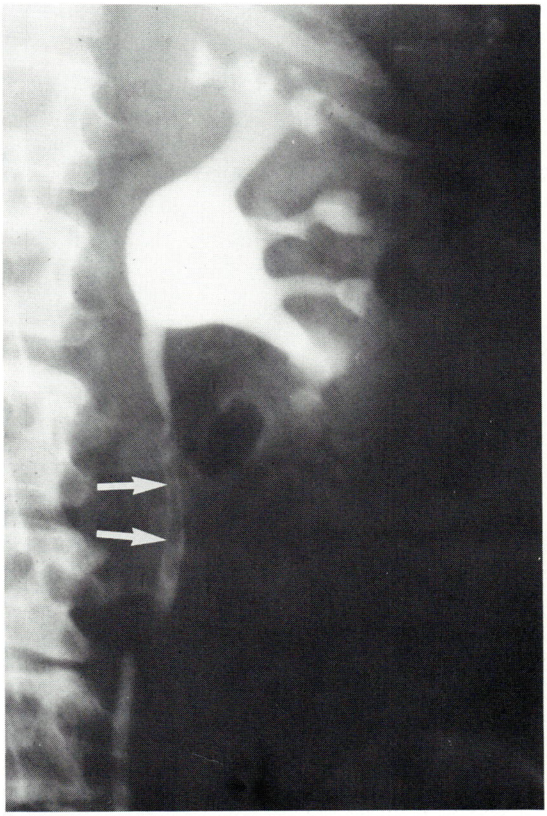

Figure 19-11. Fibroepithelial ureteral polyp. Urography shows this lesion to be a linear lucent filling defect (arrows) in the proximal ureter.

MESENCHYMAL TUMORS

Sarcomas of the ureteral wall are quite rare; leiomyosarcomas [31], spindle cell sarcomas, hemangiosarcomas, and lymphosarcomas have been described. They are usually relatively far advanced when discovered, and their imaging appearance is not significantly different from that of quite large primary ureteral carcinomas.

FIBROEPITHELIAL POLYPS

Fibroepithelial polyps are relatively unusual [9, 12]. They consist of fingerlike polyps with a central fibrovascular stroma covered by benign urothelium. They may be asymptomatic or may bleed slightly; they only rarely cause significant ureteral obstruction and have no known malignant potenial. Young or middle-aged adults are most likely to be affected.

Fibroepithelial polyps are virtually always diagnosed by intravenous or retrograde ureterography or both. Their imaging appearance is either that of a long slender smooth filling defect within the ureteral lumen (Fig. 19-11) or a bulkier lesion, which may have several fingerlike projections. Their appearance in the renal pelvis is extremely rare.

Differential diagnosis of these lesions consists of vermiform clots in the ureteral lumen (which can usually be distinguished by their tendency to resolve spontaneously) and the occasional pedunculated transitional cell carcinoma or papilloma that adopts an elongated configuration. Since fibroepithelial polyps require only local excision, distinction between them and primary transitional cell tumors is important; the distinction may be made by noting that neither exfoliative cytologic studies of the urine nor brush biopsies yield malignant cells from fibroepithelial polyps.

SECONDARY TUMORS INVOLVING THE URETER

The course of the ureter places it at risk for involvement by a number of malignancies arising in other structures [30]. The ureters may be directly invaded by tumors that arise adjacent to them, may be displaced or encased by malignant lymphadenopathy (Fig. 19-12), or may be the site of metastasis from distant tumors.

Primary carcinoma of the bladder, prostate, rectum, and cervix may all directly invade and obstruct the ureter. The specific appearances of these tumors will not be reiterated here. In patients who are known to have extensive primary carcinomas arising from these structures and in whom urography, ultrasonography or nuclear medicine demonstrates distal ureteral obstruction it is safe to assume that the tumors have directly invaded the ureters even when the imaging examination does not permit direct visualization of the neoplasm. Patients in whom follow-up examinations reveal the onset of ureteral obstruction after radiation therapy may have radiation-induced ureteral fibrosis [35], but, in general, the normal ureter is relatively radiation resistant, so postradiation ureteral obstruction much more frequently heralds recurrent tumor.

Retroperitoneal lymphadenopathy caused by metastatic malignancy is also described elsewhere in this textbook, and it may be directly demonstrated by CT, MRI or lymphangiography. Ureters that are opacified on intravenous or retrograde urography may be seen to be displaced by these enlarged nodes. Nodal enlargement rarely produces high-grade obstruction of the ureters unless the tumor has escaped from the nodes and directly invaded the ureteral walls. Ureterography may demonstrate lateral, anterolateral, or posterolateral displacement of the proximal two-thirds of the ureter by enlarged nodes; the pelvic ureter is usually displaced medially, anteromedially, or posteromedially by lymphadenopathy. In addition to carcinomas of the bladder, prostate, and cervix, lymphomas and testicular malignancies also commonly produce retroperitoneal lymphadenopathy. Less frequently, carcinoma of the lung, breast, colon, and stomach may metastasize to retroperitoneal nodes and displace the ureters.

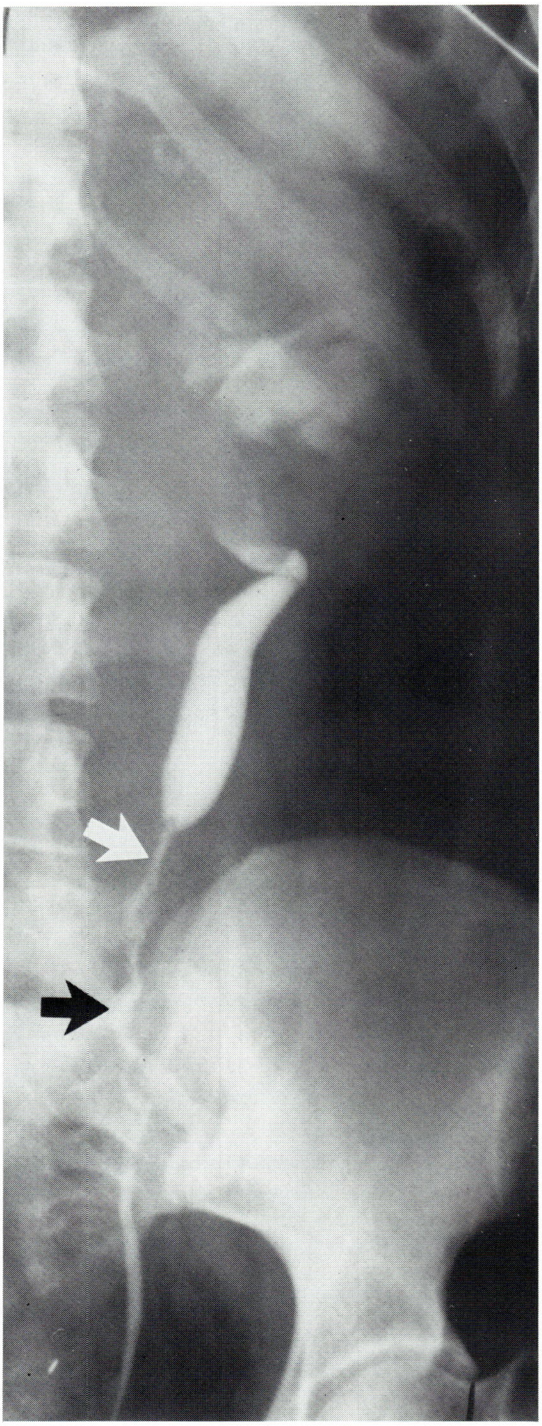

Figure 19-12. Metastatic retroperitoneal carcinoma involving the left ureter. The midureter is irregularly encased and narrowed (arrows); the proximal ureter is dilated. Insufficient contrast agent has been injected in this retrograde study to opacify the intrarenal collecting system entirely.

In addition to the tumors mentioned above, all of which may metastasize directly to the ureteral wall or immediate periureteral tissue, melanoma has also been described as occasionally metastasizing directly to the ureteral wall.

MISCELLANEOUS PERIURETERAL CONDITIONS

ENDOMETRIOSIS

Endometriosis is a condition of women of childbearing age in which endometrial tissue develops outside the endometrial cavity of the uterus. It undergoes the same cyclic changes that orthotopic endometrial tissue does, and the periodic necrosis and hemorrhage that occurs with the ectopic tissue produces hemorrhagic cystic lesions. These may appear within the myometrium; on the surface of the uterus, ovaries, or fallopian tubes; and on the peritoneal surfaces of other pelvic organs and the pelvic sidewalls. It has been proposed that the ectopic endometrial tissue represents either embryonic rests or an acquired condition in which retrograde menstruation through the fallopian tubes deposits endometrial tissues on the peritoneal surfaces. The most common presenting symptoms are infertility and severe pelvic pain with menstruation. The endometriomas themselves may be difficult to visualize if they are small; if they are of moderate or large size they display the characteristics of hemorrhagic cystic lesions or soft-tissue masses whether they are imaged by ultrasonography, CT, or MRI.

Rarely, endometriosis may involve the distal ureter [19, 22]. An endometrioma may arise near the ureter and, by expanding, obstruct it [14]; less frequently, endometriomas actually involve or invade the ureteral wall itself. Under these circumstances, if the ureter is opacified it may be seen to be obstructed; the narrowed region often reveals a short smooth tapering, and there may be evidence of ureteral displacement at the narrowed region if the endometrioma is sufficently large. If the clinical history is consistent with endometriosis, and if multiple endometriomas are seen along with a mass adjacent to the obstructed portion of the ureter, the diagnosis should be strongly suspected.

INTESTINAL INFLAMMATORY DISEASE

The pathology, clinical picture, and imaging characteristics of Crohn's disease and diverticulitis are beyond the scope of this book. Infrequently, either condition may affect the ureter, however [10, 33].

Ureteral involvement by Crohn's disease is usually on the right. Fistulae from the distal small bowel may produce abscesses that, in turn, impinge on the right ureter, displacing or obstructing it (or both). Occasionally, focal inflammation may involve the ureter even in the absence of a well-formed abscess. The ureter may be locally displaced, compressed and obstructed, or both. Ureterography usually demonstrates a smooth compression of the ureter with or without ureteral displacement by a mass. Although the specific appearance of the ureter does not permit the exact diagnosis, when the ureteral abnormality appears in a patient with known Crohn's disease the diagnosis is usually apparent.

A small fraction of patients with diverticulitis have involvement of the ureters; this usually occurs on the left side. As with Crohn's disease, there is a focus of inflammation or frank abscess that appears adjacent to the involved bowel and that, if appropriately located, may involve the ureter. Again, the ureter is displaced or compressed by the mass, and specific diagnosis depends on the clinical or imaging diagnosis of a diverticular abscess.

VASCULAR IMPRESSIONS ON THE URETER

The abdominal aorta, inferior vena cava, ovarian veins, and periureteral collaterals may all affect the ureter. The retrocaval ureter is described in Chap. 5.

Aneurysms of the abdominal aorta usually protrude to the left and may deflect the left ureter laterally. Aneurysms rarely, if ever, obstruct ureters, but if they hemorrhage and a pseudoaneurysm forms, the ureter may be involved in the wall of the pseudoaneurysm and become partially obstructed. Aneurysms or tortuosity of the common iliac arteries may deflect the more distal portions of the ureter on either side in an anterior direction.

Occasionally, intravenous or retrograde ureterography will reveal that the ureter is indented by a crossing vessel. This phenomenon usually occurs in the proximal portion of the ureter and very rarely obstructs the ureter (although, as we have seen, a crossing vessel may be the cause of partial UPJ obstruction). Usually, these crossing vessels are not of clinical significance. Occasionally, however, in patients with severe renal artery stenosis, the ureteral artery may enlarge to form a collateral for blood supply to the kidney, and the impingement of these collaterals on the ureteral wall may be a sign of renal artery stenosis. There have been reports of cases of renal vein thrombosis in which the developing collaterals produce ureteral notching (Fig. 19-13).

Ovarian Vein Syndrome
A sizable literature exists about the possibility that the right ovarian vein may compress the ureter and cause it to be mildly obstructed, that this phenomenon becomes more severe during pregnancy, that it may persist after pregnancy, and that it may be exacerbated by thrombosis of the right ovarian vein. Reasonably well documented case reports have demonstrated situations in which severe thrombosis of the right ovarian vein [1, 8, 25] have compressed the ureter and produced mild hydronephrosis, but reliable evidence that the nonthrombosed vein may significantly affect the ureter is lacking [11]. In the later stages of pregnancy it is much more likely that the gravid uterus compresses the ureter between itself and the right iliac vessels and that the ovarian veins have little or nothing to do with the ureteral dilation of pregnancy.

Figure 19-13. Vascular ureteral notching. Urography reveals multiple indentations (arrows) on the opacified ureter. This appearance could be produced either by arterial or venous periureteral collaterals that enlarged to bypass a main renal arterial or venous obstruction.

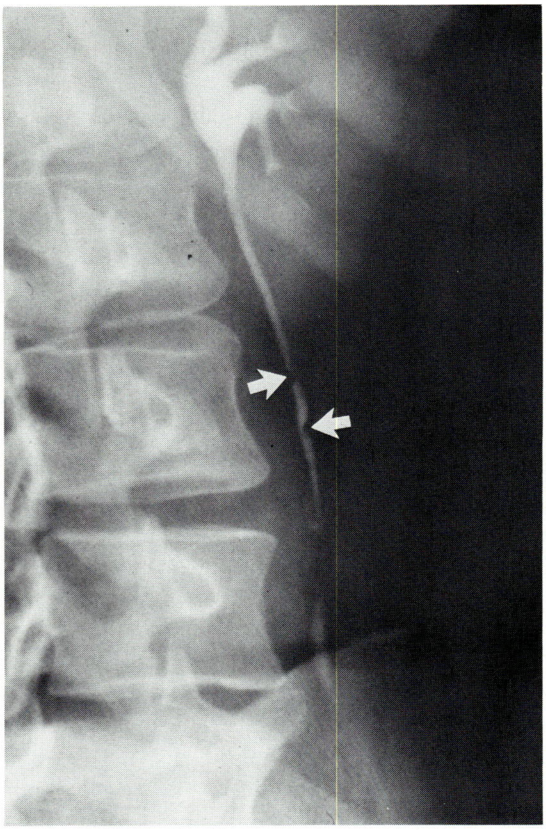

URETERAL HERNIATIONS

Herniation of the ureter, although uncommon, often has a characteristic radiographic appearance, and it may cause some obstruction of the ipsilateral collecting system. The ureter may be included in sciatic, inguinal, or femoral hernias [29]. In sciatic herniation, the middle portion of the pelvic ureter extends through the sacrosciatic notch, resulting in a lateral hairpin type of deviation on urographic or retrograde studies (Fig. 19-14). This type of herniation is only rarely obstructive and is usually an incidental finding. Ureteral herniation associated with inguinal hernias is rare; the ureter typically extends into the groin or scrotum adjacent to the

Figure 19-14. Sacrosciatic ureteral herniation. Urography shows a lateral "hairpin" deviation of the midpelvic portion of the left ureter (arrow).

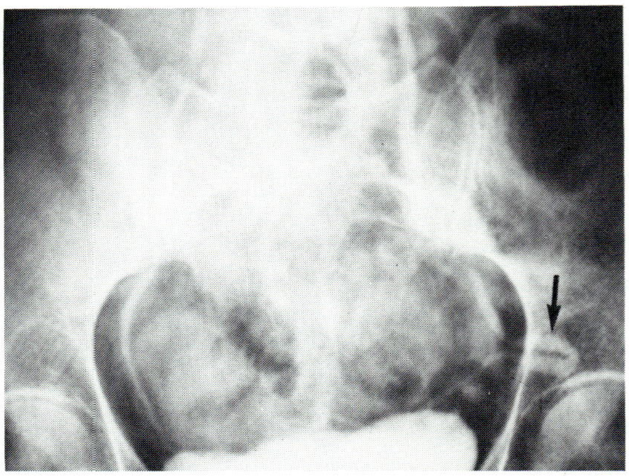

true peritoneal hernia sac (paraperitoneal). This type of herniation can be easily diagnosed if the ureter is opacified well during urography. However, there may be enough compression of the ureter to prevent its visualization. In such cases, inguinal or femoral herniation of the ureter should be suspected if there is any redundancy of the distal ureter below the level of its respective orifice. However, with significant enlargement of the prostate in men, the distal ureter may form a loop deep in the pelvis before ascending to its orifice, which has been elevated by the large prostate gland.

Yet another type of ureteral herniation is its extension into redundant folds of retroperitoneum or between the iliac vessels. These are termed internal herniations, and they result in a sharply angulated or curlique appearance of the ureter in the region of the bony pelvis or just below the pelvic brim. In women with severe uterine or bladder prolapse (or both), the pelvic ureters may be carried inferiorly with the prolapsed structures.

REFERENCES

1. Angel, J.L., and Knuppel, R.A. Computed tomography in diagnosis of puerperal ovarian vein thrombosis. *Obstet. Gynecol.* 63:61, 1984.
2. Babaian, R.J., and Johnson, D.E. Primary carcinoma of the ureter. *J. Urol.* 123:357, 1980.
3. Benson, R.C., Jr., Swanson, S.K., and Farrow, G.M. Relationship of leukoplakia to urothelial malignancy. *J. Urol.* 131:507, 1984.
4. Bree, R.L., et al. Medial deviation of the ureters secondary to psoas muscle hypertrophy. Radiology 118:691, 1976.
5. Buntley, D.W., and McDuffie, R. Pyeloureteral filling defects associated with systemic anticoagulation: A case report. *J. Urol.* 115:35, 1976.
6. Cancelmo, J.J., et al. Tumors of the ureter: Problems in diagnosis. *A.J.R.* 117:132, 1973.
7. Cochran, S.T., Waisman, J., and Barbaric, Z.L. Radiographic and microscopic findings in multiple ureteral diverticula. *Radiology* 137:631, 1980.
8. Darney, P.D., and Wilson, E.A. Intravenous pyelography in the diagnosis and management of postpartum ovarian vein thrombophlebitis: A case report. *Am. J. Obstet. Gynecol.* 127:439, 1977.
9. Debruyne, F.M.J., et al. Fibroepithelial polyp of ureter. *Urology* 16:355, 1980.
10. Demos, T.C., and Moncada, R. Inflammatory gastrointestinal disease presenting as genitourinary disease. *Urology* 13:115, 1979.
11. Dure-Smith, P. Ovarian syndrome: Is it a myth? *Urology* 13:335, 1979.
12. Eilenberg, J., Seery, W., and Cole, A. Multiple fibroepithelial polyps in the pediatric age group: Case report. *J. Urol.* 117:793, 1977.
13. Elliott, G.B. Moloney, P.J., and Clement, J.G. Malacoplakia of the urinary tract. *A.J.R.* 116:830, 1972.
14. Von Fischedick, A.R., Zaunbauer, W., and Haertel, M. Diagnose and Differential diagnose benigner ureterpolypen. *Fortschr. Röntgenstr.* 129:476, 1978.
15. Ghazi, M.R., Morales, P.A., and Al-Askari, S. Primary carcinoma of ureter. *Urology* 14:18, 1979.
16. Hanna, M.K., et al. Ureteral stucture and ultrastructure. Part II. Congenital ureteropelvic junction obstruction and primary obstructive megaureter. *J. Urol.* 116:725, 1976.
17. Hatch, T.R., Hefty, T.R., and Barry, J.M. Time-related recurrence rates in patients with upper tract transitional cell carcinoma. *J. Urol.* 140:40, 1988.
18. Hertle, L., and Androulakakis, P. Keratinizing desquamative squamous metaplasia of the upper urinary tract: Leuloplakia—cholesteatoma. *J. Urol.* 127:631, 1982.
19. Kane, C., and Drouin, P. Obstructive uropathy associated with endometriosis. *Am. J. Obstet. Gynecol.* 151:207, 1985.
20. Kenney, P.J., and Stanley, R.J. Computed tomography of ureteral tumors. *J. Comput. Assist. Tomogr.* 11:102, 1987.
21. Kossol, J.M., and Patel, S.K. Suburothelial hemorrhage: The value of preinfusion computed tomography. *J. Comput. Assist. Tomogr.* 10:157, 1986.
22. Laube, D.W., Calderwood, G.W., and Benda, J.A. Endometriosis causing ureteral obstruction. *Obstet. Gynecol.* 65:69S, 1985.
23. Loitman, B.S., and Chiat, H. Ureteritis cystica and pyelitis cystica: A review of cases and roentgenologic criteria. *Radiology* 68:345, 1957.
24. Mariani, A.J., et al. Bilateral localized amyloidosis of the ureter presenting with anuria. *J. Urol.* 120:757, 1978.
25. Mintz, M.C., et al. Puerperal ovarian vein thrombosis: MR diagnosis. *A.J.R.* 149:1273, 1987.
26. Peake, S.L., Roxburgh, H.B., and Langlois, S. Le P. Ultrasonic assessment of hydronephrosis of pregnancy. *Radiology* 146:167, 1983.
27. Pfister, R.C., and Hendren, W.H. Primary megaureter in children and adults. *Urology* 12:160, 1978.
28. Pfister, R.C., and Newhouse, J.H. Radiology of ureter. *Urology* 12:15, 1978.
29. Pollack, H.M., Popky, G.L., and Blumberg, M.L. Hernias of the ureter—an anatomic-roentgenographic study. *Radiology* 117:275, 1975.
30. Richie, J.P., Withers, G., and Ehrlich, R.M. Ureteral obstruction secondary to metastatic tumors. *Surg. Gynecol. Obstet.* 148:355, 1979.

31. Roemer, C.E., et al. Primary leiomyosarcoma of ureter. *Urology* 16:492, 1980.
32. Sethia, B., and Darke, S.G. Abdominal aortic aneurysm with retroperitoneal fibrosis and ureteric entrapment. *Br. J. Surg.* 70:434, 1983.
33. Shield, D.E., Lytton, B., Weiss, R.M., and Schiff, M., Jr. Urologic complications of inflammatory bowel disease. *J. Urol.* 115:701, 1976.
34. Shrander, D.A., and Bergreen, P.W. Cholesteatoma of ureter masquerading as ureteral tumor. *Urology* 9:556, 1977.
35. Slater, J.M., and Fletcher, G.H. Ureteral strictures after radiation therapy for carcinoma of the uterine cervix. *A.J.R.* 111:269, 1971.
36. Stanton, M.J., and Maxted, W. Malacoplakia: A study of the literature and current concepts of pathogenesis, diagnosis and treatment. *J. Urol.* 125:139, 1981.
37. Talner, L.B. Specific causes of obstruction. In H.M. Pollack (Ed.), *Clinical Urography.* Philadelphia: Saunders, 1990. Pp. 1629–1751.
38. Tokunaka, S., et al. Muscle dysplasia in megaureters. *J. Urol.* 131:383, 1984.
39. Watzer, W.C. The urinary tract in pregnancy. *J. Urol.* 125:271, 1981.
40. Wasserman, N.F., La Pointe, S., and Posalaky, I.P. Ureteral pseudodiverticulosis. *Radiology* 155:561, 1985.
41. Werth, D.D., Weigel, J.W., and Mebust, W.K. Primary neoplasms of the ureter. *J. Urol.* 125:628, 1981.
42. Willen, R., et al. Localized primary amyloidosis of the ureter. *Scand. J. Urol. Nephrol.* 17:385, 1983.
43. Wood, B.P., et al. Ureterovesical obstruction and megaloureter: Diagnosis by real-time US. *Radiology* 156:79, 1985.

The Bladder

When empty, the bladder is seen on radiography as a thin crescent of soft tissue on the pelvic floor immediately above the pubic symphysis. Masses within the pelvis that could be confused with a full bladder can usually be easily differentiated from it by the thin rim of fat surrounding the empty bladder—the perivesical fat stripe. When distended, the bladder assumes an ovoid or spherical shape as it rises into the lower abdomen. The radiographic density of the bladder on plain films is directly related to the specific gravity of the urine it contains.

When the bladder is filled with contrast medium, its inner surface is smooth and its wall is approximately 2 to 3 mm in thickness. The normal bladder mucosa on the postvoiding film, when enhanced by small residual amounts of contrast medium, has a delicate, crinkled appearance.

The relation between the urinary bladder and other pelvic structures is different in males and females. In both sexes, the anterior surface is adjacent to the lower abdominal wall, and the superior surface is invested with peritoneum and is therefore in contact with the peritoneal cavity. Loops of both small and large bowel can indent the dome of the bladder, as does the normally anteflexed uterine fundus. Posteriorly, the bladder is in contact with the upper vagina and uterine cervix in the female and with the anterior wall of the rectum and the seminal vesicles in the male. Inferiorly, the bladder is supported by the urogenital diaphragm in the female and the base of the prostate in the male.

Because of its contiguity with intraperitoneal and pelvic organs, the bladder can be involved by disease processes in these structures. Primary bladder diseases are usually inflammatory, metaplastic, or neoplastic in origin. Furthermore, the bladder may herniate, form diverticula, or be involved with fistulas to adjacent organs. Both extrinsic and intrinsic bladder pathology will be discussed in this chapter.

EXTRINSIC DISEASE RESULTING IN CHANGE OF BLADDER CONFIGURATION

DISPLACEMENT OF THE BLADDER

Lateral displacement of the bladder, as with other midline structures, implies a mass effect in the pelvis. The degree of deviation may be dramatic, or there may be subtle compression of only one wall of the bladder. After trauma or surgery, such lateral displacement may be due to a pelvic hematoma. Iliac artery aneurysms may be of sufficient size to result in lateral displacement of the bladder, as can enlargement of the pelvic lymph nodes by lymphoma or metastatic tumor. Pelvic abscesses can result from inflammatory disease of the fallopian tubes or appendix and exert a mass effect on the bladder. Tumors such as sarcomas, lipomas, or teratomas arising from the soft tissues of the pelvis can also result in this finding (Fig. 20-1), as can the soft-tissue components of primary tumors arising from the pelvic bones. Other masses extrinsic to the bladder that can result in its deviation include megacolon or primary colon carcinoma; tumors of the prostate, uterus, and adnexa; and large urachal cysts. The last are usually midline in position but with massive distention can result in eccentric displacement of the bladder. Large diverticula frequently arise posterolaterally from the bladder near the ureterovesical junction; these can usually be identified during urography or cystography as the cause of bladder displacement. However, on rare occasions the neck may be narrow or the diverticulum filled with tumor, in which case opacification of the diverticulum will not occur [14].

TEARDROP BLADDER

In some cases, pelvic abnormalities may be diffuse, resulting in circumferential compression of the bladder; this results in a "teardrop"

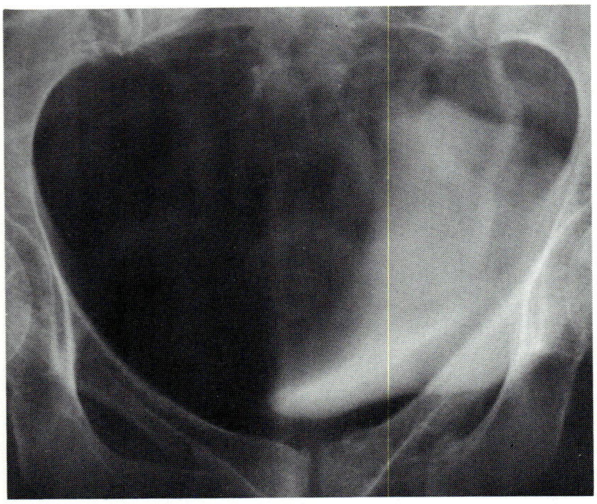

Figure 20-1. Pelvic mass displacing bladder. Coned view of bladder during urography shows marked deviation of bladder to left by a relatively lucent mass (lipoma).

configuration. This configuration can be a normal finding in black males with prominent ileopsoas muscles and a narrow pelvis [23]. The more common pathologic causes of this deformity of the bladder are given in Table 20-1. Pelvic hematoma, previously mentioned as a cause of lateral displacement of the bladder, is more commonly diffusely present in the pelvis. Such a hematoma is frequent after blunt trauma to the lower abdomen associated with pelvic fractures; it can also occur secondary to pelvic surgical procedures. On occasion, pelvic bleeding may be due to anticoagulant therapy.

When the bladder is seen to be circumferentially compressed in the absence of a history suggesting pelvic bleeding, pelvic lipomatosis is classically considered one of the primary differential diagnoses. This is a pathologic entity consisting of proliferation of mature, unencapsulated adipose tissue extraperitoneally within the pelvis. While pelvic lipomatosis generally affects men over the age of 30, it has also been reported in women and children. There is no known specific cause for this disease.

Plain films of the abdomen in patients with pelvic lipomatosis may show lucency in the pelvis due to the increased pelvic fat. Intravenous urography reveals a teardrop-shaped bladder that is often elevated out of the pelvis (Fig. 20-2). The distal ureters are deviated medially in concert with the compression of the bladder, yet the middle thirds of the ureters are often displaced laterally because of the elevation of the lower urinary tract. The ureters may, on occasion, exhibit varying degrees of obstruction. On barium studies, the sigmoid colon is also narrowed and straightened. Pelvic sonography in these cases demonstrates a tubular-shaped urinary bladder floating in the relatively echogenic pelvic fat without evidence of a definitive mass. CT and MRI are also useful in characterizing this disease process. On CT, the fat will be easily seen as negative attenuation tissue compressing the bladder. On MRI, the fat is of high signal intensity on T1 weighted images and of intermediate high signal intensity on T2 images.

Table 20-1. Common causes of the teardrop bladder

Pelvic hematoma
Pelvic lipomatosis
Pelvic adenopathy
Pelvic collateral vasculature (secondary to inferior vena cava occlusion)
Prominent ileopsoas muscles (normal variant)

Figure 20-2. Pelvic lipomatosis. Urography demonstrates a teardrop configuration of the bladder secondary to diffuse infiltration of the pelvis with fatty tissue.

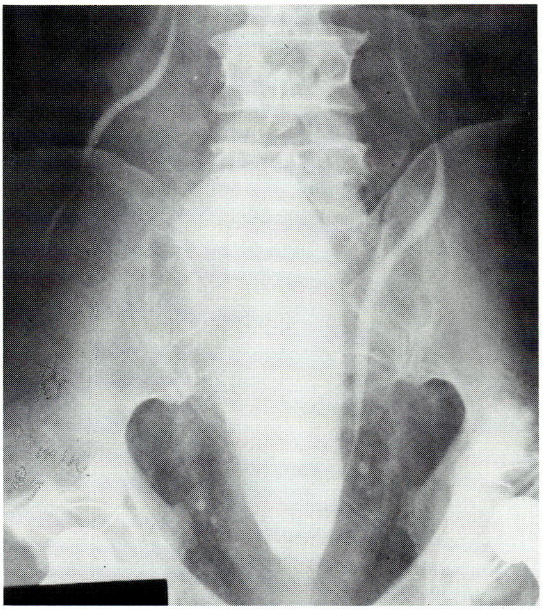

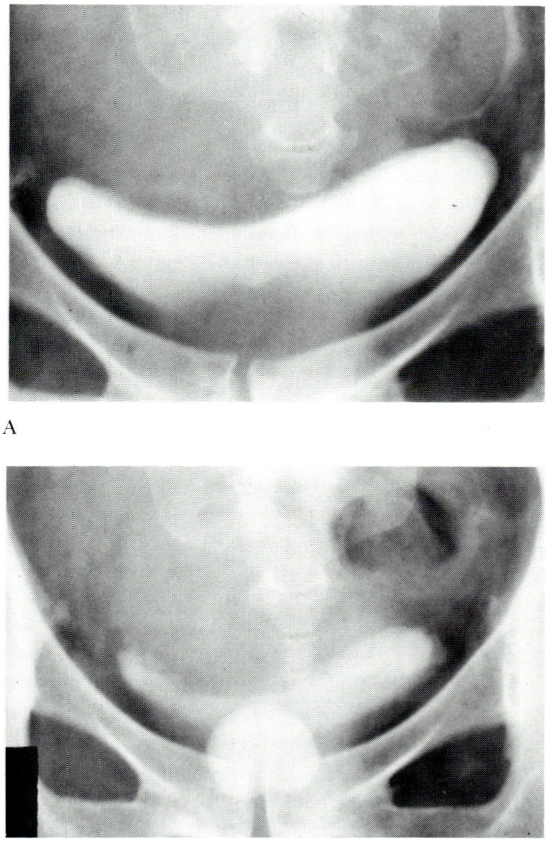

A

B

Figure 20-3. "Female prostate." A. Coned urographic view of the bladder in a woman shows impression on bladder base similar to that seen with an enlarged prostate in a man. B. Postvoiding film shows opacification of the urethral diverticulum responsible for this finding. (From E.S. Amis, Jr., J.J. Cronan, I.C. Yoder, and R.C. Pfister. Impressions on floor of the female bladder: "The female prostate." *Urology* 19(4):441–446, 1982.)

Extensive enlargement of the pelvic nodes as a cause of teardrop bladder is most commonly seen in patients with non-Hodgkin's lymphoma or, less frequently, leukemia. Thrombosis of the inferior vena cava is a rare condition that can result in extensive edema in the pelvis as well as the presence of dilated pelvic venous collaterals. Pelvic adenopathy can be easily diagnosed by CT or MRI, as can inferior vena caval occlusion. However, the latter diagnosis may be clinically suggested if lower-extremity edema is present or if venous collaterals are seen on the lower abdominal wall.

Other rare causes of the teardrop bladder include diffuse fibrosis occurring in the pelvis or lymphoceles forming in the pelvis after extensive pelvic lymph-node dissections [1].

THE FEMALE PROSTATE

The term *female prostate* has gained a bemused acceptance, denoting an impression on the base of the female bladder seen during excretory urography or cystography [3]. This radiographic appearance resembles the enlarged prostate in the male. There are a variety of pathologic processes that can produce this radiographic finding, not all of which are benign. One cause of the female prostate is a urethral diverticulum. For this to occur, the diverticulum must arise posteriorly from the proximal third of the urethra, where it can extend cephalad in the potential plane between the urethra and vagina (Fig. 20-3). These diverticula may reach diameters of up to 8 cm. On the other hand, they may be small, though surrounded by inflammatory edema, and indent the bladder base significantly. Evaluation of urethral diverticula is discussed in detail in Chap. 23, as is the female urethral syndrome, or periurethral inflammation, which can also produce a basilar impression on the bladder. Less common causes of the female prostate include benign and malignant tumors of the anterior vaginal wall, degenerative or malignant change of the pubic symphysis, urethral neoplasm, and surgical repair of urinary stress incontinence.

BLADDER HERNIATION

Virtually all bladder herniations occur in the inguinal or femoral areas, though the bladder can herniate into any pelvic or abdominal opening within its reach when distended. The presenting complaints in patients with bladder herniation are usually those related to bladder outlet obstruction. Bladder herniations in the groin are classified according to the relationship of the herniated bladder to the peritoneum. The most common one is paraperitoneal, in which the bladder remains extraperitoneal and is usually medial to the peritoneal herniation. With intraperitoneal herniation, the bladder is present in the hernia sac and completely covered by

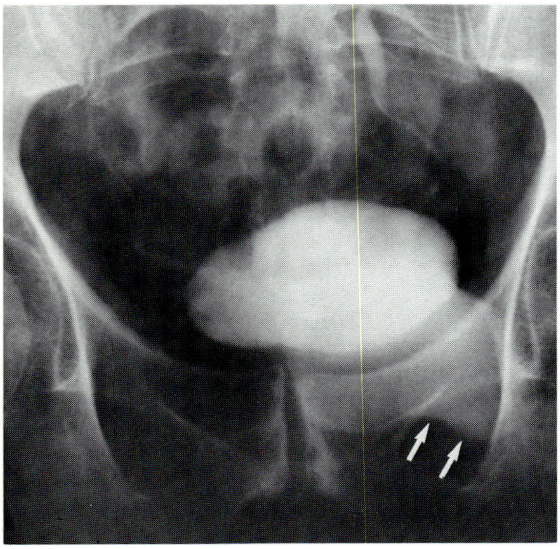

A

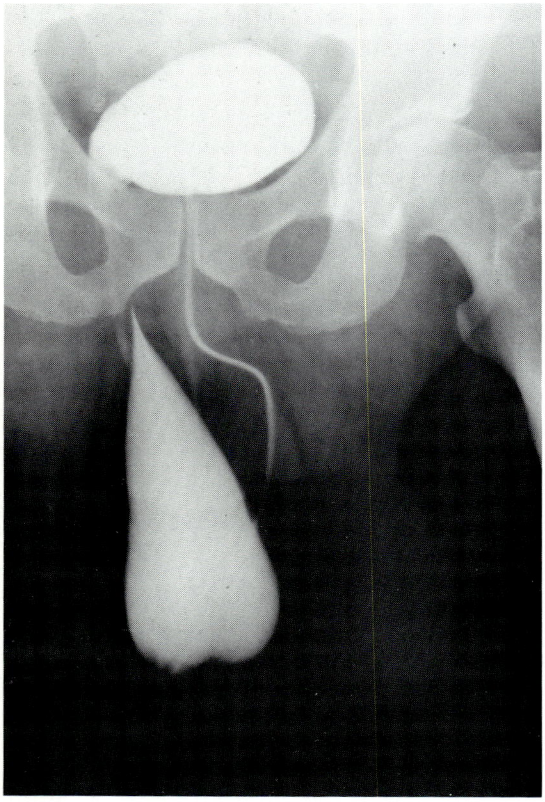

B

Figure 20-4. Bladder herniation. A. Coned urographic view of bladder demonstrates moderate inguinal herniation of bladder on left (arrows). B. Cystography shows scrotal herniation of bladder on right.

peritoneum. With extraperitoneal herniation, the rarest form, the peritoneum remains in the abdomen, and the bladder alone herniates. The type of herniation is usually determined at surgery.

Bladder herniation is found to some degree in 10 percent of all inguinal hernias in men over the age of 50 [16]. In older men, the bladder can herniate into the depths of the scrotum and may or may not be accompanied by the ipsilateral distal ureter.

Bladder hernias are most easily detected when the patient is studied in an erect position with the bladder filled with contrast agent. Since the large majority of cases are minimal herniations, only about a third of bladder hernias are seen in the supine position. Furthermore, herniation is far less obvious on a postvoiding film. Mild herniations are seen as outpouchings of the inferolateral portion of the bladder in the region of the inguinal or femoral canals. Moderate hernias are diagnosed when this bladder extension is 2.5 cm in length or longer (Fig. 20-4A), and in scrotal herniations in men, a portion of the bladder filled with contrast material can be seen in the depths of the scrotum (Fig. 20-4B).

In females, the pelvic floor musculature may lose its ability to support the bladder after multiple pregnancies or with aging. In such cases, the bladder may prolapse posteriorly into the vagina. If the bladder alone is involved, this is known as a cystocele. If this prolapse involves the urethra as well, such as occurs in stress incontinence of urine, a cystourethrocele occurs. Not uncommonly, a significant portion of the bladder may actually protrude through the vaginal introitus. Opacification of the bladder during either excretory urography or cystography in this last case will reveal an hourglass configuration of the prolapsed bladder.

BLADDER DIVERTICULA

True bladder diverticula occur when the bladder mucosa and submucosa herniate between the muscles of the bladder wall. In the case of early diverticula, which do not extend beyond the outer margin of the bladder wall, the term *cellule* is applied. As the diverticulum progressively enlarges, it protrudes beyond the outer margin of the bladder, and the serosa of the bladder becomes the outer layer of the diverticulum. While some bladder diverticula are congenital in origin, most are secondary to bladder outlet obstruction.

Bladder diverticula may be solitary or multiple. A large bladder diverticulum arising near the ureterovesical junction typically causes medial deviation of the ipsilateral ureter and of the bladder wall. If the diverticulum is opacified during contrast studies, the cause of this deviation becomes obvious. However, as previously mentioned, if the neck of the diverticulum is narrow or if the diverticulum is filled with tumor, the condition may not be so readily recognized. In many cases, bladder diverticula do not drain well, leading to stasis of urine, with chronic infection and stone formation. These secondary conditions also predispose to a higher incidence of squamous cell carcinoma within bladder diverticula. Because the wall is thin, carcinomas in diverticula tend to penetrate the wall and metastasize earlier than if they were contained within the normal vesical lumen.

A solitary diverticulum arising from the dome of the bladder should be considered urachal in origin. However, if such a diverticulum is associated with multiple other diverticula in a patient with outlet obstruction, it is probably unrelated to the urachal remnant.

Radiographically, bladder diverticula opacified during contrast studies should be evaluated for degree of emptying after the patient voids. Filling defects may represent stones or tumors (Fig. 20-5) as well as inflammatory debris. If the plain film is not helpful, CT or sonography may be required to differentiate a radiolucent calculus from a diverticular tumor. In the rare instances when the bladder or distal ureter is deviated by a nonopacifying bladder diverticulum, CT or sonography may again be required to suggest the cause of the mass. In some cases, on the postvoiding film after excretory urography or cystogaphy, small amounts of contrast material can be seen within the interstices of a tumor filling a diverticulum. In this case, the diagnosis can be suggested after careful scrutiny of this film.

The size of bladder diverticula can vary from minute to capacities exceeding what would be expected for the normal bladder. In the latter case, the radiographic pattern may be confusing, since as the diverticulum fills, it may occupy a relatively central position in the pelvis and displace the bladder laterally. The bladder may be quite contracted and small because of severe trabeculation. Communication with the urethra is the definitive finding for identifying the bladder. Otherwise, the diverticulum can usually be easily differentiated from the bladder by virtue of the appearance of its wall: The diverticulum will have a smooth wall, whereas the bladder usually exhibits an irregular appearance due to trabeculation.

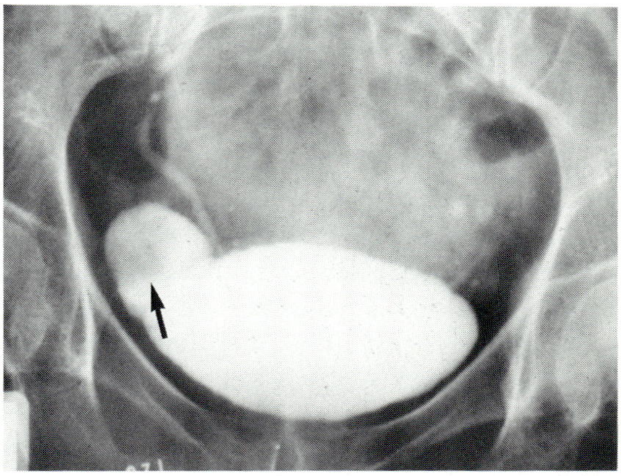

Figure 20-5. Tumor in bladder diverticulum. Coned urographic view of bladder shows moderate-sized right bladder diverticulum with filling defect (arrow) that proved to be transitional cell carcinoma.

BLADDER FISTULAS

ENTEROVESICAL FISTULAS

Demonstration of communications between the bladder and bowel are often difficult to demonstrate by conventional radiologic techniques such as excretory urography and barium enema. Furthermore, the classic presenting symptoms of fecaluria and pneumaturia are present in less than two-thirds of patients; the remainder present only with recurrent urinary infections. Therefore, a high index of suspicion is necessary in patients with disease processes predisposing to enterovesical fistula if this condition is to be accurately diagnosed.

Diverticulitis is usually considered the most common cause of these fistulas, followed by colon cancer. These conditions usually result in communications between the bladder and rectosigmoid region of the colon. Fistulas from the small bowel to the bladder are usually due to Crohn's disease. Other causes of enterovesical fistula include penetrating trauma, surgical misadventures, other inflammatory diseases in the pelvis (appendiceal abscess, pelvic inflammatory disease), and infections such as tuberculosis or schistosomiasis.

In the proper clinical setting, identification of gas within the lumen of the bladder by various imaging studies is suggestive of fistula. However, this gas may also be secondary to gas-forming organisms in the bladder (usually *Escherichia coli*) or, more commonly, to recent instrumentation or catheterization of the bladder. Air within the wall of the bladder as well as in the lumen is found only in cases of emphysematous cystitis.

Excretory urography has been one of the less useful studies in demonstrating these fistulas. Even when multiple studies are employed the actual fistula is demonstrated in only slightly over half the cases. Findings suggestive of fistula on excretory urography or cystography include focal irregularity of the bladder wall, with or without an associated mass effect. Contrast material is seen entering the bowel during cystography in only about half the cases. Similarly, the fistulous tract is identified during barium studies of the colon in an even smaller percentage of cases. However, where the fistulous tract is widely patent, radiographically dramatic demonstration of the condition may be seen (Fig. 20-6). At cystoscopy, the actual fistula is only occasionally identified; the usual cystoscopic finding is that of an isolated area of inflammation of the bladder wall.

CT has been reported as a sensitive method for documenting the presence of enterovesical fistulas. In one series, air was found in the bladder in 90 percent of patients subsequently proven to have an enterovesical fistula [9]. Furthermore, 90 percent of patients exhibited focal bladder-wall thickening (Fig. 20-7), 85 percent had focal bowel-wall thickening, and 75 percent were found to have an extravesical

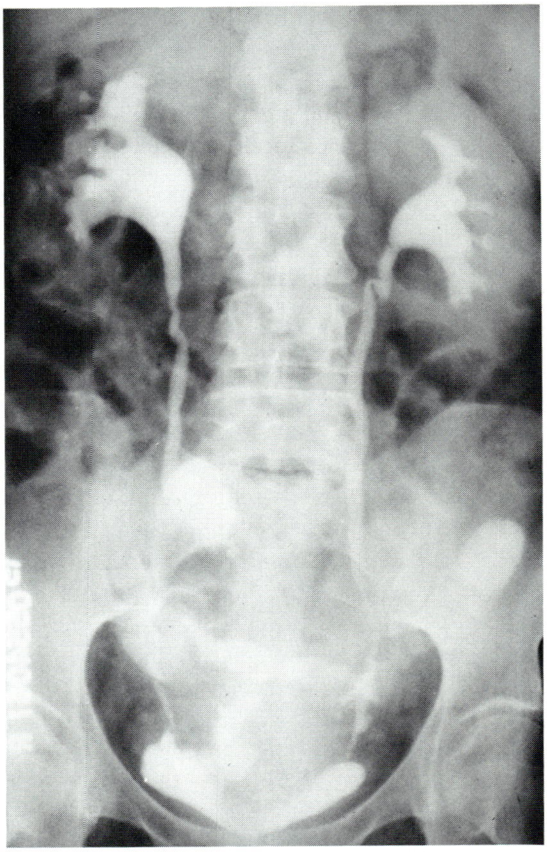

Figure 20-6. Colovesical fistula in woman with sigmoid cancer. Urography shows grossly distorted bladder with contrast material from bladder entering sigmoid colon.

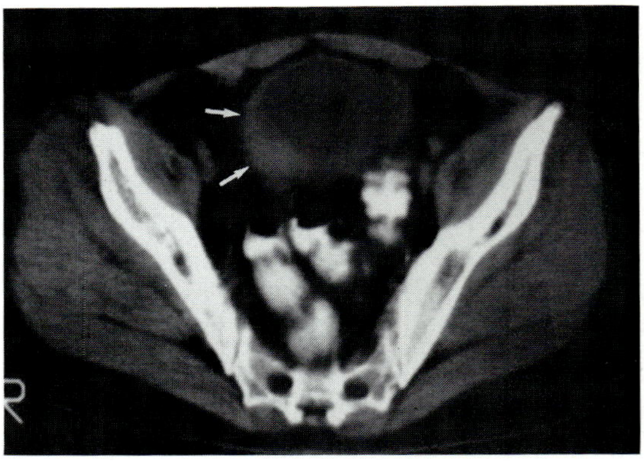

Figure 20-7. CT evidence of fistula in patient with Crohn's disease and urinary infection. Focal bladder-wall thickening (arrows) is suggestive of fistula even though no gas is seen in bladder lumen.

soft-tissue mass. As with other studies, CT is able to demonstrate passage of contrast material through the fistula from bowel to bladder or vice versa in less than half the cases.

VESICOVAGINAL FISTULAS

Vesicovaginal fistulas are usually painless and result in continual dribbling incontinence of urine via the vagina. They are most frequently the result of gynecologic surgical misadventures. In particular, this complication tends to be the result of radical surgical procedures for treatment of pelvic malignancies. Preoperative irradiation results in poor healing and is also a frequent predisposing factor in vesicovaginal fistula formation [10]. Although relatively rare, invasion of the bladder by gynecologic malignancies can result in fistulization to the uterine cavity or the vagina.

Radiographically, vescovaginal fistulas are not as difficult to demonstrate as are vesicoenteric fistulas. Cystography usually demonstrates contrast material opacifying the vagina posterior to the bladder; lateral or postdrainage films are sometimes necessary to demonstrate contrast material within the vagina. CT may be helpful in demonstrating the cause of the fistula when it is not secondary to a postoperative complication.

INFECTION OF THE BLADDER

BACTERIAL CYSTITIS

Cystitis, without modifying terms, refers to acute bacterial infection of the bladder. This is more common in women, and is often related to sexual intercourse, after which there is a transient increase in bacteriuria. In these instances, the term *honeymoon cystitis* is often applied. It is not unusual for acute cystitis in women to be accompanied by gross hematuria. The most commonly found organism is *E. coli.* Although cystitis can occur in men, usually secondary to bladder outlet obstruction, the hemorrhagic variety is distinctly uncommon. Symptoms associated with cystitis include dysuria, frequency, and urgency. Usually, there is no associated fever.

Radiographically, the acutely infected bladder may appear normal or show bullous edema of the mucosa. Furthermore, the bladder may have a decreased capacity because of irritation. When abnormal, the mucosal folds are thickened and coarse and usually exhibit a cobblestone appearance (Fig. 20-8). However, these are nonspecific findings, which can be seen with any acute inflammatory or irritative process in the bladder. With proper treatment, the mucosa will return to its normal delicate pattern within several days.

EMPHYSEMATOUS CYSTITIS

Emphysematous cystitis, in which gas is present within the wall or lumen of the bladder (or both), is also more common in females and again is usually due to *E. coli* infection. The majority of these patients have diabetes mellitus, but glycosuria from intravenous administration of glucose can also be a predisposing factor. Unlike emphysematous pyelonephritis, morbidity is not increased with this condition, and it responds well to appropriate antibiotic therapy.

Radiographically, gas is usually seen first within the bladder wall, occurring in the lamina propria or the muscularis. This is seen on plain films as a mottled radiolucency confined to the region of the bladder wall. These pockets of gas in the wall may eventually rupture, leading to the detection of gas within the bladder lumen (Fig. 20-9). Whereas gas in the bladder lumen may be secondary to vesicovaginal or vesicoenteric fistulas or may be introduced during instrumentation of the lower urinary tract, gas

Figure 20-8. Acute cystitis. Postvoiding cystography shows edematous mucosal folds. This appearance is nonspecific and can be seen with virtually any type of acute infectious or irritative bladder condition.

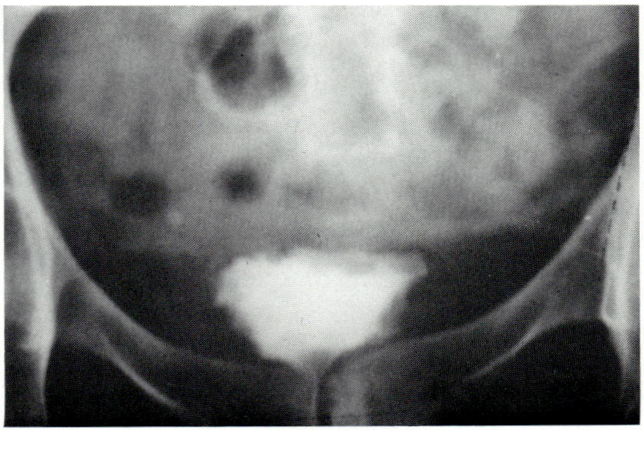

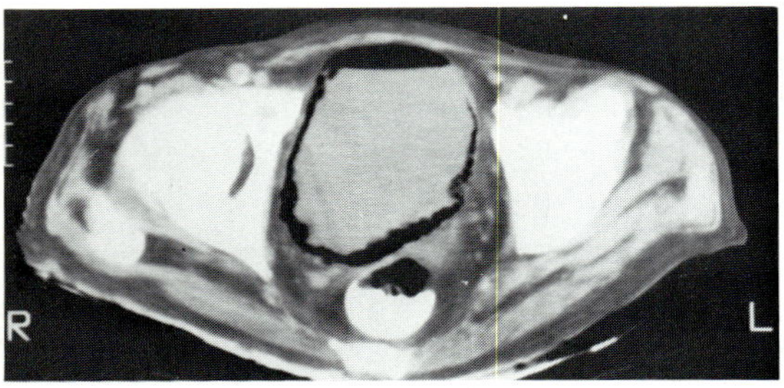

Figure 20-9. Emphysematous cystitis. CT of bladder shows gas density involving entire bladder wall and free gas in the bladder lumen anteriorly. Note the irregular mucosa. (Courtesy of Dr. Isabel C. Yoder, Massachussetts General Hospital, Boston, MA.)

within the bladder wall is always secondary to infection. Contrast studies of the bladder reveal bullous changes of the bladder mucosa.

PYOCYSTIS

Pyocystis is gross infection of a defunctionalized bladder resulting in filling of the lumen with pus. It is typically seen in patients who have undergone supravesical urinary diversion for neurogenic bladder dysfunction and in whom the chronically infected bladder has not been removed. It is a rare condition, since regular bladder irrigations usually prevent the accumulation of purulent material. However, occasionally infection can progress to the point at which the bladder becomes overdistended and septicemia occurs. Rapid treatment—either transurethral or percutaneous drainage and irrigation—is necessary, as these patients are quite ill. Parenteral antibiotics are also necessary.

Radiographically, pyocystis is seen on plain films as a soft-tissue mass in the region of the bladder that may contain varying amounts of gas. The diverted upper urinary tract usually functions normally unless septic shock supervenes.

CANDIDA CYSTITIS

Another bladder infection usually seen in patients with poorly controlled diabetes is candidiasis. This condition has also been reported in immunosuppressed patients [12]. *Candida albicans* ferments sugars in the urine, forming gas in the bladder lumen. Furthermore, the formation of fungus balls is not uncommon, and these may also contain gas. On plain films, gas within a fungus ball may have a laminated appearance. On contrast studies, a fungus ball (or balls) is seen as a discrete, irregular filling defect within the bladder.

TUBERCULOUS CYSTITIS

Tuberculosis of the bladder occurs as a descending infection of the urine after hematogenous involvement of the kidney. As with other forms of acute cystitis, early tuberculous cystitis shows bullous changes of the bladder mucosa. As the disease progresses, the bladder becomes contracted and irregular; this irregularity may be asymmetric. Rarely, calcification occurs in the bladder wall. Stiffening of the bladder wall can result in compromise of the valve mechanisms at the ureterovesical junctions, leading to vesicoureteral reflux.

SCHISTOSOMAL CYSTITIS

The bladder is involved in a large majority of patients with schistosomiasis of the urinary tract. The causative organism is *Schistosoma haematobium*. Hematuria is a common symptom in this condition, resulting from penetration of the ova (initially deposited in the bladder wall) through the bladder mucosa. In its initial stages, schistosomiasis of the bladder cannot be differentiated radiographically from other acute forms of inflammation, as it produces nonspecific bullous edematous changes of the bladder mucosa.

Schistosomiasis is the most common cause of bladder-wall calcification (Table 20-2) [17]. As

Table 20-2. Conditions associated with bladder calcification

Inflammatory
Schistosomal cystitis
Tuberculous cystitis
Alkaline encrustation cystitis
Cytoxan cystitis
Neoplastic
Transitional-cell carcinoma
Squamous-cell carcinoma
Urachal adenocarcinoma
Tumors of bladder muscle
Miscellaneous
Nephrogenic adenoma
Enlarged prostate with calcifications
Bladder calculi

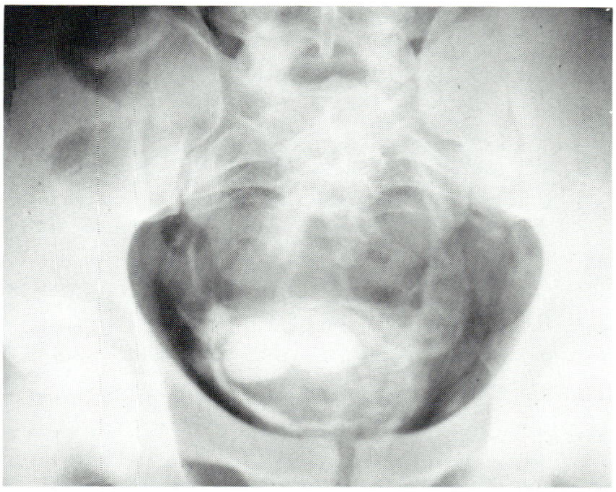

Figure 20-10. Bladder-wall calcification in schistosomiasis. Plain film of pelvis shows calcification outlining the wall of the bladder and distal ureters. Bladder calculi are also seen.

the disease progresses, calcification of the entire bladder wall can occur (Fig. 20-10). However, as the bladder initially begins to calcify, segmental linear or amorphous calcification is not unusual. There is an increased incidence of squamous cell carcinoma in these patients, and neoplasm should be suspected when follow-up films of the calcified bladder wall reveal areas where the calcification is no longer present.

INFLAMMATION OF THE BLADDER

There are multiple noninfectious types of cystitis. These include catheter-induced cystitis as well as conditions such as eosinophilic, granulomatous, interstitial, chemical, drug-induced, and radiation cystitis. As with cystitis of infectious causes, the bladder in any of these conditions often acutely shows bullous edematous change. With progression of the disease, the chronic variety presents with a small-capacity, thick-walled bladder that has an irregular mucosal pattern. The more common of these conditions are discussed below.

CATHETER CYSTITIS

Catheter-induced irritation of the bladder wall is the most common cause of noninfectious cystitis. An indwelling Foley catheter can result in bullous edema of the bladder wall in a matter of hours. Radiographically, the bullous changes may be localized (where the catheter tip touches the bladder wall) or generalized. This condition resolves completely after removal of the catheter.

INTERSTITIAL CYSTITIS

The cause of interstitial cystitis is unknown. This condition usually occurs in postmenopausal women, and it is marked by a relentless contraction of the bladder to the point at which its capacity may be 30 ml or less. These patients complain of severe urgency and frequency and usually have pain with any degree of bladder distention, which is relieved when the patient voids. Histologically, there is a nonspecific chronic inflammatory cell infiltration of the bladder wall. On cystoscopy, a reddened area that tends to crack and bleed with bladder distention may be seen in the region of the bladder dome (Hunner's ulcer). Radiographically, these patients are difficult to study becaue of their very small bladder capacity (Fig. 20-11) and the pain experienced with distention of the bladder.

CYCLOPHOSPHAMIDE (CYTOXAN) CYSTITIS

A severe hemorrhagic cystitis can occur in up to 40 percent of patients treated with cyclophosphamide. The hematuria is due to exposure of the bladder mucosa to the metabolites of cyclophosphamide and may be so severe as to require multiple transfusions. This condition occurs in both acute and chronic forms. The acute form usually follows intravenous injections of large doses of cyclophosphamide within a matter of days, though it tends to be a self-limiting process. The chronic variety occurs several months after long-term oral therapy with cyclophosphamide and has a tendency to progress to chronic cystitis. Calcification in the bladder wall can occasionally be found in the chronic variety.

RADIATION CYSTITIS

Radiation cystitis also occurs in both acute and chronic forms. Acute radiation cystitis is usually seen after external-beam radiation doses of greater than 3000 rads. Symptoms include

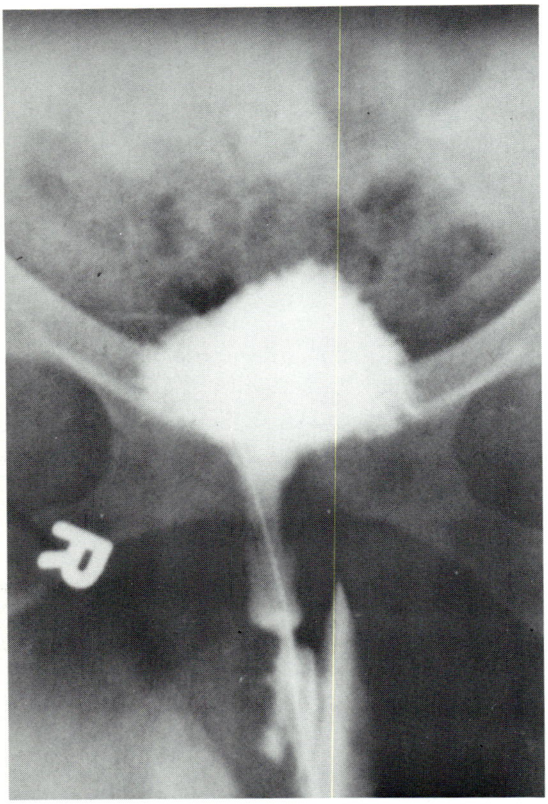

Figure 20-11. Interstitial cystitis. Cystography shows a tiny bladder (30 ml capacity) with irregular mucosa. Patient had severe pain during procedure.

dysuria and frequency. This condition is usually self-limiting. When chronic radiation cystitis occurs, it is usually seen from several months to years after irradiation. Fortunately, it occurs in only a small minority of irradiated patients. Presentation is usually with painless hematuria. In the acute phase, bullous edema may be seen. As with other chronic forms of cystitis, a contracted bladder may be the end result; this is more likely when a bladder operation has been performed in conjunction with the irradiation.

ALKALINE ENCRUSTATION CYSTITIS

Alkaline encrustation cystitis, in which amorphous sheets of calcification are deposited on damaged bladder urothelium, occurs in the presence of an alkaline urine. Typically, chronic proteus infection is a precursor, though this condition has also been reported in patients with bladders compromised by irradiation.

PROLIFERATIVE DISEASES OF THE BLADDER

Injuries to the bladder mucosa, such as can occur with recurrent or chronic infection, may result in several varieties of proliferative change of the bladder mucosa [5].

CYSTITIS CYSTICA

Cystitis cystica is a benign condition that does not undergo malignant degeneration. It occurs most commonly in females in the setting of chronic or recurrent urinary tract infection, usually caused by *E. coli.* Degeneration of subepithelial clusters of transitional cells (Brunn's epithelial nests) results in cystic bubbles; these are seen cystoscopically as multiple small domed lesions containing a clear yellow fluid primarily involving the bladder floor. Radiographically, the cysts, which can range from a few millimeters to over a centimeter in diameter, are seen as discrete smooth lesions, usually involving the bladder base but occasionally extending throughout the bladder.

CYSTITIS GLANDULARIS

Cystitis glandularis, also associated with chronic or recurrent infection, results from the change of Brunn's nests into glandular structures resembling intestinal epithelium. This is considered a premalignant lesion, as it has occasionally been reported to undergo metaplasia to adenocarcinoma. Grossly, there are one or more irregular lesions of the bladder that can mimic transitional cell carcinoma. Radiographically, single or multiple irregular defects, which can be quite large, are seen. The resemblance to transitional cell carcinoma is often striking, resulting in the necessity for biopsy to confirm the diagnosis.

NEPHROGENIC ADENOMA

Nephrogenic adenoma is a rare proliferative response of the urothelium to irritation or chronic infection. Histologically, this lesion resembles the proximal tubules of the nephron. Although it can occur throughout the urinary tract, it is more common in the bladder, exhibiting diverse radiographic appearances including mucosal irregularities or masses arising from the bladder wall [29]. There are no distinctive radiographic features that allow its differentiation from tumor or other proliferative lesions such as cystitis glandularis. Therefore biopsy is necessary to establish the diagnosis. Although this is considered a benign lesion with no potential for malignant degeneration, bladder involvement may be extensive, and eradication of the lesion may be difficult.

SQUAMOUS METAPLASIA AND LEUKOPLAKIA

Metaplasia of the normal urothelium in the trigonal area to a squamous variety is not uncommon. This condition can progress to the formation of leukoplakia (white plaques), which can slough epithelial debris into the bladder lumen and form cholesteatomas (keratin balls). As with the other proliferative disorders, it usually occurs in response to chronic infection or irritation. On rare occasions, malignant degeneration to squamous cell carcinoma can occur. When advanced enough to produce radiographic changes, leukoplakia is difficult to differentiate from other proliferative or neoplastic conditions.

MALACOPLAKIA

Malacoplakia is an uncommon response of the urinary tract to chronic or recurrent infection. Although it can occur throughout the urinary system, it is most common in the bladder. The incidence is much higher in females than in males. Cystoscopically, multiple round or ovoid yellowish plaques are seen to involve the bladder, usually in the region of the bladder base. Although this is considered a benign process in the bladder, diffuse involvement of both kidneys can result in renal failure. Radiographically, the bladder lesions are difficult to distinguish from cystitis cystica—they are seen as multiple smooth defects, usually in the region of the bladder base and trigone. On occasion, malacoplakia may be difficult to differentiate from neoplasm.

BENIGN INFILTRATIVE CONDITIONS OF THE BLADDER

ENDOMETRIOSIS

Endometriosis denotes the presence of endometrial tissue in locations other than the uterine cavity. It is a condition of the reproductive years, frequently presenting in the fourth decade. The typical site of occurrence of endometriosis is the pelvic cavity. The bladder is involved in about 1 percent of patients; this is usually a result of contiguous spread from other sites of pelvic endometriosis. On occasion, however, primary infiltration of the bladder wall can occur. Symptoms include frequency, dysuria, hematuria, and suprapubic pain, all of which are usually cyclic and related to the menstrual periods. The dome of the bladder is most commonly involved.

On contrast studies of the bladder, a smooth ovoid filling defect can be seen protruding into the bladder. (Fig. 20-12A). On CT, the primarily intramural location of the lesion is usually

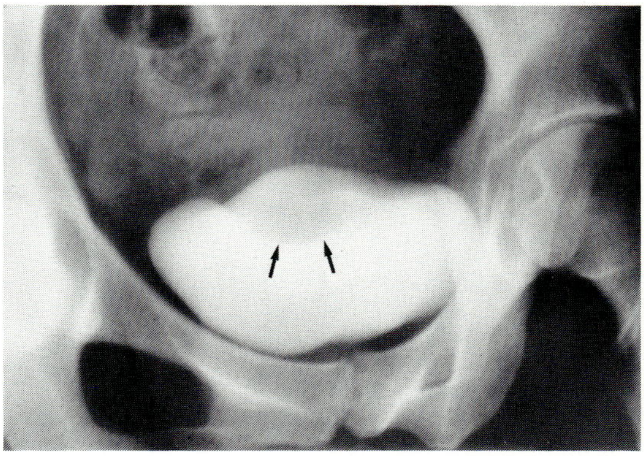

A

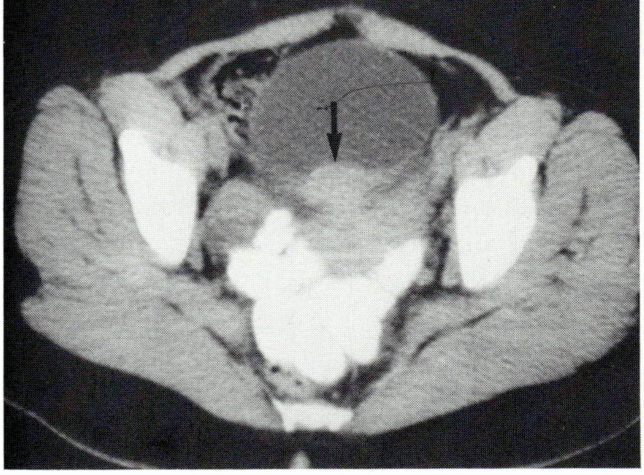

B

Figure 20-12. Endometriosis of bladder. A. Coned urographic view of bladder shows smooth mural defect in dome (arrows). B. CT section through bladder shows mural nodule (arrow) extending from irregular pelvic mass (endometriosis).

well demonstrated (Fig. 20-12B). Sonography typically shows a mildly echogenic, smooth, or lobular soft-tissue mass in the bladder wall, usually near the dome. The combination of cyclic symptoms and the relatively benign appearance of the lesion should suggest the diagnosis of endometriosis.

AMYLOIDOSIS

In amyloidosis, a proteinaceous starchlike material infiltrates the bladder wall [22]. This may occur as a primary bladder process, or be associated with primary systemic amyloidosis or secondary amyloidosis in which there are known predisposing causes. It affects males and females equally and is usually seen in the sixth decade. Irritative lower urinary tract symptoms are common, as is gross hematuria. The most frequent site of bladder involvement is the lateral wall; the base is usually spared. Radiographically, the irregular filling defect seen with amyloidosis cannot be differentiated from bladder neoplasm.

INTRALUMINAL BLADDER DEFECTS

Aside from the benign and malignant mural or epithelial conditions that can protrude into the lumen and present as filling defects in the bladder filled with contrast material, there are multiple causes of free intraluminal masses. The most common of these are bladder calculi, which are discussed in Chap. 15. As previously noted, fungus balls can be seen in diabetics with candida cystitis. Large smoothly lobular defects are usually blood clots resulting from bleeding from the bladder or prostate, but they often must be differentiated from tumor. Bleeding from the upper tracts may result in clots that are vermiform or "spaghettilike" because of their formation in the ureter.

Other defects include sloughed papillae and epithelial debris; the latter can aggregate into cholesteatomalike masses. Finally, foreign bodies, such as stent or catheter fragments, can result from instrumentation of the bladder. Other foreign bodies, usually introduced through the urethra for sexual gratification, depend entirely on the ingenuity and determination of the patient. The authors have seen dice (in a female), balls of wax, the skeleton of a small snake, various types of wire, and coiled tubing in the bladder lumen. Any of these may act as a nidus for stone formation.

NEOPLASMS OF THE BLADDER

A variety of tumors can occur in the urinary bladder. This is probably due to the fact that the bladder derives from the cloaca, which subsequently differentiates into various organs. Tumors involving the bladder are classified as primary (lesions arising from either the mucosa or other layers of the bladder wall) and secondary. Tumors of the urothelium constitute approximately 95 percent of bladder neoplasms. Similar lesions may affect any part of the urinary tract lined with transitional epithelium. However, the bladder is the most commonly involved portion of the urinary tract because of its greater surface area and because it functions as a reservoir allowing carcinogenic substances longer contact with the mucosa [4].

EPITHELIAL BLADDER TUMORS

Of the epithelial tumors, 1 percent are adenocarcinomas, 4 percent are squamous cell carcinomas, and 95 percent are transitional cell carcinomas. Grossly and radiographically, these neoplasms are not easily differentiable, and biopsy is therefore required to establish the definitive diagnosis.

Adenocarcinoma

Although isolated occurrences of adenocarcinoma can be seen anywhere in the bladder, this neoplasm is typically found in patients with exstrophy of the bladder or arising from the urachal cord connecting the bladder and umbilicus, thus involving the dome of the bladder. As previously noted, it can also arise as a further metaplastic transformation of cystitis glandularis. The prognosis when this tumor occurs in an exstrophic bladder is relatively good. However, urachal adenocarcinoma, spreading by extensive local invasion, has a worse prognosis than transitional cell neoplasms—the reported 5-year survival rates do not exceed 15 percent.

Ninety percent of urachal adenocarcinomas arise in the juxtavesical segment. Males are affected three to four times more frequently than females, typically between the ages of 40 and 70 [15]. The majority of patients present clinically with hematuria. While the passage of mucus in the urine is characteristic of this tumor, this occurs in only 10 percent of patients. Calcification has been reported in about 4 percent of urachal carcinomas.

Radiographically, adenocarcinoma of the bladder cannot be differentiated from other epithelial tumors. However, a tumor occurring in the dome of the bladder that is found on biopsy to be adenocarcinoma must be considered urachal in origin, especially when accompanied by an extrinsic mass effect on the dome of the bladder (Fig. 20-13A). Such lesions must be further studied by cross-sectional imaging techniques. CT or ultrasonography are ideal in this regard, and they demonstrate a soft-tissue mass extending anteriorly from the dome of the bladder, which, when extensive, may reach the umbilicus (Fig. 20-13B, C). Treatment involves surgical excision of the entire urachus, including the umbilicus and the dome of the bladder.

Squamous Cell Carcinoma

As with squamous cell carcinoma elsewhere in the urinary tract, the majority of patients with this disorder have a history of chronic or recurrent urinary tract infection, stone disease, or both. There is a higher incidence of squamous cell carcinoma in bladder diverticula because of the stasis of urine seen in these structures.

Schistosomiasis is an important factor in the development of bladder carcinoma. Two-thirds of tumors found in patients with this infection are poorly differentiated squamous cell lesions. The tumors are multiple in 25 percent of cases and commonly involve the bladder dome or anterior bladder wall. Whatever the cause, squamous cell carcinomas tend to occur in a younger age group than other bladder neoplasms, they are usually infiltrating, and the patients have a 5-year survival rate of less than 10 percent.

Radiographically, squamous cell carcinoma presents as an irregular filling defect in the bladder or thickening of the bladder wall that cannot be differentiated from other urothelial tumors.

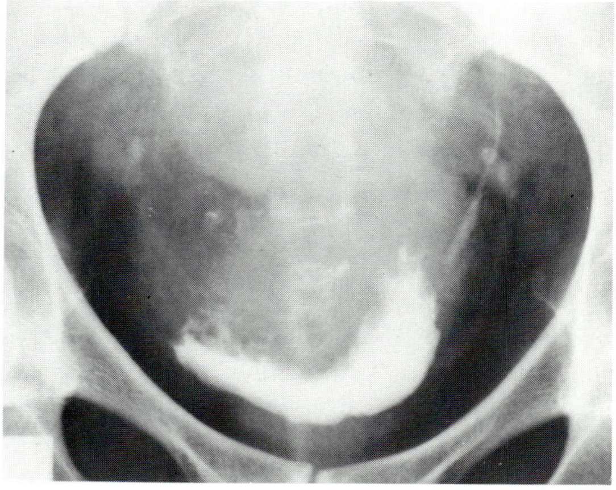

A

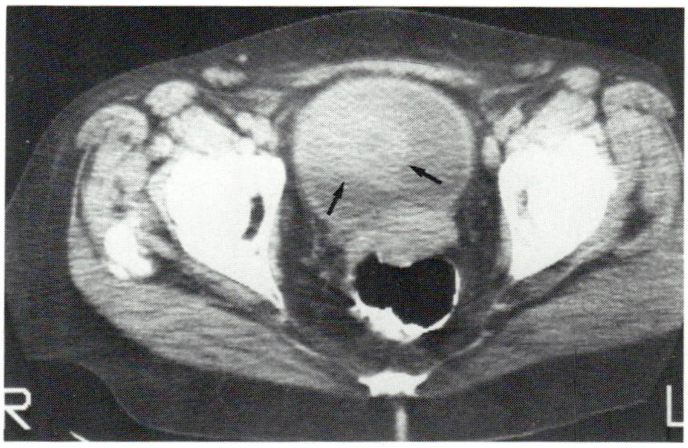

B

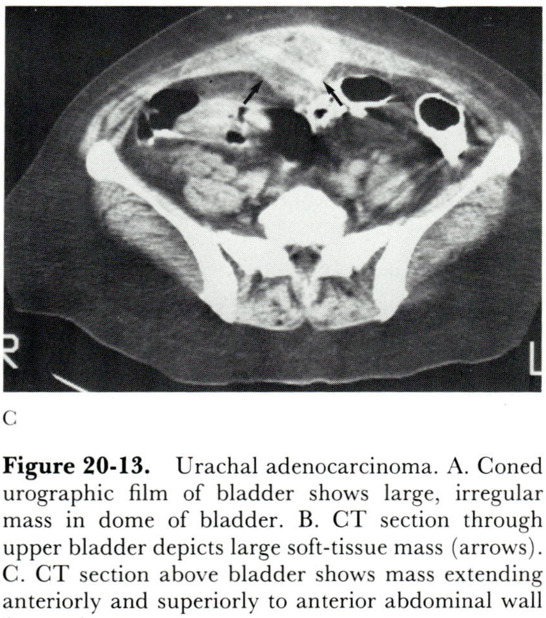

C

Figure 20-13. Urachal adenocarcinoma. A. Coned urographic film of bladder shows large, irregular mass in dome of bladder. B. CT section through upper bladder depicts large soft-tissue mass (arrows). C. CT section above bladder shows mass extending anteriorly and superiorly to anterior abdominal wall (arrows).

As with other tumors, staging is best accomplished with CT.

Transitional Cell Carcinoma

Although it usually occurs in the seventh and eighth decades, transitional cell carcinoma (TCC) has been reported in children as young as 6 years of age [13]. Fortunately, the behavior of these tumors occurring in young patients appears more benign than those in older patients. At all ages, TCC is about four times more common in males than in females. Multiple agents and conditions have been associated with an increased incidence of bladder cancer; these have been discussed in Chap. 9.

Patients with TCC most commonly present with hematuria, lower urinary tract irritative symptoms such as frequency and dysuria, or both. Occasionally, there may be a superimposed urinary tract infection. If the tumor has obstructed a ureteral orifice, the patient may present with symptoms referable to upper tract obstruction, though this obstruction is usually silent. The lateral wall is the most common area of the bladder affected by TCC (40 to 50%), followed by the trigone (including the ureteral orifices and bladder neck) (25%), and the dome of the bladder (5 to 10%) [4].

TCC spreads by direct extension through the bladder wall and subsequently via the lymphatics and bloodstream. Direct extension into the prostate and seminal vesicles in the male and the vagina in the female is not uncommon. Hematogenous spread most frequently results in involvement of the liver or lungs. Bony metastases are uncommon but are typically lytic when they do occur. Pelvic lymph-node extension is frequently seen because of the large number of interconnecting submucosal lymphatics in the bladder wall. There are two staging classifications for urothelial tumors in fairly common use. These are illustrated in Figure 20-14. Recently, the tumor–node–metastasis (TNM) classification seems to be replacing the Jewett–Strong–Marshall staging system.

In slightly over 2 percent of patients with TCC of the bladder, metachronous upper tract lesions can be expected to develop after an average delay of 70 months [28]. Furthermore, about 20 percent of patients with upper-tract TCC will have had an antecedent primary bladder lesion. Of all newly diagnosed tumors, about 70 percent are superficial (T_a, T_{is}, T_1), 25 percent will infiltrate muscle (T_2, T_3), and 5 percent are metastatic. Therefore, most patients present with clinically localized tumors. In this group, the major risk is that of subsequent new tumor formation, which occurs in more than 50 percent of cases [26]. This high incidence of recurrence mandates the need for close follow-up. The overall 5-year survival rate in the group with superficial tumors is about 70 per-

Figure 20-14. Staging of transitional cell carcinoma of the bladder. Both Jewett–Strong–Marshall (A, B, C, D) and tumor–node–metastasis (TNM) systems are shown.

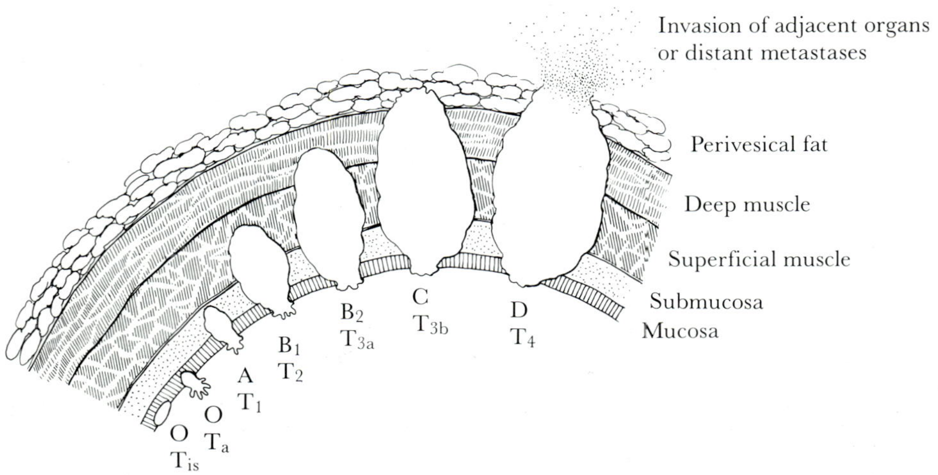

cent. For muscle-invading tumors, survival drops to about 50 percent, and with metastatic disease, to a dismal 10 percent. The diagnosis of transitional cell carcinoma of the bladder is best made cystoscopically, since in some cases there is no distortion of the bladder mucosa that would produce radiographic findings.

The role of radiography in the detection of TCC is to suggest the diagnosis when bladder lesions are seen in patients undergoing excretory urography or cystography for other reasons. On plain films of the abdomen, faint stippled calcifications can be seen in urothelial bladder tumors in less than 1 percent of cases; these calcifications are also easily seen on CT sections obtained using no contrast agent (Fig. 20-15).

Figure 20-15. Calcification in transitional cell carcinoma of bladder. A. Plain film of pelvis shows faint calcifications in bladder region (arrows). B. CT section through bladder demonstrates bladder mass with calcifications on luminal surface.

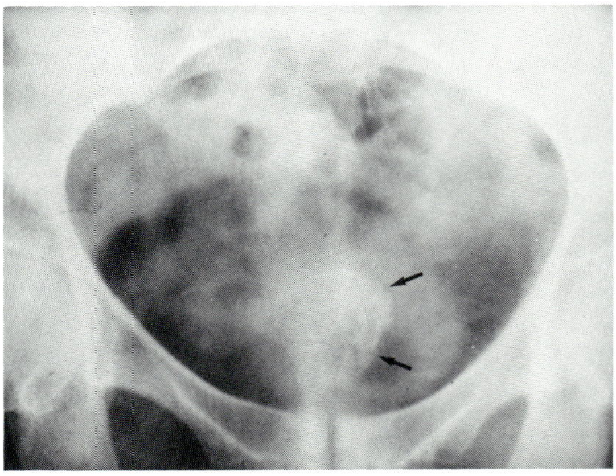

A

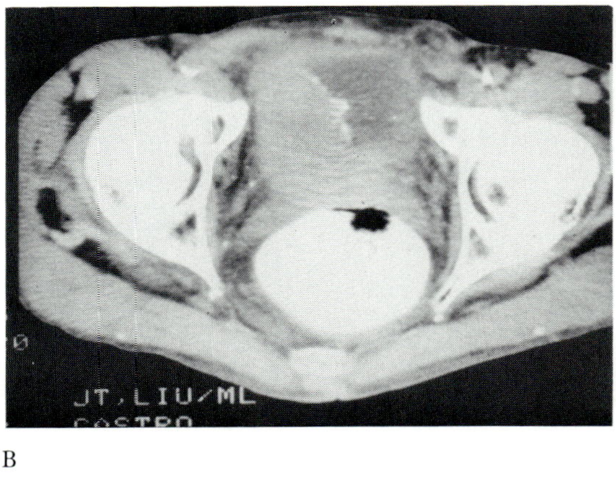

B

During excretory urography, TCC should be suspected when an irregular sessile or polypoid filling defect is seen within the bladder (Fig. 20-16A). The diagnosis can also be suggested when focal irregular thickening of the bladder wall is demonstrated (Fig. 20-16B). If, at the time of presentation of TCC, there is unilateral or bilateral ureteral obstruction, it can be presumed that the tumor is at least somewhat invasive, and this portends a significant decrease in the 5-year survival rate as compared with the group with no obstruction [8].

When suspicious filling defects are observed in the bladder during excretory urography,

Figure 20-16. Presentations of transitional cell carcinoma in bladder. A. Coned urographic view of bladder shows large fronded filling defect arising from right bladder wall. Elevation of bladder base is due to an enlarged prostate. B. Coned urographic view of bladder shows a focal thickening of left inferolateral bladder wall (arrows).

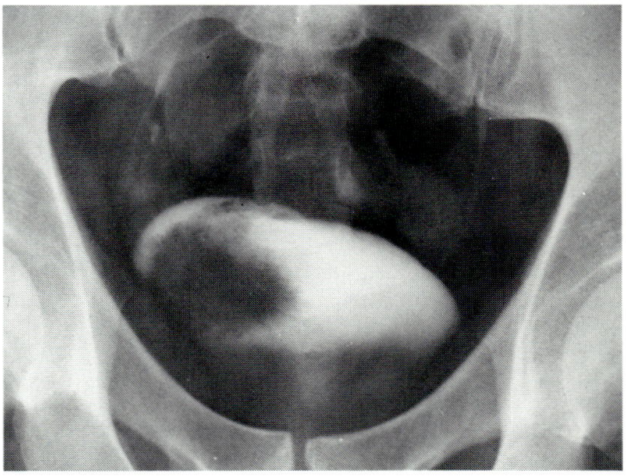

A

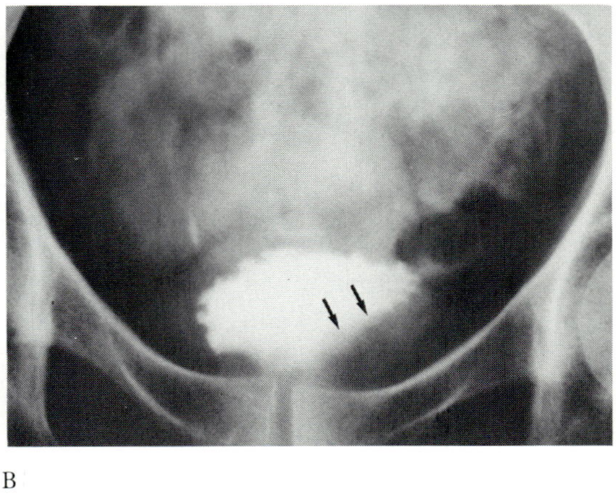

B

coned oblique views may be helpful in demonstrating that the lesion is real and not rectal gas seen through the bladder filled with contrast material. Postvoiding radiography is also valuable, and it can provide the correct diagnosis in a significant number of cases in which the lesion was not detected on other views during urography. As with TCC anywhere in the urinary tract, great care should be taken to evaluate the entire urinary tract for multifocal lesions.

Although transabdominal sonography is not primarily used for the detection of bladder tumors, a soft-tissue mass of moderate echogenicity protruding into the bladder lumen or focal thickening of the bladder wall seen during study of the bladder for other reasons should suggest this diagnosis. Reports indicate that the ability of sonography to detect the presence or absence of bladder tumors varies from 58 to 94 percent [6]. The lower figures are probably more correct, since small (less than 0.5 cm) or flat lesions, especially those located in the dome, on the anterior wall, or at the bladder neck, are usually not seen by sonography.

Once the diagnosis of TCC has been established, accurate staging becomes of paramount importance in determining the treatment regimen. Clinically, determination of muscle invasion is accomplished by transurethral biopsy of the tumor, including a full-thickness biopsy of the underlying bladder wall. However, understaging with this procedure occurs in up to 50 percent of cases. It has been suggested that intravesical ultrasonography may be the best method for determining the extent of spread through the musculature of the bladder wall [21]. However, this technique is not universally available and has not gained wide acceptance as the staging method of choice. Currently, further staging is usually accomplished by CT, though MRI is probably also accurate in staging this neoplasm.

The extent to which TCC has invaded the muscular layers of the bladder cannot be determined on CT. Its main benefits are the ability to detect direct extension beyond the bladder wall and to image pelvic and retroperitoneal nodes, enlargement of which may suggest malignant involvement. Infiltration through the bladder wall (Stage T_{3b}) is suggested by localized thickening of the bladder wall without sharp delineation of its outer contour or by the observance of soft-tissue masses or stranding in the perivesical fat adjacent to the tumor (Fig. 20-17).

Unfortunately, since the patient may have undergone recent transurethral biopsy of the tumor in order to establish the diagnosis, these findings may be secondary to surgery and result in overstaging of the tumor [20]. Contrast-enhanced CT scans through the region of the tumor have been recommended to overcome this difficulty, assuming that only tumor extending beyond the bladder wall will enhance [19]. However, it has been shown that inflammatory tissue and dilated perivesical veins also enhance, somewhat limiting the usefulness of this technique. The reported sensitivity for CT in detecting this direct spread has been reported as 25 to 90 percent. The sensitivity for detecting nodes involved with metastatic neoplasm is about 60 percent, reflecting the inability of CT to detect tumor in nonenlarged nodes [24]. Generally speaking, for pelvic nodes the upper limit of normal is 1.5 cm. Perhaps the main value of CT is to provide the urologist with an estimation of the approximate clear margin around the bladder prior to cystectomy in the absence of gross lymphadenopathy [25].

Reports have indicated that the accuracy of MRI staging of TCC varies from 50 to 88 percent [2, 7, 27]. As with CT, MRI demonstrates tumor invasion of the perivesical fat, prostate, and seminal vesicles. The intraluminal portion

Figure 20-17. Stage T_{3b} (Stage C) transitional cell carcinoma of bladder. CT section through bladder shows soft-tissue mass on left extending through the bladder wall into the perivesical fat (arrows).

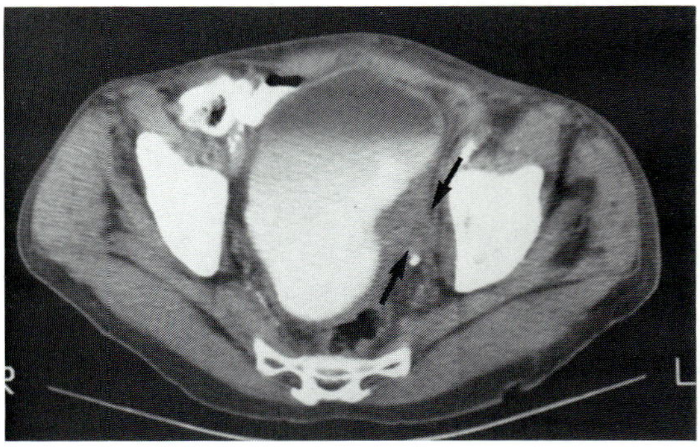

of a TCC, by virtue of its intermediate signal intensity, is best seen on T1 weighted images because of the inherent contrast between the tumor and urine. On T2 weighted images, the normal bladder wall appears as a thin, low-signal-intensity structure; disruption of this low-intensity line in the region of a known tumor is thought to indicate deep-muscle invasion, whereas visualization of this line implies a more localized lesion [18]. The ability of MRI to image enlarged nodes seems to be roughly equivalent to that of CT.

NONEPITHELIAL BLADDER TUMORS

Tumors of Bladder Muscle

As previously noted, primary tumors of the bladder wall are relatively rare lesions. The most common benign bladder-wall neoplasms are leiomyoma and rhabdomyoma. These usually present as smooth, well-demarcated masses in the bladder wall, though they may occasionally be pedunculated. The more common malignant bladder-wall lesions are leiomyosarcoma and rhabdomyosarcoma. Leiomyosarcomas tend to be quite large and may ulcerate. If the lesion is undifferentiated, it becomes difficult to distinguish from a rhabdomyosarcoma. Leiomyosarcomas tend to occur in patients over the age of 40.

Rhabdomyosarcoma of the bladder occurs in two forms—adult and embryonal. As with leiomyosarcoma, the adult form of rhabdomyosarcoma is usually seen in older patients. As with rhabdomyosarcomas elsewhere, the prognosis is poor. Embryonal rhabdomyosarcoma of the bladder occurs primarily in the first few years of life. This is similar to the embryonal rhabdomyosarcoma that involves the prostate in boys and the vagina in girls. This tumor often has a lobulated appearance, resembling a cluster of grapes, resulting in the name sarcoma botryoides. These are highly malignant lesions, and the cure rate is low even after extensive surgical resection.

Radiographically, smooth mural defects seen on excretory urography or cystography should suggest the possibility of a benign bladder-wall tumor. CT or MRI can demonstrate these benign lesions as smooth, soft-tissue masses in the bladder wall, without evidence of extension. The sarcomas, being more aggressive, are usually irregular and may be ulcerated. In some cases, it is difficult to ascertain the exact point of origin of these lesions, as extension through the bladder wall and into adjacent pelvic organs or to the pelvic sidewall is not uncommon. As noted above, sarcoma botryoides has a rather characteristic radiographic appearance, and the lesion may occasionally be large enough to almost fill the bladder. Both benign and malignant mural tumors are somewhat vascular and tend to enhance when studied by CT after administration of an intravenous contrast agent.

Pheochromocytoma

Pheochromocytoma occurring primarily in the bladder wall is a rare lesion. This tumor is usually small, averaging about 2 cm in diameter; most frequently it is seen in the region of the trigone. Though these lesions have been reported to occur between the ages of 14 and 78, the average age at presentation is about 40. More than half the patients give a classic clinical history of experiencing a hypertensive episode during or immediately after voiding. The large majority of these tumors (95%) are benign.

Radiographically, pheochromocytomas in the bladder are difficult to differentiate from other benign bladder-wall tumors. All of these lesions can result in a relatively small smooth filling defect on contrast studies (Fig. 20-18) or an intramural soft-tissue lesion on cross-sectional methods. However, pheochromocytomas, being quite vascular, enhance significantly on CT after administration of an intravenous contrast agent, and on MRI they exhibit a fairly characteristic homogeneous low signal on T1 images and a very high signal on T2 images. These findings in association with the typical clinical history should lead to the correct diagnosis.

Lymphoma

Though very rare, lymphoma can primarily involve the bladder wall, usually occurring in the region of the bladder base or trigone. It is three times more common in women than in men, and it is usually seen after the age of 40 [11]. Arising as a slightly nodular, slow-growing focus in the bladder wall, it is difficult to distinguish radiographically from other mural malignancies.

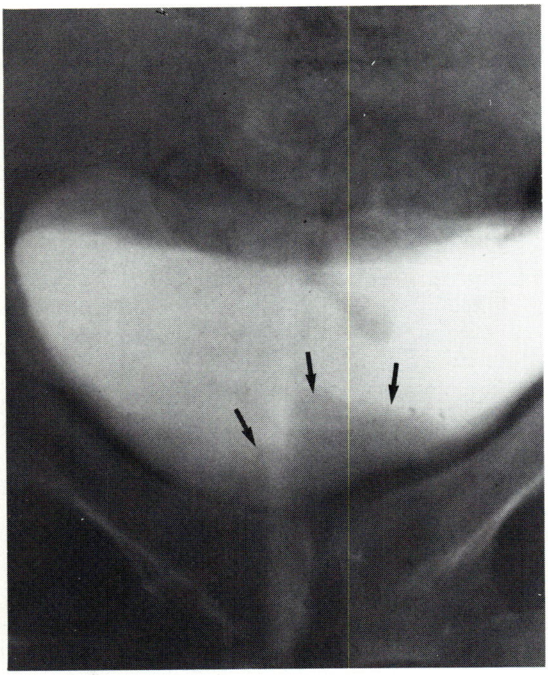

Figure 20-18. Pheochromocytoma of bladder. Coned urographic view of bladder shows smooth mural-based mass in region of left trigone (arrows).

Other Primary Neoplasms

Other nonepithelial tumors of the bladder have been reported but are extremely rare. These include hemangioma, neurofibroma, plasmacytoma, lipoma, myxoma, osteosarcoma, osteochondrosarcoma, and angiosarcoma.

SECONDARY BLADDER TUMORS

Slightly more than 1 percent of all neoplastic lesions involving the bladder are metastatic in origin. Furthermore, the bladder is involved in about 3.5 percent of patients dying from generalized carcinomatosis. The most frequent metastatic lesion to involve the bladder is malignant melanoma, usually occurring as multiple metastatic foci. Other tumors that commonly involve the bladder via hematogenous spread are stomach, pancreatic, ovarian, colon, breast, kidney, and lung cancers. The bladder can also be involved by metastatic tumor via intraperitoneal seeding to the bladder dome.

More commonly, tumors of other pelvic structures adjacent to the bladder can involve the bladder by direct extension. Prostate cancer frequently involves the bladder floor, sigmoid carcinoma can invade the lateral or posterior wall in both sexes, and cervical carcinoma is the most common gynecologic malignancy to spread to the bladder.

Radiographically, most metastatic lesions of the bladder present as single or multiple filling defects within the bladder lumen on contrast studies. This finding, coupled with the clinical history of primary tumor elsewhere in the body, should suggest the diagnosis of metastatic disease. In cases of direct extension from adjacent tumors, the earliest radiographic sign may be mild irregularity of the bladder wall. In end-stage disease, large fungating masses may be seen to involve the bladder.

REFERENCES

1. Ambos, M.A., et al. The pear-shaped bladder. *Radiology* 122:85, 1977.
2. Amendola, M.A., et al. Staging of bladder carcinoma: MRI-CT-surgical correlation. *A.J.R.* 146:1179, 1986.
3. Amis, E.S., Jr., et al. Impressions on floor of the female bladder: "The female prostate." *Urology* 19:441, 1982.
4. Bosniak, M.A., Siegelman, S.S., and Evans, J.A. *The Adrenal, Retroperitoneum and Lower Urinary Tract: An Atlas of Tumor Radiology*. Chicago: Year Book, 1976. Pp. 440–450.
5. Dann, R.H., Arger, P.H., and Enterline, H.T. Benign proliferative processes presenting as mass lesions in the urinary bladder. *A.J.R.* 116:822, 1972.
6. Dershaw, D.D., and Scher, H.I. Serial transabdominal sonography of bladder cancer. *A.J.R.* 150:1055, 1988.
7. Fisher, M.R., Hricak, H., and Tanagho, E.A. Urinary bladder MR imaging. Part II. Neoplasm. *Radiology* 157:471, 1985.
8. Gloding, R.P., et al. Intravenous urography as a prognostic indicator in vesical carcinoma. *Cancer* 60:883, 1987.
9. Goldman, S.M., et al. CT in the diagnosis of enterovesical fistulae. *A.J.R.* 144:1229, 1985.
10. Hattery, R.R. Imaging of the bladder. In H.M. Pollack, and G.W. Hartman (Eds.), *ARRS Categorical Course Syllabus (Uroradiology)*. Reston, Va.: American Roentgen Ray Society, 1989.
11. Heiken, J.P., McClennan, B.L., and DiSantis, D.J. Nontransitional cell tumors of the bladder. In J.M. Taveras, and J.T. Ferrucci (Eds.), *Radiology: Diagnosis-Imaging-Intervention*. Philadelphia: Lippincott, 1988.

12. Imray, T.J., and Kaplan, P. Lower urinary tract infections and calculi in the adult. *Semin. Roentgenol.* 18:276, 1983.
13. Javadpour, N., and Mostofi, F.K. Primary epithelial tumors of the bladder in the first two decades of life. *J. Urol.* 101:706, 1969.
14. Korobkin, M., Minagi, H., and Palubinskas, A.J. Lateral displacement of the bladder. *A.J.R.* 125:337, 1975.
15. Kwok-Liu, J.P., Zikman, J.N., and Cockshott, W.P. Carcinoma of the urachus: The role of computed tomography. *Radiology* 137:731, 1980.
16. Liebeskind, A.L., Elkin, M., and Goldman, S. Herniation of the bladder. *Radiology* 106:257, 1973.
17. Pollack, H.M., et al. Diagnostic considerations in urinary bladder wall calcifications. *A.J.R.* 136:791, 1981.
18. Rholl, K.S., et al. Primary bladder carcinoma: Evaluation with MR imaging. *Radiology* 163:117, 1987.
19. Sager, E.M., et al. Contrast-enhanced computed tomography to show perivesical extension in bladder carcinoma. *Acta Radiol.* 28:307, 1987.
20. Sager, E.M. et al. The role of CT in demonstrating perivesical tumor growth in the preoperative staging of carcinoma of the urinary bladder. *Radiology* 146:443, 1983.
21. Salo, J.O., Kivisaari, L., and Lehtonen, T. Comparison of magnetic resonance imaging with computed tomography and intravesical ultrasound in staging bladder cancer. *Urol. Radiol.* 10:167, 1988.
22. Spataro, R.F. Benign conditions of the bladder. In J.M. Taveras and J.T. Ferrucci (Eds.), *Radiology: Diagnosis-Imaging-Intervention.* Philadelphia: Lippincott, 1988.
23. Wechsler, R.J., and Brennan, R.E. Teardrop bladder: Additional considerations. *Radiology* 144:281, 1982.
24. Weinerman, P.M., et al. Pelvic adenopathy from bladder and prostate carcinoma: Detection by rapid-sequence computed tomography. *A.J.R.* 140:95, 1983.
25. Weinerman, P.M., Arger, P.H., and Pollack, H.M. CT evaluation of bladder and prostate neoplasms. *Urol. Radiol.* 4:105, 1982.
26. Whitmore, W.F., Jr. Bladder cancer: An overview. *CA* 38:213, 1988.
27. Wood, D.P., Jr., et al. The role of magnetic resonance imaging in the staging of bladder carcinoma. *J. Urol.* 140:741, 1988.
28. Yousem, D.M., et al. Synchronous and metachronous transitional cell carcinoma of the urinary tract: Prevalence, incidence, and radiographic detection. *Radiology* 167:613, 1988.
29. Zimmermann, K., Amis, E.S., Jr., and Newhouse, J.H. Nephrogenic adenoma of the bladder: Urographic spectrum *Urol. Radiol.* 11:123, 1989.

Neurogenic Bladder Dysfunction and Urinary Incontinence

The normal urinary bladder both stores and periodically expels urine. During storage the urethra remains closed while the bladder becomes progressively distended; when the bladder is distended to capacity, a need to void is transmitted to sensory centers in the brain. During voluntary micturition the detrusor muscle of the bladder contracts in response to motor impulses originating in parasympathetic neurons in the sacral spinal cord. Simultaneously, the bladder neck (internal sphincter) funnels, and the smooth muscle (intrinsic) sphincter around the urethra relaxes. The striated (external) sphincter in the urogenital diaphragm also relaxes, and voiding occurs through a completely open urethra. Additional neurologic input from the sympathetic and pudendal nerves is necessary for totally coordinated voiding. During both the storage and expulsion phases the valve mechanisms at the ureterovesical junctions prevent vesicoureteral reflux.

Normally, there is perfect coordination between the bladder and urethra during voiding. This coordination requires an intact "brainstem micturition center" in the pons, which is under conscious cortical control, and intact neural pathways in the spinal cord connecting this upper center to the "sacral micturition center." The sacral micturition center lies in the second through fourth sacral cord segments and is connected to the bladder via the sacral reflex arc. Thus, lesions anywhere from the brain to the neural pathways of the sacral reflex arc can cause disintegration of coordinated voluntary voiding and result in neurogenic bladder dysfunction (Fig. 21-1). Urinary incontinence can be secondary to neurogenic dysfunction of the lower urinary tract, but there are multiple other causes. This chapter will discuss neurogenic bladder dysfunction and urinary incontinence, including areas in which these two conditions overlap.

NEUROGENIC BLADDER DYSFUNCTION

Multiple classifications for neurogenic bladder dysfunction have been proposed [18]. These are generally based on anatomic or functional changes. Some classifications have been based on the principle of the upper-motor-neuron lesion versus the lower-motor-neuron lesion with respect to the innervation of the detrusor muscle of the bladder. The upper-motor-neuron reflex bladder results from a lesion that separates the sacral micturition center from higher control mechanisms. On the other hand, the lower-motor-neuron autonomous bladder is produced by a lesion functionally separating the bladder from the sacral micturition center. A more appropriate classification, derived in light of present-day knowledge, redefines the upper-motor-neuron bladder as hyperreflexive and the lower-motor-neuron bladder as areflexive [10].

A third pattern of neurogenic bladder dysfunction is the uninhibited neurogenic bladder. In the infant, voiding is a reflex occurrence. As neuromuscular maturation occurs with aging, the higher cortical centers gain control over voiding. Uninhibited bladder activity represents a failure of normal development of this cortical regulation of micturition or an acquired lesion of the central nervous system, resulting in a persistence or reappearance of the incompletely controlled bladder [9].

Although in the past it was predicted that an upper-motor-neuron lesion would always produce a hyperreflexive bladder and, conversely, that a lower-motor-neuron lesion would always result in an areflexive bladder, it has been shown that this simple classification is not always true. In other words, lesions may overlap various portions of the micturition control centers or pathways, lesions may be multiple and involve various parts of the centers or pathways,

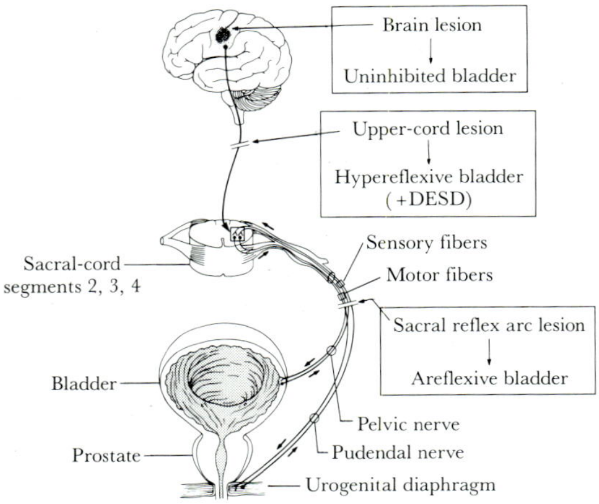

Figure 21-1. Simplified diagram of nerve pathways controlling bladder function. Failure of proper development or diseases affecting the inhibitory center in the brain result in an uninhibited bladder. Lesions of the suprasacral cord cause a hyperreflexive bladder. Lesions of the sacral reflex arc result in an areflexive bladder. (DESD = detrusor–external sphincter dyssynergia.)

or a lesion may be single and involve only motor or sensory portions of the centers or pathways. This can result in mixed types of neurogenic bladder dysfunction. However, there is enough correlation between location of lesions and expected neurogenic dysfunction to recommend the simple classification of neurogenic bladder dysfunction shown in Table 21-1. The main categories of neurogenic bladder dysfunction will be discussed in more detail below.

UNINHIBITED NEUROGENIC BLADDER

Uninhibited neurogenic bladder in its milder idiopathic form occurs because of a persistence of the infantile pattern of voiding, usually as a result of incomplete or delayed neuromuscular maturation. This results in uninhibited, involuntary bladder contractions, which may be spontaneous or provoked by rapid filling, alterations of posture, coughing, walking, jumping, or other triggering procedures. These contractions are sensed by the patients as an urge to void followed, on occasion, by some degree of urge

Table 21-1. Simplified classification of neurogenic bladder dysfunction

Type	*Mechanism*	*Common Causes*	*Incontinence*	*Coordination of Voiding*
Uninhibited bladder unstable bladder infantile bladder immature bladder	Idiopathic	Delayed or incomplete maturation of inhibitory mechanism	Urge	Normal
	Central nervous system lesion above brain-stem micturition center	Cerebrovascular accident Brain tumor Parkinson's disease Normal pressure hydrocephalus	Reflex	Normal
Hyperreflexive bladder spastic bladder upper-motor-neuron bladder	Spinal cord lesion (suprasacral)	Multiple sclerosis Myelodysplasia Spinal cord trauma Spinal cord tumors Herniated intervertebral disk Arteriovenous malformations of cord	Reflex	Abnormal (DESD)
Areflexive bladder flaccid bladder autonomous bladder lower-motor-neuron bladder	Lesions of conus medullaris or sacral nerve outflow	Herniated intervertebral disk Diabetic neuropathy Multiple sclerosis Lower spinal cord tumors Pelvic surgery	Overflow	Abnormal

incontinence before voluntary control of the external urethral sphincter can be exerted. In children, recurrent urinary tract infections, vesicoureteral reflux, or episodic incontinence may suggest this condition. In adults, symptoms include frequency and urgency of urination.

A more serious form of uninhibited bladder occurs when disease of the central nervous system compromises voluntary control of the micturition reflex. The patient simply loses the ability either to initiate or prevent voiding; uninhibited contractions, when they occur, are not sensed and thus are not counteracted. Because the micturition centers remain intact, coordinated, physiologically normal voiding occurs reflexly without patient awareness in these cases. Lesions that can result in this type of uninhibited voiding include cerebrovascular accident, brain tumor, Parkinson's disease, normal pressure hydrocephalus, and other miscellaneous conditions [3]. In both types of uninhibited bladder, since micturition is well coordinated, radiographic evaluation of the urinary tract is often normal.

HYPERREFLEXIVE NEUROGENIC BLADDER

Hyperreflexive neurogenic bladder is caused by interruption of the neural pathways in the suprasacral spinal cord connecting the brain-stem micturition center to the sacral micturition center. This often results in detrusor–external sphincter dyssynergia (DESD)—incoordination between the bladder detrusor and the external urethral sphincter at the level of the urogenital diaphragm, especially when the cord lesion is at the level of T-5 or higher. In these patients there is no perception of bladder filling or emptying, and voluntary micturition is not possible. Reflex bladder contractions can occur at any volume of filling, and during these contractions there is frequently a simultaneous contraction of the external urethral sphincter. This results in an obstruction to bladder emptying. As a result of the chronically increased intravesical pressure, upper urinary tract deterioration can occur. Common neurologic disorders that result in this type of dysfunction include multiple sclerosis, myelodysplasia, spinal cord tumors, spinal cord trauma, and herniated intervertebral disks.

If these patients are untreated, or if treatment has been inadequate, urography often reveals bilateral upper tract dilation, either as a result of vesicoureteral reflux or functional obstruction of the ureters due to hypertrophy of the bladder wall and increased intravesical pressure (Fig. 21-2). These patients are prime candidates for urinary infection and stone disease. On voiding cystourethrography, vesicoureteral reflux may or may not be present. The bladder frequently has a vertical configuration with significant trabeculations, resulting in the so-called Christmas-tree bladder. During the voiding phase of the study, the external sphincter at the level of the urogenital diaphragm may be seen to contract inappropriately (DESD). This lack of coordination between bladder detrusor and external sphincter contractions may also result in massive reflux into the prostatic ducts due to the high pressures present in the posterior

Figure 21-2. Hyperreflexive bladder with upper tract changes in patient with upper spinal cord injury. Intravenous urography shows bilateral moderate hydronephrosis and trabeculated, vertically oriented ("Christmas-tree") bladder.

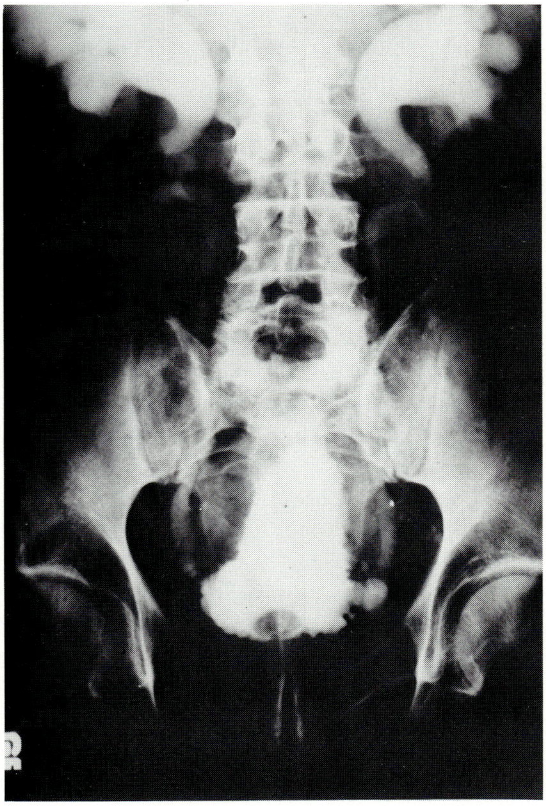

urethra during voiding (Fig. 21-3). Intraprostatic reflux may lead to the presence of multiple prostatic calculi. Also seen is poor distention of the anterior urethra distal to the external sphincter. Finally, emptying of the bladder is usually significantly compromised.

AREFLEXIVE BLADDER

In this condition the bladder may also be termed *hyporeflexive*, because there are often weak or poorly sustained detrusor contractions. Areflexive bladder dysfunction is secondary to neurologic lesions that affect the sacral micturition center or reflex arc; these include herniated disks, multiple sclerosis, diabetic neuropathy, and lower spinal cord tumors. When the spinal cord is involved, the level is usually either at the conus medullaris or the cauda equina. The sacral reflex arc can also be affected by trauma or by pelvic surgery such as radical hysterectomy or abdominoperineal resection of the rectum.

In cases of areflexive neurogenic dysfunction of the bladder, the urethral sphincter mechanism may remain competent. Since there is no perception of bladder distention, the bladder will fill until intravesical pressure exceeds that exerted by the urethral sphincter. At this point overflow incontinence occurs until the pressures are equalized.

On occasion, for unknown reasons, there may be a significant rise in intravesical pressure during bladder filling. As in cases of hyperreflexive bladder, this can result in deterioration of the upper urinary tract. In yet other cases, the urethral sphincter mechanism may be totally compromised, resulting in continual dribbling incontinence of urine. Patients in whom some sphincter activity is preserved may retain a degree of continence.

In most patients with areflexive bladders, urography reveals normal upper tracts and occasionally a large bladder (Fig. 21-4). Voiding cystourethrography shows a thin-walled bladder with generous capacity, a smooth contour, and poor emptying. Vesicoureteral reflux is rare because of the low pressures usually encountered within the bladder lumen. On removal of the filling catheter, the patient may exhibit total incontinence of urine. On the other hand, if some urethral sphincter activity remains, the patient will be continent and able to void only with

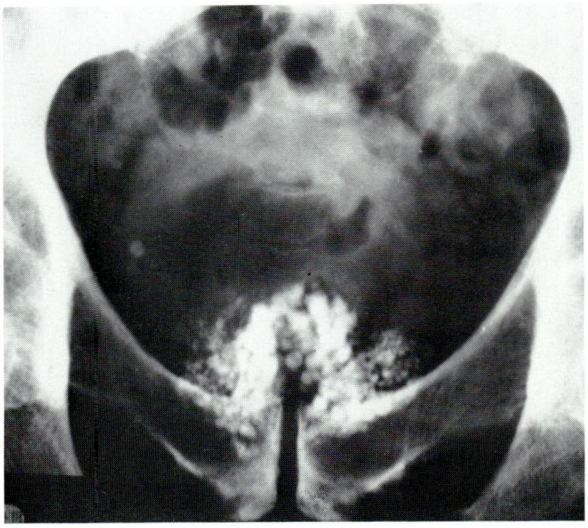

A

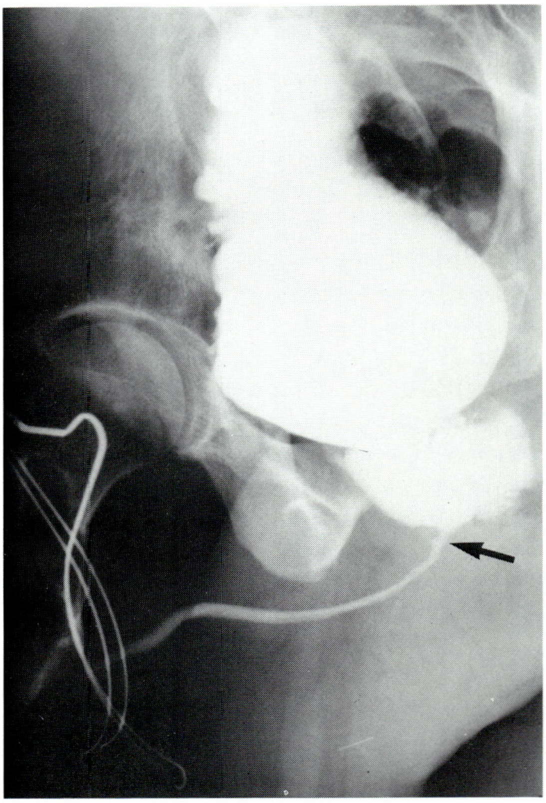

B

Figure 21-3. DESD in man with high thoracic cord injury. A. Coned radiography of pelvis shows prostatic calculi. B. Voiding cystourethrography demonstrates Christmas-tree bladder. The external sphincter (arrow) is contracted, resulting in massive reflux into the prostatic ducts and poor distention of the anterior urethra even though a Zipser clamp has been applied to the distal penis.

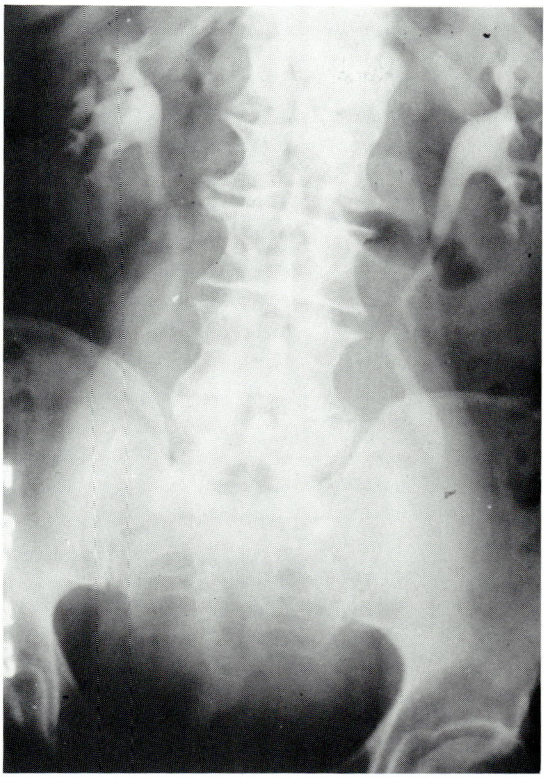

Figure 21-4. Areflexive bladder in patient with compromise of sacral reflex arc. Intravenous urography shows that the bladder is greatly distended, but because of relatively low intravesical pressure, the upper tracts are normal.

straining or the Credé maneuver. The amount of residual urine is dependent on the effectiveness of these ancillary voiding mechanisms.

EVALUATION OF NEUROGENIC BLADDER DYSFUNCTION

Urodynamic studies play a vital part in the examination of the patient with a known or suspected neurogenic dysfunction of the bladder [12]. These studies require sophisticated equipment for performing cystometrics and for documenting results of the cystometrogram and the electromyogram of the periurethral striated sphincter muscle. Additionally, simultaneous transrectal ultrasonography has been recommended as a useful correlative study in evaluating the bladder neck and urethra during cystometrics [16]. As the bladder neck and external sphincter are easily visualized during transrectal evaluation of the urethra, uncoordinated contraction of the bladder neck or external sphincter in response to increased pressure in the bladder can be easily documented.

The typical radiographic findings associated with the various types of neurogenic bladder dysfunction have been described above. Plain abdominal radiography is useful in initially evaluating these patients, since abnormalities such as sacral agenesis or spinal dysraphism are frequently associated with neurogenic bladder dysfunction. Urography is usually performed on a regular basis, especially in patients with hyperreflexive bladders, to document the status of the upper urinary tract. On the other hand, voiding cystourethrography is often used as part of the initial evaluation of the patient with symptoms possibly referable to neurogenic dysfunction of the bladder. Care should be taken while performing this study in patients with cord lesions above T-5, as they may manifest autonomic dysreflexia when the bladder is distended. Such patients can have diaphoresis, headache, hypertension, and bradycardia and should be treated with an alpha-adrenergic blocker before the bladder is studied [7].

It is important to note that in patients with early or partial lesions affecting the micturition reflex, the urinary tract may appear completely normal. This is also true if there has been adequate treatment of a diagnosed neurogenic dysfunction.

Voiding cystourethrography can be modified to study the bladder for uninhibited contractions. In this technique, the bladder is catheterized with a small feeding tube and dilute contrast medium is instilled into the bladder through a gravity drip from a constant height of 30 cm above the level of the bladder [6]. An abnormal bladder contraction is manifested by slowing or cessation of the contrast drip. Fluoroscopically, these contractions are usually accompanied by an opening of the bladder neck of variable duration and degree. This finding, combined with cessation of the drip or backup of contrast material in the tubing, suggests the presence of an uninhibited bladder. During the voiding phase of the study, girls with uninhibited bladders are often seen to have a "spinning-top" urethra, a term used to describe a widened posterior urethra [15]. This configuration of the urethra most likely results from a chronic increase in external sphincter tone in response to unstable bladder contractions in an attempt to prevent leakage of urine. In the past the spinning-top urethra was commonly regarded as a normal variant.

At some point during their disease process, many patients with neurogenic dysfunction of the bladder are treated with an indwelling Foley catheter for variable periods. The catheter remains a source of infection until an intermittent catheterization program is instituted or voiding problems are corrected by surgical or medical means. Urethral changes such as diverticula, strictures, or extravasation of contrast material outside the urethra may be seen in a third of these patients [5]. Bladder calculi are also common; it has been estimated that 10 to 15 percent of patients with spinal cord injuries will develop urinary tract calculi, with the bladder being the most common site of stone formation. Causes of stones other than an indwelling catheter include immobilization, urinary stasis, and infection.

Clean (nonsterile) intermittent catheterization (CIC) has proved to be a safe technique for the treatment of neurogenic disease of the bladder, and it is currently widely used when catheter drainage is necessary. Even CIC is not without complications, however, as a pubic hair can be inadvertently introduced into the bladder during this procedure and may act as a nidus for stone formation [2]. These calcifications have a vermiform appearance radiographically, and this configuration of bladder calculi should suggest the probability of hair as a nidus.

URINARY INCONTINENCE

Urinary incontinence is an involuntary loss of urine that is objectively demonstrable and a social or hygienic problem [1]. There are several different types and many causes of urinary incontinence. As noted in the previous section, various types of neurogenic bladder dysfunction result in different patterns of incontinence. On the other hand, one of the more common types of urinary incontinence is that of stress incontinence in women, which is due to anatomic urethral dysfunction rather than a neurogenic lesion. Table 21-2 gives a classification of urinary incontinence, including the most common associated causes.

Table 21-2. Classification of urinary incontinence

Stress incontinence
Urethral dysfunction
Urge incontinence
Uninhibited neurogenic bladder
Bladder irritation or infection
Overflow incontinence
Areflexive neurogenic bladder
Bladder-outlet obstruction
Reflex incontinence
Hyperreflexive neurogenic bladder
Uninhibited bladder (central nervous system disease)
Total incontinence
Congenital abnormalities
Ectopic ureteral orifice
Epispadias
Vesicovaginal or ureterovaginal fistula
Surgery or trauma affecting sphincters
Psychological incontinence

STRESS INCONTINENCE

The original theory emphasizing an anatomic basis for stress incontinence points to an altered posterior urethrovesical angle as a cause. It has been shown that women with stress incontinence have an altered anatomic position of the urethra below the confines of the abdomen. Thus, increased intraabdominal pressure during activities such as laughing or coughing will be differentially transmitted to the bladder and urethra. This results in elevated intravesical pressure without a comparable rise in urethral pressure [13]. This combination of events will produce incontinence until the external sphincter can be consciously contracted to prevent urine flow. Anatomic change in the position of the urethra is often due to multiparity and results from a downward and posterior rotation of the bladder neck. Displacement of the urethra correlates well with the loss of the posterior urethrovesical angle.

Far less commonly, the female urethra partially loses its sphincter capability. Because of low urethral pressure, in these patients urinary leakage occurs with the slightest provocation. Additionally, usually after multiple pelvic surgical procedures, the female urethra can becomes fibrotic and rigid and hence incapable of continually maintaining complete continence.

In Green's original classification of stress incontinence, Type I was characterized by loss of the posterior urethrovesical angle and Type II by a posterior, inferior, and rotational descent of the bladder base and urethra in addition to loss of the angle [8]. Type II corresponds to a cystourethrocele. This classification has now been modified to include Type III stress incontinence, which is characterized by a urethra that no longer functions as a sphincter, as discussed earlier [11]. Type III stress incontinence is seen in approximately 75 percent of patients with recurrent stress incontinence who have had two or more urethropexy operations [4]. When surgical correction is tailored to the specific cause of stress incontinence, the reported cure rate is in excess of 90 percent.

URGE INCONTINENCE

Urge incontinence may, at times, resemble stress incontinence. This type of incontinence occurs in patients who have an overwhelming desire to void and cannot totally suppress this urge. It may be neurogenically induced or may be caused by nonneurogenic diseases such as acute or chronic cystitis or carcinoma of the bladder. The major neurogenic cause of this type of incontinence is uninhibited contraction of the bladder detrusor. Whatever the cause, the incontinence is usually manifested as episodic loss of small amounts of urine.

OVERFLOW INCONTINENCE

Overflow incontinence occurs in the areflexive bladder. It can also be caused by nonneurologic processes that produce bladder outlet obstruction, such as benign hyperplasia of the prostate in older men. As with urge incontinence, on occasion overflow incontinence may resemble loss of urine as a result of stress such as coughing or straining. This is true because the bladder is never emptied, and increased abdominal pressure may result in leakage. Generally speaking, with overflow incontinence there is a large-capacity bladder with a relatively low intravesical pressure. As the bladder fills beyond the point of normal compliance of the bladder wall, the increased intravesical pressure becomes higher than that generated by the urethral sphincters, and leakage of urine follows. The volume of urine leaked is only that necessary to reequilibrate the bladder pressure with the urethral sphincteric pressure.

REFLEX INCONTINENCE

Reflex incontinence is generally seen in patients with lesions of the suprasacral spinal cord that result in a hyperreflexive bladder. With lesions of this type, there is no transmission of the sensation of bladder filling to the cortex, and the patient does not perceive a desire to void. Furthermore, there is no perception of bladder contraction. Therefore, the patient voids urine without any awareness that this is occurring. With central nervous system lesions above the brain-stem micturition center, complete physiologic reflux voiding occurs randomly because of loss of consciously controlled inhibition.

TOTAL INCONTINENCE

Constant dribbling incontinence is most often seen in males after trauma to the urethral sphincter during prostatectomy. In females, after multiple procedures to correct stress incontinence, the urethra may be reduced to a fibrotic nonresistant tube, resulting in total incontinence. Ureterovaginal or vesicovaginal fistulas secondary to previous surgery or pelvic neoplasms result in a constant loss of urine.

Total incontinence in children should prompt a thorough evaluation for congenital anomalies such as ectopic insertion of the ureter (often in association with complete duplication) into the cervix, vagina, or vestibule. In young girls, minor degrees of epispadias may not be readily clinically apparent, though the urethra may be sufficiently compromised to allow urine loss.

PSYCHOLOGICAL INCONTINENCE

Only on very rare occasions is urinary incontinence a symptom of a psychiatric disorder. These patients are usually voluntarily able to control their voiding but void at an inappropriate time and in an improper place.

RADIOLOGIC EVALUATION OF URINARY INCONTINENCE

Prior to radiologic evaluation of the patient with urinary incontinence, a careful history and physical examination should provide a clue as to the type of dysfunction present and its cause. However, there may be significant overlap in the incontinence patterns of various disease processes. In these cases, radiologic evaluation may be helpful in differentiating the various types of incontinence.

As in the patient with neurogenic bladder, intravenous urography is often performed to evaluate the upper tracts. In cases in which incontinence is caused by a hyperreflexive bladder, upper tract dilation and parenchymal scarring are not uncommon, and the bladder is frequently thick-walled and trabeculated. Voiding cystourethrography, which should be performed prior to intravenous urography, is the mainstay in evaluating incontinence radiographically. This is usually performed in conjunction with, or in addition to, cystometric studies of the lower urinary tract. Fluid should be instilled into the bladder at low pressure using gravity drip. The patient is asked to note the first sensation of filling or the urge to void. As the bladder becomes nearly filled, its contour and wall thickness should be assessed for the suggestion of trabeculation. With hyperreflexive bladders, reflux may occur. The volume required to fill the bladder to capacity should be recorded; with the uninhibited bladder, this should average 300 to 500 ml. With the hyperreflexive bladder, the capacity may be somewhat reduced, and voiding around the catheter may occur at virtually any level of filling on a reflex basis. Areflexive bladders may have capacities approaching several liters.

In patients with hyperreflexive bladders and DESD, the bladder contracts, the bladder neck opens, and there is narrowing of the distal urethra in females or the membranous urethra

Figure 21-5. Diagram of urethrovesical relationships in female stress incontinence (lateral projections with pubis shown anterior to bladder). A. Normal—Posterior urethrovesical angle approximately 90 degrees. B. Type I stress incontinence—Mild downward and posterior rotation of the bladder results in an increased posterior urethrovesical angle. C. Type II stress incontinence—Further rotation has resulted in a cystourethrocele. D. Type III stress incontinence—Previous surgeries have resulted in an overcorrected posterior urethrovesical angle, but the urethra is fixed and fibrotic and has lost its ability to maintain continence. E. True cystocele—The urethrovesical angle is normal, and these patients are usually continent.

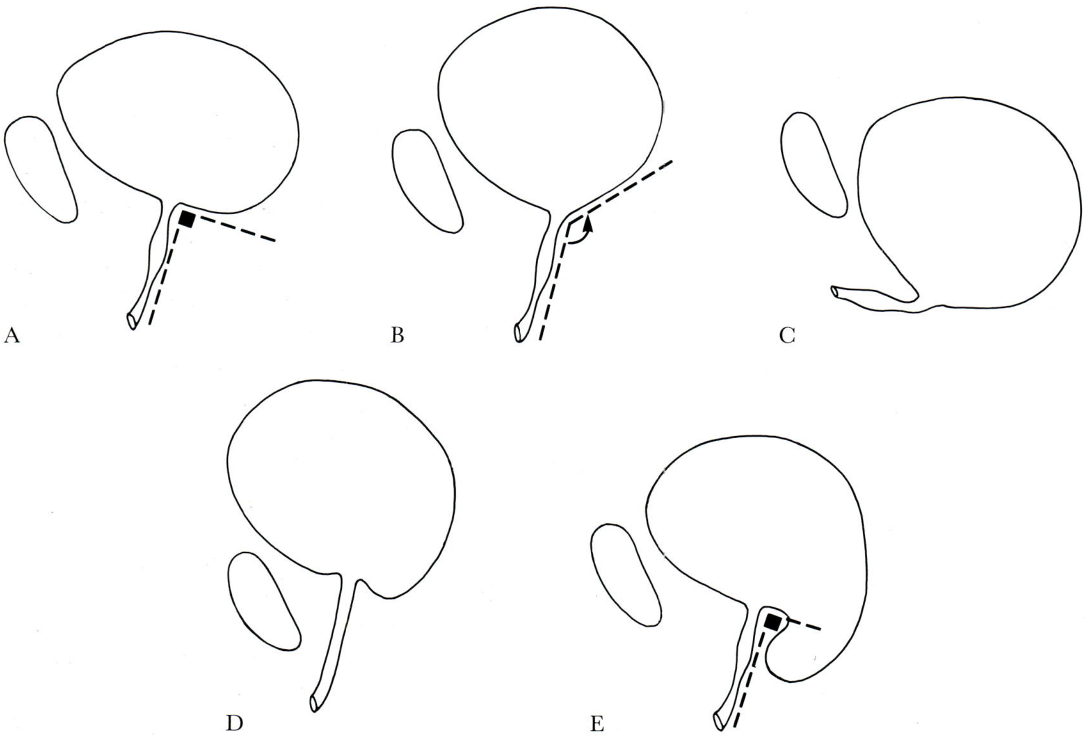

in males that resists the outflow of urine during voiding. In males, reflux into prostatic ducts may be seen during voiding. Hyporeflexive bladders have large capacities and, when filled, may exhibit an overflow dribbling incontinence of urine immediately after removal of the catheter. In all cases, the ability (or inability) to initiate voiding and the amount of residual urine after voiding (whether reflex or voluntary) should be noted.

With the bladder full, standing cystography demonstrates a continence level at the bladder neck in normal patients. Straining or coughing in a woman with stress incontinence may show descensus of the bladder and leakage of urine. On the other hand, increasing abdominal pressure may also induce a contraction in hyperreflexive or uninhibited bladders, resulting in urine leakage. Standing, straining lateral views in a woman with stress incontinence may reveal the posterior and downward rotation of the bladder typical of this condition. In the past "chain cystography" has been performed to allow determination of the posterior urethrovesical angle. In this technique, a small, flexible metal chain is placed in the urethra and into the opacified bladder, allowing clear definition of this angle on lateral views of the patient while standing and straining. Figure 21-5 diagrammatically depicts the urethrovesical relationships in female stress incontinence. A true cystocele, as opposed to the cystourethrocele seen in Type II stress incontinence, leaves the urethrovesical angle intact. Descensus of the bladder base below its normal position just above the pubic symphysis in supine views in women does not correlate well with stress incontinence, as the urethrovesical relationship may remain normal in many of these cases.

In all cases of incontinence the bladder should be evaluated for mucosal edema or irregularities that may suggest infection or tumor. Vesicovaginal fistulas may require oblique or lateral views to demonstrate contrast material leaking into the vagina during cystography, or they may be readily apparent (Fig. 21-6). Small ureterovaginal fistulas, on the other hand, may be difficult to see during urography. In some cases, the ureter may appear slightly irregular or may be partially obstructed at the point of fistulization. Retrograde studies will usually demonstrate the leak.

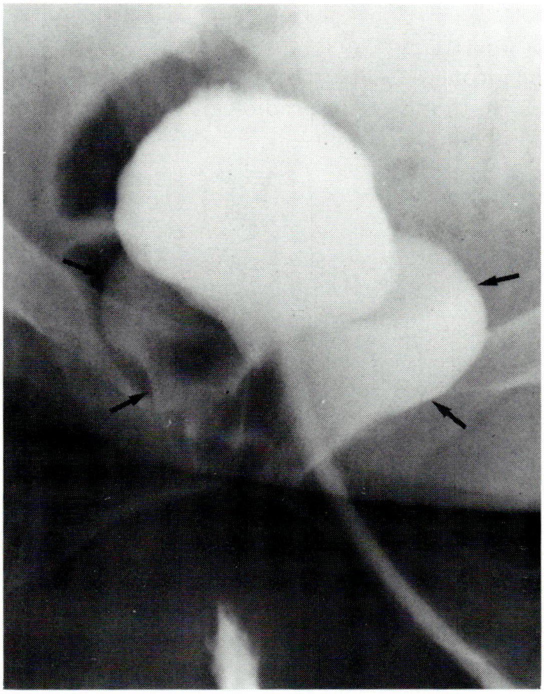

Figure 21-6. Vesicovaginal fistula occurring as a complication of radical pelvic surgery. Cystography via suprapubic tube shows free flow of contrast medium into vagina (arrows) and out the vaginal introitus.

In children with incontinence there is frequently no underlying structural abnormality. However, as previously noted, there are anatomic defects that can result in incontinence [17]. The preliminary film may reveal a widened interpubic distance, suggesting undiagnosed epispadias in a female; normally, this separation should not exceed 1 cm. On urography, a poorly functioning or obstructed duplicated upper-pole system should suggest the possibility of ectopic ureteral insertion outside normal sphincter control. This diagnosis may also be suggested if a nonfunctioning kidney is seen. Voiding cystourethrography might reveal significant vaginal reflux in young girls, which may explain postvoiding dribbling incontinence as urine subsequently drains from the vagina.

When incontinence has been treated by insertion of a prosthetic sphincter, radiographic evaluation of its function may be requested. The

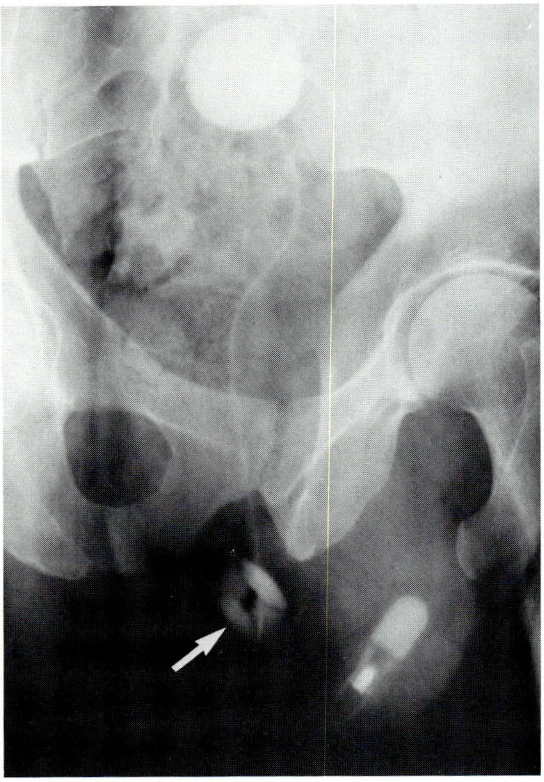

Figure 21-7. Prosthetic urethral spincter. Low pelvic radiography reveals the reservoir in the pelvis, the valve in the scrotum, and the inflated cuff (arrow) around the urethra.

typical prosthesis used is comprised of an inflatable cuff surrounding the urethra; inflation is controlled by a valve, implanted in the scrotum or one labium, that directs flow between the cuff and a reservoir located in the pelvis (Fig. 21-7). Because the fluid usually contains contrast material, the integrity of the system can be determined by pelvic radiographs taken during the inflated and deflated phases.

INCONTINENCE IN ELDERLY PATIENTS

Little is known about the causes of incontinence in the 1 million institutionalized elderly persons with this condition. A study of a representative sample of this group of patients indicated that incontinence was due to an overactive detrusor in 61 percent of cases [14]. Among women, stress incontinence accounted for 21 percent of cases of incontinence. In men, bladder outlet obstruction, usually due to prostate enlargement, was the cause of incontinence in 29 percent. In fully 35 percent of patients, at least two coexisting probable causes of incontinence were identified.

REFERENCES

1. Abrams, P., et al. Standardization of terminology of lower urinary tract function. *Neurourol. Urodynam.* 7:403, 1988.
2. Amendola, M.A., et al. Bladder calculi complicating intermittent clean catheterization. *A.J.R.* 141:751, 1983.
3. Blaivas, J.G. Neurologic dysfunctions. In S.V. Yalla et al. (Eds.), *Neurourology and Urodynamics.* New York: Macmillian, 1988.
4. Blaivas, J.G., and Olsson, C.A. Stress incontinence: Classification and surgical approach. *J. Urol.* 139:727, 1988.
5. Calenoff, L., Foley, M.J., and Hendrix, R.W. Evaluation of the urethra in males with spinal cord injury. *Radiology* 142:71, 1982.
6. Fotter, R., et al. Unstable bladder in children: Functional evaluation by modified voiding cystourethrography. *Radiology* 161:811, 1986.
7. Friendland, G.W., and Perkash, I. Neuromuscular dysfunction of the bladder and urethra. *Semin. Roentgenol.* 18:255, 1983.
8. Green, T.H., Jr. Urinary stress incontinence: Differential diagnosis, pathophysiology, and management. *Am. J. Obstet. Gynecol.* 122:368, 1975.
9. Koff, S.A., Diokno, A.C., and Lapides, J. Neurogenic bladder dysfunction. *Am. Fam. Physician* 19:100, 1979.
10. Krane, R.J., and Siroky, M.B. Classification of neurologic disorders. In R.J. Krane and M.B. Siroky (Eds.), *Clinical Neuro-Urology.* Boston: Little, Brown, 1979.
11. McGuire, E.J., Jr. Evaluation of urinary incontinence. In S.V. Yalla et al. (Eds.) *Neurourology and Urodynamics.* New York: Macmillan, 1988.
12. Perkas, I., and Friedland, G.W. Principles of modern urodynamic studies. *Invest. Radiol.* 22:279, 1987.
13. Raz, S. Evaluation of the incontinence patient. In R.J. Krane and M.B. Siroky (Eds.), *Clinical Neuro-Urology.* Boston: Little, Brown, 1979.
14. Resnick, N.M., Yalla, S.V., and Laurino, E. The pathophysiology of urinary incontinence among institutionalized elderly persons. *N. Engl. J. Med.* 329:1, 1989.
15. Saxton, H.M., et al. Spinning top urethra: Not a normal variant. *Radiology* 168:147, 1988.
16. Shapeero, L.G., Friedland, G.W., and Perkash, I. Transrectal sonographic voiding cystourethrography: Studies in neuromuscular bladder dysfunction. *A.J.R.* 141:83, 1983.
17. Stannard, M.W., and Lebowitz., R.L. Urography in the child who wets. *A.J.R.* 130:959, 1978.
18. Wein, A.J. Classification of neurogenic voiding dysfunction. *J. Urol.* 125:605, 1981.

22

The Prostate and Seminal Vesicles

THE PROSTATE

In males the prostate is one of the more common organs to be affected by disease. Many diseases can involve the prostate, but it is the triad of prostatitis, benign prostatic hypertrophy (BPH), and carcinoma of the prostate (CAP) that regularly involve this small organ. BPH is the most common benign proliferative abnormality found in any male organ [29]; CAP is equaled in incidence only by pulmonary malignancies; and prostatitis is one of the staples of any busy urologic practice. In an organ that is inherently inhomogeneous to begin with, the superimposition of the above conditions results in difficulties in detection and categorization of diseases even when the best imaging practices are employed.

BLADDER OUTLET OBSTRUCTION

Bladder outlet obstruction, whatever the cause, results in a complex of symptoms known as prostatism. The symptoms of prostatism are hesitancy, weak urinary stream, postvoiding dribbling, a feeling of incomplete emptying, frequency, and nocturia. The last three are due to a progressively increasing residual urine as the bladder musculature eventually fails to overcome outlet resistance; with the bladder continually partially filled by chronic residual urine, its functional capacity is decreased. Furthermore, chronic residual urine and a hypertrophied bladder detrusor result in higher intravesical pressure, which decreases the frequency and effectiveness of ureteral peristalsis and therefore increases pressure in the upper urinary tract. Over the long term, the result is hydronephrosis, which is usually bilateral and symmetrical. Rarely, the valve mechanism at the ureterovesical junction fails because of increased bladder pressure, and reflux occurs, which may also result in either unilateral or bilateral dilation of the upper urinary tract.

The prostate surrounds the proximal urethra and can interfere with normal urinary outflow. While BPH is the most common cause of prostatism, CAP and prostatitis (particularly the granulomatous form) may also be culprits. Other causes of bladder outlet obstruction include urethral stricture, bladder-neck contracture, and dyssynergia between contraction of the bladder detrusor and urethral sphincters.

As does the heart, the bladder compensates for increased resistance to outflow with hypertrophy of the muscular wall. Initially, this hypertrophy provides higher voiding pressures to overcome the increased outlet resistance. As pressure continues to rise, the bladder mucosa begins to herniate between the hypertrophied muscle bands, initially resulting in cellules—mucosal outpouchings that do not extend beyond the outer wall of the bladder. As time passes, this herniation progresses to the formation of frank bladder diverticula that are not invested with muscle and are therefore unable to empty on voiding. Diverticula, coupled with chronic residual bladder urine, predispose to urinary stasis with the sequelae of infection and stone formation. Eventually, if obstruction persists, the bladder detrusor fails and urinary retention occurs. The sequence is variable enough that there is no direct correlation between bladder failure and upper tract dilation. Treatment of obstructing disease of the prostate is undertaken for the amelioration of the symptoms of prostatism and for the prevention or relief of associated upper tract changes.

IMAGING OF THE NORMAL PROSTATE

On urography, the bladder base is parallel to and immediately above the superior margin of the symphysis; the normal prostate is located behind the symphysis and is not seen. CT of the normal prostate reveals a small, rounded, homogeneous soft-tissue density on the sections immediately below the bladder base (Fig. 22-1).

On transrectal ultrasonography and MRI, the internal anatomy of the prostate can be seen. Transrectal ultrasonography can image in axial

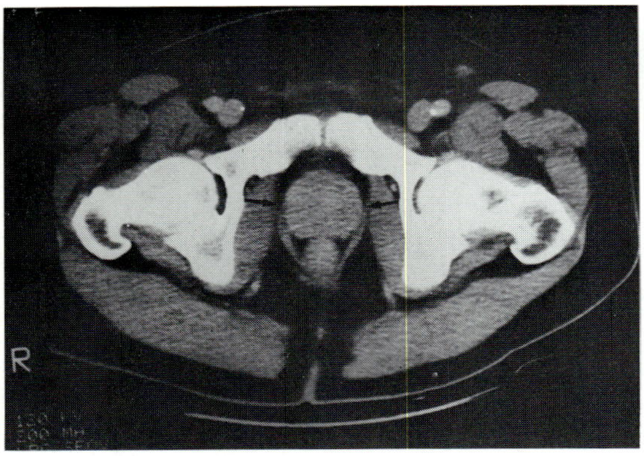

Figure 22-1. CT appearance of normal prostate. Section below bladder base shows the prostate to have smooth margins and homogeneous texture (arrows).

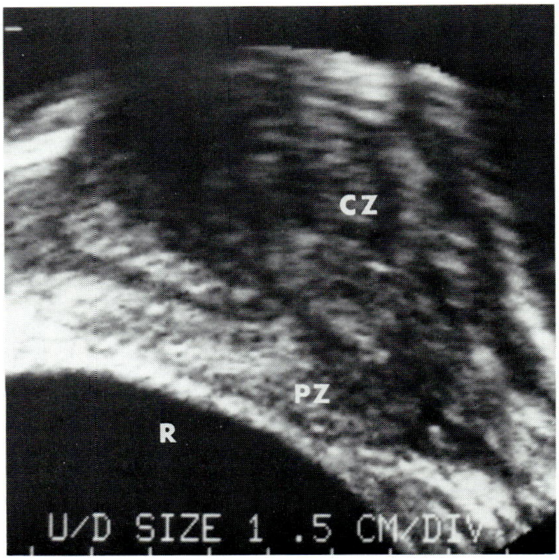

A

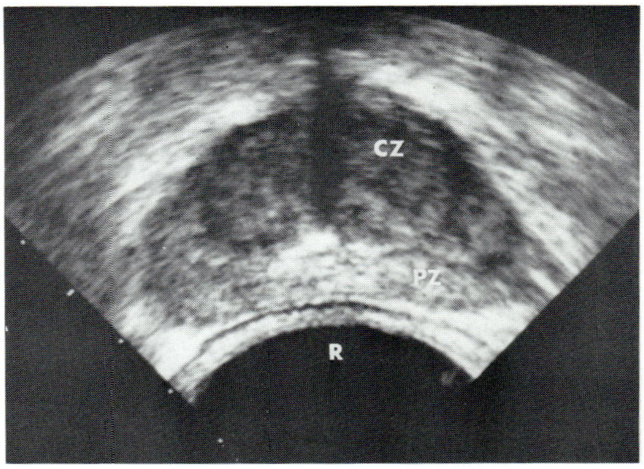

B

Figure 22-2. Transrectal sonogram of normal prostate. A. Longitudinal view (patient's head to right). B. Transverse view. (Note the clear demarcation of the central and peripheral zones.) (CZ = central zone; PZ = peripheral zone; R = rectum.) (Courtesy of Dr. John J. Cronan, Rhode Island Hospital, Providence, R.I.)

and longitudinal planes, the former showing a semilunar section of the prostate and the latter a triangular shape tapering from the base at the bladder neck to the apex at the urogenital diaphragm (Fig. 22-2). The combined transitional and central zones can often be seen as a globular, somewhat sonolucent area surrounding the urethra near the bladder base. The peripheral zone exhibits a homogeneous echogenicity, which is considered the reference echotexture by which the echogenicity of various lesions is classified. For example, a nodule that is hypoechoic is one that is less echogenic than the peripheral zone. Anterior to the prostate, the periprostatic venous plexus can often be seen as anechoic, oval-shaped structures; posteriorly, the rectal wall is a hyperechoic band.

With MRI, T1 weighted sections show the prostate as a homogeneous organ of intermediate signal intensity. However, on most T2 weighted scans internal architecture of the gland becomes apparent; the combined transitional and central zones exhibit an intermediate signal and the peripheral zone a high signal.

PROSTATITIS

Prostatitis affects a large group of men, who present with irritative complaints referable to the lower urogenital tract, including urinary frequency, urgency, dysuria, and perineal discomfort. Prostatitis can be acute or chronic, and bacteria may or may not be found in the prostatic secretions. The terms prostatosis and prostatodynia refer to prostatic pain without the finding of inflammation; this syndrome usually has a significant psychological overlay but is often included in the general category of prostatitis. It has been estimated that 50 percent of men will experience symptoms of prostatitis at some time in their lives [19].

Granulomatous prostatitis may occur and be nonspecific or caused by organisms such as *Mycobacterium tuberculosis*, *Treponema pallidum*, various fungi, metazoa, or *Brucella abortus* [27]. The significance of granulomatous involvement of the prostate lies in its ability to mimic the firmness or nodularity often found with CAP on rectal examination.

Prostatic abscess usually occurs in the fifth and sixth decades of life and presents with high fevers and perineal or rectal pain (or both) often associated with difficult voiding. As with other infections, diabetes seems to be a major predisposing factor. Prostatic abscesses can frequently be diagnosed by rectal examination, but the diagnosis may be overlooked when signs and symptoms have been masked by previous or current antibiotic therapy.

Urographically, prostatitis may result in enlargement of the prostate and be manifested as a mass impression on the bladder base such as that seen with BPH. In fact, as previously noted, these diseases often occur simultaneously. Like other longstanding causes of bladder outlet obstruction, granulomatous prostatitis may result in upper tract dilation, which regresses with proper treatment of the primary disease. The diagnosis of prostatitis is usually made on the basis of clinical examination and laboratory tests. Therefore, little has been written about its appearance on imaging with ultrasonography, CT, or MRI. Suffice it to say that there do not appear to be characteristic changes that would enable the diagnosis to be made with any degree of certainty. This nonspecificity, however, does not pertain in cases in which infection has progressed to frank abscess formation. Although a prostatic abscess is often diagnosed on the basis of clinical examination of the patient, CT or transrectal ultrasonography may be used to determine the extent of the lesion. CT typically shows a single or multilocular low-attenuation area within the prostate (Fig. 22-3). Sections should be obtained through the level of the urogenital diaphragm because on rare occasions the abscess may penetrate into the root of the penis. Transrectal or suprapubic ultrasonography can also demonstrate an abscess as a relatively anechoic area within the prostate. Drainage of a prostatic abscess is usually accomplished via transurethral unroofing.

Although the cause of prostatic calculi is often thought to be prior episodes of prostatitis, in

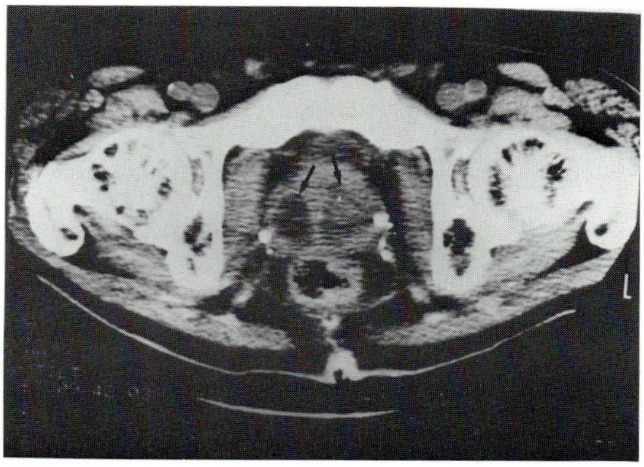

Figure 22-3. Prostatic abscess. CT section through prostate reveals a multiloculated, low-attenuation lesion in the prostate (arrows).

many cases calculi are incidental findings and are not associated with symptoms or clinically evident disease [28]. They are seen in the suprapubic region as a cluster of small calcifications in about 14 percent of adult males on abdominal plain films (Fig. 22-4), though on CT they are more frequently found. Ultrasonography shows them as small echogenic foci in the prostate, which may shadow if large enough. They usually surround centrally located nodules of BPH and rarely occur in the peripheral zone. Just as their presence does not presume prior prostatitis, they are not considered predicators of diseases such as BPH or CAP; their incidence in men with CAP has been reported as 6.4 percent and in men with BPH as 7.9 percent [10].

Figure 22-4. Prostatic calcifications. Coned view of pelvis shows a collection of small calcifications in the suprapubic area.

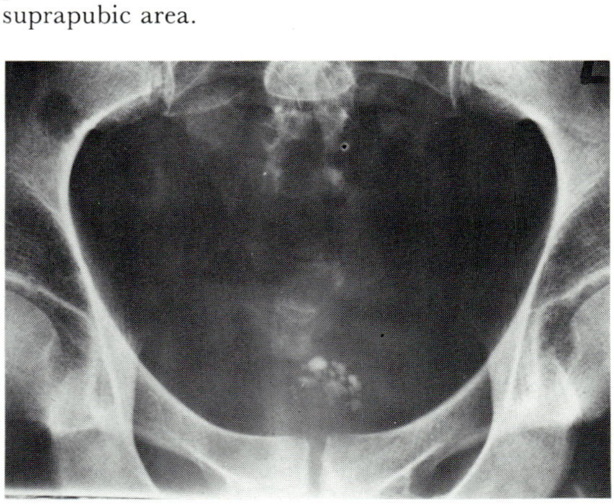

BENIGN PROSTATIC HYPERTROPHY

The normal prostate attains a weight of 15 to 20 g in young adults and remains stable unless BPH supervenes. The prevalence of BPH has been reported as 8 percent in the fourth decade of life; however, this increases dramatically with increasing age, affecting 50 percent of the male population during their sixth decade [3]. The average autopsy weights of prostates containing BPH is 33 g, with only 4 percent of glands reaching weights over 100 g. The largest recorded prostate was 820 g. Prostatic weight has clinical significance: Smaller glands with BPH are amenable to transurethral resection (TURP), whereas open prostatectomy may be required for glands weighing 60 g or more.

In cases of outflow obstruction due to BPH, there is a general, though inconstant, agreement between the size of the gland and the severity of symptoms. In spite of the commonness of the disease, only 10 percent or so of men with BPH will require surgery to relieve symptoms or establish proper drainage of the urinary tract. However, in one large series of patients with this disease, 14.5 percent were found to have some degree of azotemia due to their outlet obstruction [2]. Certainly, this group requires immediate catheter drainage, usually followed by surgical excision of the obstructing adenomatous tissue.

Excretory urography is usually performed in men with prostatism and almost always in men for whom prostatic surgery is anticipated, though there is an ongoing debate about the efficacy of this practice. Reasons for ordering urography include the desire to evaluate the status of the upper urinary tract for secondary changes and the possibility of detecting unsuspected renal lesions such as renal cell or transitional cell carcinomas; on the other hand, the yield of significant abnormalities is low. Talner [34] has summarized the literature on this subject. He found that in almost 4,000 reported cases, the prevalence of renal tumors in men with prostatism was 0.4 percent. He concludes that, even if we were to acknowledge a slightly increased incidence of renal tumors in men with prostatism, it would not be sufficient to condone routine urography in such patients. Furthermore, there is no evidence linking bladder outlet obstruction with upper tract neoplasia. However, the practice of routine urography continues in many institutions, and is often the only imaging study of the urinary tract performed when benign prostate disease is suspected.

Imaging of BPH

The preliminary film obtained prior to urography should be scrutinized for prostatic calculi; these may influence the surgical approach, since TURP can be difficult when many calculi are present. A full bladder suggests significant outlet obstruction, as patients are routinely directed to void before the scout film is obtained. Bladder calculi should also lead to the suspicion of outlet obstruction.

After injection of contrast medium, the upper tracts should be evaluated for hydronephrosis. With functional obstruction due to bladder outlet problems, upper tract dilation is usually bilateral and symmetrical. While unilateral or asymmetric dilation is possible with benign prostate disease, CAP extending into the retrotrigonal area and involving one or both distal ureters should be considered when this pattern is seen.

The normal bladder base parallels the superior pubic margin; enlargement of the prostate results in a smooth, dome-shaped indentation of the base. On rare occasions, BPH may have irregular or nodular margins, but such a finding should suggest the possibility of CAP. There is a loose correlation between the size of this indentation and the weight of the resected prostate. With progressive enlargement, significant elevation of the trigone occurs, resulting in "J-ing" or "hooking" of the distal ureters (Fig. 22-5); this characteristic ureteral appearance is one of the more reliable urographic signs of significant enlargement of the prostate.

With hypertrophy of vestigial prostatic tissue behind the bladder neck and trigone, posterior protrusion of the prostate into the bladder occurs. This presents as a smooth, round filling defect that appears to lie within the bladder lumen (Fig. 22-6), even though the prostate is extravesical and simply protrudes from the posterior side. This is classically termed the lobe of

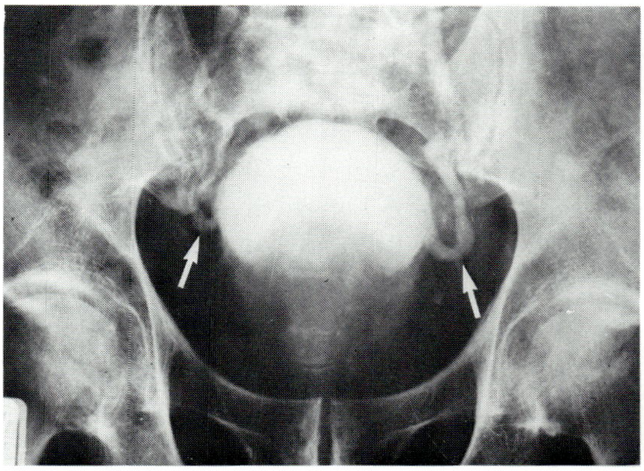

Figure 22-5. Benign prostatic hypertrophy. Coned view of bladder shows a moderately enlarged prostate with "J-ing" of the distal ureters (arrows) due to elevation of the trigone by the prostate.

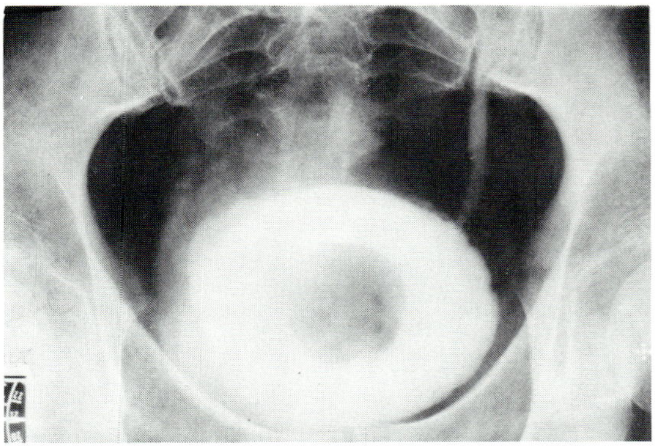

Figure 22-6. Intravesical prostate (lobe of Albarrán). Coned view of bladder shows a smooth round filling defect that appears to have no connection to the prostate. Note similarity to an inflated Foley ballon.

Albarŕan, and it should be differentiated from hypertrophy of the median lobe, which may be more completely rounded than the standard case of BPH, yet is seen to extend into the bladder inferiorly (Fig. 22-7). Other differentials of the lobe of Albarrán include an inflated Foley ballon, a müllerian duct cyst (which is midline and also invaginates the bladder posteriorly), and a single, large bladder calculus; the last is usually seen on the preliminary film. Clots within the bladder or a bladder neoplasm usually have irregular margins. CT and lower abdominal ultrasonography are useful in con-

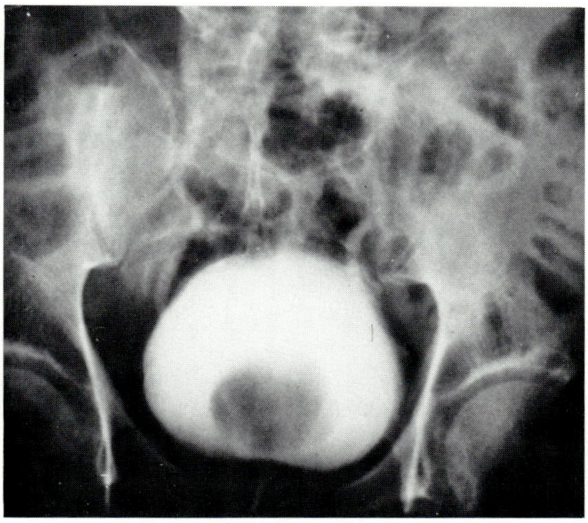

Figure 22-7. Median-lobe hypertrophy. Coned view of bladder shows rounded appearance of the enlarged prostate in the bladder base. Compare with the more typical pattern of enlargement seen in Fig. 22-5.

firming the retrovesical origin of the lobe of Albarrán.

In the normal full bladder, the detrusor measures only 2 to 3 mm in thickness, and the wall outlined by contrast medium is smooth. When detrusor hypertrophy occurs, its thickness increases, and the enlarged muscle bands result in an irregularity of the wall known as trabeculation. This is difficult to diagnose radiographically, especially in the partially filled bladder, but a feathery appearance of the filled bladder, coupled with visible thickening of the wall, is highly suspicious for trabeculation. It should be noted, however, that various types of cystitis may result in similar findings. When cellules or frank diverticula are seen, the diagnosis of trabeculation can be made with confidence (Fig. 22-8). As noted in Chap. 19, a severe medial deviation of either distal ureter can be caused by a large, laterally placed bladder diverticulum. It is important to be aware of this finding, as the diverticulum may not opacify because it has a small orifice or, less likely, because it is filled with tumor.

CT generally depicts BPH as a homogeneously enlarged gland with smooth margins. Transrectal ultrasonography, on the other hand, may show discrete central nodules of varying

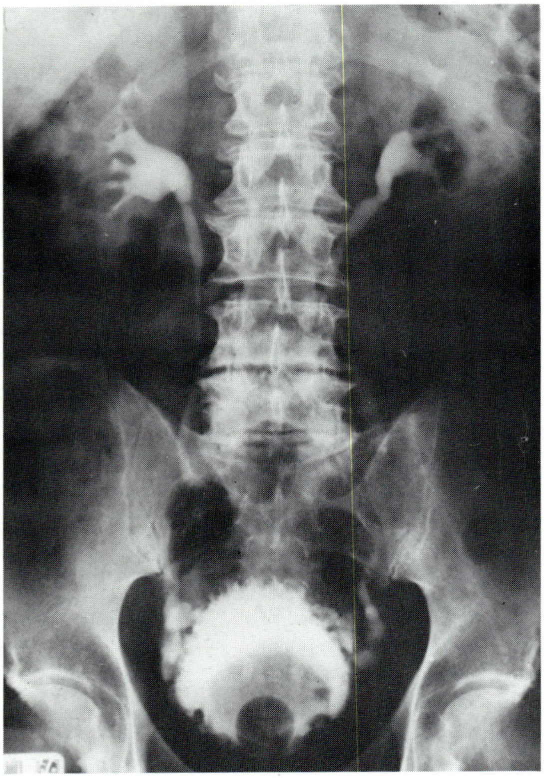

Figure 22-8. Trabeculated bladder secondary to bladder outlet obstruction. Urography shows irregular bladder mucosa and several small diverticula. The prostate is moderately enlarged, and a Foley balloon is seen at the bladder base. Note that the upper urinary tract has not yet been compromised.

echogenicity, though these are rarely purely hypoechoic. T1 weighted MRI often shows a heterogeneous prostate with discrete nodules, or the gland may be homogeneous. T2 weighted sections typically show central nodules of varying signal intensity, which probably reflect a mixture of fibrous tissue, glandular lumina, and epithelium. Growth of these nodules can obliterate the normally seen peripheral zone.

Classic treatment for BPH continues to be TURP or open prostatectomy. However, some reports have indicated that balloon dilation of the prostatic urethra in benign disease may provide long-term symptomatic relief. Initially performed in cadavers and dogs, use of the procedure in human volunteers has found resolution of obstructive symptoms over follow-up periods of up to 8 months [6].

MALIGNANT NEOPLASMS OF THE PROSTATE

Although most prostatic neoplasms occur in older men, rhabdomyosarcomas may rarely arise from the prostate in young boys, the large majority occurring before the age of 5 years. This lesion may also originate from the bladder base, and difficulty in determining the site of origin has been reported. However, sarcoma of the prostate tends to show earlier spread than the vesical variety, with distant dissemination found in about 40 percent of patients at the time of diagnosis. Presenting symptoms are usually related to bladder outlet obstruction. Progressive renal failure indicates ureteral involvement by the tumor. If renal function allows, urography depicts a lobular mass protruding into the bladder or elevating the bladder base (Fig. 22-9). This lobular or polypoid appearance has resulted in the

Figure 22-9. Sarcoma botryoides (rhabdomyosarcoma arising from prostate) in young boy. Urography shows a nodular mass elevating the bladder base and filling two-thirds of the bladder.

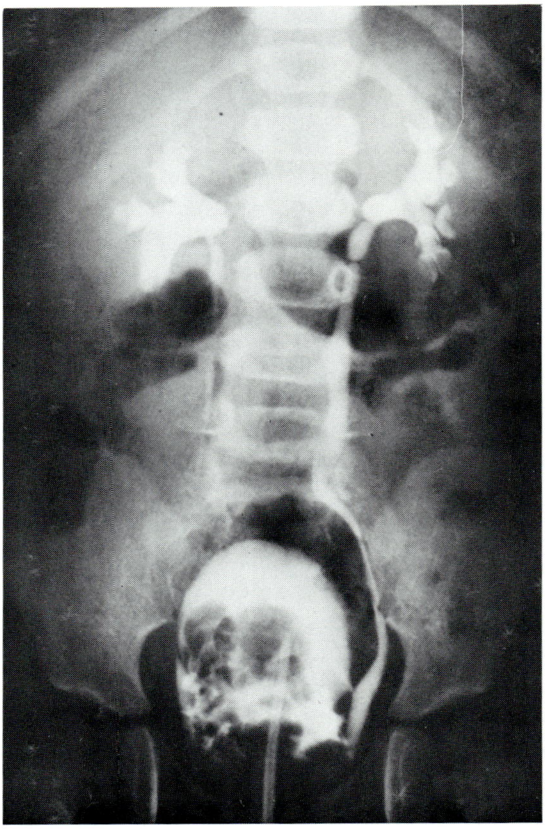

term *sarcoma botryoides*, referring to the resemblance of the tumor to a cluster of grapes. This is a highly malignant lesion.

Sarcomas of the prostate can rarely occur in older men, as can carcinosarcomas; both have a rather poor prognosis. Other uncommon malignant tumors include endometrioid carcinomas arising from the prostatic utricle, transitional cell carcinomas originating from the prostatic urethra or distal prostatic ducts, and squamous cell carcinomas. While endometrioid cancers tend to grow slowly and metastasize late, the squamous and transitional cell varieties are more aggressive lesions. Though the prostate is an uncommon site for secondary tumors, melanoma and lung cancer can metastasize there. The remainder of this discussion will involve only CAP, which comprises 95 percent of all prostate malignancies and is the most common tumor of the male genitourinary system.

As with BPH, cancerous cells in the prostate may develop in response to circulating androgens. This theory is supported by the facts that CAP does not occur in eunuchs and regresses rapidly when endogenous circulating androgens are reduced. Environmental, viral, and hereditary factors have also been postulated.

CAP almost always occurs after the age of 50, and now comprises 20 percent of all neoplasms diagnosed in men. The diagnosis is usually based on the results of transperineal or transrectal needle biopsy of a palpable prostatic abnormality or on the histologic examination of tissue removed during TURP or open prostatectomy for presumed benign disease. In one series, CAP was found in over 17 percent of patients undergoing TURP for presumed BPH [26]. Autopsy figures are even more dramatic, with a summary of 10 such studies reporting a 20 percent incidence of CAP in men over 50 years of age [11]. In one of these studies over 50 percent of men above age 80 had unsuspected CAP, confirming that incidence increases with age.

The above data indicate that CAP can occur in the asymptomatic patient and lie dormant for years, perhaps never becoming clinically overt. It has been speculated that perhaps there are two varieties of CAP, one that grows progressively and one that is latent. However, current thinking is that there is only a single species of CAP, which exhibits an initial slow growth rate and then shows a logarithmic growth curve. Predictors of growth include the size of the primary tumor, stage of the disease when discovered, and histologic differentiation (grade) of the tumor.

These predictive factors are closely intertwined. Poorly differentiated tumors are far more likely to spread beyond the prostatic capsule and are usually larger when detected than are more well-differentiated tumors. Furthermore, it has been reported that CAP undergoes a gradual increase in malignant potential that is closely linked to tumor size; metastases are usually found only in cases in which the volume of the primary tumor exceeds 4 ml [23].

The grade, or degree of histologic differentiation, of CAP is a significant predictor of aggressive potential, regardless of the stage or size at the time of detection. The Gleason grading system is widely employed; it is based on the microscopic study of tumors at low magnification to identify predominant and secondary growth patterns [13]. Standardized patterns of growth are recognized and are numbered from 2 to 10 in order of increasing malignancy. Clinical experience with the Gleason grading system has found it to be reliable and reproducible. One reported series found that of patients with Gleason grade 8, 9, or 10, 93 percent had regional nodal metastases, while patients with grade 4 or less showed no nodal spread [18]. Table 22-1 shows the relationship between grade and stage of CAP.

Table 22-1. Relation between grade and stage in CAP

	Stage			
	A	*B*	*C*	*D*
Well differentiated	61.9%	41.0%	30.0%	18.3%
Moderately differentiated	18.5	32.7	31.5	32.1
Poorly differentiated	5.4	13.0	23.0	30.2
Undifferentiated	0.3	1.0	2.5	3.1
Not graded or unknown	13.9	12.3	13.0	16.3

Based on data from National Survey of Prostate Cancer in the United States by the American College of Surgeons [25].

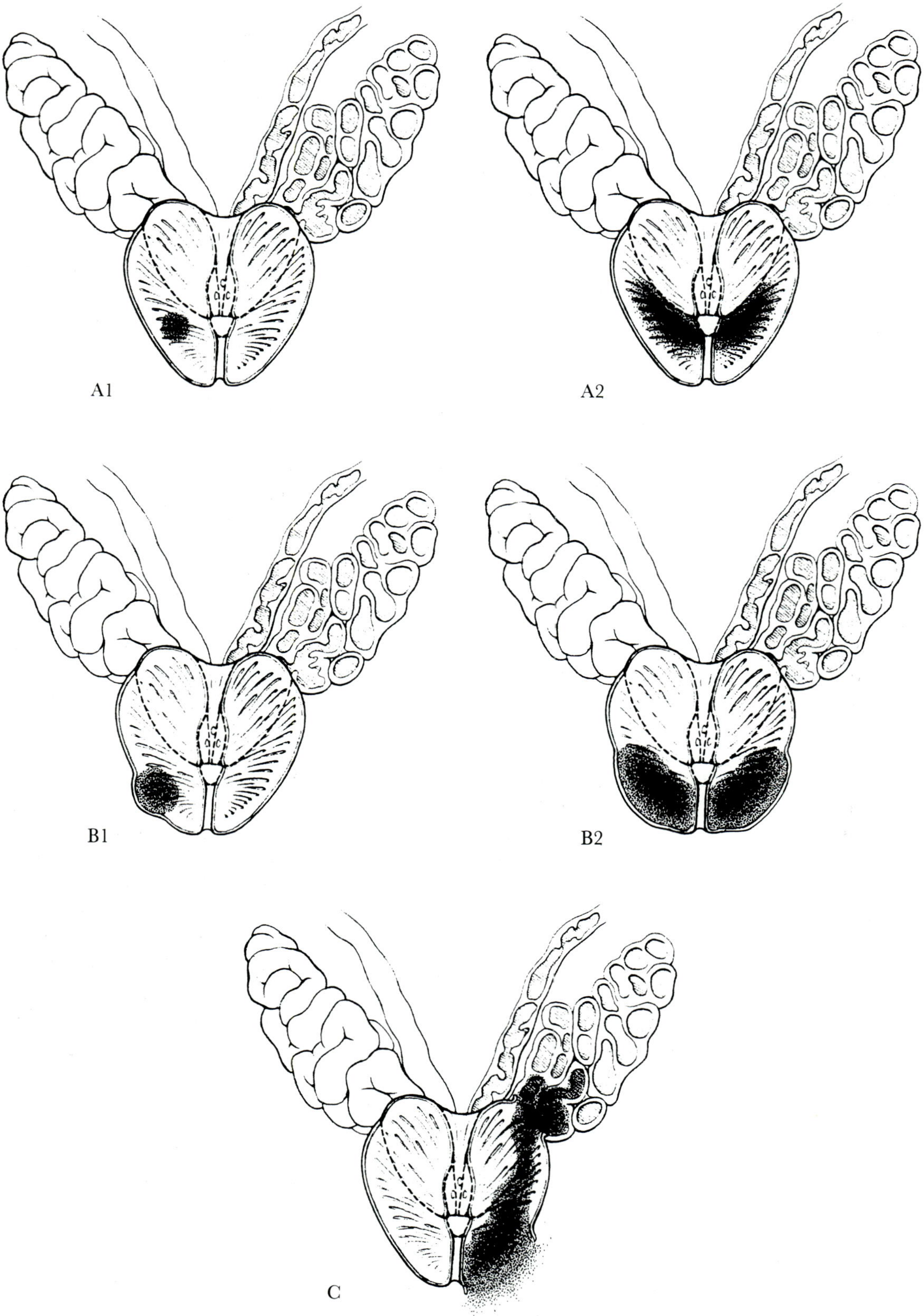
A1
A2
B1
B2
C

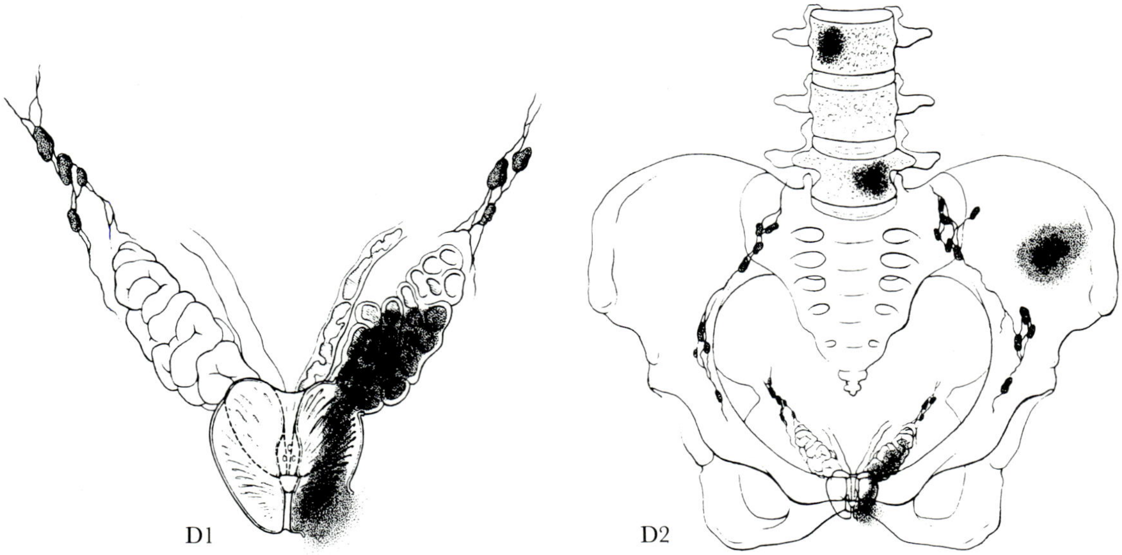

Figure 22-10. Staging of prostate cancer. Note that Stage A cancer is not palpable. In Stage D cancer, nodal and bony metastases can be seen regardless of the local extent of tumor spread, though in most cases invasive local disease (as shown) is found. (From E.S. Amis, Jr. Epidemiology and natural history of carcinoma of the prostate. American Roentgen Ray Society Categorical Course Syllabus on Uroradiology, 1989, 87–92. Copyright 1989, American College of Radiology.)

The staging of CAP is based on the extent of growth of the tumor within the prostate, invasion into the periprostatic tissues, or distant spread. Accurate staging is important, as evidenced by the dramatic decrease in 5-year survival with increasing stage of the disease. An alphabetical staging system is widely used in the United States (Fig. 22-10). Initial staging is performed clinically and then modified as necessary based on imaging evaluation of the patient. Histologic examination of excised tissue remains the gold standard for final staging.

Stage A CAP has two substages—A1 and A2—neither of which is palpable on rectal examination. This stage is diagnosed on the basis of histologic examination of tissue removed during prostatectomy for presumed benign disease or by needle biopsy of suspicious lesions initially detected by transrectal ultrasonography. A small nonpalpable lesion is generally staged A1, while A2 lesions are more diffuse or highly undifferentiated lesions of any size. The difference is important, as A2 lesions have a worse prognosis than B1 tumors. However, even patients with A1 tumors are not free from risk, as an 8-year follow-up of such patients found a 16 percent incidence of progression of the disease [9].

Stage B CAP also has two categories. B1 tumors are palpable nodules less than 1.5 cm in diameter that have not invaded the capsule of the prostate; B2 denotes larger, more diffuse palpable tumors also confined to the prostate. Some investigators have shown that small stage A tumors tend to occur more anteromedially in the peripheral zone, while stage B tumors are more posterior [24]. This helps explain the difference in palpability of these two stages. With stage B disease, understaging is a major problem, as it is often difficult to separate lesions contained within the gland from those that have microscopically spread into the periprostatic area.

Stage C CAP has invaded the periprostatic tissues or spread to the seminal vesicles. At this stage, the tumor is thought by many not to be amenable to cure by radical prostatectomy, and the patient may be treated with radiation therapy if there is no evidence of more distant spread. Thus the importance of accurate staging can be seen, especially between localized tumors (stage A or B) and those exhibiting local spread (stage C). However, it has been reported that as many as two-thirds of patients initially staged as A or B have microscopic spread into adjacent tissues at the time of prostatectomy [33]. This fact highlights the difficulty in selecting patients for surgical cure, especially since over 50 percent of patients are clinically found to have stage A or B lesions.

Stage D1 indicates tumors that have spread to regional pelvic nodes, while D2 denotes widespread metastatic disease. These patterns of spread can occur regardless of the size or extent of local spread of the primary tumor in the prostate, though there is often a logical progression of increasing size of the primary tumor, local invasion, and then more distant spread. Treatment in these advanced cases is usually by hormonal manipulation, accompanied by local radiation of bone metastases for symptomatic relief. CAP most commonly metastasizes to regional pelvic lymph nodes with spread to bone a slightly less common event. In nodal spread, there is usually a predictable predilection for various pelvic node groups: The obturator nodes are initially involved, followed by external and internal iliac groups [12]. Bone involvement by CAP is found in about 70 percent of patients with advanced disease. The bones involved, in decreasing frequency, are the spine, femur, pelvis, ribs, sternum, skull, and humerus [15]. Early spread to the lower spine and pelvis occur via communications of the prostatic veins with the venous plexus of Batson, which invests these bony areas. Visceral metastases are most common to the lung, liver, and adrenal, though any organ can be involved.

Considering the weaknesses of clinical and radiographic staging of CAP, patients initially thought to be good candidates for radical prostatectomy (stage A or B disease) will usually undergo a staging pelvic lymphadenectomy with frozen sections prior to removal of the prostate. Many urologists consider this procedure diagnostic rather than therapeutic. The patient with negative histology then undergoes curative surgery.

The incidence of CAP appears to be on the increase. While 60,000 new cases were identified yearly during the 1970s, estimates for 1990 are for over 100,000. This increase is more than would be expected based on population increases and is probably due to detection of small, asymptomatic lesions that previously would not have been found. During this same time, however, the death rate from CAP has remained relatively stable. The increased incidence, in conjunction with the flat death rate, has resulted in an increased overall 5-year survival rate to 70 percent. Notably, the survival for black men is significantly lower than for whites, whereas for orientals it is higher [25]. The overall improvement in survival is probably due to the increased detection of early tumors, which have only minimal aggressive potential. As transrectal ultrasonography and MRI become more accurate in detecting smaller tumors, the prediction of the malignant potential of these early lesions becomes of great importance in determining which patients should be subjected to radical prostatectomy. Although current evidence indicates that surgery provides the best chance for total eradication of the tumor, it is not without complications such as impotence or urinary incontinence. Fortunately, surgical technique has been modified to allow preservation of the nerve plexus that innervates the corpora cavernosa, thus preserving erectile function in 70 percent of patients [35].

Imaging of CAP

Imaging of CAP has two basic functions: initial detection of the disease and, once the diagnosis is confirmed, staging of the tumor. Excretory urography and CT have nothing to offer in detecting intraprostatic disease. Urography may suggest CAP when the prostate gland is grossly irregular or nodular (at which time it will usually have spread), when there is local invasion obstructing one or both ureters, or when blastic bony metastases are seen. CT is primarily useful in staging CAP once the diagnosis has been established.

There has been controversy regarding the possible role of transrectal ultrasonography as a screening method for subclinical CAP. Controversy notwithstanding, men are referred for transrectal ultrasonography for several reasons, including equivocal rectal examination, elevated tumor markers or bone metastases in patients with a normal digital examination, and for characterization and guided biopsy of palpable prostatic abnormalities. There has been universal agreement that a meticulous search for hypoechoic lesions occurring in the peripheral zone (or elsewhere in the prostate) is the most important part of the examination [17] (Fig. 22-11). Sonographic–pathologic correlation studies have shown that CAP is hypoechoic in approximately 60 percent of cases, the remainder being essentially isoechoic with the peripheral zone and thus camouflaged within the prostate. However, not all hypoechoic lesions prove to be CAP; other causes include BPH, prostatitis, fibrosis, cyst, or normal structures such as the ejaculatory duct or a dilated prostatic duct. Overall, about 20 to 40 percent of hypoechoic nodules prove on biopsy to be CAP [20, 32].

MRI is not generally used for the detection of CAP, though the tumor may be incidentally suspected during MRI performed for other reasons. CAP presents as a lower-signal-intensity defect in the otherwise bright peripheral zone on T2 weighted images [5] (Fig. 22-12). However, the size of the defect seen may not correlate well with the actual size of the tumor. Furthermore, BPH and prostatitis may mimic CAP in producing peripheral zone lesions.

Figure 22-11. Hypoechoic prostate cancer (arrows) on transrectal sonography (tranverse view). Note the erosion of the bright white line of periprostatic fat posteriorly (arrowhead) indicating capsular invasion by this stage C tumor (R = rectum). (Courtesy of Matthew Rifkin, M.D., Thomas Jefferson University Hospital, Philadelphia, Pa.)

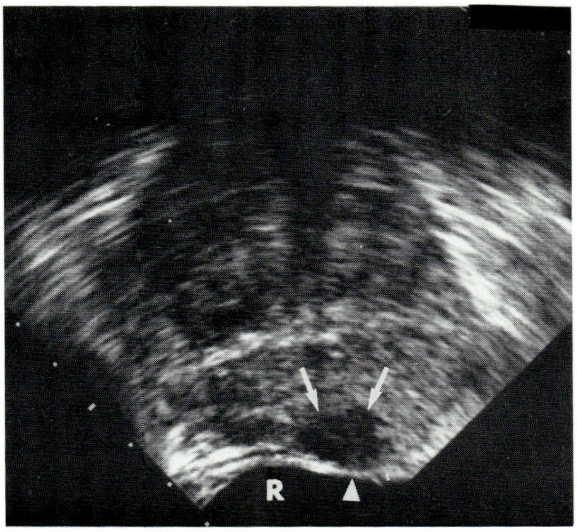

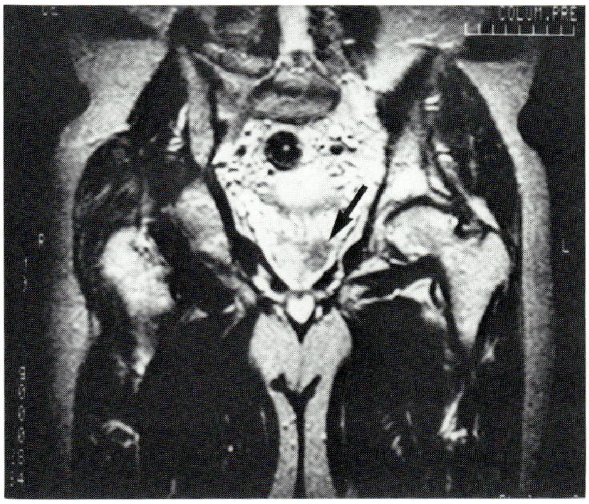

Figure 22-12. Prostate cancer on MRI. Coronal T2 weighted section through the bright posterior peripheral zone shows a medium-intensity nodule (arrow). Although this lesion appears confined to the prostate, stage C disease was found at surgery.

Although the capabilities of various methods are more clearly defined in staging CAP, the choice of studies employed varies from hospital to hospital and depends largely on the preference of the referring urologist and the capabilities of the radiology department.

A patient with presumed stage A or B disease who is being considered for radical prostatectomy as a curative procedure must have more advanced disease excluded by imaging, since even a diagnostic staging pelvic lymphadenectomy will not be performed if conclusive evidence of spread exists. Thus, some studies are done routinely to visualize the areas of common metastatic involvement—the periprostatic area, the pelvic lymph nodes, and the bones.

Transrectal ultrasonography is showing some promise in detecting the local extent of CAP, though reported sensitivities and specificities are still highly variable. Capsular invasion is seen as an asymmetric bulge with thinning or absence of the adjacent hyperechoic periprostatic fat. Invasion of the seminal vesicle by CAP is manifested by enlargement and increased echogenicity of the seminal vesicle and loss of the normal fatty angle between the prostate and seminal vesicle.

More commonly, CT is used for staging. The CT criterion for capsular invasion is focal alteration in the normally smooth contour of the prostate. Invasion of the seminal vesicles is suspected when there is asymmetry or enlargment of these organs or when there is loss of the normal acute angle between either or both seminal vesicles and the bladder (Fig. 22-13). However, neither of these signs has proven uniformly accurate. More specifically, the loss of the normal seminal vesicle angle can occur with a full bladder, when the patient is in the prone position, or even with benign disease of the prostate. CT is most useful in detecting enlarged pelvic lymph nodes. Its weakness in this area is that microscopic foci of tumor in normal-sized nodes are missed, and enlarged nodes may be so because of hyperplasia, inflammation, or fatty infiltration rather than tumor involvement. Some data suggest that equivocal CT examinations should not be used to influence decisions concerning surgical versus nonsurgical treatment in patients clinically staged as having local disease [30]. On a practical basis, CT is used primarily to exclude macroscopic pelvic nodal involvement. Patients without enlarged nodes will usually undergo a staging pelvic lymphadenectomy in a search for microscopic tumor foci in nodes before definitive therapy is carried out. If CT shows massive nodal involvement, surgery is precluded. It is the in-between cases, in which perhaps a single marginally enlarged node is seen, that create difficulty in making the decision whether to operate. This is complicated even further by the varying criteria for nodal enlargement. Nodes are considered positive by some investigators when they are over 1 cm in diameter, by others when over 1.5 cm, and by still others only when over 2.0 cm.

Figure 22-13. Stage D1 prostate cancer. CT section at level of seminal vesicles shows loss of the normal seminal vesicle angle on the left (arrow). On the right, enlarged nodes can be seen in the external iliac and obturator chains (arrowheads). The seminal vesicles are seen as a bowtie-shaped soft-tissue structure immediately behind the bladder.

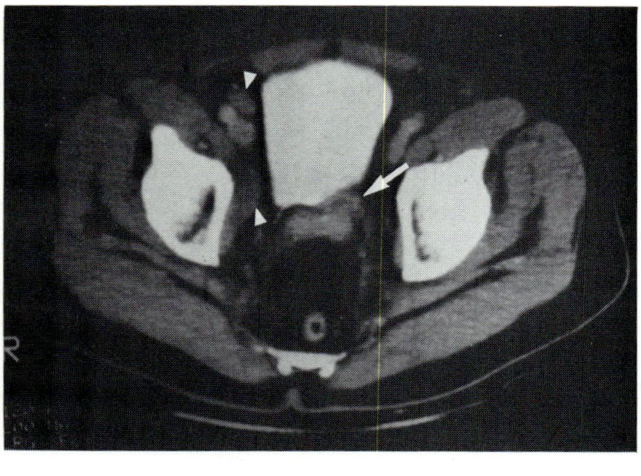

MRI suffers much the same limitations in staging CAP as those mentioned for CT. However, the unique ability of MRI to image rapidly in multiple planes provides some advantage. One report states that the accuracy of clinical staging of CAP is 61 percent, the accuracy of CT is 65 percent, and the accuracy of transverse T1 weighted MRI is 61 percent [14]. However, when transverse T1 and T2 weighted images, supplemented by additional T2 weighted coronal or sagittal images, are obtained, the accuracy increases to 83 percent. The axial T1 sections allow assessment for adenopathy, as the enlarged nodes, exhibiting medium signal intensity, stand out against the surrounding bright fat. T2 images in multiple planes allow better evaluation for direct extension of CAP into the periprostatic tissues or seminal vesicles [4]. The use of endorectal coils seems to hold promise for greatly increased accuracy in staging CAP.

Pedal lymphangiography is used routinely in some medical centers for staging CAP. Normal nodes have a diffuse, homogeneous stippled appearance. Metastatic foci in nodes are seen as well-demarcated negative defects (Fig. 22-14). Tumor-bearing nodes may also be significantly enlarged and, if totally replaced by tumor, may not be seen on lymphangiography. Unfortunately, as previously discussed, the same benign processes that can cause nodal enlargement as seen on CT can also result in nodal defects resembling CAP. Furthermore, some metastatic deposits may be so small that they are undetectable by lymphangiography. Overall, lymphangiography has a reported accuracy rate of 60 to 90 percent in detecting nodal involvement by CAP. To overcome these inherent weaknesses, lymphangiography may be

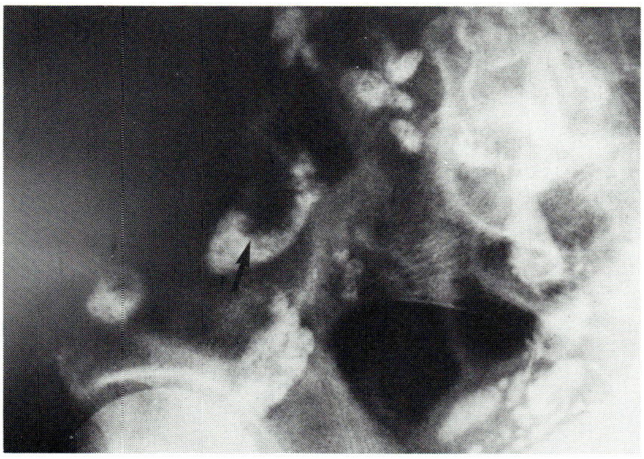

Figure 22-14. Stage D1 prostate cancer. Lymphangiography (oblique view of pelvis) shows a discrete filling defect in a right external iliac node (arrow).

augmented by percutaneous needle biopsy of filling defects in nodes, or even of normal-appearing opacified nodes, to confirm or exclude metastatic disease, but this has not been uniformly successful. Perhaps the best studies for determining the accuracy of lymphangiography are those in which the histology and radiographic appearance of excised nodes are compared. One study of 17 histologically positive nodes from a total of 587 excised during multiple radical prostatectomies performed after lymphangiography found that only 5 showed a radiographic defect [17].

More than 90 percent of bone metastases in CAP are osteoblastic, and these usually present a characteristic smudgy, sclerotic appearance on plain-film radiography. However, it may occasionally be difficult to distinguish blastic metastases from benign lesions such as bone islands or infarcts, degenerative disease of the spine, and Paget's disease. While bone islands or infarcts are usually smaller, fewer, and more well defined than metastatic lesions, degenerative disease and metastases may coalesce in such a way that definitive diagnosis becomes radiographically impossible. Paget's disease should be suspected in preference to CAP when there is widening of the bone, thickening of the cortex, and a prominent trabecular pattern. Reliance on the radiographic approach alone for the detection of bone metastases is unwise, as the lesion must be well established to be visible. A more sensitive method is bone scintigraphy, which may detect changes 3 to 6 months earlier than conventional radiography.

The usual abnormal bone scan associated with metastatic CAP is typified by asymmetric skeletal uptake of the radioisotope (Fig. 22-15A). However, this is a nonspecific finding, and it may be produced by a variety of conditions, including degenerative joint disease, healing fractures, metabolic skeletal disorders, and Paget's disease. It is therefore necessary in most such cases to supplement the interpretation of the bone scan with plain radiography of the area in question. Another appearance is that of the "super" bone scan, in which there is diffuse and symmetric increased uptake of radioisotope by all the bones without obvious focal abnormalities (Fig. 22-15B). However, in the super scan, there is absent isotope activity in the kidneys, which normally excrete about 15 percent of the injected radiopharmaceutical. Lack of visualization of the kidneys confirms more avid uptake of isotope by bone, usually secondary to diffuse metastatic spread. In these cases, radiographic examination of the skeleton will often confirm the blastic involvement of most, if not all, of the bones.

Other studies useful in evaluating osseous disease in CAP include serum alkaline phosphatase, which is elevated in 80 percent of patients with skeletal metastases, and serum acid phosphatase, which is increased in 60 to 70 percent of patients with distant metastases [22]. Prostate-specific antigen, a protein that is immunologically distinct from acid phosphatase, has been identified as another useful serum tumor marker.

It should be obvious from the preceding discussion that the radiographic staging of CAP may follow several pathways varying from simple to involved. It is our experience that a common imaging system after the initial diagnosis of CAP would include intravenous urography for evaluation of the upper tracts, followed by CT and bone scintigraphy to assess the status of pelvic nodes and the bony skeleton. CT has also proved useful in follow-up of patients subjected to radical prostatectomy for stage A or B disease or undergoing radiotherapy for stage C disease in whom there was no pretreatment evidence of nodal involvement. Furthermore, CT has been

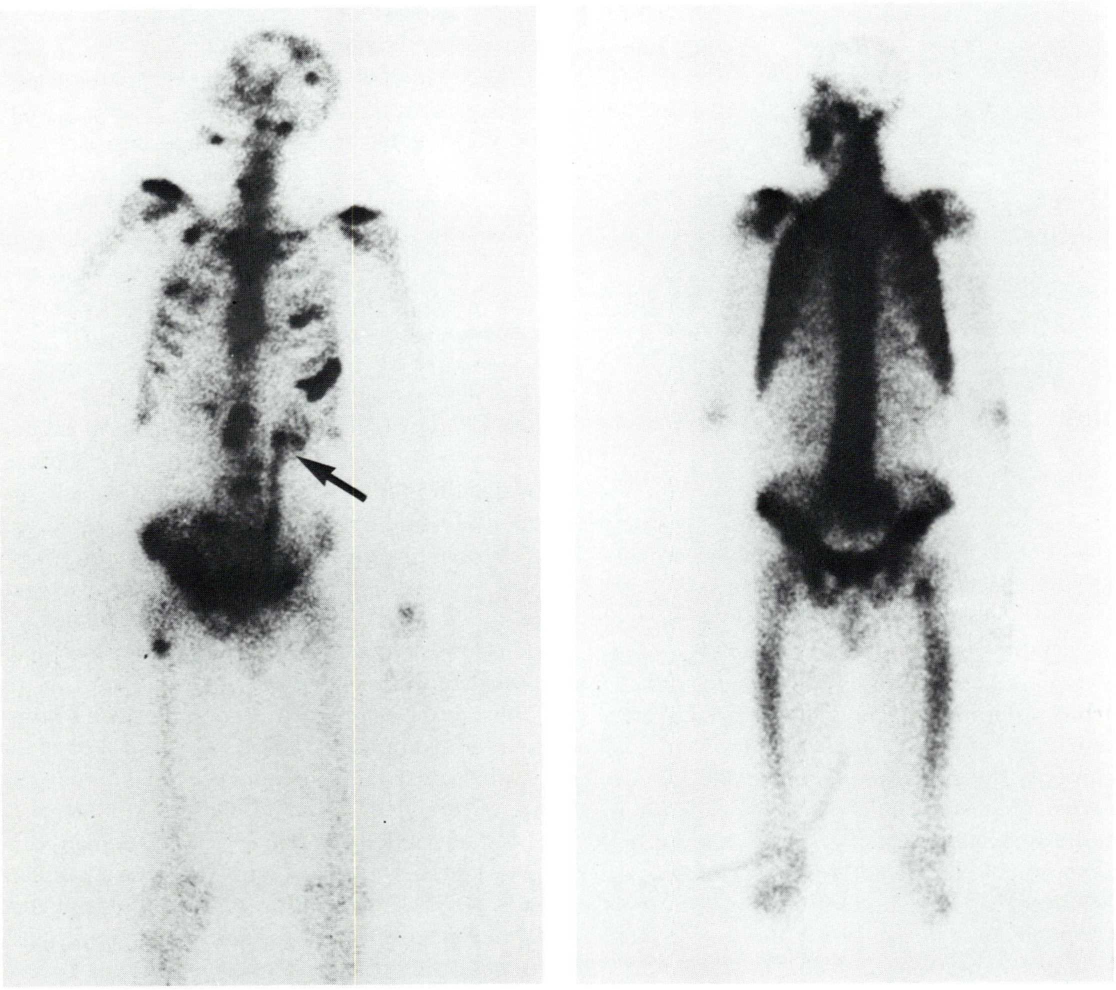

A B

Figure 22-15. Stage D2 prostate cancer. A. Bone scan shows multiple, asymmetric areas of increased pharmaceutical uptake by the osseous metastases. Note the obstructed right kidney in this posterior view (arrow). B. "Super" bone scan shows symmetrical increased uptake of radiopharmaceutical in patient with diffusely metastatic disease. It is significant that the kidneys are not seen.

employed to monitor the regression of known nodal involvement by CAP during and after hormonal therapy. MRI, with its proven capability for detecting nodal enlargement, is similarly useful.

SEMINAL VESICLES

Symptoms secondary to seminal vesicle disease are difficult to differentiate from those due to some prostate abnormalities; these include painful ejaculation, bloody semen (hematospermia), and perineal discomfort. Imaging of normal and diseased seminal vesicles will be discussed in the following sections.

NORMAL SEMINAL VESICLES

The seminal vesicles are paired structures lying just above the prostate and posterior to the bladder. They are best imaged by transrectal sonography, CT, and MRI [16]. The normal seminal vesicles are seen on transverse sonographic sections as a uniformly echogenic bow-tie-shaped structure just superior to the prostate (Fig. 22-16); on longitudinal images they present as cephalad soft-tissue extensions of the posterolateral prostate bilaterally. On CT, they also have a bowtie configuration and soft-tissue density, seen best on the sections immediately above the prostate (see Fig. 22-13). MRI shows the seminal vesicles to be medium-signal-intensity structures on T1 weighted images that become bright on T2 sections. Each seminal vesicle is about 3 cm long and 1.5 cm in diameter and has a tubular or ovoid configuration.

SEMINAL VESICLE STONES

Seminal vesicle stones are uncommon, and when they occur they are often related to stone disease elsewhere in the urinary tract or ectopic insertion of a ureter into the involved seminal vesicle. Reflux of urine into the seminal vesicle via the ejaculatory ducts has also been postulated as cause. Radiographically, the stones are usually opaque (calcium phosphate and calcium carbonate) and may range in size from 1 mm to 2 cm [1]. They may be single or multiple. On transrectal sonography, acoustic shadowing usually is seen with most stones, and on CT, the calculi can be easily identified as high-attenuation lesions within the seminal vesicles. Passage of smaller stones may result in pain and hematospermia. Calcium carbonate lithiasis may be seen as milk of calcium in the seminal vesicles. Calculus disease should not be confused with the calcifications of the walls of the seminal vesicles that can be found in diabetic men.

Figure 22-16. Normal seminal vesicles on transrectal sonography. Transverse section above the prostate shows a uniformly echogenic "bowtie" structure extending to both sides of the midline (arrows). (R = rectum.) (Courtesy of Matthew Rifkin, M.D., Thomas Jefferson University Hospital, Philadelphia, Pa.)

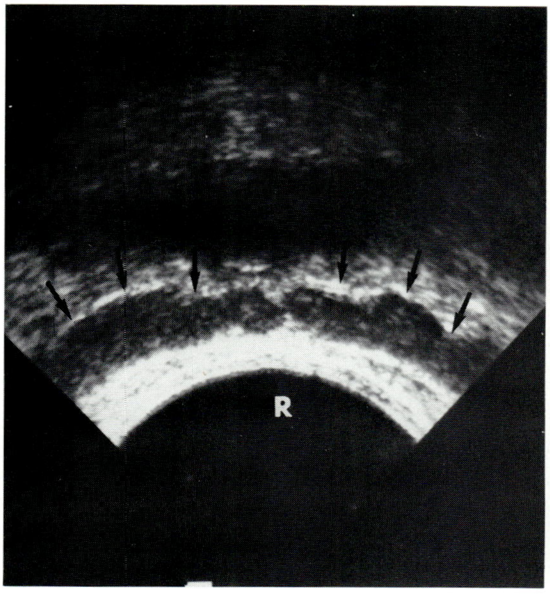

SEMINAL VESICLE CYSTS

Cysts of the seminal vesicles are rare. At least two-thirds of them are associated with ipsilateral renal agenesis and are congenital in origin. Acquired cysts are usually less than 5 cm in diameter and may have an obstructive or inflammatory cause. On CT or ultrasonography, these cysts have a thick wall. If hemorrhage has occurred into the cyst, they may appear as solid masses on CT (Fig. 22-17) and exhibit internal echoes or dependent debris on sonography.

SEMINAL VESICLE INFECTION

Isolated seminal vesiculitis seems to be rare. On the other hand, infection of the seminal vesicles in conjunction with prostatitis is probably not uncommon. This condition is difficult to diagnose because abnormal imaging findings of the seminal vesicles are often nonspecific. A frank abscess has a similar imaging pattern to a seminal vesicle cyst, as described above, though

Figure 22-17. Seminal vesicle cyst. CT shows a somewhat solid-appearing rounded mass in the right seminal vesicle (arrows).

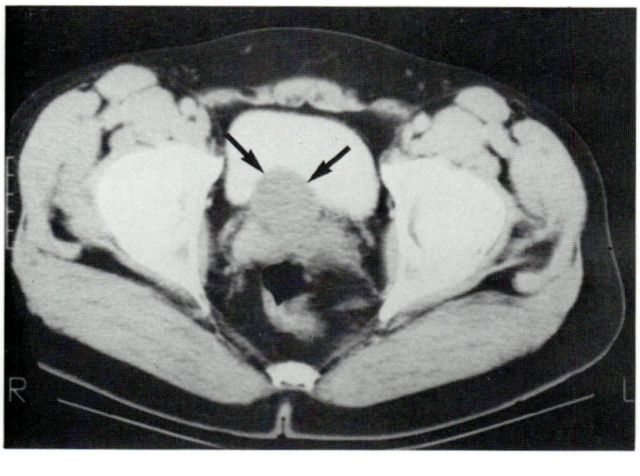

in the clinical setting of fever, leukocytosis, and lower urinary tract irritative symptoms the correct diagnosis can be suggested. Seminal vesiculitis may be secondary to obstruction of the ejaculatory ducts as they traverse an inflamed prostate; in this case, cystic dilation of the seminal vesicles may be seen [21]. With chronic infection, histopathologic examination of excised seminal vesicles reveals replacement fibrosis.

In the past seminal vesiculography has been used to diagnose disease. This technique is indentical to that of vasography, which will be described in Chap. 28. The vas is surgically exposed near the scrotal neck and its lumen injected with contrast medium in a cephalad direction using a small-gauge needle; this results in opacification of the vas and ipsilateral seminal vesicle. Although this examination is useful in diagnosing obstruction of the ductal system as a cause of seminal vesiculitis, it is otherwise often nonspecific because dilation of the gland, the most typical finding, does not always indicate current infection [8]. Cystic dilation of the seminal vesicles without infection can occur with aging or may be found on an obstructive basis after prostatectomy.

Of special note, tuberculosis of the seminal vesicles can result from primary involvement of the genital tract, or as a descending infection in the urine after infection of the kidney. Unfortunately, the imaging findings in this condition are also nonspecific, including thick-walled, cystic dilation of the seminal vesicles [31] (Fig. 22-18). However, with end-stage disease the seminal vesicles may calcify.

Figure 22-18. Tuberculosis of the seminal vesicles. CT shows irregularly enlarged seminal vesicles with a small, ill-defined area of low attenuation (arrow).

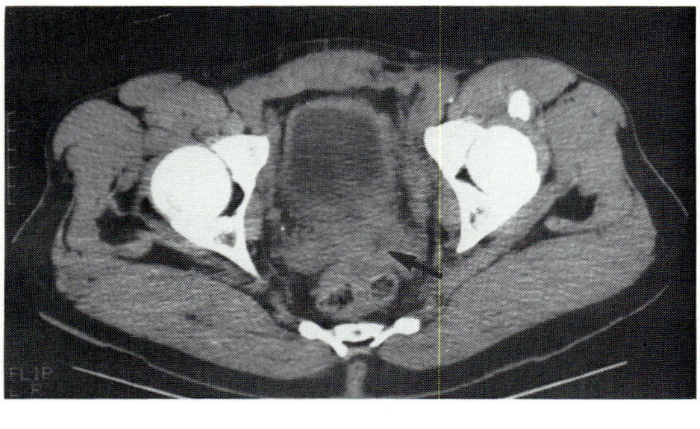

SEMINAL VESICLE NEOPLASMS

Direct invasion of the seminal vesicles by prostate cancer is by far the most common cause of neoplastic involvement; bladder and rectal carcinomas can also involve them secondarily. Imaging findings with invasion by prostate cancer have already been described; a similar pattern can be expected with involvement by bladder tumors, though a posterior intravesical mass in association with loss of the seminal vesicle angles or asymmetric enlargement of the ipsilateral seminal vesicle should aid in the differentiation. Invasion by rectal cancer is seen as an encroaching posterior soft-tissue mass.

Primary tumors of the seminal vesicles are very rare; these can be mesenchymal or carcinomatous. Although enlargement of or mass in a seminal vesicle in conjunction with a normal prostate may suggest this diagnosis on imaging studies, the finding is often nonspecific, as it may also indicate infection or hemorrhagic cyst.

REFERENCES

1. Banner, M.P., and Pollack, H.M. Urolithiasis in the lower urinary tract. *Semin. Roentgenol.* 17:140, 1982.
2. Beck, A.D. Benign prostatic hypertrophy and uraemia. *Br. J. Surg.* 57:561, 1970.
3. Berry, S.J., et al. The development of human benign prostatic hyperplasia with age. *J. Urol.* 132:474, 1984.
4. Bezzi, M., et al. Prostatic carcinoma: Staging with MR imaging at 1.5T. *Radiology* 169:339, 1988.
5. Carrol, C.L., et al. The abnormal prostate: MR imaging at 1.5T with histopathologic correlation. *Radiology* 163:521, 1987.
6. Castaneda, F., and Reddy, R. Benign prostatic hypertrophy: Retrograde transurethral dilation of the prostatic urethra in humans. *Radiology* 163:649, 1987.
7. Dahnert, W.F. Ultrasonography of carcinoma of the prostate: A critical review. *Appl. Radiol.* 7:39, 1988.
8. Dunnick, N.R., et al. Seminal vesiculography: Limited value in vesiculitis. *Urology* 20:454, 1982.
9. Epstein, J.I., et al. Prognosis of untreated stage A1 prostatic carcinoma: A study of 94 cases with extended follow-up. *J. Urol.* 136:837, 1986.
10. Fox, M. The natural history and significance of stone formation in the prostate gland. *J. Urol.* 89:716, 1963.
11. Franks, L.M. Latent carcinoma of the prostate. *J. Pathol. Bacteriol.* 68:603, 1954.

12. Friedland, G.W. Staging of genitourinary cancer. *Cancer* 60:450, 1987.
13. Gleason, D.F., Mellinger, G.T., and the VA Cooperative Urological Research Group. Prediction of prognosis for prostatic adenocarcinoma by combined histological grading and clinical staging. *J. Urol.* 111:58, 1974.
14. Hricak, H., et al. Prostatic carcinoma: Staging by clinical assessment, CT, and MR imaging. *Radiology* 162:331, 1987.
15. Jacobs, S. C. Spread of prostatic cancer to bone. *Urology* 21:337, 1983.
16. King, B.F., et al. Seminal vesicle imaging. *RadioGraphics* 9:653, 1989.
17. Komatsu, H., et al. Evaluation of early metastatic lesions of pelvic lymph nodes from carcinoma of the bladder or prostate. *J. Urol.* 138:341, 1987.
18. Kramer, S.A., et al. Experience with Gleason's histopathologic grading in prostatic cancer. *J. Urol.* 124:223, 1980.
19. Krieger, J.N. Prostatitis syndromes: Pathophysiology, differential diagnosis, and treatment. *Sex. Transm. Dis.* 11:100, 1984.
20. Lee, F., et al. Hypoechoic lesions of the prostate: Clinical relevance of tumor size, digital rectal examination and prostate-specific antigen. *Radiology* 170:29, 1989.
21. Littrup, P.J., et al. Transrectal US of the seminal vesicles and ejaculatory ducts: Clinical correlation. *Radiology* 168:625, 1988.
22. Lote, K., Walloe, A., and Bjersand, A. Bone metastases: Prognosis, diagnosis and treatment. *Acta Radiol. Oncol.* 25:227, 1986.
23. McNeal, J.E., et al. Patterns of progression in prostate cancer. *Lancet* 1:60, 1986.
24. McNeal, J.E., et al. Stage A versus stage B adenocarcinoma of the prostate: Morphological comparison and biological significance. *J. Urol.* 139:61, 1988.
25. Murphy, G.P., et al. The national survey of prostate cancer in the United States by the American College of Surgeons. *J. Urol.* 127:928, 1982.
26. Murphy, W.M., et al. Incidental carcinoma of the prostate: How much sampling is adequate? Am. *J. Surg. Pathol.* 10:170, 1986.
27. Ney, C., Miller, H.L., and Levy, J.L. Granulomatous prostatis. *Urology* 21:320, 1983.
28. Meares, E.M. Infection stones of prostate gland. *Urology* 6:560, 1974.
29. Phillips, M.E., et al. Prostatic disorders: MR imaging at 1.5T. *Radiology* 164:386, 1987.
30. Platt, J.F., Bree, R.L., and Schwab, R.E. The accuracy of CT in the staging of carcinoma of the prostate. *A.J.R.* 149:315, 1987.
31. Premkumar, A., and Newhouse, J.H. Seminal vesicle tuberculosis : CT appearance. *J. Comput. Assist. Tomogr.* 12:676, 1988.
32. Rifkin, M.D., and Choi, H. Implications of small, peripheral hypoechoic lesions in endorectal US of the prostate. *Radiology* 166:619, 1988.
33. Spirnak, J.P., and Resnick, M.I. Clinical staging of prostatic cancer: New modalities. *Urol. Clin. North Am.* 11:221, 1984.
34. Talner, L.B. Routine urography in men with prostatism. *A.J.R.* 147:960, 1986.
35. Walsh, P.C., and Lepor, H. The role of radical prostatectomy in the management of prostatic cancer. *Cancer* 60:526, 1987.

23

The Urethra

Interpretation of urethrographic studies is usually straightforward in normal patients. However, the multiplicity of disease processes and the possibility of their involving periurethral structures, especially in the male, can result in complex radiographic patterns. These require a thorough knowledge of urethral anatomy for deriving the correct diagnosis.

With the exception of tumors, there is a considerable difference between the disease processes affecting the male and female urethras. These will be discussed in the following sections.

MALE URETHRA

The male urethra is divided into posterior (3 to 3.5 cm) and anterior (12 to 15 cm) portions by the 1-cm membranous urethra coursing through the urogenital diaphragm (Fig. 23-1). The membranous urethra is radiographically defined proximally by the distal end of the verumontanum and distally by the tip of the cone of the bulbous urethra. The bulbous, or proximal anterior, urethra extends from the tip of the cone to the angle at the penoscrotal junction. The penile (or pendulous) portion of the anterior urethra then continues through the penis to the urethral meatus. The distal 2 cm of the anterior urethra, which is slightly dilated, is known as the fossa navicularis.

The most common acquired urethral conditions are inflammatory, neoplastic, or traumatic in origin. Many of these conditions result in narrowing of the urethral lumen either acutely or chronically and produce symptoms referable to the obstruction of urine flow (Table 23-1). The prostatic urethra is narrowed and lengthened in direct relation to benign prostatic enlargement.

INFECTION

Urethritis may be nonspecific or caused by a variety of agents. Probably the most common of the specific infections is gonorrheal urethritis. This is a clinically significant disease in that in the United States approximately 40 percent of all male urethral strictures are gonorrheal in origin. This is primarily a disease of the anterior urethra, though on rare occasion it can extend through the membranous urethra. The bacteria become sequestered in the glands of Littre, where the inflammation, if not properly treated, results in formation of granulation tissue that can progress to fibrous scarring. Periurethral involvement may also result in thrombosis of the corpus spongiosum. The proliferation of fibrous tissue results in stricture formation. The majority of these strictures involve the bulbous urethra because of the abundance of the glands of Littre in this area and its dependent position.

Radiographically, the typical postgonorrheal stricture is several centimeters in length and has a beaded, irregular appearance. These strictures may also be multiple or involve the entire anterior urethra (Fig. 23-2). They are frequently accompanied by opacification of the adjacent glands of Littre, which appear as small collections of contrast material dorsally paralleling the involved segment of the urethral lumen.

Other venereally contracted varieties of urethritis are caused by chlamydia or mycoplasma. Although these are generally more benign conditions, urethral strictures form in a small percentage of these patients.

Tuberculosis is a rare cause of urethritis. It most commonly is a descending form of infection resulting from tuberculous involvement of the kidneys. It may result in prostatic abscess, urethral strictures, and periurethral abscess or fistula formation. Fistulas may be numerous, resulting in the so-called watering-can perineum (Fig. 23-3).

Schistosoma haematobium, prevalent in Africa along the Nile valley, is not found in North America. Urethral involvement is not uncommon, and scrotal and perineal fistulas are frequently seen. Repeated infection and chronic fistulas almost invariably lead to urethral stricturing. As

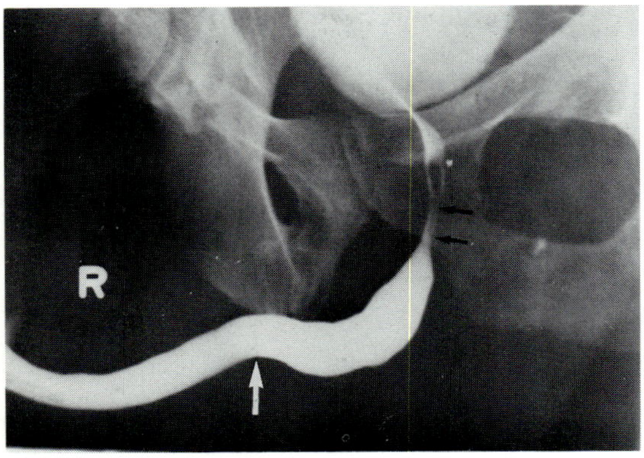

A

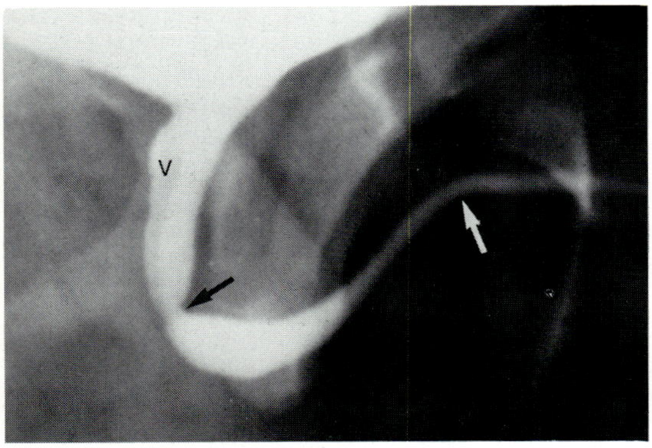

B

Figure 23-1. Normal male urethra. A. Retrograde urethrography shows entire urethra, though the prostatic urethra is poorly distended. The membranous urethra (black arrows) is delineated proximally by the distal end of the verumontanum (ovoid filling defect in prostatic urethra) and distally by the tip of the cone of the bulbous urethra. The penoscrotal junction (white arrow) divides the anterior urethra into proximal bulbar and distal penile segments. B. Voiding urethrography shows normal distention of the prostatic and membranous (black arrow) segments of the urethra. The verumontanum (V) is well seen in the prostatic urethra, as is the penoscrotal junction (white arrow).

Table 23-1. Causes of male urethral strictures

Postgonococcal
Bulbous and penile urethra
Postinstrumentation (TURP)
Membranous urethra/penoscrotal junction
Bladder-neck contracture
Postcatheterization (indwelling)
Penoscrotal junction
Neoplastic
Anterior urethra
Other inflammatory diseases (tuberculosis, schistosomiasis, chlamydia, etc.)
Anterior urethra
Posttraumatic
Bulbous urethra ("straddle injury")
Prostatomembranous urethra (pelvic fracture)

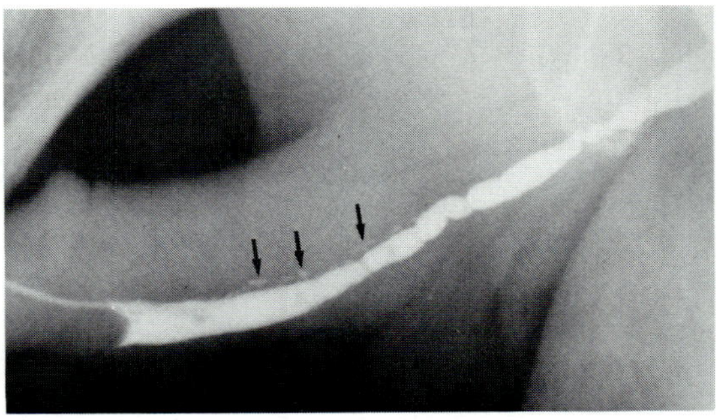

Figure 23-2. Postgonorrheal stricture. Retrograde urethrograpy shows irregular narrowing (beading) of the entire anterior urethra. Note contrast material in glands of Littre along dorsum of urethra (arrows).

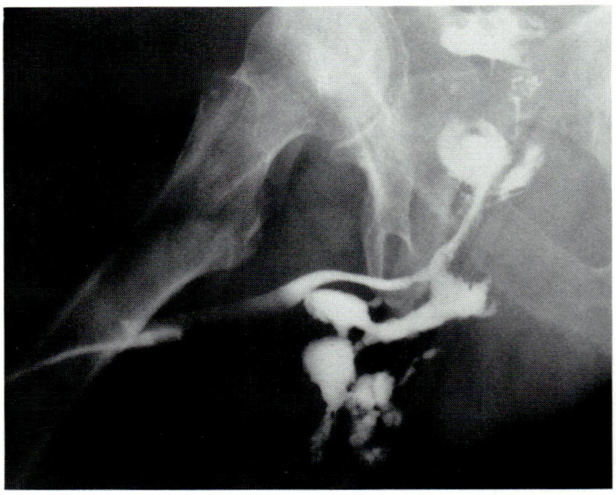

Figure 23-3. Tuberculous fistulas and sinuses ("watering-can perineum"). Retrograde urethrography demonstrates irregular narrowing of the bulbar urethra associated with multiple sinuses and cutaneous fistulas involving the urethra from bulb to bladder neck.

with tuberculosis, urethrography reveals irregular strictures, with multiple fistulas draining to the perineum or scrotum.

Condyloma accuminata is a condition in which virus-induced verrucae occur on the shaft or glans of the penis or both. In up to 5 percent of these patients, intraurethral extension of the disease can be found. Rarely, these verrucae may involve the entire urethra and extend into the bladder. They do not usually cause obstruction, but irritative voiding symptoms and penile discharge are common. Intraurethral verrucae can be seen on urethrography as multiple nonobstructive filling defects.

NEOPLASMS

Benign tumors of the urethra are rare. Congenital fibroepithelial polyps of the posterior urethra, usually seen in young boys, have been discussed in Chap. 5. These can also be seen in young men as an acquired condition. They are usually on stalks and seen as linear or oval filling defects in the posterior urethra on urethrography. On occasion, they may prolapse into the bladder or through the membranous and into the bulbous urethra.

Other benign tumors include transitional cell papillomas and adenomatous polyps, both occurring in the posterior urethra [5]. Inflammatory "tags" resembling polyps can form in response to posterior urethritis. Any of these can present as a filling defect in the posterior urethra.

Malignant tumors of the urethra are also rare, and they are usually heralded by obstructive symptoms or initial hematuria (hematuria that clears with voiding). As the tumor progresses, a periurethral mass may be palpable, or the tumor may present with abscess or fistula formation. Over half these tumors occur in the bulbous urethra, while a third are seen in the penile urethra and only 10 percent in the prostatic urethra. Almost three-fourths of these tumors are squamous cell carcinomas, and over 70 percent of these are associated with a history of longstanding urethral stricture or a previous history of venereal disease [8].

Transitional cell carcinoma usually occurs in the prostatic urethra in association with bladder carcinoma. On the other hand, adenocarcinomas usually occur in the bulbomembranous urethra, where they are thought to arise from either Cowper's glands or the glands of Littre. Other primary tumors that can occur in the urethra include rhabdomyosarcomas, fibrosarcomas, and malignant melanomas. The last usually arise de novo in the fossa navicularis near the meatus. On very rare occasions, amyloidosis can involve the male urethra and mimic neoplasm symptomatically and radiographically.

Metastatic spread of urethral tumors is usually via lymphatics to inguinal, external and internal iliac, and obturator nodes. Hematogenous metastases are less common.

The most common secondary tumors involving the urethra are from transitional cell carcinomas of the bladder or adenocarcinoma of the prostate. Tumors from the bladder usually seed the urethral mucosa directly, whereas other neoplasms metastasize to the periurethral tissues hematogenously.

Radiographically, a urethral tumor may present as a filling defect or luminal narrowing (Fig. 23-4). When they occur in an area of previous stricturing, the stricture may retain its benign appearance, but more commonly will show an irregular or ulcerated contour [3]. Change in a preexisting urethral stricture, especially increasing irregularity or ulceration, should therefore lead to the suspicion of neoplasm. Secondary tumors may also present as single filling defects within the urethra but commonly, especially in the case of transitional cell carcinoma, may present as multiple defects in the urethral lumen. CT is useful for staging urethral tumors by imaging the nodes in the pelvis and inguinal areas.

URETHRAL CHANGES DUE TO INSTRUMENTATION

Indwelling urethral catheters, especially if not properly positioned and cared for, may result in urethral inflammation and stricture formation within a matter of days. The shaft of an indwelling Foley catheter should be taped to the lower abdomen to allow a smooth curve as it passes through the urethra. Otherwise, pressure necrosis can occur where the urethra angles at the penoscrotal junction. This necrosis can result in abscess formation and stricture in this area, though catheter-induced strictures can occur at any point in the urethra. Strictures secondary to pressure necrosis alone are usually short, while those due to necrosis with infection are usually long [7].

Transurethral resection of the prostate or of bladder tumors is frequently conducted using a large-caliber (26 to 28 French) sheath. This can be traumatic to the urethra, especially during

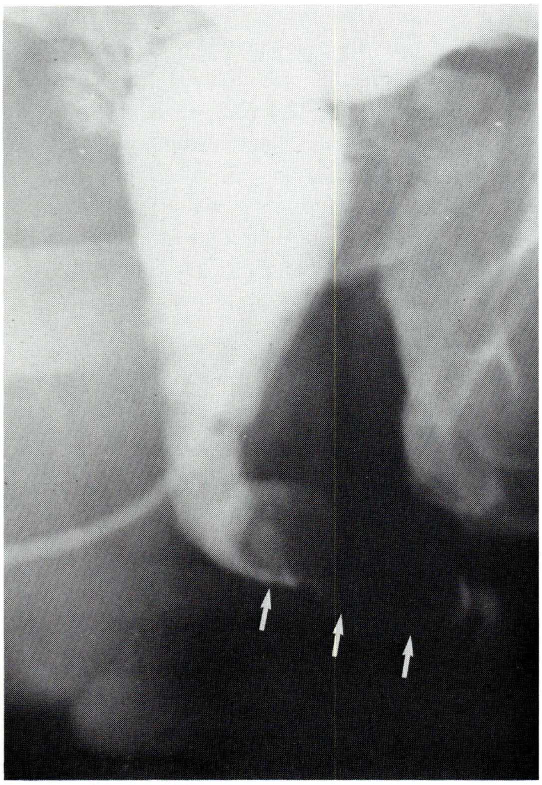

A

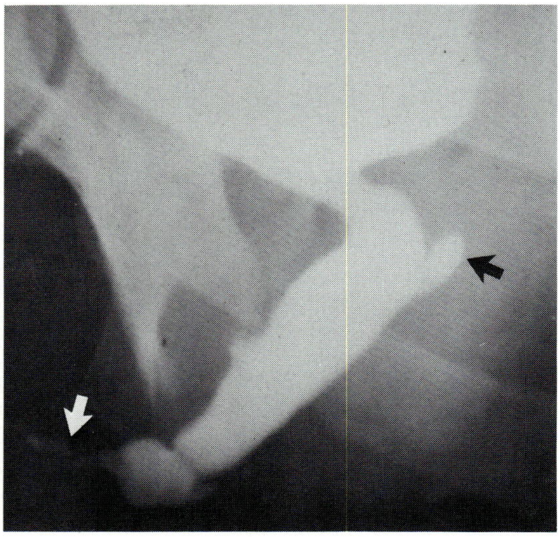

B

Figure 23-4. Primary urethral tumors (squamous cell carcinoma). A. Voiding cystourethrography shows filling defect in bulbar urethra (arrows). The urethra proximal to the tumor is dilated, and reflux is seen into prostatic ducts. B. Voiding cystourethrography shows long, irregular stricture of bulbar urethra (white arrows). Again, the urethra proximal to the tumor is dilated, and the utricle is prominent and filled with contrast material (black arrow). (Fig. 23-4B from E.S. Amis, Jr., J.H. Newhouse, and J.J. Cronan. Radiology of male periurethral structures. *A.J.R.* 151:321–324. © by American Roentgen Ray Society, 1988.)

long procedures. The incidence of strictures after transurethral surgery has been reported to be as high as 14 percent [9]. External trauma to the urethra is also a frequent precursor of urethral stricture formation, and will be discussed in Chap. 25.

OPACIFICATION OF PERIURETHRAL STRUCTURES

The urethra is surrounded by several structures that may be opacified during urethrography and produce confusing images. Stricture of the urethra is the most common associated finding in these patients [2].

On urethrography, the glands of Littre appear as small linear collections of contrast material parallel to the superior margin of the anterior urethra. These glands are usually opacified in association with chronic infection or urethral strictures. Strictures can also result in opacification of Cowper's ducts and glands. A stricture proximal to the point at which the ducts insert in the bulbous urethra causes high intraurethral pressure during retrograde studies, which in turn can produce reflux into the ducts and glands (Fig. 23-5). A distal stricture may result in dilation of the ducts due to elevated urethral voiding pressure, and the ducts may then opacify during voiding urethrography.

Membranous or anterior urethral strictures or poorly synchronized contractions of the bladder detrusor muscle and the external sphincter (detrusor–external sphincter dyssynergia) may elevate voiding pressures within the prostatic urethra. In these circumstances it is common to see a dilated posterior urethra. Furthermore, contrast material may fill a dilated utricle (posterior to the verumontanum) or reflux into the prostatic ducts. Dilation of the prostatic ducts may be severe, and multiple prostatic calculi are not uncommon in this condition.

On occasion, prostatic abscesses may drain spontaneously into the prostatic urethra or be unroofed transurethrally. Either type of drainage may result in a periurethral cavity that opacifies during urethrography (Fig. 23-6). In fact, periurethral abscesses adjacent to any part of the urethra may cause irregular collections of

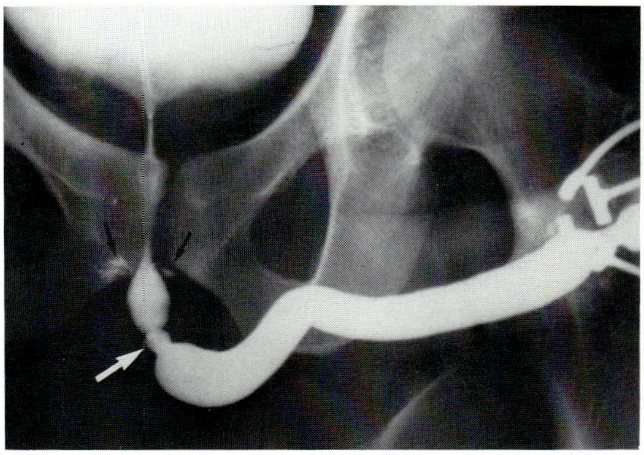

Figure 23-5. Proximal bulbar stricture secondary to previous "straddle injury". There is reflux into Cowper's glands. Retrograde urethrography shows typical short bulbar stricture (white arrow) and contrast material in Cowper's glands (black arrows). The ducts of the glands insert distally to the stricture, and high pressure in the anterior urethra during this retrograde study has resulted in reflux into the ducts. (From E.S. Amis, Jr., J.H. Newhouse, and J.J. Cronan. Radiology of male periurethral structures. *A.J.R.* 151:321–324. © by American Roentgen Ray Society, 1988.)

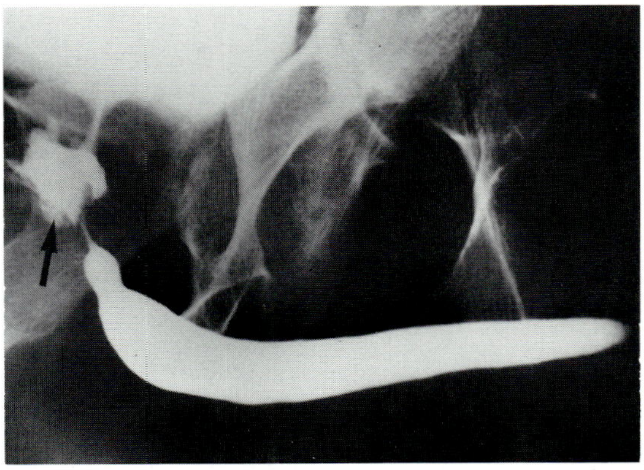

Figure 23-6. Prostatic abscess cavity. Retrograde urethrography shows abscess cavity (arrow) that previously drained into prostatic urethra. (From E.S. Amis, Jr., J.H. Newhouse, and J.J. Cronan. Radiology of male periurethral structures. *A.J.R.* 151:321–324. © by American Roentgen Ray Society, (1988.)

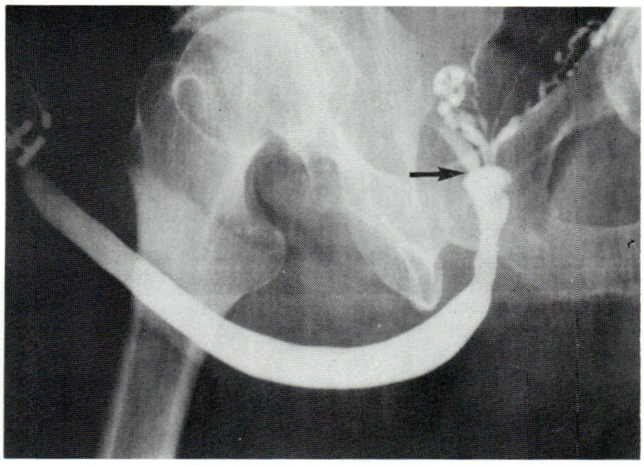

Figure 23-7. Bladder-neck contracture. Retrograde urethrography demonstrates tight bladder neck (arrow) with resultant reflux into the ejaculatory ducts, seminal vesicles, and vasa deferentia. (From E.S. Amis, Jr., J.H. Newhouse, and J.J. Cronan Radiology of male periurethral structures. *A.J.R.* 151:321-324. © by American Roentgen Ray Society, 1988.)

contrast material or fistulous tracts that can be seen during urethrography.

Partial or complete contracture of the bladder neck usually occurs as a complication of open or transurethral prostatectomy and may result in elevation of intraurethral pressure sufficient to cause reflux into the ejaculatory ducts, seminal vesicles, and vasa deferentia during retrograde urethrography (Fig. 23-7). On the other hand, these structures may be demonstrated during voiding urethrography in patients with distal urethral strictures.

FEMALE URETHRA

The female urethra is significantly different anatomically from that of the male. It is only 2.5 to 4.0 cm long, roughly equivalent to the length of the posterior urethra in the male, and is less fixed in the pelvis than that portion of the male urethra. On voiding studies there is a wide range of configurations that can be considered normal. Typically, however, the female urethra is ovoid or tubular, and its average diameter is 6 mm. On sonography, the sphincter surrounding the closed urethra is routinely seen as a hypoechoic structure below the bladder base, measuring 1.0 to 1.3 cm in diameter [4] (Fig. 23-8A).

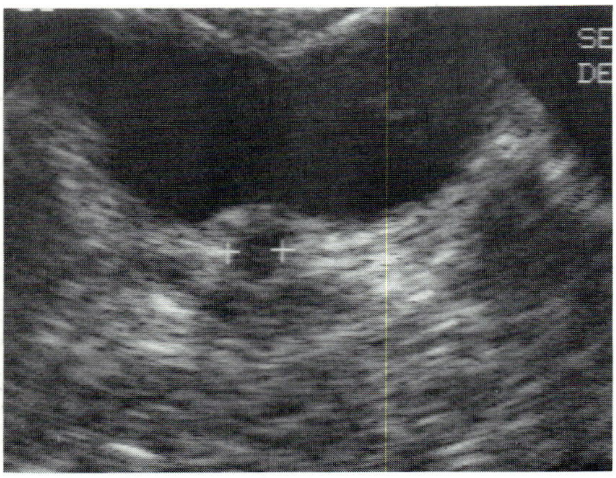

A

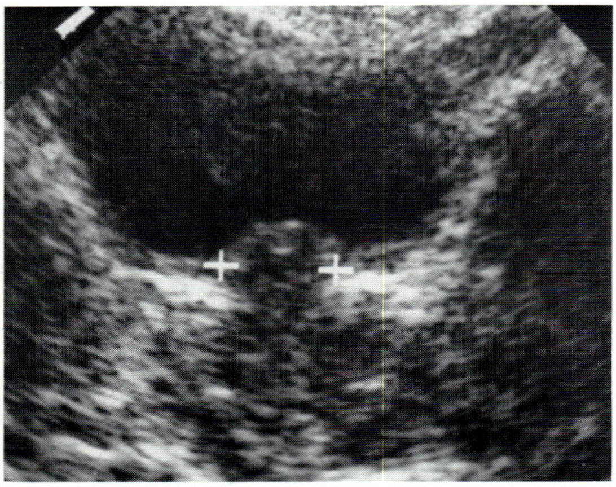

B

Figure 23-8. Normal and abnormal female urethra. A. Sonography shows the normal urethral sphincter as a hypoechoic area below the bladder base (markers indicate 9-mm diameter). B. Sonography in woman with female urethral syndrome shows enlarged hypoechoic periurethral area (markers show 1.8-cm diameter).

This should not be confused with a pathologic condition.

INFECTION

Venereal diseases almost never affect the urethra primarily in the female, being transmitted instead by way of the vagina, uterine cavity, and fallopian tubes to the pelvic cavity. Other isolated urethral infections are also rare, although urethritis in conjunction with acute cystitis is common. Malacoplakia, a rare granulomatous response to *Escherichia coli* infection, affects the urethra in 2 percent of patients with urinary tract involvement by this condition. However, nonspecific chronic infection of the urethra is more common and can result in periurethral inflammation and inflammatory edema and polyps in the region of the bladder neck. This is known as the female urethral syndrome, and it results in chronic irritative voiding symptoms. Sonography in these cases reveals hypoechoic tissue of increased thickness surrounding the urethra. This inflammatory tissue is larger than the normal sphincter (Fig. 23-8B) and may be prominent enough to elevate the bladder floor on urography. Stricturing of the female urethra in response to inflammation is extremely rare, though mucosal irregularity in cases of acute or chronic infection can occasionally be seen during voiding cystourethrography.

NEOPLASMS

Although carcinoma of the female urethra is uncommon, it nonetheless has an incidence five times greater than that found in males. Primary carcinoma of the urethra often presents with symptoms of chronic urinary tract infection, including frequency, dysuria, urinary retention, and pain. Hematuria may, on occasion, be a presenting symptom. The distal two-thirds of the female urethra is lined with squamous epithelium, and 90 percent of tumors occur in this region. As in the male, the large majority (70%) are squamous cell carcinomas. Transitional cell carcinoma usually involves the posterior portion of the urethra. Adenocarcinoma, also as in the male, appears to originate in the periurethral glands, which in the female are known as Skene's glands. Very rarely, female urethral neoplasms may be undifferentiated carcinomas or malignant melanomas. Metastatic spread is via pelvic and inguinal lymphatics.

Diagnosis is difficult and often delayed because the clinical symptoms and laboratory data are similar to those found with chronic infection. Furthermore, the radiographic findings on cystourethrography are nonspecific. The diagnosis is usually made on the basis of biopsy of a urethral mass discovered on physical examination. MRI, with its superior soft-tissue contrast-material resolution and its capability of imaging in multiple planes, may overcome some of the limitations found with CT and be able to show involvement of adjacent viscera, fat, or musculature by the urethral tumor [6].

DIVERTICULA

Diverticula are a well known clinical entity. An acquired cause for most female urethral diverticula is currently favored. Infection of the periurethral Skene's glands is probably the initial event, followed by obstruction of the gland and abscess formation. Subsequent rupture of the abscess into the urethra results in formation of a diverticulum. Symptoms include dyspareunia, postvoiding dribbling, frequency, and dysuria.

Calculi are found within these diverticula in 5.7 to 10 percent of cases [10]. The detection of stones is important, as there is an increased morbidity in these patients after sugical removal of the diverticulum. In addition, there appears to be an increased incidence of carcinoma arising within stone-containing diverticula.

Although squamous cell carcinoma is the most common urethral neoplasm in the female, adenocarcinoma is the most common neoplasm arising within a urethral diverticulum. It has been suggested that the same factors leading to stone formation, notably chronic infection and urinary stasis, could also act as inciting agents for these diverticular neoplasms.

An unobstructed urethral diverticulum can be detected on the postvoid film obtained during urography in approximately 75 percent of cases. This is seen as a small rounded or ovoid collection of contrast material located behind the pubic symphysis. With the denser contrast material used in voiding cystourethrography, identification of the diverticulum occurs in approximately 90 percent of cases. The remainder require positive-pressure urethrography with a double-balloon catheter for radiographic visualization. Although the majority of diverticula occur in the distal urethra or midurethra, a diverticulum arising in the proximal portion of the urethra may extend cephalad and cause elevation of the bladder base during urography not unlike that seen with an enlarged prostate in the male [1].

Sonography has been advocated for evaluation of female urethral diverticula. This may show that the diverticulum is partially filled with inflammatory debris or has a thickened wall surrounded by inflammatory edema. CT has also been reported to be useful in diagnosing this condition, showing a soft-tissue or fluid-filled mass below the bladder. A filling defect within a urethral diverticulum on contrast studies should suggest stone or tumor (Fig. 23-9). If the plain film does not show a calcification, CT or sonography should be used to differentiate a calculus from a soft-tissue tumor mass.

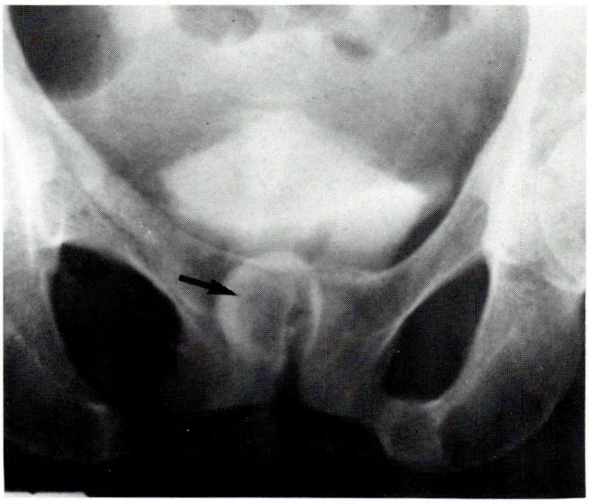

Figure 23-9. Tumor in female urethral diverticulum. Coned postvoiding urography shows rounded collection of contrast material below the bladder base. Filling defect (arrow) proved to be tumor.

REFERENCES

1. Amis, E.S. Jr., et al. Impressions on the floor of the female bladder: "The female prostate." *Urology* 19:441, 1982.
2. Amis E.S., Jr., Newhouse, J.H., and Cronan J.J. Radiology of male periurethral structures. *A.J.R.* 151:321, 1988.
3. Bosniak, M.A., Siegelman, S.S., and Evans, J.A. *Atlas of Tumor Radiology: The Adrenal, Retroperitoneum and Lower Urinary Tract.* Chicago, Year Book, 1976. Pp. 450–451.
4. de Gonzalez, E.L., et al. The appearances on ultrasound of the female urethral sphincter. *Br. J. Radiol.* 61:687, 1988.
5. DiSantis, D.J., McClennan, B.L., and Heiken, J.P., Acquired disorders of the urethra. In J.M. Taveras and J.T. Ferrucci (Eds.), *Radiology: Diagnosis-Imaging-Intervention.* Philadelphia: Lippincott, 1988.

6. Fisher, M., et al. Female urethral carcinoma: MRI staging. *A.J.R.* 144:603, 1985.
7. McCallum, R.W. The urethra and seminal vesicles. In C.E. Putman and C.E. Ravin (Eds.), *Textbook of Diagnostic Imaging*. Philadelphia: Saunders, 1988. Pp. 1351–1360.
8. McCallum, R.W. The adult male urethra: Normal anatomy, pathology, and method of urethrography. *Radiol. Clin. North Am.* 17:227, 1979.
9. Shaver, W.A., Richter, P.H., and Orandi, A. Changes in the male urethra produced by instrumentation for transurethral resection of the prostate. *Radiology* 116, 623, 1975.
10. Tines, S.C., Bigongiari, L.R., and Weigel, J.W. Carcinoma in diverticulum of the female urethra. *A.J.R.* 138:582, 1982.

The Scrotum

In the past, indeterminate results of clinical examination in patients with acute scrotal pain resulted in the necessity for surgical exploration to rule out testicular torsion. Similarly, testicular tumors could not always be differentiated from benign scrotal lesions, also resulting in the need for surgical intervention. Currently, in many of these instances, imaging is able to provide an accurate diagnosis rapidly, thus obviating the need for surgery.

For effective scrotal imaging, the radiologist must be familiar with the anatomic details of this area, the imaging techniques useful in delineating this anatomy, and the various pathologic processes that can occur in the scrotum. This chapter will address these topics.

SCROTAL ANATOMY

Figure 24-1 depicts the anatomy of the scrotum and testis. The scrotum is composed of several layers. Immediately beneath the skin is found the dartos muscle, whose fibers also form the scrotal septum. The dartos muscle is separated from the cremaster muscle by a layer of loose connective tissue. Beneath the cremaster muscle lies the tunica vaginalis, which has parietal and visceral layers forming a potential cavity around the testis. A few milliliters of lubricating fluid are normally found within this space. The layers of the tunica vaginalis are joined on the posterolateral aspect of the testis in the region of its mediastinum.

The normal testis measures approximately 3 cm × 3 cm × 4 cm. It is covered by a thick fibrous capsule—the tunica albuginea. The testis is divided into multiple small lobules, which are wedge-shaped and converge toward the superior part of the testis in its posterolateral aspect. Each lobule contains one or more seminiferous tubules, in which sperm are produced. These seminiferous tubules form an interconnecting network of small cystic spaces—the rete testis—in the area where thin fibrous septae dividing the lobules converge on the mediastinum of the testis. The rete testis is connected to the head of the epididymis by a series of efferent ductules that penetrate the tunica albuginea in the mediastinum testis. The multiple tubules in the head of the epididymis eventually coalesce into a single coiled tube that forms the body and tail of the epididymis, which are loosely applied to the posterolateral surface of the testis. The tail of the epididymis connects with the vas deferens.

The appendix testis, a müllerian remnant, is a tiny nodule attached to the superior pole of the testis. The appendix epididymis, thought to be an isolated efferent ductule, is similar in size, and it arises from the head of the epididymis.

The major blood supply of the testis is via the testicular artery. The paired testicular arteries arise from the anterior aspect of the aorta slightly below the level of the renal arteries. Each testicular artery joins the ipsilateral spermatic cord at the level of the internal inguinal ring. As it reaches the testis, the testicular artery divides into multiple branches that pierce the tunica albuginea and then run peripherally around the testis. These peripheral arteries give off centripetal branches that traverse the testicula parenchyma as they course toward the mediastinum testis. The deferential and cremasteric arteris also supply a small amount of blood to the testis, though they primarily supply the epididymis and scrotal tissues.

The spermatic cord contains the arteries noted above, the pampiniform venous plexus, the vas deferens, lymphatics, cremaster muscle fibers, and fat.

SCROTAL IMAGING TECHNIQUES

Radionuclide scanning, MRI, and various applications of sonography are the primary methods useful in imaging the scrotum and its contents [21]. Although CT has no direct application in imaging the scrotum itself, it is extremely useful in imaging pelvic and retroperitoneal nodes in staging testis tumors.

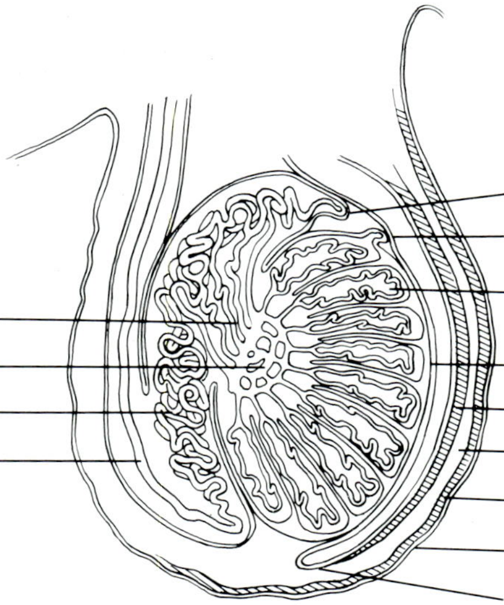

Figure 24-1. Diagram of scrotal and testicular anatomy.

SCROTAL SONOGRAPHY

Scrotal sonography is the most commonly used technique for evaluating the scrotal contents. Its primary capabilities lie in differentiating cystic and solid lesions and localizing disease as being intratesticular or extratesticular. For imaging the small structures within the scrotum a 7.5-to-10.0-MHz, high-resolution transducer is usually necessary. An acoustic gel is required for proper coupling of the transducer to the scrotum. Both longitudinal and transverse scans are routinely obtained.

The normal testis exhibits a homogeneous, moderately echogenic texture (Fig. 24-2). The mediastinum testis is even more echogenic and, as previously noted, is seen superiorly in the posterolateral aspect of the testis. The echotexture of the epididymis is similar to that of the testis.

Doppler sonography, either pulsed or color flow, has been show to be effective in evaluating the blood supply to the testis. Doppler used in conjunction with sonographic imaging is known as duplex sonography. This system permits direct visualization of the source of any detected vascular signal. Color Doppler has been reported to be capable of reliably imaging intratesticular as well as supratesticular cord arteries. In the cord, the testicular artery exhibits a low-impedance-type wave form, although some high-impedance patterns can be seen originating from the deferential or cremasteric arteries [16]. Intratesticular wave forms are consistently of a low-impedance variety.

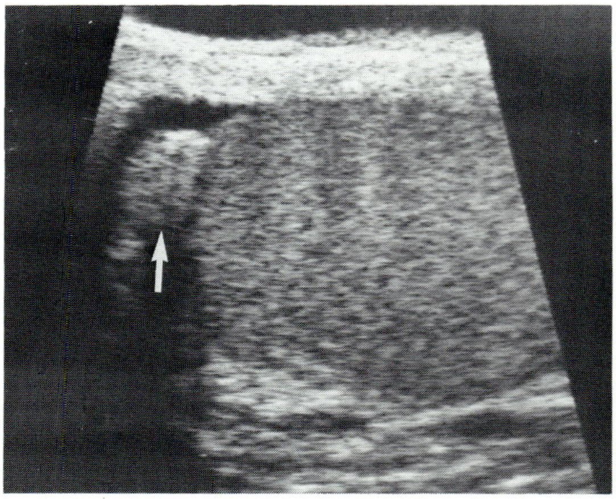

Figure 24-2. Longitudinal sonogram of normal testis, including head of epididymis (arrow). Note the homogeneous echotexture.

RADIONUCLIDE SCANNING

Radionuclide scanning is currently used only for evaluation of blood flow to the testes. Therefore, it is usually employed in the clinical setting of acute scrotal pain in which torsion must be differentiated from an inflammatory condition such as epididymitis. Using a gamma camera, both dynamic and static images are obtained after the injection of a bolus of technetium-99m pertechnetate (5 to 20 mCi). In this technique, both testes are evaluated simultaneously, with the penoscrotal junction serving as the center of the imaged field. A cold area in the region of one testis is presumed to indicate loss of normal arterial supply. Because this technique cannot identify the absolute location of the testes, sonography is a valuable adjunctive technique for this task.

MAGNETIC RESONANCE IMAGING

Experience indicates that MRI can produce high-resolution images of the scrotal contents [1, 8, 18, 24]. However, MRI is not widely used for imaging the scrotum at present, as it is significantly more expensive than scrotal sonography and has not yet been proven to yield significantly greater information.

The testis exhibits a homogeneous, intermediate signal on T1 weighted images and shows high signal intensity on T2 weighted images. The signal intensity of the fibrous tunica albuginea is low on both image sequences.

SCROTAL PATHOLOGY

TESTICULAR TORSION

Either the appendix testis or the appendix epididymis can twist and result in acute onset of scrotal pain; however, the pain is usually more moderate than that seen with true testicular torsion, and tenderness on clinical examination is often localized to the upper pole of the testis. The torsed appendage may be palpable as a firm lump the size of a pea in some instances.

Testicular torsion can be a cause of scrotal pain in patients of all ages, ranging from the newborn to the elderly. However, the most typical clinical presentation is that of a boy or young man with painful scrotal swelling of acute onset. The differential diagnoses include epididymitis, orchitis, acute hydrocele, strangulated inguinal hernia, hemorrhage into a testicular tumor, or fat necrosis in the spermatic cord [17].

In normal men, the testis is somewhat fixed at the point where the leaves of the tunica vaginalis converge posteriorly, thereby preventing the testis from twisting on the spermatic cord. However, there is an anomalous situation in which the testes are not fixed in the scrotum—the so-called bell-clapper deformity; this allows twisting of the testis on the spermatic cord, resulting in compromise of its blood supply. If spontaneous untwisting does not occur, surgical intervention is required. The testicular salvage rate approaches 100 percent if surgery is performed within 6 hours of the onset of pain. If surgery is delayed for more than 12 hours, a 20 percent salvage rate has been reported. Beyond 24 hours, the testis in all cases is found to be necrotic; this is known as a "missed" torsion. Because the deformity allowing torsion is bilateral, an orchiopexy, or fixation of the testis within the scrotum, is required for both testes. Even with missed torsion, this diagnosis should be established so that orchiopexy of the contralateral testis can be performed.

Radionuclide scans have been the standard method for evaluating patients with acute onset of scrotal pain, though Doppler sonography has been reported as capable of showing decreased blood flow in cases of acute testicular ischemia [15]. Scintigraphy relies on the finding of decreased perfusion to the symptomatic testis during dynamic imaging and demonstration of a central cold defect in the region of the testis on static images for establishing the diagnosis of torsion (Fig. 24-3A). If these criteria are followed, scintigraphy is approximately 95 percent accurate in diagnosing torsion. In missed torsions, static scintigraphy often shows a peripheral rim of increased activity surrounding the central void [6]. However, this finding is nonspecific, as it has been reported in association with tumor, trauma, and inflammation [27].

On sonography, the torsed testis characteristically becomes inhomogeneous and hypoechoic (Fig. 24-3B). However, the testis may appear sonographically normal during the first 6 hours after torsion of the cord [5]. Extratesticular findings include epididymal enlargement, thickening of the scrotal skin, and formation of a reactive hydrocele. On occasion, extratesticular hemorrhage can occur secondary to torsion, resulting in an echogenic or complex extratesticular mass in addition to the classic findings described above [26]. With longstanding torsion,

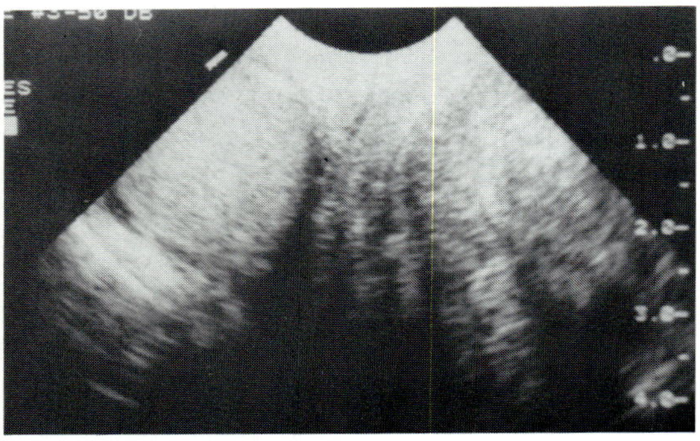

A

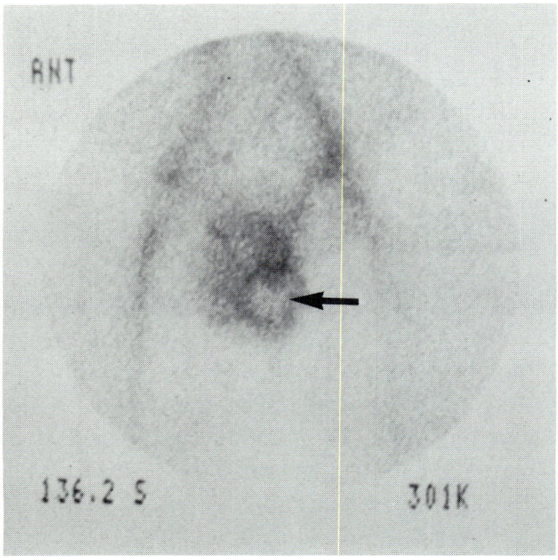

B

Figure 24-3. Acute testicular torsion. A. Transverse scrotal sonography shows the left testis to be slightly inhomogeneous and hypoechoic as compared with the normal right testis. B. Static scintigraphy demonstrates a "cold" defect in the region of the left testis (arrow).

the typical sonographic finding is a small echopenic testis.

INFLAMMATORY CONDITIONS

Epididymitis commonly presents with relatively rapid onset of scrotal pain and swelling, usually in adolescents and middle-aged men. It may be idiopathic or bacterial in origin, the most common infective agents being *Escherichia coli* and pseudomonas and aerobacter species [20]. Gonococcal urethritis may also progress to epididymitis through retrograde flow of infected urine down the vas. The epididymis may be affected by tuberculosis in patients with urinary tract involvement by this disease. A diffuse or focal orchitis may accompany epididymitis; orchitis without epididymal involvement is often due to the mumps virus or syphilis.

On radionuclide studies, acute epididymitis presents as increased perfusion through the spermatic cord vessels. Subsequent increased hemiscrotal radioactivity is usually concentrated in the region of the epididymis; this is seen as a linear or curvilinear area of increased activity corresponding to the hyperemic, inflamed epididymis. On sonography, the epididymis is enlarged, and its echogenicity is usually decreased (Fig. 24-4). Reactive hydroceles are commonly seen. Focal orchitis is seen as an area of decreased echogenicity within the testis, whereas with diffuse orchitis, the testis is swollen and generally hypoechoic. Focal testicular inflammation is sonographically similar to a testis tumor. This mandates imaging follow-up after resolution of the acute symptoms. Not uncommonly, severe acute epididymitis can lead to obstruction of the blood supply to the testis, resulting in testicular infarction [4].

CYSTIC LESIONS

Cystic lesions can occur in the testicular parenchyma, the tunica albuginea, and the epididymis. Testicular parenchymal cysts, once thought to be rare, have been reported in 8 to 10 percent of asymptomatic men studied by scrotal so-

Figure 24-4. Epididymitis. Transverse sonography shows the testis (defined by markers) to be normal. The epididymis (arrows) is grossly enlarged and inhomogeneous.

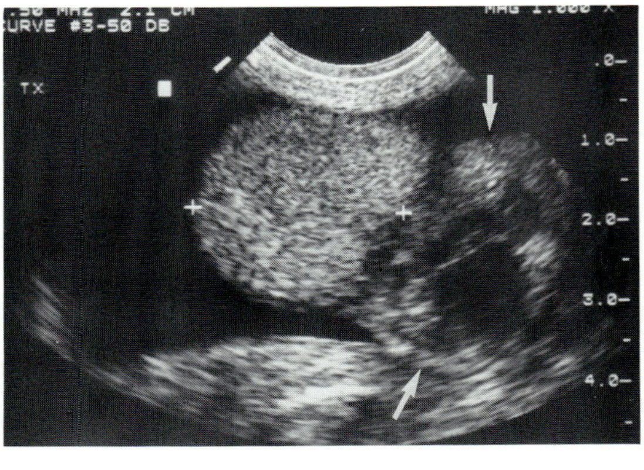

nography. These cysts can also occur in the pediatric population, and they present a diagnostic problem at all ages since testis tumors may also have cystic components. Among testis tumors, cysts are most commonly seen in association with teratomas. Epidermal cyst (a variety of benign neoplasm) can also occur in the testicular parenchyma.

On ultrasonography, simple parenchymal cysts are seen as well-circumscribed, anechoic areas with imperceptible walls and distal acoustic enhancement [11] (Fig. 24-5). These are usually small and thus nonpalpable. They tend to be located near the mediastinum of the testis. Epidermal cysts are typically larger and therefore often palpable. On sonography, they present as solitary cystic structures with an echogenic rim [13]. Cysts of the tunica albuginea are palpable as small masses because of their peripheral location. By contrast, the cysts associated with teratoma are usually multiple or loculated and seen in conjunction with lesions of marked inhomogeneity [22].

Within the epididymis, two types of cystic structures can be identified. Simple cysts are filled with clear serous fluid, whereas spermatoceles contain sperm, and on gross examination the fluid is thick and creamy. However, these two cystic lesions often cannot be distinguished by sonography. Generally speaking, spermatoceles are usually found in the head of the epididymis and can occasionally be multiloculated,

Figure 24-5. Testis cyst. Sonographically, this 1.3-cm cyst defined by markers is seen as a well-circumscribed, anechoic area in the parenchyma of the testis.

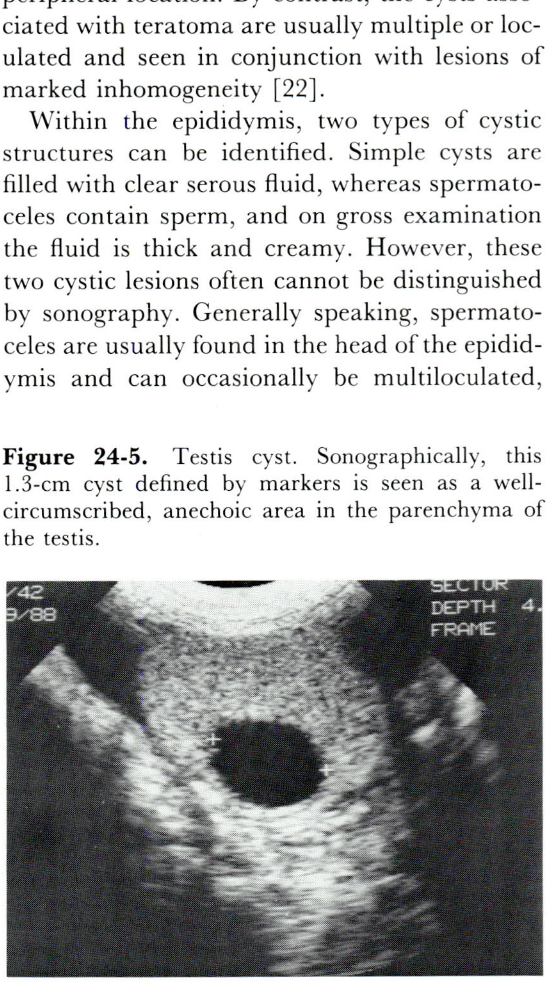

whereas simple cysts are unilocular and can be found throughout the epididymis. The size of either lesion can vary between 0.2 and 9.0 cm in diameter [19].

Cystic lesions in the scrotum, as with cystic lesions elsewhere in the body, exhibit fairly characteristic findings on MRI when large enough to be successfully imaged. These are of low signal intensity on T1 weighted and high signal intensity on T2 weighted images.

TESTIS TUMORS

Testis tumors are rare neoplasms, which gain significance by affecting men in the prime of life. These neoplasms may be either primary or secondary. Primary testis tumors arising from germinal epithelium, the so-called germ-cell tumors, are by far the most common, accounting for 95 percent of all neoplasms of the testis. The remainder include tumors arising from the nongerminal cells in the testis (Sertoli- and Leydig-cell tumors), adrenal rest tumors, adenomatoid tumors, and metastatic lesions from reticuloendothelial neoplasms or various carcinomas.

Germ-Cell Testis Tumors

The germ-cell tumors of the testis exhibit one or a combination of five basic histologic patterns: seminoma, embryonal carcinoma, teratoma, choriocarcinoma, and yolk-sac tumor. Although these tumors constitute only 1 to 2 percent of malignant growths in males, they are the most common solid tumors of men between the ages of 20 and 34 years [3].

In children, about 70 percent of testis tumors are of germ-cell origin. Of these, yolk-sac tumors and pure teratoma constitute 85 percent. In the adult, pure seminoma accounts for about 45 percent of germ-cell tumors, followed by embryonal carcinoma (20 to 25%), teratocarcinoma (25 to 30%), teratoma (5 to 10%), and pure choriocarcinoma (less than 1%).

The association between testis tumors and cryptorchidism has been well documented. Approximately 10 percent of testis tumors occur in cryptorchid testes; furthermore, the chance of a tumor occurring in an undescended testis is over 30 times greater than for a testis located normally in the scrotum.

Spread of testis tumors is by direct invasion of the epididymis or spermatic cord, by lymphatic involvement of the retroperitoneal lymph nodes, and by hematogenous spread, usually to the lungs. Stage I tumors are those confined to the testis, with or without spread to other scrotal structures. In Stage II disease there is involvement of the retroperitoneal lymph nodes below the diaphragm. Stage III tumors have metastasized to sites other than the retroperitoneal nodes.

Certain tumor markers produced by testis tumors are useful in both staging and monitoring these neoplasms; these include alpha-fetoprotein (AFP) and human chorionic gonadotropin (HCG). Over three-fourths of patients with metastatic nonseminomatous germ-cell neoplasms exhibit an elevated AFP level, while about one-half of these patients are positive for HCG.

Once the primary testis lesion has been detected, either by physical examination or scrotal imaging, the use of CT for evaluating the lungs and retroperitoneum in conjunction with the tumor markers results in staging errors of less than 10 percent for these malignancies. Various combinations of retroperitoneal lymphadenectomy, external-beam radiation, and chemotherapy are used for treating testis tumors. Seminomas are extremely radiosensitive, and even large nodal masses are curable by irradiation; lymphadenectomies are generally not used. In contrast, nonseminomatous germ-cell tumors of the testis are less radiosensitive and usually require a combined therapeutic approach. Early therapy for all types of primary testis tumors is a radical removal of the involved testis via an inguinal incision (radical orchiectomy). Generally speaking, the 5-year survival rate for patients with Stage I disease approaches 90 percent, whereas it is less than 70 percent for the higher stages.

Clinically, testis tumors present as a mass in the testis or painless scrotal swelling in the majority of cases. The acute onset of scrotal pain, occurring in about 10 percent of patients, usually indicates intratumoral bleeding. In 25 percent or less of patients, the presenting symptoms may be secondary to metastatic disease; these include supraclavicular-node masses, dyspnea secondary to multiple lung metastases, or unilateral lumbar back pain secondary to retroperitoneal nodal involvement. On initial scrotal examination of the patient with a suspected testis tumor, the diagnosis may be unclear in approximately one-fourth of patients.

Scrotal sonography has become an accepted adjunctive examination in assessing scrotal abnormalities, specifically because of its ability to differentiate extratesticular from intratesticular masses. Unfortunately, sonography of testis tumors, although highly sensitive, is not specific in differentiating among cell types. Generally speaking, a large majority of testis neoplasms exhibit a predominantly decreased echogenicity as compared with the echotexture of a normal testis. However, in some cases the specific diagnosis can be suggested. Pure seminomas are characterized as hypoechoic, reasonably well-marginated lesions (Fig. 24-6). Teratomas tend to be inhomogeneous with cystic areas; there may also be dense echogenic foci that are thought to be due to calcification, cartilage, or immature bone. Embryonal-cell carcinoma, however, may also demonstrate these echogenic foci (Fig. 24-7), and up to one-third of these tumors also have cystic components, though in general the tumor texture tends to be more homogeneous than that found in teratomas. Overall, the most consistently found sonographic changes suggesting testis tumor include hypoechoic mass, bright echogenic foci with or without shadowing, and diffuse parenchymal

Figure 24-6. Seminoma. Longitudinal sonography of testis shows a well-defined, hypoechoic nodule (defined by markers) in an otherwise normal testis.

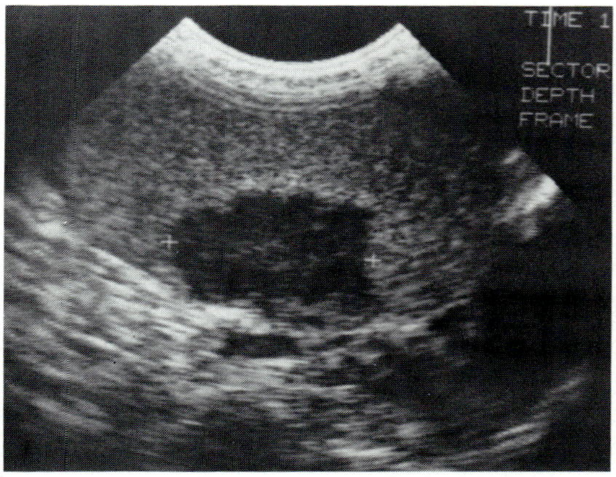

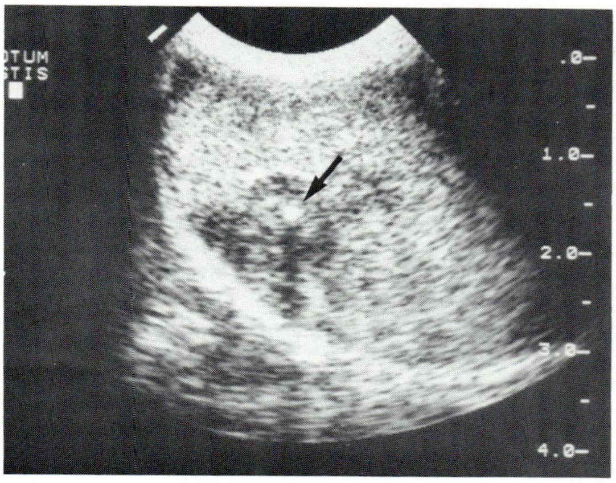

Figure 24-7. Embryonal cell carcinoma. Longitudinal sonography of testis shows an irregular, hypoechoic tumor nodule with a small, bright echogenic focus (arrow) and faint acoustic shadowing.

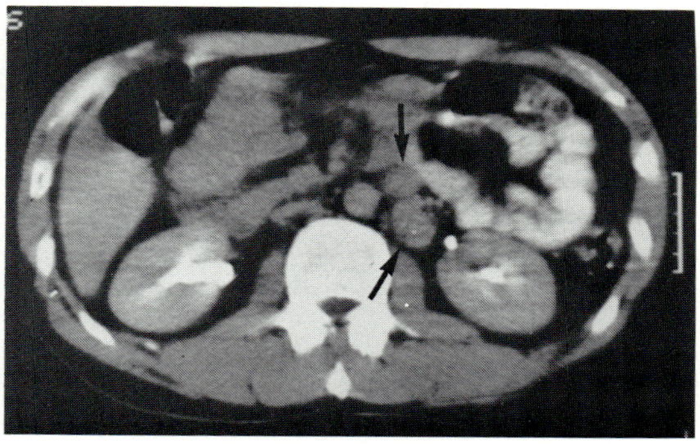

Figure 24-8. Seminoma metastatic to retroperitoneal nodes. CT section at level of kidneys shows two enlarged nodes in the left paraaortic region (arrows).

texture change [12]. Bright echogenic foci seen without an associated mass have been considered to represent regressed germ-cell tumors in patients with known distant metastases. In these patients, histologic examination may reveal a scar but no viable tumor cells. This may represent autoinfarction of a tumor that has outgrown its blood supply.

T2 weighted images are most useful in depicting testicular lesions during MRI of the scrotum [2, 25]. Some reports indicate a relatively uniform appearance of testicular tumors (low signal intensity in comparison with that of normal testis), and others indicate that testis tumors can exhibit a spectrum of findings on either T1 or T2 weighted images. Like ultrasonography, MRI demonstrates excellent sensitivity for tumor detection but poor specificity in characterizing various tumors and differentiating them from other lesions. Unfortunately, as with sonography, focal orchitis or infarct of the testis can result in an imaging picture similar to that seen with testis tumor.

The predominant route of spread of testis tumors is via the regional lymphatics rather than by hematogenous dissemination. The testicular lymphatics, following the course of the spermatic vessels, drain primarily into the node groups in the region of the renal hilum (Fig. 24-8). After involvement of the retroperitoneum, spread to the mediastinum and supraclavicular nodes occurs, following which hematogenous dissemination is seen. Hematogenous dissemination tends to occur more often and earlier with the nonseminomatous germ-cell tumors.

As previously mentioned, CT is the method most commonly used for the detection of retroperitoneal, mediastinal, and pulmonary parenchymal metastatic lesions. As in the staging of other urologic malignancies, the major limitation of CT is its inability to detect metastatic spread in normal-sized nodes. Pedal lymphangiography was once widely advocated for the staging of testis tumors, but it is not as commonly used today. Some investigators suggest that CT be performed first, followed by lympangiography in negative or equivocal cases in an effort to detect metastatic foci in normal-sized nodes. MRI is roughly equivalent in accuracy to CT in detecting nodal metastases.

Nongerminal Testis Tumors

Nongerminal testis neoplasms are distinctly uncommon. When primary in the testis, these arise from the sustentacular cells of the testis, the rete testis, adrenal rests, or the tunica albuginea. They include Leydig- and Sertoli-cell tumors, gonadoblastoma, adenocarcinoma of the rete testis, adrenal rest tumors, and mesenchymal neoplasms such as fibromas and leiomyomas. Sarcomas in the scrotum almost always involve the muscle tissue in the spermatic cord rather than the testis. Adenomatoid tumors, which are small and benign, may occur in the testis, but are usually found in the epididymis. Secondary tumors to the testis can be of diverse cell types. Most of the above lesions lack clinical and imaging findings that would allow establishing the definitive diagnosis preoperatively. However, a few deserve brief discussion because of their association with systemic disease.

Adrenal rest tumors occur in conditions associated with increased circulating adrenocorticotropic hormone (ACTH), including congenital adrenal hyperplasia, Addison's disease, and Cushing's syndrome. Probably arising from aberrant adrenal tissue that migrated with gonadal tissue in fetal life, they are usually multiple and bilateral [23]. Sonographically, they are seen as multiple, round hypoechoic nodules near the hilus of the testis. During therapy with glucocorticoids, these lesions may regress or remain stable. If they regress, they may become fibrotic, resulting in increased echogenicity and even acoustic shadowing. Because the potential for malignant degeneration is rare, sonographic follow-up without biopsy is probably sufficient, given the clinical setting of the typical associated endocrinopathy.

Of the secondary testis neoplasms, those of the reticuloendothelial variety are by far the most common. The ones most frequently seen are reticulum-cell sarcomas, though any type of non-Hodgkin's lymphoma or leukemic infiltrate can also be found. Infiltrates can be focal or diffuse, and both testes can be involved in up to half of cases. In patients with leukemia, the testes may be the first site of extramedullary relapse and their involvement usually precedes hematologic relapse [14]. On sonography, the testis lesions are hypoechoic and thus similar to primary testis tumors (Fig. 24-9). However, in patients with known lymphoma or leukemia, metastatic involvement of the testis by these conditions should be strongly suspected when hypoechoic intratesticular lesions are seen.

Other tumors metastatic to the testes are usually discovered at autopsy. The common primary sites are prostate, lung, gastrointestinal tract, malignant melanoma, and kidney.

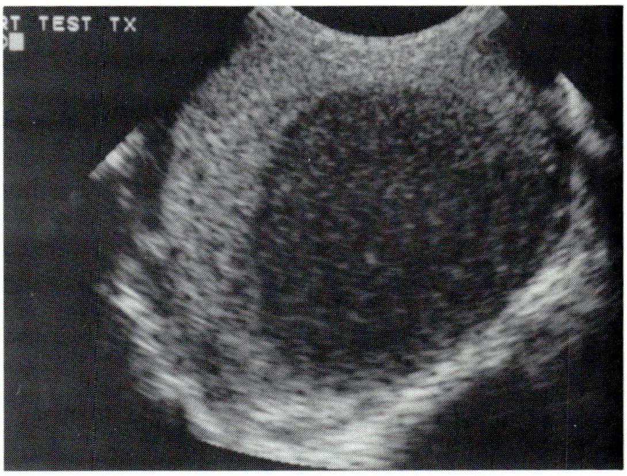

Figure 24-9. Leukemic nodule in testis. Longitudinal sonography shows large, hypoechoic nodule almost replacing testis in patient with chronic myelogenous leukemia.

EXTRATESTICULAR SCROTAL PATHOLOGY

Hydroceles are the most common cause of scrotal swelling. Fluid collecting between the visceral and parietal layers of the tunica vaginalis is responsible for their formation. They are usually insidious in onset, and they may be idiopathic or secondary to inflammatory disease of the testis or epididymis, torsion, neoplasm, or trauma. Sonographically, a simple hydrocele is seen as an echo-free fluid collection almost completely surrounding the testis (Fig. 24-10). Fluid is not seen posterolaterally where the tunica vaginalis invests the testis and epididymis. On occasion, thin septa can be demonstrated within an otherwise simple hydrocele. Diffuse low-level echoes should suggest hematocele or pyocele, which are usually secondary to trauma or epididymal and testis inflammation, respectively.

Figure 24-10. Large hydrocele. Longitudinal sonography shows large, echo-free fluid collection around a normal testis. Small nodule at upper pole of testis is the appendix testis (arrow).

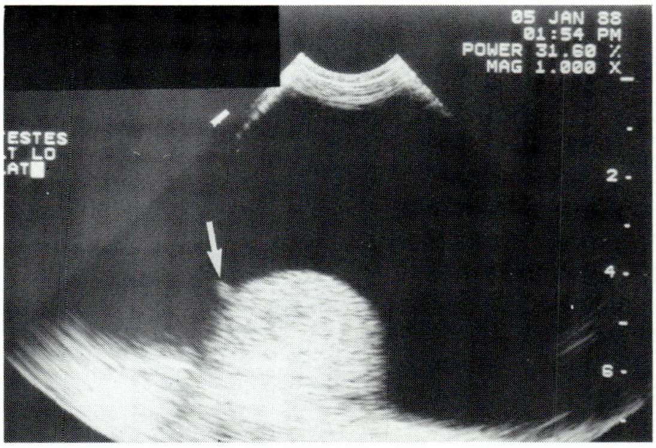

An inguinal hernia containing bowel loops may extend into the depths of the scrotum. This is usually easy to distinguish from a simple hydrocele, as air within the bowel and mesenteric fat are highly echogenic. Scrotal herniation of the bladder, on the other hand, may be difficult to differentiate from a hydrocele, since it can present as a fluid collection in the scrotum.

Varicoceles result from dilation of the pampiniform plexus of veins in the spermatic cord due to absent or incompetent values in the internal spermatic vein. These are discussed in detail in Chap 28. Sonographically, they are seen as tortuous, intercommunicating, fluid-filled tubular structures usually measuring 3 mm or more in diameter. This diameter increases when the patient performs the Valsalva maneuver.

Lesions of the spermatic cord, other than varicocele, are rare. After vasectomy or inguinal surgery, hematomas of the cord can occur. These are characterized by varying echotextures of the disorganized soft tissues extending the length of the cord. The most common tumor of the spermatic cord is the lipoma [10]. Lipomas present as pliable nontender masses with medium echointensity. An infarcted lipoma should be considered when a mass is felt in the region of the inguinal cord in a patient who has not had surgery; however, a rhabdomyosarcoma, the most common malignant lesion of the cord, should also be considered.

CRYPTORCHIDISM (UNDESCENDED TESTIS)

Cryptorchidism has also been discussed in Chap. 5. In the past, sonography has been the method of choice for localizing the impalpable undescended testis, characteristically showing a small ovoid or elongated mass with a homogeneous, fine echotexture [28]. However, since sonography is consistently able to image only testes that are in the region of the external iliac vessels, the inguinal ring, or inguinal canal, there has been a trend toward using MRI when sonography fails to identify a low-lying cryptorchid testis. Like the normally located testis, the cryptorchid one is of low signal intensity on T1 weighted images and has a high signal on T2 images [9]. In some institutions, testicular venography or arteriography are used for localizing an impalpable undescended testis. Neither study is definitive, and both have the disadvantage of exposing the young patient to ionizing radiation. In adult men, in whom the use of ionizing radiation is of less concern, CT has been shown to be accurate in localizing many undescended testes. These are seen as round or ovoid nonenhancing masses whose attenuation is slightly lower than adjacent soft tissue. In general, imaging of undescended testes offer little new information that can directly influence the decision to operate or the surgical approach [7]. This is due to the unfortunate inability of all imaging methods to be consistent in finding undescended testes located high in the retroperitoneum.

REFERENCES

1. Baker, L.L., et al. MR imaging of the scrotum: Normal anatomy. *Radiology* 163:89, 1987.
2. Baker, L.L., et al. MR imaging of the scrotum: Pathologic conditions. *Radiology* 163:93, 1987.
3. Barzell, W.E.I., and Whitmore, W.F., Jr. Neoplasms of the testis. In J.H. Harrison, et al. (Eds.), *Campbell's Urology* (4th ed.). Philadelphia: Saunders, 1979.
4. Bird, K., and Rosenfield, A.T. Testicular infarction secondary to acute inflammatory disease: Demonstration by B-scan ultrasound. *Radiology* 152:785, 1984.
5. Bird, K., Rosenfield, A.T., and Taylor, K.J.W. Ultrasonography in testicular torsion. *Radiology* 147:527, 1983.
6. Dunn, E.K., Macchia, R.J., and Solomon, N.A. Scintigraphic pattern in missed testicular torsion. *Radiology* 139:175, 1981.
7. Friedland, G.W., and Chang, P. The role of imaging in the management of the impalpable undescended testis. *A.J.R.* 151:1107, 1988.
8. Fritzsche, P.J. MRI of the scrotum. *Urol. Radiol.* 10:52, 1988.
9. Fritzsche, P.J., et al. Undescended testis: Value of MR imaging. *Radiology* 164:169, 1987.
10. Gooding, G.A.W. Sonography of the spermatic cord. *A.J.R.* 151:721, 1988.
11. Gooding, G.A.W., Leonhardt, W., and Stein, R. Testicular cysts: US findings. *Radiology* 163:537, 1987.
12. Grantham, J.G., et al. Testicular neoplasms: 29 tumors studied by high-resolution US. *Radiology* 157:775, 1985.
13. Hamm, B., Fobbe, F., and Loy, V. Testicular cysts: Differentiation with US and clinical findings. *Radiology* 168:19, 1988.
14. Lupetin, A.R., et al. Ultrasound diagnosis of testicular leukemia. *Radiology* 146:171, 1983.

15. Middleton, W.D., and Melson, G.L. Testicular ischemia: Color Doppler sonographic findings in five patients. *A.J.R.* 152:1237, 1989.
16. Middleton, W.D., Thorne, D.A., and Melson, G.L. Color Doppler ultrasound of the normal testis. *A.J.R.* 152:293, 1989.
17. Mueller, D.L., et al. Acute scrotal abnormalities in children: Diagnosis by combined sonography and scintigraphy. *A.J.R.* 150:643, 1988.
18. Rholl, K.S., et al. MR imaging of the scrotum with a high-resolution surface coil. *Radiology* 163:99, 1987.
19. Rifkin, M.D. Scrotal ultrasound. *Urol. Radiol.* 9:119, 1987.
20. Rifkin, M.D., Kurtz, A.B., and Goldberg, B.B. Epididymis examined by ultrasound. *Radiology* 151:187, 1984.
21. Rosenfield, A.T., and Bird, K. Scrotal imaging. In H.M. Pollack and G.W. Hartman (Eds.), *ARRS Categorical Course Syllabus on Uroradiology*. Reston, Va.: American Roentgen Ray Society, 1989.
22. Schwerk, W.B., Schwerk, W.N., Rodeck, G. Testicular tumors: Prospective analysis of real-time US patterns and abdominal staging. *Radiology* 164:369, 1987.
23. Seidenwurm, D., et al. Intratesticular adrenal rests diagnosed by ultrasound. *Radiology* 155:479, 1985.
24. Seidenwurm, D., et al. Testes and scrotum: MR imaging at 1.5 T. *Radiology* 164:393, 1987.
25. Thurnher, S., et al. Imaging the testis: Comparison between MR imaging and US. *Radiology* 167:631, 1988.
26. Vick, C.W., et al. Extratesticular hemorrhage associated with torsion of the spermatic cord: Sonographic demonstration. *Radiology* 158:401, 1986.
27. Vieras, F., and Kuhn, C.R. Nonspecificity of the "rim sign" in the scintigraphic diagnosis of missed testicular torsion. *Radiology* 146:519, 1983.
28. Wolverson, M.K., et al. Comparison of computed tomography with high-resolution real-time ultrasound in the localization of the impalpable undescended testis. *Radiology* 146:133, 1983.

25

Urologic Trauma

Trauma is the most common cause of death in persons under 38 years of age. Furthermore, more than 60 percent of trauma victims are under the age of 20 [5]. Approximately 10 percent of injuries seen in emergency departments involve the genitourinary system. Even though hematuria occurs in 90 percent of patients with urologic trauma, its presence does not correlate well with the extent of damage to the urinary tract: 25 percent of patients with gross hematuria are found to have a significant renal injury after blunt abdominal trauma, whereas only 1 to 2 percent of patients with microhematuria have severe kidney damage [13].

Comprehensive radiographic evaluation of suspected occult urologic trauma is expensive, and it can be time consuming in the clinical setting, where time is of the essence. Studies have indicated that in both penetrating and blunt urologic injuries, simultaneous involvement of both the upper and lower urinary tract is rare, occurring in only 0.5 percent of cases [12]. Therefore, evaluation may be expediently limited to the area of maximal injury in most cases.

TRAUMA TO THE ADRENAL

Cross-sectional imaging of the abdomen after trauma has resulted in an increased frequency of identification of traumatic hemorrhage of the adrenal gland. In fact, traumatic adrenal hemorrhage has been reported to occur in up to 25 percent of severely traumatized patients [11]. Trauma to the adrenal may be an isolated injury or may be associated with injury of adjacent organs.

The right adrenal, lying medial to the right hepatic lobe and lateral to the spine, is especially vulnerable; it is involved in 85 percent of cases of adrenal trauma. It has been postulated that traumatic hemorrhage in the right adrenal may be secondary to direct compression of the gland between the spine and liver or an acute rise in intraadrenal venous pressure due to compression of the inferior vena cava, in which case hemorrhage is a secondary reaction [22]. Either adrenal may be affected by deceleration forces, which cause shearing of small vessels perforating the adrenal capsule. Bilateral involvement is found in 20 percent of cases of adrenal injury.

IMAGING OF ADRENAL TRAUMA

CT is the imaging method of choice for evaluation of the adrenal after blunt abdominal trauma. Adrenal involvement by trauma is seen as an adrenal mass associated with stranding of the periadrenal fat and possibly thickening of the adjacent diaphragmatic crus.

On sonography, adrenal hemorrhage is seen as a mass in the adrenal region that is slightly hyperechoic with respect to the liver. As with other adrenal masses, MRI is a potentially useful imaging method. Adrenal hemorrhage is similar to hemorrhage in other body parts in that the intensity depends on the age of the hematoma as well as the field strength and pulse sequences. The hematomas may be dark on T1 weighted images and bright in T2 weighted images, or they may be bright on both. Bright rings and dark hemosiderin rims may be seen.

As with other organs, preexisting pathologic change predisposes the gland to hemorrhage after even minor trauma. Therefore, the diagnosis of an underlying primary or secondary neoplasm should always be excluded on follow-up studies.

TRAUMA TO THE KIDNEY

Renal trauma represents about two-thirds of all genitourinary injuries [18]. Blunt injuries—commonly due to automobile accidents, direct blows to the flank, or falls—account for 80 percent of renal trauma. Penetrating injuries, either gunshot or stab wounds, can also directly involve the kidney.

In renal contusion, the kidney is intact, though the patient presents with either microscopic or gross hematuria. Interstitial edema is present, often leading to reduced renal blood flow. Incomplete laceration and intrarenal hematoma are renal cortical injuries that do not extend into the caliceal system. Complete lacerations extend into the collecting system and are usually associated with extravasation of urine. Renal fracture indicates separation of renal fragments. If the renal capsule remains intact after laceration of the kidney, subcapsular collections of blood and urine are not uncommon. Once the capsule is disrupted, perirenal collections of blood and urine typically accompany the injury.

Subintimal tears resulting in partial or complete occlusion of the renal artery are not uncommon after blunt trauma. These are due to a sudden stretching of the renal artery. If left untreated, this type of injury usually progresses to renal artery thrombosis and ischemic necrosis of the kidney. Severe blunt trauma or penetrating injury may also result in severing of the main renal vessels. Furthermore, penetrating renal injury may result in traumatic arteriovenous fistulas, which can cause parenchymal ischemia as a result of the siphoning effect of such fistulas [8].

In the large majority of cases of renal injury (85%), the lesions are relatively minor, and consist of contusion or small cortical lacerations with no disruption of the caliceal system. Moderate injuries (about 10 percent of cases) are comprised of fractures or cortical lacerations that communicate with the collecting system. Finally, only about 5 percent of cases are classified as severe; these consist of shattered kidneys and renal pedicle injuries [4]. Figure 25-1 diagrammatically depicts these injuries. Minor injuries are usually best managed conservatively, whereas renal pedicle injuries or shattered kidneys require urgent surgical intervention. In patients with intermediate injuries, assessment of the degree of function of the involved kidney and hemodynamic stability of the patient are important factors in determining the necessity for surgical repair.

Kidneys that are abnormal because of congenital anomaly (fusion or ectopy), obstruction, or underlying tumor are more susceptible to traumatic injury than normal kidneys [14]. It has been estimated that 10 percent of renal injuries in adults and up to 25 percent of these injuries in children involve abnormal kidneys. Simple cysts or tumors of the kidney may bleed or rupture spontaneously or as a result of minor trauma. In some cases, the traumatic incident may be so minor as to not be remembered by the patient. Of the renal tumors, angiomyolipomas and hypernephromas have a particular tendency to hemorrhage. Congenital renal anomalies predispose to traumatic injury because of their size, shape, or location. For example, a horseshoe or pelvic kidney lies in an area unprotected by the ribs and therefore may be driven against the vertebral column by blunt abdominal trauma (Fig. 25-2). The distended collecting system found in a hydronephrotic kidney is predisposed to laceration or rupture, often without major renal parenchymal damage. In these cases, massive extravasation of opacified urine may be seen.

IMAGING OF RENAL TRAUMA

The initial radiographic evaluation of the patient with upper abdominal trauma should be a plain film of the abdomen. Perirenal hematoma tends to obscure the upper third of the psoas muscle. Furthermore, fluid within the closed perirenal space forms a mass that can displace adjacent viscera in a characteristic fashion [10]. On the right side, most cases of perirenal hemorrhage localize above the right transverse colon and displace it downward. The ascending colon will be displaced medially, and the second and third portions of the duodenum may be compressed. On the left side, perirenal hemorrhage is usually inframesocolic, resulting in displacement of the transverse colon superiorly. The descending colon is compressed against the lateral abdominal wall, while the small bowel is displaced medially. Pneumoperitoneum or hemoperitoneum are further signs of significant intraabdominal injury. Fractures of the lower ribs or upper lumber transverse processes may be associated with renal injuries, whereas pelvic fractures should suggest the possibility of bladder or urethral disruption.

In many cases of suspected trauma to the urinary tract, excretory urography is the next

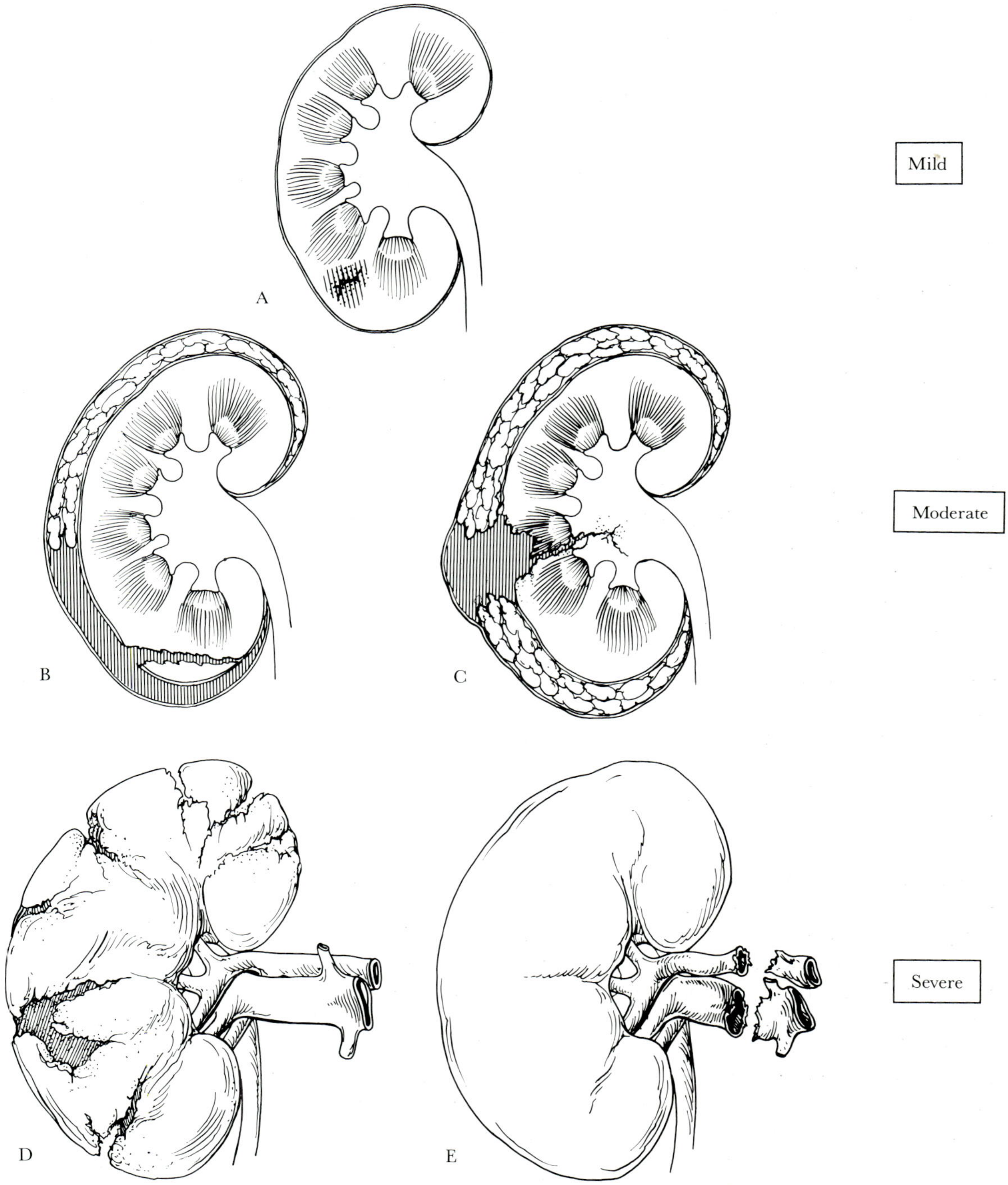

Figure 25-1. Classification of renal injury caused by blunt trauma. A. Small cortical laceration with associated hematoma (mild injury). B. Parenchymal fracture with perirenal hematoma (moderate injury). C. Cortical laceration extending into collecting system and associated with urine extravasation and perirenal hematoma (moderate injury). D. Shattered kidney (severe injury). E. Pedicle injury (severe injury).

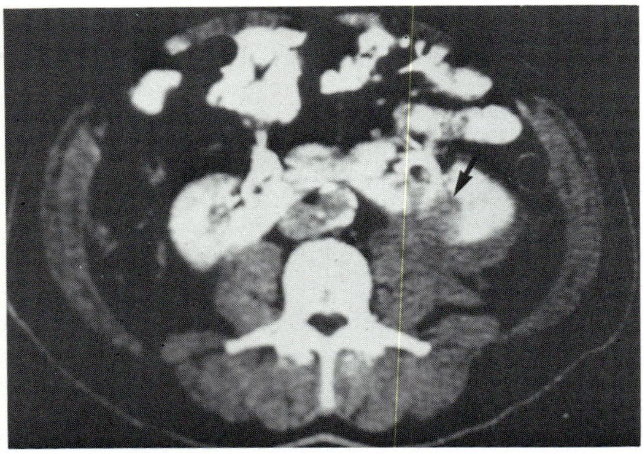

Figure 25-2. Fractured horseshoe kidney resulting from blunt abdominal trauma. CT of horseshoe kidney shows that the left side is fractured (arrow); there are associated intrarenal and perirenal hematomas.

examination to be obtained, though CT is a more definitive study. When performed, urography should be accompanied by nephrotomography immediately after bolus injection in all cases. In cases of renal contusion, urographic abnormalities may be minimal or even absent. When abnormalities are present, they usually consist of a mild decrease or delay in opacification of the kidney secondary to interstitial edema and reduced blood flow. The decreased density can involve both the nephrographic and pyelographic phases of the urogram. Attenuation of the intrarenal collecting system may also be seen as a result of the interstitial edema. Renal laceration with associated hematoma produces a mass effect on the collecting system and a defect in the nephrogram. A renal laceration without significant hematoma formation may appear as a fissure in the nephrographic phase. Associated subcapsular hematomas present as extrinsic pressure defects on the nephrogram and perinephric hematoma frequently obscures part or all of the renal outline.

If the pyelocaliceal system has been disrupted, extravasation of contrast material may be intrarenal, subcapsular, or perinephric (Fig. 25-3). Blood clots in the intrarenal collecting system cause filling defects, and these may pass down the ureter, resulting in urinary obstruction. Retroperitoneal hematoma and urine extravasation can both cause extrinsic compression of the proximal ureter, further aggravating extravasation. Complete nonfunction of the affected kidney is the most significant urographic finding, usually indicating a pedicle injury or massive parenchymal damage. This finding requires urgent arteriography for further evaluation of the renal pedicle.

Whereas a normal urogram generally indicates minor or no injury, the abnormal urogram may frequently be nonspecific. In acute injury, excretory urography that includes nephrotomography accurately depicts the extent of renal trauma in only about 70 to 85 percent of cases. This probably occurs because the patient with multiple system injuries is usually poorly prepared for urography or may be so hemodynamically unstable that the quality of the urogram is marginal at best.

Ultrasonography is not routinely used for evaluation of the patient suspected of having renal trauma; however, fresh hematoma within the kidney is visible sonographically and usually has a characteristic appearance of a rounded echogenic focus. Perinephric hematoma presents acutely as echogenic tissue surrounding all or part of the kidney (see Fig. 25-3B).

CT is now recognized as the examination of choice for studying severely injured patients with suspected renal trauma. This is especially true given that excretory urography is inconclusive in up to 30 percent of cases of renal trauma. If used as the primary diagnostic method in renal trauma, the CT scanner must be located in proximity to the emergency department and available around the clock. CT is also advocated as the initial diagnostic procedure in patients with evidence of injuries of other intraabdominal organs. By providing precise anatomic detail, ease of performance and interpretation, and the ability to image other intraabdominal structures simultaneously, CT scanning is thought to be superior to other diagnostic studies [3]. Furthermore, a film of the abdomen can be obtained after a contrast-enhanced CT study to define the collecting system better when necessary.

All CT scans for the evaluation of trauma should be performed after a bolus injection of 75 to 100 ml of contrast material. With renal contusion there may be a mild decrease in opacification of the renal parenchyma or an inhomogeneous nephrogram as compared with the normal kidney; however, there will be no

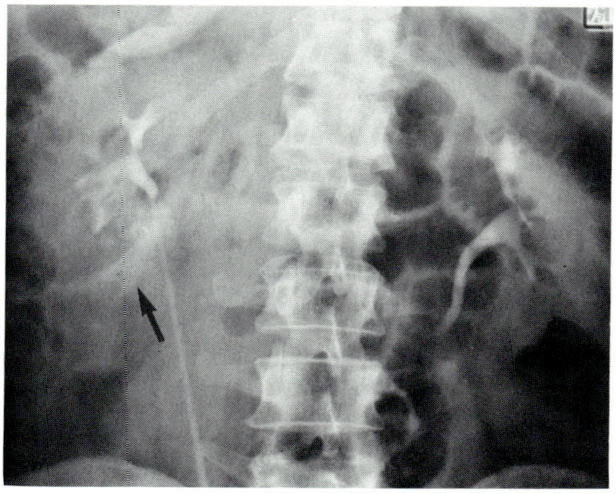

A

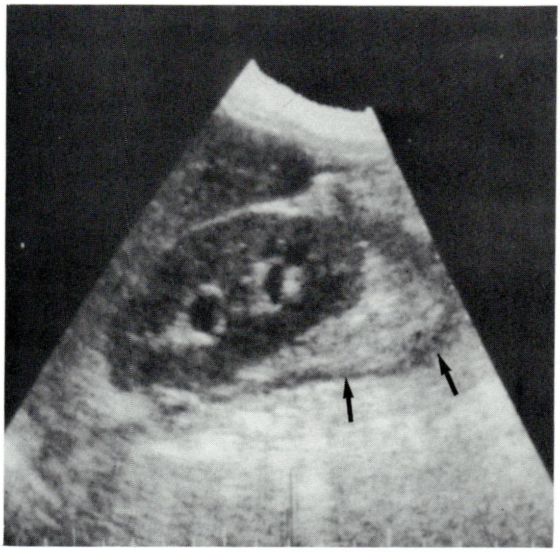

B

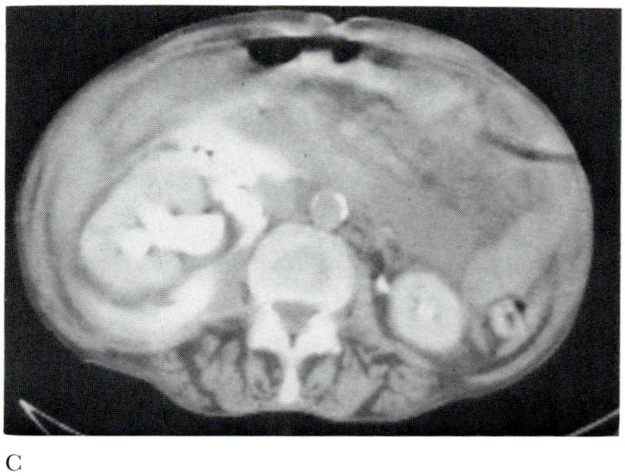

C

evidence of parenchymal disruption. Intrarenal hematomas are demonstrated by CT as rounded areas of decreased attenuation with poorly marginated borders. Depending on the time between injury and CT examination, the attenuation coefficients of these hematomas can vary from approximately 50 to 60 Hounsfield units acutely to water attenuation in the later phases [17]. With renal fracture, the fragments of the kidney may be separated, though still functioning (Fig. 25-4B).

With perinephric hematomas, the blood tends to infiltrate the fat, producing a streaky or bubbly appearance (Fig. 25-4). These are usually easily distinguished from subscapular hematomas, in which the kidney parenchyma is compressed and deformed because of the high pressure of the collection (Fig. 25-5).

As noted previously, contrast material extravasation from the collecting system can be seen intrarenally or in the subcapsular or perinephric spaces (see Fig. 25-3C). However, the absence of a fluid collection does not exclude a significant renal injury. Furthermore, the presence of a perirenal fluid collection does not always correlate with the extent of renal trauma. However, fluid infiltrating Gerota's fascia or the psoas muscle or involving the anterior pararenal space seems to be a more consistent indicator of renal fracture or pedicle disruption [21].

With disruption of polar arterial branches, focal renal infarcts represented by wedge-shaped areas of low attenuation may be found. However, global infarction is more commonly seen after trauma because of the typical involvement of major renal arteries. In these cases, the cortical rim sign (high attenuation of peripheral renal tissue) is frequently seen. This is thought

Figure 25-3. Perirenal contrast material extravasation and hematoma after blunt trauma to right flank. A. Ten-minute film from intravenous urogramphy shows contrast medium in the perirenal space medial to the lower pole of the right kidney (arrow). The kidney is displaced superiorly and laterally by hematoma in this area. B. Sonography of right kidney demonstrating echogenic hematoma (arrows) around lower pole of kidney. C. CT obtained after administration of intravenous contrast agent shows extravasation of agent into perirenal space around right kidney.

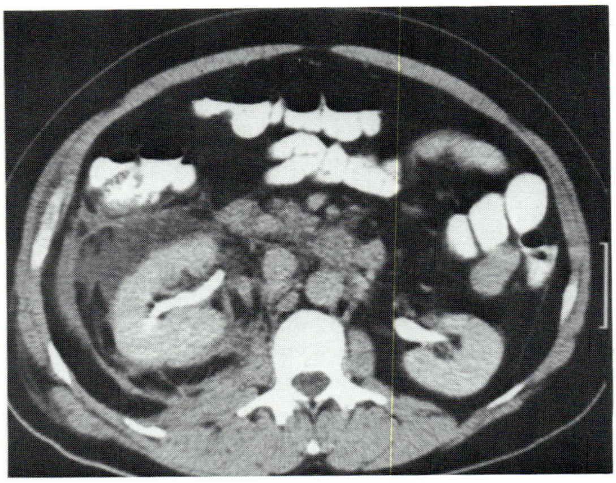

A

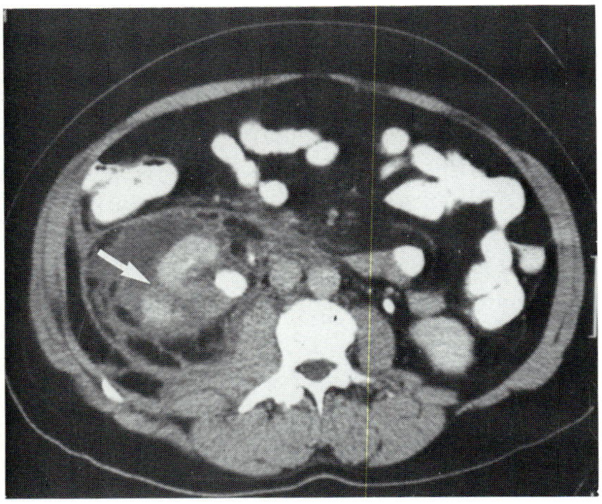

B

Figure 25-4. Renal fracture with perirenal hematoma after blunt abdominal trauma. A. CT after administration of intravenous contrast agent shows blood in the right perirenal space infiltrating the fat in this area. B. CT section through lower poles of kidneys demonstrates fracture on right (arrow). Even though fragments are separated, function is still present.

to be due to perfusion of the preserved outer rim of the renal cortex by collateral vessels via the renal capsular artery. Renal infarct can sometimes be differentiated from intrarenal hematoma by virtue of the infarct's clear margination from adjacent functioning tissue. Furthermore, mass effect is rare with infarct and is common with hematoma, although subcapsular hematomas can occur in 21 percent of patients with infarcts [23].

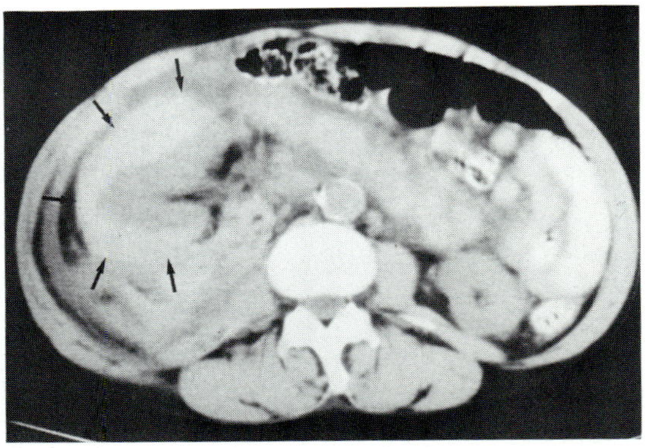

Figure 25-5. Subcapsular and perirenal hematomas after blunt trauma. CT section through kidneys with no contrast agent shows relatively high attenuation hematoma (60 Hounsfield units) within right renal capsule (arrows) distorting renal margin. Blood is also seen in the perirenal space posteriorly.

CT is able to diagnose a renal pedicle injury by showing minimal or no function of the involved kidney, rim enhancement, abrupt termination of an enhanced renal artery, or hematoma in the renal hilar area [20]. Shattering of the renal parenchyma is also easily demonstrated.

Dynamic computed tomography, which involves acquisition of 6 to 12 sections over a period of approximately 1 minute after intravenous bolus injection of 100 ml of contrast material, has been advocated to assess perfusion of the entire kidney or of questionable areas within the kidney [8]. This is thought to be especially useful since perfusion of the kidney is the gold standard for assessment of renal parenchymal viability.

Although CT is highly accurate in delineating the extent of most renal injuries, in patients with preexisting renal lesions that bleed after trauma, CT may not be able to detect the original abnormality. This is especially true in cases in which small peripheral tumors or cysts are the cause of the bleeding. In such cases, the mass may not be seen as distinct from the adjacent hemorrhage.

Angiographic evaluation of the traumatized kidney is usually reserved for cases in which minimal or no function is demonstrated on CT or excretory urography (Fig. 25-6A). In these cases, selective renal arteriography may demonstrate an intimal tear; this presents as a luminal

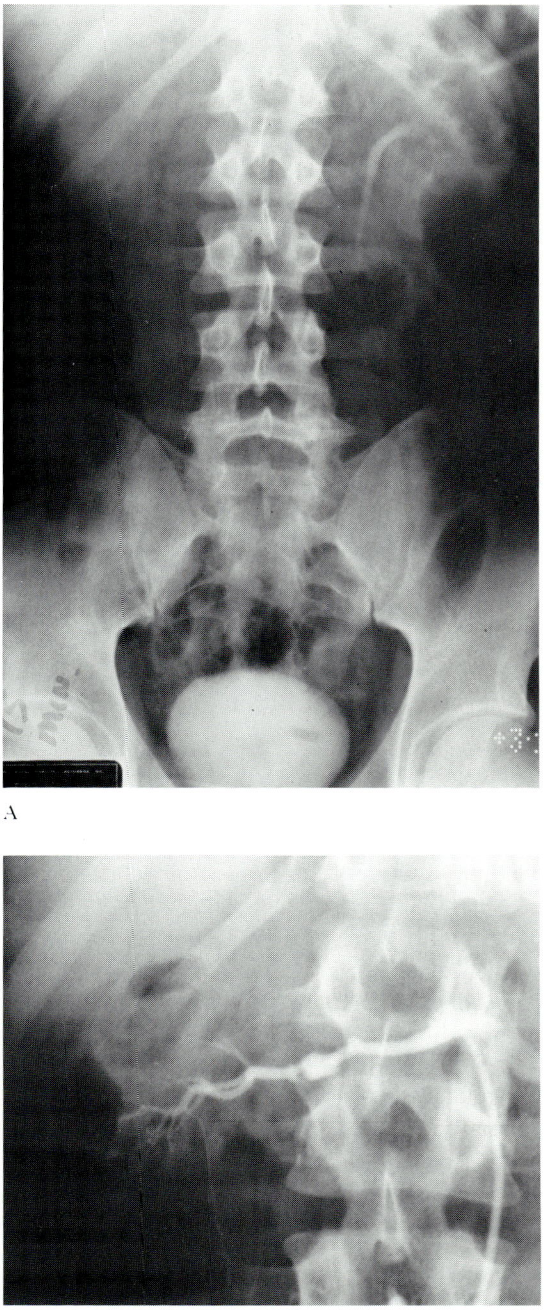

A

B

Figure 25-6. Intimal tear of right renal artery after blunt abdominal trauma. A. Fifteen-minute film from intravenous urogramphy shows no function on right. B. Selective right renal arteriography demonstrates irregular narrowing of renal artery with only minimal opacification of the intrarenal arterial tree.

irregularity that partially or completely occludes the flow of contrast material (Fig. 25-6B). Unfortunately, renal arteriography cannot always differentiate between renal artery thrombosis resulting from an intimal tear and complete avulsion of the renal pedicle. A completely disrupted renal artery that is still bleeding into the retroperitoneum can be easily diagnosed by this study, however.

In the past, retrograde pyelography was routinely used for determining that the collecting system was intact in a patient with nonfunctioning kidneys. Currently, CT findings of an intact kidney are accepted.

Radionuclide renal scanning with a cortical labeling agent such as technetium-99m glucoheptanate has been advocated by some as an accurate method of assessing the traumatized kidney. Generally speaking, however, this study is usually reserved for follow-up of renal injuries that are treated conservatively. In these cases, a base-line study is obtained after the initial diagnosis is established by other methods and then used for comparison with serial studies. With this method, contusion is seen as a generalized decrease in radioactivity over the involved kidney. With renal laceration, hematoma, or infarct, discrete areas of low radioactivity are seen.

TRAUMA TO THE URETER

The ureter is freely mobile in the retroperitoneum and thus is rarely traumatized. When trauma does occur, it is about equally divided between external and iatrogenic causes. Blunt trauma to the abdomen almost never involves the ureter; the few cases reported consist of usually disruption near the level of the ureteropelvic junction. Of penetrating trauma, the blast effect of a gunshot wound is far more likely to injure the ureter than a stab wound. In these cases, the midureter is most likely to be involved.

Iatrogenic causes of ureteral trauma include ureteral instrumentation and open surgery. The lower ureter is most commonly involved. Urologic endoscopic procedures such as stone extraction or fragmentation can injure the ureter. Open procedures are most commonly gynecologic. Colonic surgery and aortic vascular procedures are responsible for the majority of proximal ureteral injuries.

IMAGING OF URETERAL TRAUMA

Excretory urography is the procedure of choice for diagnosing ureteral injury. A periureteral hematoma may show displacement of the ureter medially or laterally. Mucosal injuries from endoscopic surgery are seen as luminal irregularities, which in some cases may be significantly obstructive. Contrast material extravasation from an otherwise intact ureter indicates only partial tear, whereas visualization of the ureter only above an area of extravasation usually indicates complete disruption. Pelvic surgery can result in partial or complete disruption of the distal ureter, obstruction (secondary to ligature or devascularization), or fistula formation between the ureter and vagina.

TRAUMA TO THE BLADDER

Bladder trauma comprises about one-fourth of all urologic injuries (Table 25-1). Though the bladder can be injured by a penetrating wound, blunt trauma is the more common cause. Most bladder injuries result from perforation or tearing of the bladder by pelvic fractures or from compression of the distended bladder. Bladder trauma is almost always accompanied by hematuria.

Bladder contusion implies an intact bladder wall with hematuria. This is the most common injury of the bladder. Though there is no extravasation of urine, the bladder may be elevated, deviated, or circumferentially compressed (teardrop bladder) by a pelvic hematoma.

There is an approximately equal incidence of intraperitoneal and extraperitoneal rupture of the bladder. In about 10 percent of cases, a combined type of rupture is found. It is unusual to find an extraperitoneal rupture of the bladder without an associated pelvic fracture. Typical fractures resulting in lower urinary tract injury include the double vertical pubis fracture and the Malgaigne fracture. The first involves bilateral superior and inferior pubic rami fractures, allowing posterior displacement of the pubis and injury of the bladder by sharp fragments of the superior rami. With the Malgaigne fracture there is a pubic separation or unilateral pubic fracture associated with an ipsilateral posterior pelvic arch fracture or sacroiliac joint separation, resulting in a shearing tear of the bladder base or prostatic urethra [2]. Rupture of the bladder occurs in only 10 percent of patients with fractures of the bony pelvis; however, approximately 83 percent of patients with extraperitoneal bladder rupture secondary to blunt trauma have associated pelvic fractures [15]. The most common cause of this type of trauma is motor vehicle accident. When full, the bladder may be injured by a direct blow to the lower abdomen without an associated pelvic fracture. This type of injury usually results in intraperitoneal rupture of the bladder dome.

Table 25-1. Categories of bladder injury

Bladder contusion (most common)
Bladder disruption
Intraperitoneal (approx. 45%)
Extraperitoneal (approx. 45%)
Combined intraperitoneal and extraperitoneal (10%)

IMAGING OF BLADDER TRAUMA

The possibility of bladder rupture should be considered in any patient suffering lower abdominal trauma, especially if there is an associated pelvic fracture seen on plain films. Suprapubic pain, hematuria, and difficulty in voiding or inability to void also indicate the possibility of a significant bladder injury. Excretory urography is often performed in these patients, but it is inadequate for evaluating the bladder because the normal pressure within the bladder may be too low to demonstrate even a large laceration.

Retrograde cystography is needed to evaluate the traumatized bladder. However, up to 10 percent of bladder disruptions may be missed even with this examination unless the bladder is overfilled. A catheter should be passed through the urethra into the bladder only if there is no suspicion of urethral injury. The bladder is then filled under fluoroscopic control using 30 percent contrast material. The examination is halted if extravasation is seen. Otherwise, the bladder is filled to at least 400 ml. Alternatively, the bladder can be filled to the level of discomfort, at which point another 50 to 60 ml are added. Anteroposterior and both oblique views are then obtained. A post drainage film is imperative because a small posterior extraperitoneal rupture of the bladder may otherwise be missed (Fig. 25-7). If urethral injury is suspected, retrograde urethrography should be performed as the initial examination.

With bladder contusion, no extravasation of contrast material is seen; however, as previously mentioned, the bladder may be deformed by a pelvic hematoma. Intraperitoneal rupture is seen as extravasation of contrast material into the peritoneal cavity. This results in the characteristic appearance of contrast material outlining loops of bowel and intraperitoneal viscera and layering in the paracolic gutters (Fig. 25-8). With extraperitoneal rupture of the bladder, contrast material tends to streak in the perivesical area in a "sunburst" type of pattern. In the case of large extraperitoneal tears, this extravasation may be massive (Fig. 25-9). With a small bladder tear, only minimal amounts of extravesical

Figure 25-7. Small, posterior bladder rupture after blunt suprapubic trauma. A. Filled phase of cystography shows no abnormality (extravasation obscured by full bladder). B. Postdrainage view demonstrates small amount of posterior extraperitoneal extravasation.

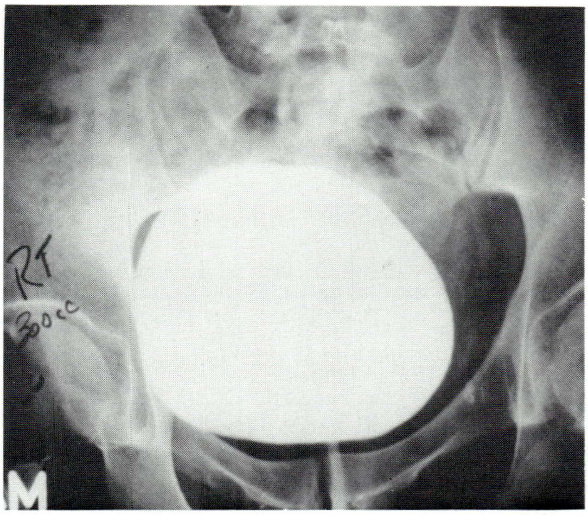

A

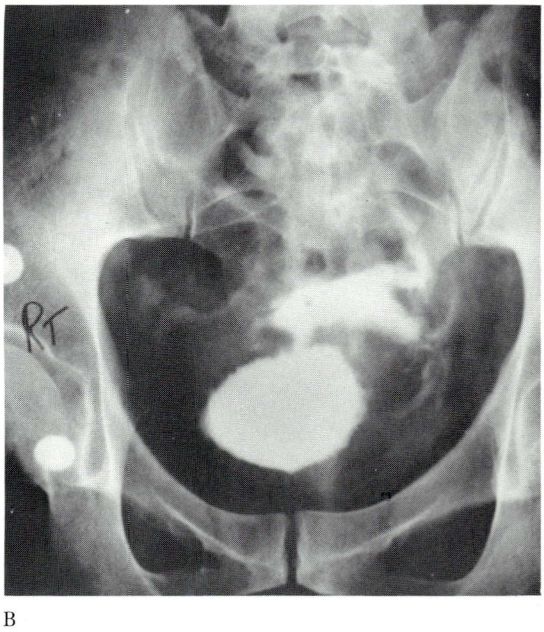

B

Figure 25-8. Intraperitoneal bladder rupture after blunt trauma to lower abdomen. Cystography shows contrast material outlining the liver margin and bowel loops and filling inferior peritoneal recess (arrows). An intrauterine contraceptive device is seen above the bladder.

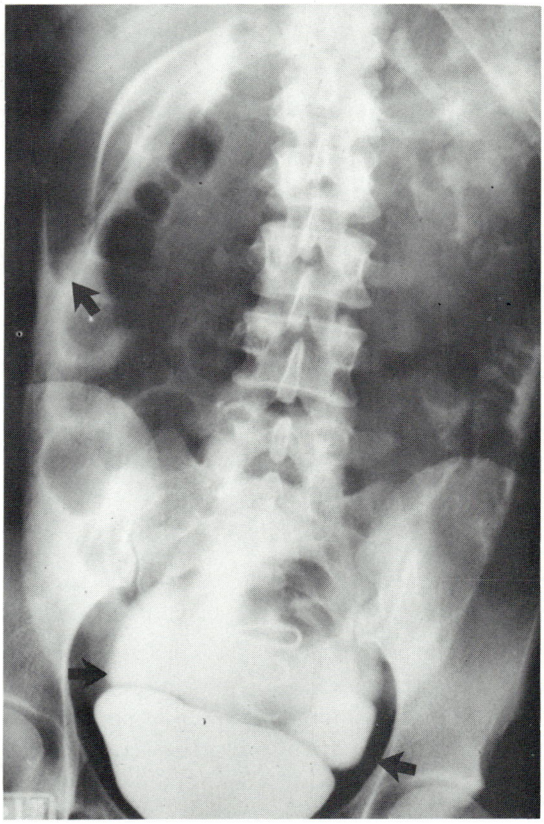

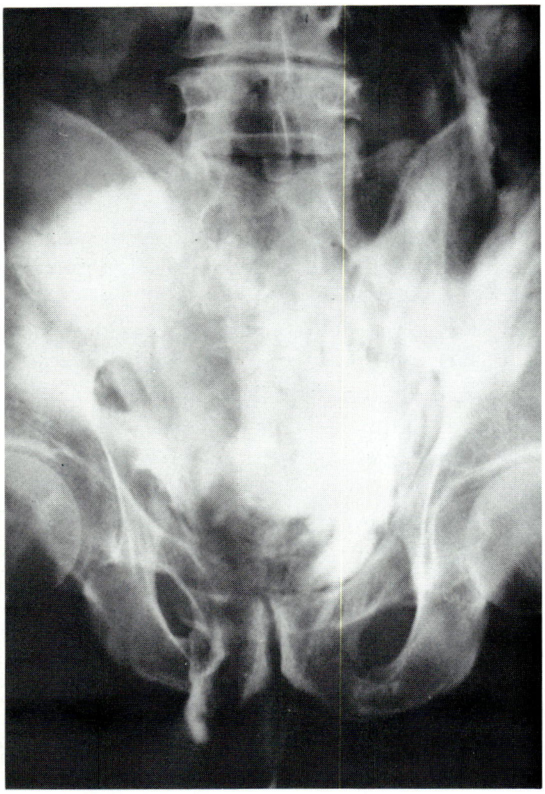

Figure 25-9. Extraperitoneal bladder rupture associated with pelvic fracture. Cystography shows "sunburst" pattern of massive extraperitoneal extravasation of contrast agent.

contrast material may be seen. In cases with extensive extravasation, the streaky appearance of extraperitoneal contrast material may rarely be lost, and an intraperitoneal rupture may thus be simulated. Combined intraperitoneal and extraperitoneal bladder ruptures usually demonstrate both classical sets of findings.

If the bladder is torn near the bladder neck, the urogenital diaphragm may also disrupted, resulting in extravasation of contrast material into the scrotum. In severe cases, contrast material may extravasate into the thigh and penis. In these cases, it is difficult to differentiate bladder from urethral disruptions.

In patients with bladder disruption, CT can easily distinguish the extravasation patterns for the various types of ruptures. In addition, with extraperitoneal rupture of the bladder, contrast medium may dissect upward within the retroperitoneum; this is also easily detectable by CT.

TRAUMA TO THE URETHRA

The female urethra, because of its relative shortness and lack of fixation, is rarely injured except during birth trauma. In the male, however, urethral injuries are more common than bladder injuries and can involve any part of the urethra (Table 25-2).

Table 25-2. Categories of urethral injury in males

Prostatomembranous urethra (associated with pelvic fracture)
Type I—stretching without tear
Type II—partial or complete disruption of prostatomembranous junction
Type III—complete disruption in region of membranous urethra extending through urogenital diaphragm
Anterior urethra
Straddle injury—partial or complete disruption of proximal or midbulbous urethra
Iatrogenic—urethral tear secondary to instrumentation
Self-induced—intraurethral masturbation

Figure 25-10. Classification of posterior urethral injuries in males (modified from R.W. McCallum [9]) A. Normal. B. Type I—Stretched, but intact, prostatomembranous urethra. C. Type II—Disruption of prostatomembranous urethra above urogenital diaphragm. D. Type III—Disruption of prostatomembranous urethra extending through urogenital diaphragm.

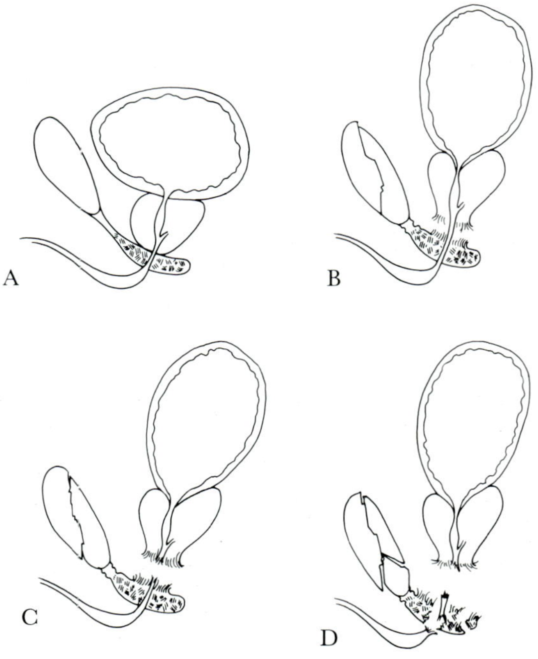

PROSTATOMEMBRANOUS URETHRAL INJURY

Fixation of the prostate by the puboprostatic ligaments and the membranous urethra by the urogenital diaphragm results in immobility of the prostatomembranous junction. Significant injury in this area occurs in up to 11 percent of patients with pelvic fracture [16]. Tears in this region are usually secondary to shearing of the urethra as the pelvis destabilizes at the moment of trauma.

Posterior urethral injury should be strongly suspected in the patient with a pelvic fracture who presents with blood at the urethral meatus and who is unable to void or is able to void only with difficulty. In such cases, retrograde urethrography is indicated before any attempt is made to catheterize the bladder. If a catheter is passed through an injured urethra, a minor tear might be converted into a significant laceration or complete disruption, and a sterile extravasation might be contaminated, resulting in an infected urinoma.

IMAGING OF PROSTATOMEMBRANOUS URETHRAL TRAUMA

Figure 25-10 diagrams the categories of posterior urethral injury [9]. In Type I injuries, retrograde urethrography reveals no extravasation, though the posterior urethra is elongated and narrowed. Type II injuries result in extravasation of contrast material at the prostatomembranous junction without dissection below the level of the intact urogenital diaphragm. Type III injuries are the most common urethral disruptions associated with pelvic fracture; the urethral disruption extends both above and below the urogenital diaphragm. In the last case,

Figure 25-11. Pericatheter retrograde urethrogram. Patient has disrupted pubic symphysis, and Foley catheter placed shortly after trauma is not draining. Contrast material in bladder is from previous intravenous urography. A. Normal anterior urethra opacified by 8 French feeding tube (arrow) placed alongside shaft of Foley catheter. B. Feeding tube has been advanced into posterior urethra. Injection of contrast agent shows significant disruption. Note that Foley balloon is inflated in posterior urethra.

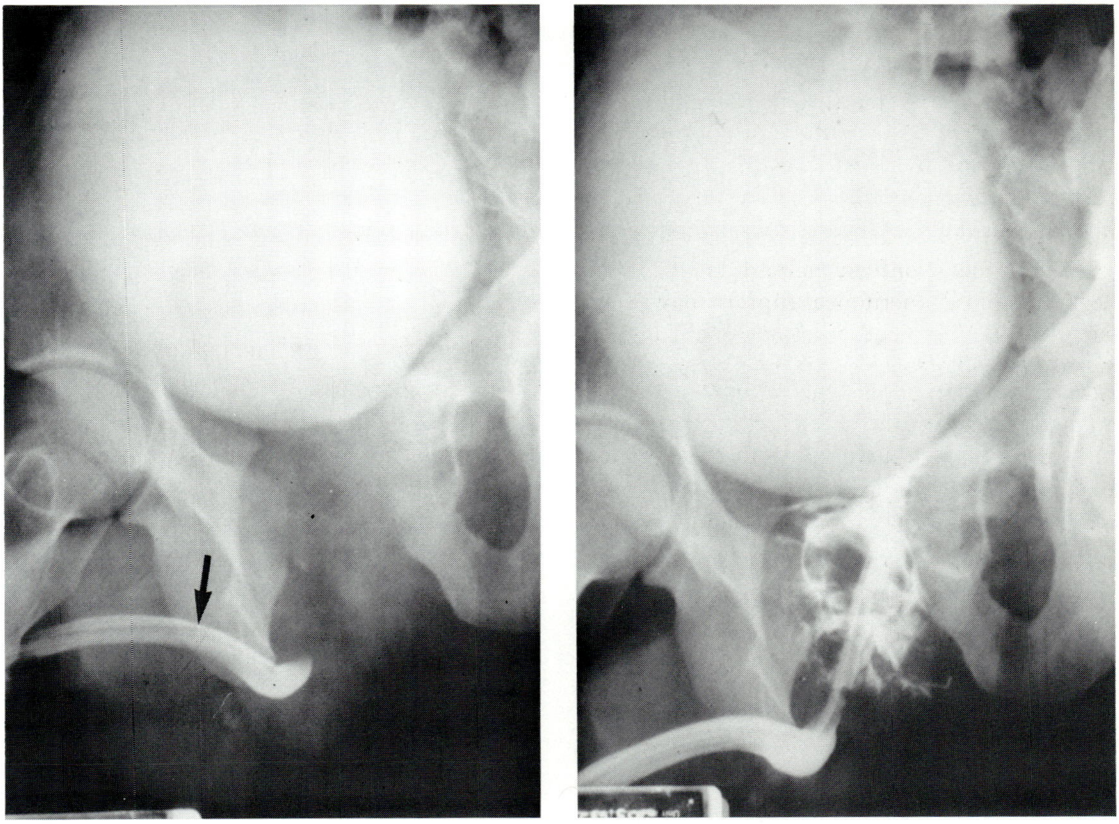

as expected, extravasation is seen both above and below the diaphragm on retrograde urethrography. Massive extravasation of contrast material in the region of the prostatomembranous urethra may track superiorly around the bladder base and make the differentiation between posterior urethral and bladder disruptions difficult.

In some cases, a urethral catheter will have been placed through an injured urethra into the bladder prior to radiographic evaluation of the urethra. In such cases, if urethral injury is strongly suspected based on the presence of a pelvic fracture, the urethra can be evaluated without removal of the catheter. This is accomplished by pericatheter retrograde urethrography. In this technique, an 8 French pediatric feeding tube with opaque marker is lubricated and passed through the urethra alongside the indwelling catheter. Beginning just inside the meatus, small amounts of contrast medium are injected under fluoroscopic control. The catheter is incrementally advanced, followed by small injections, until either the entire urethra has been cleared of injury or the point of disruption is determined (Fig. 25-11).

ANTERIOR URETHRAL INJURY

Injuries of the anterior urethra are much less common than those of the posterior urethra. Injuries in this area are almost never seen with pelvic fracture. The most common cause of injury of the bulbous portion of the urethra is a "straddle" injury, in which the patient falls astride a narrow beam or bar, thus compressing the bulbous urethra against the inferior margin of the pubic arch. A resultant tear may be partial or complete. This type of injury, if severe enough, subsequently results in a rather characteristic, short, well-defined stricture of the proximal or midbulbous urethra.

Injury of the penile urethra by external trauma is uncommon. Internal causes of urethral trauma include passage of potentially damaging instruments such as dilating sounds by a urologist or passage of foreign bodies into the urethra by the patient for sexual gratification.

As with posterior urethral injuries, the combination of a traumatic event involving the anterior urethra and blood at the meatus should strongly suggest injury and mandate retrograde urethrography. The patient should not be instructed to void, since with complete disruption of the urethra massive extravasation of urine into the scrotum or penis may occur.

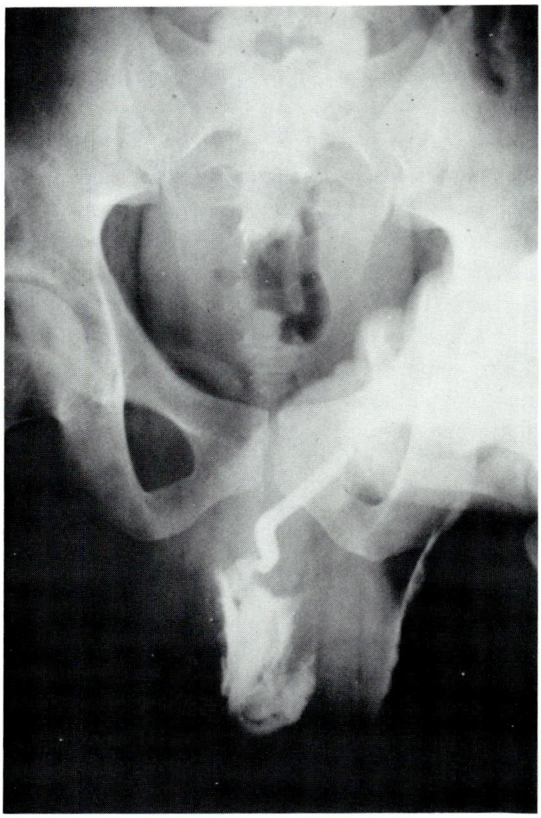

Figure 25-12. Complete tear of bulbous urethra after "straddle" injury. Retrograde urethrography demonstrates contrast medium extravasating into scrotum at site of disruption.

IMAGING OF ANTERIOR URETHRAL TRAUMA

In patients with partial tears of the anterior urethra, extravasation at the site of the tear is seen, but the continuity of the urethra is maintained. With complete disruption of the urethra, the portion proximal to the tear is not opacified, and extravasation into the penis or scrotum is seen (Fig. 25-12).

TRAUMA TO THE PENIS

Acute penile "fracture," or rupture of the corpus cavernosum, is fortunately an unusual surgical emergency. Trauma to the penis during excessive sexual activity accounts for approximately one-third of these cases of acute rupture. Other reported causes include gunshot wounds, industrial accidents, or forcible "breaking" of an erection by excessive manipulation or even rolling over in bed [6]. Clinically, the patient will complain of severe penile pain after a cracking or snapping noise. The resultant hematoma causes swelling and ecchymosis of the penis. Although conservative treatment has been employed in the past, early surgical intervention is the current approach to this problem. This involves evacuation of the hematoma with repair of the torn tunica albuginea.

IMAGING OF PENILE TRAUMA

Cavernosography is the preferred diagnostic technique in evaluating penile trauma. The penis is sterilely prepared and a 23-gauge butterfly needle is inserted directly into the midlateral portion of one of the corpora cavernosa. Because there is free communication between the corpora cavernosa, only the single puncture is required. Under fluoroscopic control, 30 percent contrast material is injected slowly, and the penis is filmed in frontal, lateral, and both oblique positions. Although extravasation can often be identified at the point of disruption, on occasion a hematoma may occlude the tear and prevent contrast material from extravasating. In such cases, a filling defect in one of the corpora cavernosa should suggest that a tear has occurred (Fig. 25-13). Retrograde urethrography is also indicated, as associated urethral injuries occur in 22 percent of cases [19].

Figure 25-13. Penile "fracture." Corpora cavernosography shows filling defect in one corpus (arrows) secondary to clot in this area. This finding strongly suggests tear of the tunica albuginea. Contrast medium in urethra ventrally is from retrograde urethrography performed immediately before this study.

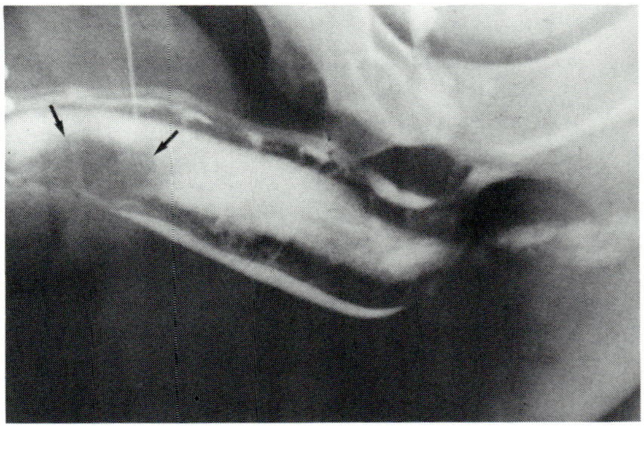

TRAUMA TO THE TESTES

Prompt diagnosis and treatment of testicular injuries is essential. Repair of a testis rupture delayed beyond 3 days increases the chance for ischemic necrosis and abscess formation in the injured testis. Fortunately, blunt trauma to the testicle is uncommon. However, clinical examination of the scrotum after this type of injury is limited in its ability to differentiate uncomplicated hematocele from testis rupture. Furthermore, testis fractures may occur without an accompanying hematocele.

IMAGING OF TESTIS TRAUMA

Sonography is useful in evaluating testicular trauma. Although discrete fracture planes are not usually identified in cases of testis rupture, focal alterations of normal testis echogenicity have been found to correspond with areas of intratesticular hemorrhage or infarction [7] (Fig. 25-14). These sonographic features are nonspecific and often cannot be differentiated from other testis lesions, such as neoplasms or abscesses. However, in traumatized patients, any area of abnormal testis echogenicity should suggest disruption and is an indication for surgical exploration. Low-level echoes within a surrounding fluid collection are consistent with

Figure 25-14. Testis rupture. Sonography shows irregular hypoechoic area in testis consistent with hematoma. This finding strongly suggests rupture of the testis.

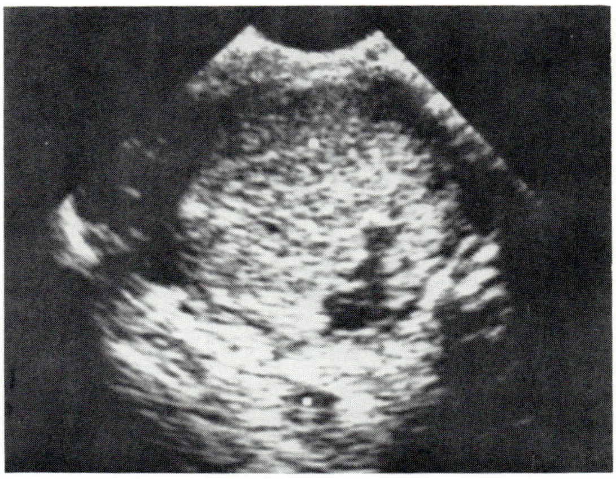

hematocele, and they help to differentiate this entity from an uncomplicated hydrocele.

MRI has recently been advocated for studying the scrotum. The normal tunica is visualized as a band of low signal intensity surrounding the testis on both T1 and T2 weighted images. Thus MRI is able to show disruption of the tunica clearly. The normal testis is of low signal intensity on T1 weighted images and high signal intensity on T2 weighted images. Intratesticular hemorrhage is seen as an area of high or low signal intensity, depending on its age, in comparison with the normal testis tissue. This results in an overall inhomogeneity of the traumatized testis [1].

REFERENCES

1. Baker, L.L., et al. MR imaging of the scrotum: Pathologic conditions. *Radiology* 163:93, 1987.
2. Bonavita, J.A., and Pollack, H.M. Trauma of the adult bladder and urethra. *Semin. Roentgenol.* 18:229, 1983.
3. Erturk, E., et al. Renal trauma: Evaluation by computerized tomography. *J. Urol.* 133:946, 1985.
4. Federle, M.P., et al. The role of computed tomography in renal trauma. *Radiology* 141:455, 1981.
5. Godec, C.J. Genitourinary trauma. *Urol. Radiol.* 7:185, 1985.
6. Grosman, H., et al. The role of corpus cavernosography in acute "fracture" of the penis. *Radiology* 144:787, 1982.
7. Jeffery R.B., et al. Sonography of testicular trauma. *A.J.R.* 141:993, 1983.
8. Lang, E.K., Sullivan, J., and Frentz, G. Renal trauma: Radiological studies. *Radiology* 154:1, 1985.
9. McCallum, R.W. The adult male urethra: Normal anatomy, pathology, and method of urethrography. *Radiol. Clin. North Am.* 17:227, 1979.
10. McCort, J.J. Perirenal fat infiltration by hemorrhage: Radiographic recognition and CT confirmation. *Radiology* 149:665, 1983.
11. Murphy, B.J., Casillas, J., and Yrizarry, J.M. Traumatic adrenal hemorrhage: Radiologic findings. *Radiology* 169:701, 1988.
12. Peterson, N.E., and Schulze, K.A. Selective diagnostic uroradiography for trauma. *J. Urol.* 137:449, 1987.
13. Pollack, H.M., and Wein, A.J. Imaging of renal trauma. *Radiology* 172:297, 1989.
14. Rhyner, P., Federle, M.P., and Jeffery, R.B. CT of trauma to the abnormal kidney. *A.J.R.* 142:747, 1984.
15. Sandler, C.M., et al. Bladder injury in blunt pelvic trauma. *Radiology* 158:633, 1986.
16. Sandler, C.M., et al. Posterior urethral injuries after pelvic fracture. *A.J.R.* 137:1233, 1981.
17. Sandler, C.M., and Toombs, B.D. Computed tomographic evaluation of blunt renal injuries. *Radiology* 141:461, 1981.
18. Sclafani, S.J.A, and Becker, J.A. Radiologic diagnosis of renal trauma. *Urol. Radiol.* 7:192, 1985.
19. Sclafani, S.J.A., and Becker, J.A. Radiologic diagnosis of extrarenal genitourinary trauma. *Urol. Radiol.* 7:201, 1985.
20. Sclafani, S.J.A., et al. CT diagnosis of renal pedicle injury. *Urol. Radiol.* 7:63, 1985.
21. Siegel, M.J., and Balfe, D.M. Blunt renal and ureteral trauma in childhood: CT patterns of fluid collections. *A.J.R.* 152:1043, 1989.
22. Wilms, G., et al. CT and ultrasound features of post-traumatic adrenal hemorrhage. *J. Comput. Assist. Tomogr.* 11:112, 1987.
23. Wong, W.S., et al. Renal infarction: CT diagnosis and correlation between CT findings and etiologies. *Radiology* 150:201, 1984.

The Postoperative Urinary Tract

It is impossible to describe all postoperative appearances of the urinary tract because of the wide diversity of procedures available to the urologist. Furthermore, urologists continually invent new procedures to solve old problems. However, in many instances, long-accepted procedures are performed in standard fashion and result in easily recognizable postoperative radiographic patterns. This chapter will address this latter group.

The evaluation of patients after surgery requires that the radiologist be familiar with the exact nature of the procedure performed in order to anticipate the altered anatomy. This may require reference to standard operative textbooks, or a rough drawing of the procedure may be requested from the urologist. Another important factor in the evaluation is the time between surgery and the radiographic study, since in the immediate postoperative period there may be edema, hematoma formation, or inflammation resulting in obstruction or further distortion of already altered anatomy. Healing, with resolution of acute changes, usually occurs over a period of approximately 6 weeks.

It is further incumbent on the radiologist to become familiar with the various stents, tubes, and drains placed at the time of operation, and these should be described in the radiographic report. In addition, when injecting contrast medium directly into the postoperative urinary tract, it is of particular importance to avoid stressing fresh suture lines when searching for leaks of contrast material or obstruction at the sites of recent incisions or anastomoses. Finally, familiarity with surgical word endings, such as *-ectomy, -otomy,* and *-ostomy,* is important in formulating credible reports. The suffix *-ectomy* refers to excision of an organ or portion thereof, as in nephrectomy; *-otomy* indicates that an organ has been opened and then closed, as in ureterotomy, and if stone removal was involved, the term becomes ureterolithotomy; and *-ostomy* denotes the creation of a opening that is not closed, for example cutaneous ureterostomy indicates that the ureter has been brought to the skin for drainage, and ureteroureterostomy indicates the anastomosis of the end of one ureter to the side of the other (transureteroureterostomy) or the free ends of the same ureter after disruption or excision of an intervening portion.

RENAL SURGERY

The retroperitoneal operative approach via a flank incision is commonly employed for renal surgery. If the kidney is high riding, or if upper-pole surgery is planned, the incision will be over the eleventh or twelfth rib, and the distal portion of the rib is excised, leaving the periosteum intact. This results in a truncated appearance of the involved rib, and on occasion there may be calcification of the distal remaining periosteum.

NEPHRECTOMY

After nephrectomy for any cause, compensatory hypertrophy of the remaining kidney may be found, especially if the surgery was performed before the age of 40. This hypertrophy has also been reported as occurring to a lesser degree in the older patient. If the left kidney has been removed through a transperitoneal approach, the anatomic splenic flexure can usually be seen occupying the left renal fossa. This is because of mobilization of the left colon in exposing the kidney. However, there are other reasons for colon to be seen in the renal fossa—notably, ectopy or agenesis of the left kidney. Displacement of the hepatic flexure has not proven to be a reliable sign of excision, ectopy, or agenesis of the right kidney.

Simple nephrectomy is performed for benign disease of the kidney, such as advanced chronic infection or stone disease. Nephroureterectomy, which involves the excision of the ureter and a cuff of bladder along with the kidney, is reserved for treatment of transitional cell carcinoma of the intrarenal collecting system, renal pelvis, or ureter. The findings after either operation are absence of the kidney on that side, unlike radical nephrectomy for renal cell carcinoma, during which a localized node dissection is performed in addition. After radical nephrectomy, metallic surgical clips in the region of the renal hilum are common findings. The ipsilateral adrenal may or may not be removed during this procedure.

PARTIAL NEPHRECTOMY

Partial nephrectomy has many indications, including calculous disease, chronic inflammation, benign neoplasms (e.g., oncocytoma, angiomyolipoma), and duplicated systems with obstructed upper moieties or pyelonephritic lower moieties. The amount of tissue removed determines the final radiographic appearance, which is usually that of flattening of one pole and truncation of the adjacent major calix.

WEDGE EXCISION

Wedge excisions of renal lesions are usually reserved for benign conditions such as angiomyolipoma, oncocytoma, or an obstructed caliceal diverticulum. On occasion, local excision of renal cell carcinoma may have been performed, as in patients with von Hippel–Lindau disease who have many such tumors. After wedge resection, the renal parenchymal defect is usually raw and bleeding; surgical filling of these defects with vascularized perinephric or retroperitoneal fat provides hemostasis and promotes healing. This results in postoperative sonographic and CT appearances that may simulate a focal renal fat-containing mass such as angiomyolipoma [12] (Fig. 26-1). The history of surgical intervention is helpful in the correct identification of this abnormality in order to avoid unnecessary further evaluation to exclude renal tumor.

STONE SURGERY

Since the advent of extracorporeal shock-wave lithotripsy (ESWL), indications for surgery to remove renal calculi are few. In general, it is safe to say that renal parenchymal or renal pelvic incisions for stone removal may only rarely leave scars. The renal findings of caliceal clubbing and parenchymal scarring seen postoperatively are due in large part to the longstanding calculous disease rather than surgical intervention. This is true even in the case of anatrophic nephrolithotomy, in which the kidney is bivalved along its avascular coronal plane for removal of a staghorn calculus, the so-called kidney split.

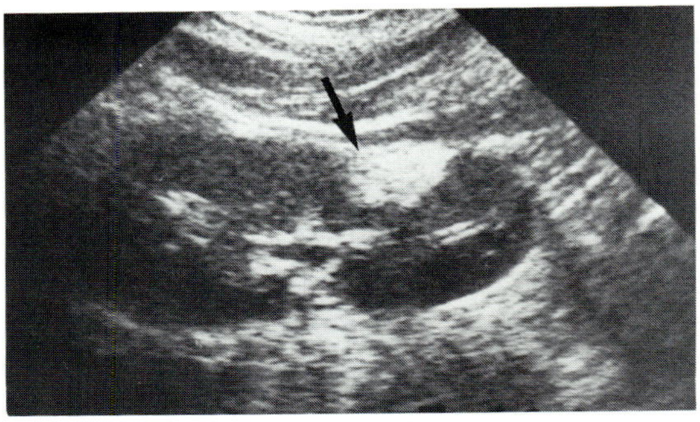

Figure 26-1. Fat-filled renal cortical defect occurring after removal of benign adenoma. Renal sonography shows hyperechoic mass (arrow) resembling angiomyolipoma.

PYELOPLASTY

Treatment of ureteropelvic junction (UPJ) obstruction has been attempted by many different techniques in the past. Currently, however, the Anderson–Hines dismembered pyeloplasty enjoys wide acceptance; it often results in a typical postoperative appearance of the renal pelvis. In this procedure, the excess renal pelvis, including the pathologic UPJ, is excised. The remaining edges of the pelvis are then sutured together medially and the spatulated proximal ureter anastomosed to the most dependent portion of the reconfigured pelvis. The result is flattening of the medial side of the renal pelvis, which can be irregular in the acute postoperative period because of the healing suture line (Fig. 26-2). Furthermore, edema at the ureteropelvic anastomosis may result in some degree of obstruction that may persist for up to 6 weeks. Postoperative study via a surgically placed nephrostomy tube or ureteral stent may be requested. While leakage of contrast material is not expected, a small amount of leakage is not cause for alarm, since it will usually resolve in a few days. Even without nephrostomy or stent drainage, extravasation will usually clear if a drain has been left in the retroperitoneum.

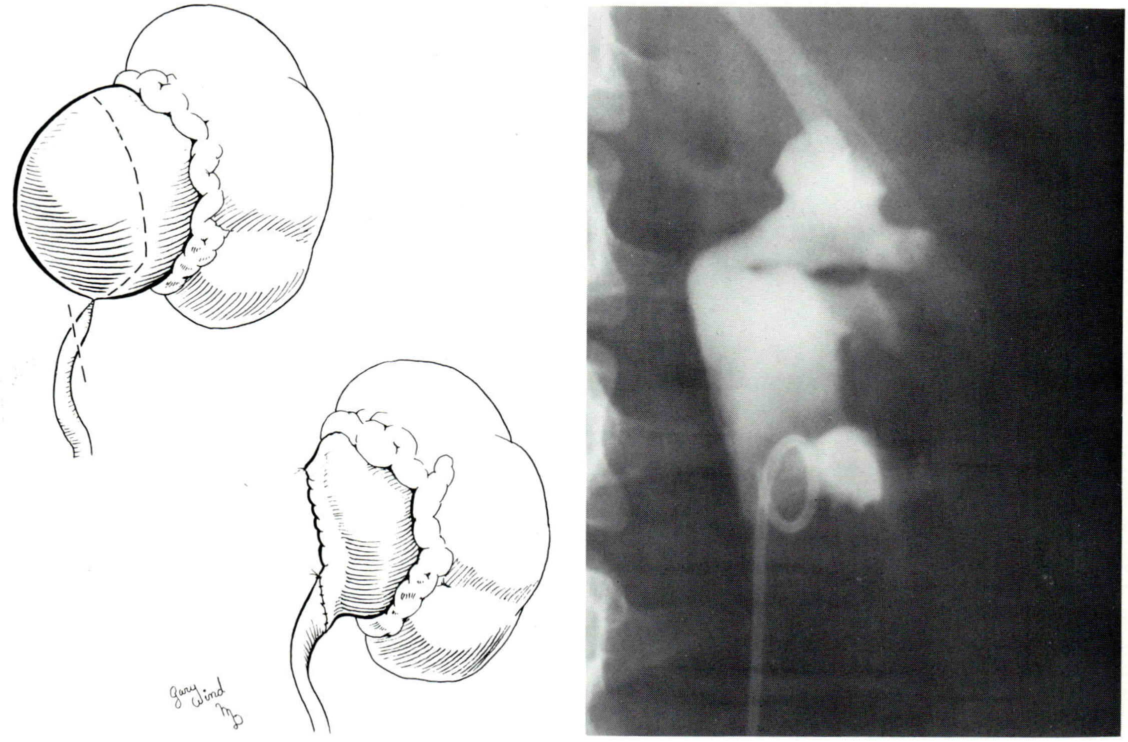

A B

Figure 26-2. Anderson–Hines pyeloplasty for ureteropelvic junction obstruction. A. Diagram of surgical technique. B. Stent study 7 days postoperatively shows flattening and minimal irregularity of medial renal pelvic margin. (From E.S. Amis, Jr. Postoperative changes in the urinary tract. In *Radiology: Diagnosis-Imaging-Intervention*, ed. J.M. Taveras and J.T. Ferrucci, 1–9. Philadelphia: J.B. Lippincott, 1988.)

URETERAL SURGERY

URETEROLYSIS

Ureterolysis, or freeing up of the ureter, is standard surgical treatment for the ureter trapped by benign retroperitoneal fibrosis. In this procedure, the ureter is dissected from its fibrotic bed, then transposed intraperitoneally, and often wrapped with omentum. This usually results in a gentle, lateral bowing of the operated ureter(s). The ureter may be stented during the acute postoperative period. After removal of a ureteral stent, with this procedure or after being left indwelling for any reason, obstruction may ensue because of spasm of the ureter. This obstruction is transient and usually resolves in a day or two.

ABDOMINOPERINEAL RESECTION (EFFECT ON URETERS)

Abdominoperineal resection of a rectal neoplasm typically results in medial deviation of both ureters over the sacral promontory (Fig. 26-3). This may be due in part to the ureters following the normal pelvic curvature, but it is more likely secondary to reapproximation of the posterior peritoneum after removal of a segment of this peritoneum with the surgical specimen. This reapproximation retracts the ureters, which are loosely adherent to the posterior peritoneum, toward the midline. The deviation seen can vary from a mild medial curvature of both ureters toward the midline to acute medial angulation of the ureters in the sacral area. If obstruction of one or both ureters is seen, postsurgical fibrosis or recurrent tumor are the most likely causes; when ureteral obstruction appears months or years after surgical therapy for malignant disease, the cause is more likely to be recurrent tumor than benign fibrosis. CT is usually able to resolve this differential, showing a presacral soft-tissue mass in cases of tumor recurrence and nontumefactive fibrous tissue strands with benign stricturing.

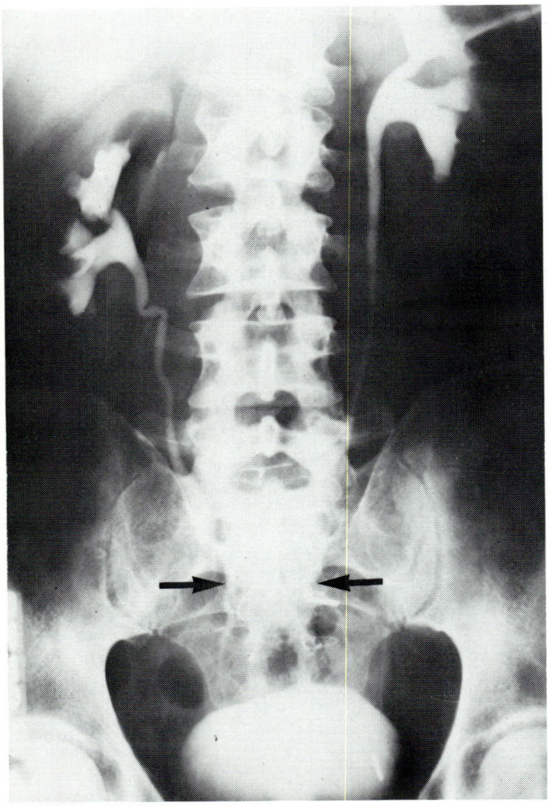

Figure 26-3. Abdominoperineal resection for rectal cancer. Urography demonstrates medial deviation of both ureters over the midsacrum (arrows). (From E.S. Amis, Jr. Postoperative changes in the urinary tract. In *Radiology: Diagnosis-Imaging-Intervention*, ed. J.M. Taveras and J.T. Ferrucci, 1-9. Philadelphia: J.B. Lippincott, 1988.)

Table 26-1. Ureteral replacements

Loss of short segment	
	Boari flap
	Psoas hitch
Loss of moderate segment	
	Transureteroureterostomy
	Transureteropyelostomy
Loss of entire ureter	
	Bowel substitution
	Autotransplantation of kidney

URETERAL SUBSTITUTION

In cases in which there has been loss of all or part of a ureter, bridging of the resultant gap becomes necessary to restore continuity of the urinary tract. Multiple techiques have been developed for treating ureteral loss (Table 26-1). The most common cause of such a loss is devascularization of a segment of the ureter; this can occur even during the most meticulously performed procedure. Absence of only the distal portion of the ureter can be overcome by a Boari flap or psoas-hitch procedure, the latter being more commonly employed. Both of these procedures result in rather typical findings postoperatively. The Boari flap refers to the creation of a large oblique anterior bladder flap, which is then rotated 180 degrees superiorly and rolled into a tube for bridging the distal ureteral defect. This results radiographically in a fingerlike tube several centimeters in length projecting from the bladder and connecting with the ureter. The psoas-hitch procedure involves mobilization of the bladder followed by stretching it superiorly on the side of ureteral deficit and suturing its posterior wall to the ileopsoas fascia. This results in a superiorly elongated bladder deviated to the side of repair (Fig. 26-4). Not only can this procedure compensate for some ureteral loss, it can also provide a long, fixed posterior bladder wall for antirefluxing reimplantation of the ureter.

More severe ureteral loss can be handled by transureteroureterostomy (TUU) or transureteropyelostomy (TUP). The remaining ureteral segment is brought across the midline and anastomosed to the contralateral normal renal pelvis or ureter for reestablishment of urine drainage. TUU is the more commonly employed of these techniques, and the donor ureter can be seen sweeping obliquely across the midline to its anastomosis with the normal, or recipient, ureter. Angulation and proximal obstruction as the donor ureter crosses the midline may indicate that it is trapped in the angle formed by the inferior mesenteric artery and the aorta.

In cases in which there has been loss of most, if not all, of the ureter, small-bowel segments may be used to bridge the deficit. If reflux is to be prevented, the bowel segment can be tapered and reimplanted into the bladder by an antirefluxing technique. In some patients who chronically pass stones that obstruct the normal-sized ureter, a bowel segment may be used to replace the normal ureter in an effort to pro-

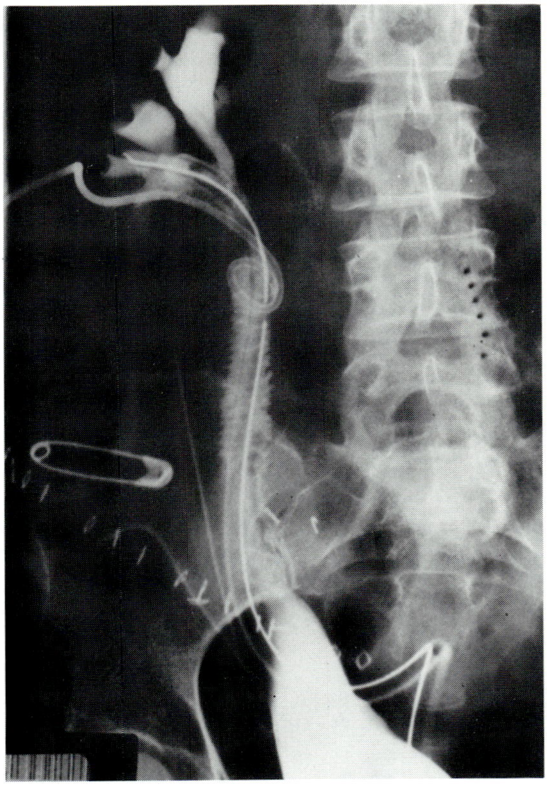

Figure 26-4. Ileal substitution and psoas-hitch procedure for replacement of right ureter. Nephrostography 7 days postoperatively demonstrates ileal pattern of the ureteral substitution and superiorly elongated bladder typical of a psoas hitch.

vide a lumen of increased diameter connecting the kidney to the bladder. Bowel segments thus used are usually ileum, and they are easily recognized radiographically as such (see Fig. 26-4). As an alternative to replacing the lost or compromised ureter, autotransplantation of the involved kidney may be considered. This involves moving the kidney to the ipsilateral iliac fossa and reanastomosing the renal vessels to the iliac vessels. No rejection phenomena are encountered in this procedure. Again, if the patient is a chronic stone-former, the renal pelvis may be anastomosed directly to the bladder wall to provide a wide opening for stone passage.

BLADDER SURGERY

In children with exstrophy of the bladder, primary closure is being performed more frequently, whereas in the past urinary diversion was the more common treatment. When successfully reconstructed, the bladder has a rather typical appearance, which results from the creation of a continent, proximal urethra from basilar bladder flaps. Radiographically, there is an indented bladder base with an elongated, very narrow posterior urethra. Furthermore, the bladder, if initially small, may be augmented by large- or small-bowel segments; the typical mucosal pattern of these is usually recognizable. These findings may be accompanied by healed iliac osteotomies and midline wiring together of the pubic bones, although in some cases no attempt is made to correct the bony abnormality of widely separated pubes. Unfortunately, neoplastic change in the reconstructed bladder has been reported in from 4.0 to 7.5 percent of cases [17].

Vesical-neck suspension in women for the treatment of stress urinary incontinence recreates the posterior urethrovesical angle. This can also result in an elevation of the bladder base.

Other bladder procedures, such as ureteral reimplantation for the correction of reflux (ureteroneocystostomy) or partial cystectomy for tumor, often result in significant contour or mucosal irregularities of the bladder in the weeks immediately after surgery (Fig. 26-5). These findings are due to edema, inflammation, hematoma formation, or all of the above, and

Figure 26-5. Bilateral ureteroneocystostomies (ureteral reimplants for reflux). Cystography performed 7 days postoperatively shows no reflux, but the contour of the bladder is grossly deformed bilaterally secondary to edema or hematoma formation or both.

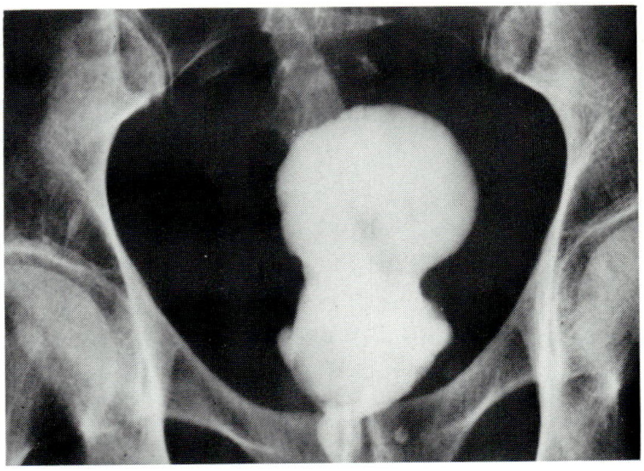

usually resolve by 6 weeks, leaving no evidence that surgical intervention had occurred. On occasion, however, after ureteroneocystostomy the reimplanted ureter can be seen entering the bladder superiorly and medially to its expected insertion site [10].

PROSTATE SURGERY

TRANSURETHRAL AND OPEN RESECTION

Benign prostatic hypertrophy is the most common cause of bladder outlet obstruction and is usually treated by transurethral resection (TURP) or open removal of the obstructing adenomatous tissue. This almost always results in the finding of variable-sized collections of contrast material in the region of the prostatic urethra on static urography or cystography (Fig. 26-6). This is due to loss of the internal sphincter mechanism at the bladder neck, which is resected as part of the prostatectomy. After prostatectomy, passive continence is maintained by the intrinsic sphincter at the level of the membranous urethra. Since TURP is performed through a large-caliber sheath, other urethral abnormalities can result. Postoperative urethral strictures have been reported in 14 percent of such patients, and urethral contour irregularities or serrations have been found in 30 percent [14]. Regrowth of residual prostatic adenoma after TURP may present as round or ovoid nodules in the widened posterior urethra on urethrography. These are commonly found near the apex of the prostate just above the urogenital diaphragm.

RADICAL PROSTATECTOMY

Radical prostatectomy for carcinoma of the prostate can be accomplished through a transperineal or retropubic approach. The latter is currently favored because it allows the performance of a staging pelvic lymphadenectomy prior to excision of the prostate. With either approach, the entire prostate and both seminal vesicles are removed. The bladder neck must then be anastomosed to the stump of urethra protruding from the urogenital diaphragm, resulting in funneling of the bladder base behind the pubic symphysis (Fig. 26-7). Multiple surgical clips in the pelvis are frequently seen in

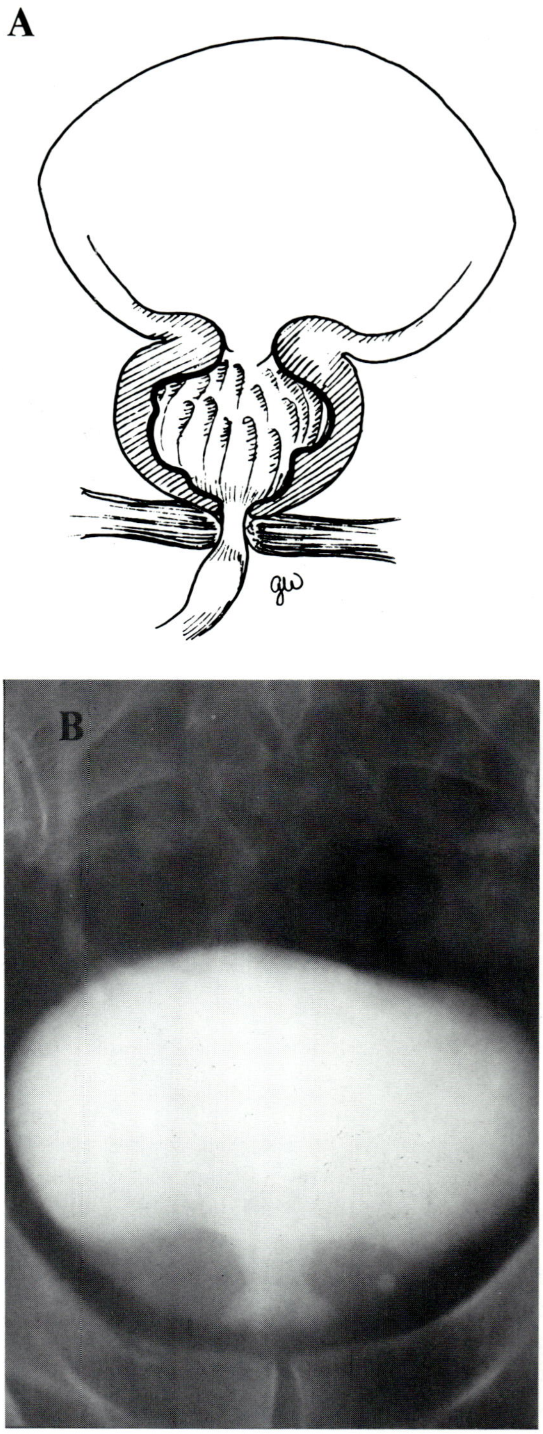

Figure 26-6. TURP defect. A. Diagram of resected prostate. B. Bladder phase of urography showing irregular collection of contrast material in prostatic urethra. (From E.S. Amis, Jr. Postoperative changes in the urinary tract. In *Radiology: Diagnosis-Imaging-Intervention,* ed. J.M. Taveras and J.T. Ferrucci, 1-9. Philadelphia: J.B. Lippincott, 1988.)

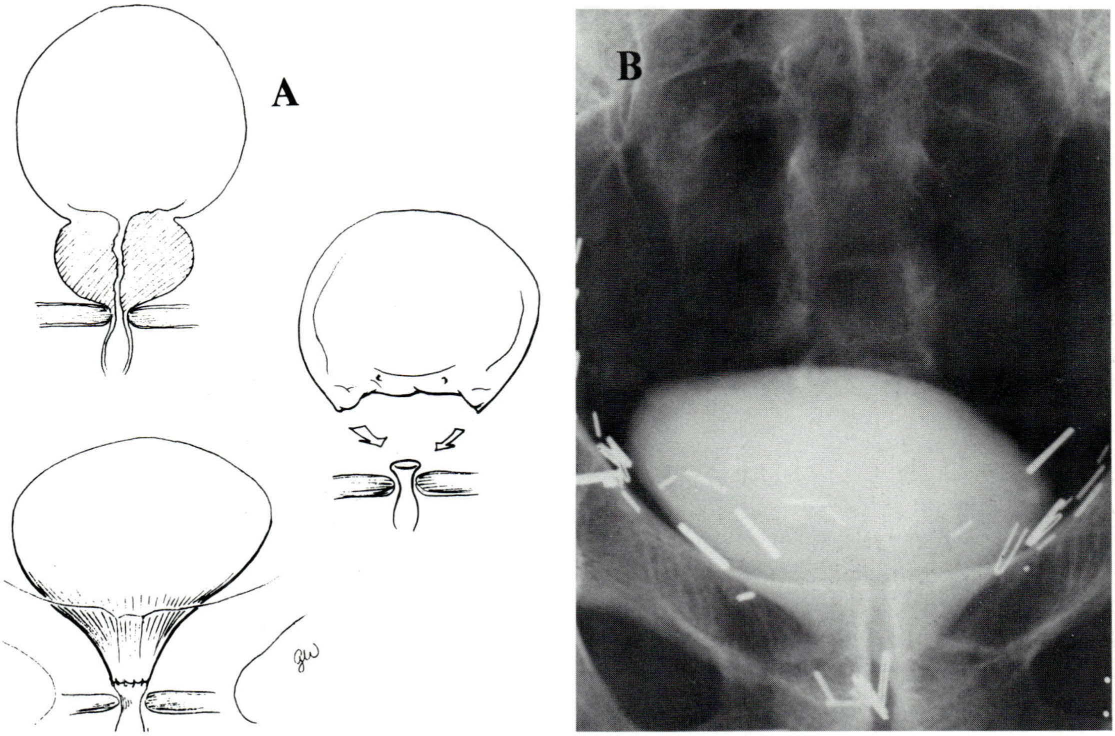

Figure 26-7. Radical prostatectomy for carcinoma of the prostate. A. Diagram of surgical procedure. B. Bladder phase of urography several months postoperatively shows funneling of bladder base behind pubis. (From E.S. Amis, Jr. Postoperative changes in the urinary tract. In *Radiology: Diagnosis-Imaging-Intervention*, ed. J.M. Taveras and J.T. Ferrucci, 1–9. Philadelphia: J.B. Lipincott, 1988.)

association with this finding and indicate that a lymphadenectomy preceded the prostatectomy.

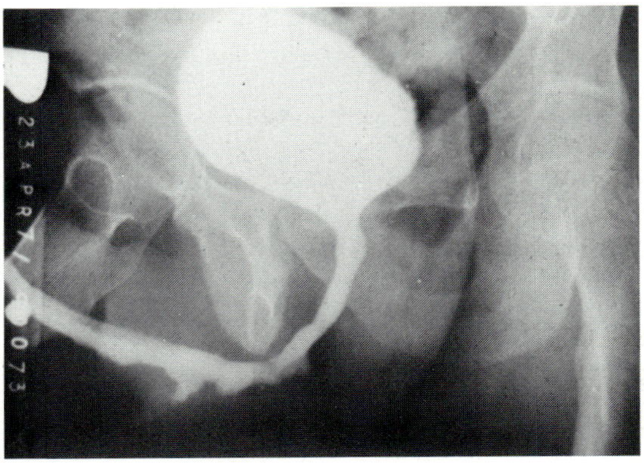

Figure 26-8. Posturethroplasty sacculations after repair of bulbar urethral stricture. Voiding cystourethrography demonstrates patent bulbar urethra with gross sacculations.

URETHRAL SURGERY

Urethral surgery is usually performed for hypospadias and for strictures that recur after more conservative means of treatment. Multiple operative techniques have been described, but most result in typical findings postoperatively for both stricture and hypospadias repair. Although the region of repair should be widely patent, irregularities in the caliber of the lumen are commonly found. On occasion, sacculations of the urethra are seen after the repair, usually at the proximal and distal ends, though they may occur throughout the area of the urethroplasty (Fig. 26-8). One procedure, the Waterhouse transpubic repair of prostatomembranous strictures, results in a classic postoperative appearance. In this technique, the bulbar urethra is mobilized, brought through the urogenital diaphragm posterior to the membranous urethra, and anastomosed end-to-side to the prostatic urethra proximal to the stricture. This angled anastomosis is easily recognizable.

URINARY DIVERSION

The need for diversion of urine may be temporary or permanent. Temporary diversion is often indicated to allow return of renal function in cases in which the bladder is expected to recover some degree of normal function, as with posterior urethral valves. This is usually accomplished by bilateral nephrostomies, loop cutaneous ureterostomies, or vesicostomy. Loop cutaneous ureterostomy involves bringing a loop of intact ureter to the skin and creating an opening in the exposed portion for drainage of urine. The radiographic appearance of severe lateral deviation of the midureters is typical. Vesicostomy is an anterior bladder incision that is sutured to the skin for drainage; a collecting appliance is usually seen in the suprapubic region. Permanent urinary diversions are required when the bladder has been irrevocably damaged or when cystectomy has been performed for malignant disease. This is most frequently accomplished by contruction of an ileal conduit [4], though large-bowel conduits or implantation of the ureters into the intact colon (ureterosigmoidostomy) have also been used. Figure 26-9 depicts the various types of diversions.

ILEAL CONDUIT

In the ileal conduit, the ureters are anastomosed by various techniques to an isolated short segment of terminal ileum, the distal end of which is brought to the anterior abdominal wall. The ileal segment acts as a conduit rather than a reservoir, and thus it drains continuously into a collecting appliance that the patient wears over the stoma. Loopography, described in Chap. 3, is required for study of the conduit. These are almost always freely refluxing systems, the absence of reflux into one or both ureters indicating postsurgical fibrotic stricturing or recurrent tumor in the region of the ureteroileal anastomoses. In up to 20 percent of conduits that have been constructed by the commonly employed Bricker technique (both ureters anastomosed end-to-side to the conduit and the proximal end of the conduit closed), a filling defect can be seen in the proximal end of the bowel loop [1]. This is caused by a multilayer closure of the proximal end of the conduit in which each successive layer is "turned in" during closure. Other filling defects, however, may indicate stones or tumor—either primary or metastatic—in the conduit, and they should be investigated further. With other techniques for construction of ileal conduits, both ureters may be spatulated and sutured to the proximal end of the conduit (Wallace technique), or one ureter may be anastomosed end-to-side to the conduit and the remaining ureter attached to the proximal end (Pyrah technique).

Figure 26-9. Various types of urinary diversions. A. Vesicostomy. B. End-cutaneous ureterostomies. C. Loop-cutaneous ureterostomies. D. Bowel conduit. E. Ureterosigmoidostomies. (From E.S. Amis, Jr., R.C. Pfister, and W.H. Hendren. Radiology of urinary undiversion. *Urol. Radiol.* [Springer-Verlag, N.Y.] 3:161-169, 1981.)

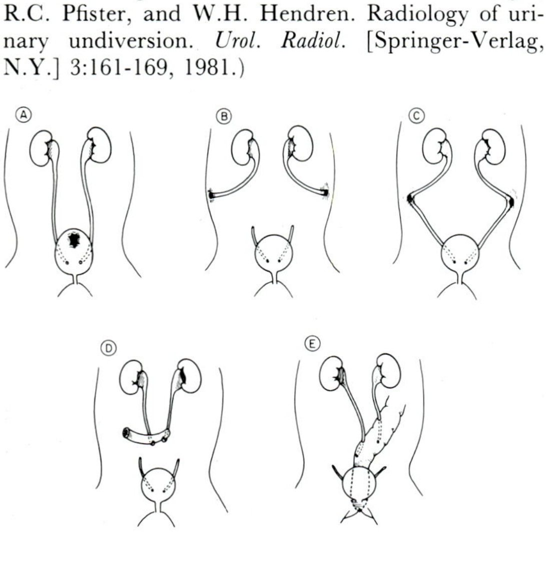

Because ileal conduits are freely refluxing, it is not unusual to find mild to moderate dilation of the upper urinary tracts on urography, although significant dilation most frequently represents obstruction and requires loopography for further evaluation. One study reported that with mild dilation of the upper tracts, only 20 percent were obstructed, whereas with severe dilation 80 percent were obstructed [6]. Long-term complications of ileal conduits include stomal stenosis, fibrosis and stricturing of the conduit (Fig. 26-10), and obstruction of the ureteroileal anastomoses. Furthermore, deterioration of the upper tracts has been found in up to 41 percent of patients [11].

CONTINENT URINARY DIVERSIONS

Continent urinary diversions have been gaining wide acceptance as an alternative to the ileal conduit. This has been facilitated by the proven safety of clean intermittent catheterization,

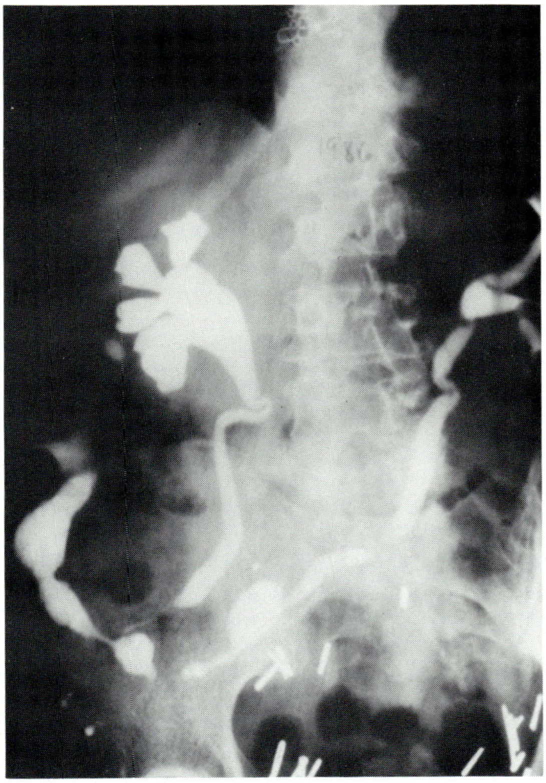

Figure 26-10. Stenosis and stricturing of ileal conduit 7 years after urinary diversion. Loopography shows grossly irregular and segmentally narrowed conduit. Although there is free reflux bilaterally, the right distal ureter is stenotic also.

which allows the patient to empty the urine reservoir every 3 to 6 hours by self-catheterization, with continence being maintained during the intervening time. An external collecting device is not needed. These procedures are being performed more frequently as patients choose this form of diversion or seek conversion of ileal conduits because of inability to maintain dryness or because of the psychosocial stigmata of wearing an external appliance. Furthermore, the trend away from radiotherapy before cystectomy for bladder cancer allows better healing of these more technically complex diversions. Several procedures have been described for creation of a continent urine reservoir [2]. This discussion will include only those in common use.

Most continent diversions open on the anterior abdominal wall; however, some are adaptable for replacement of the bladder if the urethra and its sphincters are intact. The former are classified as cutaneous and the latter as orthotopic. Orthotopic pouches are contraindicated for patients in whom cystectomy has been performed for multifocal transitional cell carcinoma or those in whom carcinoma extended into the prostatic urethra. Also, orthotopic diversions have a significant incidence of nocturnal incontinence. Patients with orthotopic pouches void by voluntary relaxation of the urethral sphincters coupled with abdominal straining. In some cases, self-catheterization will be necessary because of chronic residual urine after voiding.

Continent urinary pouches are constructed from either ileum alone or a combination of terminal ileum and ascending colon. For proper function, the ideal reservoir must have a consistently low pressure and high capacity. The cutaneous pouch should require catheterization by the patient no more frequently than every 3 to 6 hours. Furthermore, the upper tracts should be protected from the effects of reflux or obstruction by special techniques for implanting the ureters into the pouch. Finally, continence between catheterizations and ease of insertion of the catheter must be achieved.

Low pressure in the urinary reservoirs is obtained by "detubularization" of the bowel segment used. This detubularization, or interruption of normal bowel continuity, prevents organized contractions that might result in intermittent high pressures that can cause incontinence or reflux. This concept is especially important in reservoirs composed primarily of large bowel. Metallic staples, which have been used in the construction of some pouches, may act as nidi for stone formation; techniques have been devised that eliminate this potential complication.

Camey Pouch

Named after its originator, the Camey pouch is used only for orthotopic replacement of the bladder. It is composed of an isolated U-shaped loop of distal ileum located in the true pelvis. An opening is created in the most dependent portion of the loop, which is then anastomosed to the urethral stump. Continence is provided by the sphincter surrounding the membranous urethra, and the ureters are implanted in a mucosal trough at each end of the loop in an effort to prevent reflux. Camey has reported that in 176 patients undergoing this procedure, the average voided volume was 300 ml, and reflux was avoided in 80 percent [5].

Mainz Pouch

The Mainz pouch derives its name from Mainz, Germany, where it was developed. An ovoid pouch is constructed from two connected opened limbs of terminal ileum folded into the opened cecum. The ureters are tunneled into the posterior taenia of the cecum to prevent reflux, and continence is obtained by intussuscepting an intact ileal segment that is in continuity with the pouch and that becomes the catheterizing port. Reflux has not been a problem, and the average capacity has been reported as 500 ml [16].

Kock Pouch

The Kock pouch is named for its originator, Dr. Nils Kock, who introduced it in the United States in 1982 [9]. Constructed entirely from a long segment of terminal ileum, it is probably the most technically difficult continent pouch to construct. Both ends of the original isolated ileal segment are retained intact and intussuscepted; the ureters are attached to the proximal segment, and the distal segment acts as a continent catheterizing port. The pouch itself is constructed from the opened central segment of ileum (Fig. 26-11). In a series of 250 patients, the average pouch capacity was 800 to 1000 ml, and reflux and incontinence were rare [15].

Indiana Pouch

Named after its place of development (the University of Indiana) the Indiana pouch uses the cecum as the reservoir and the intact terminal ileum, which is narrowed by plication, as the continence mechanism and catheterization port [13]. Reflux is prevented by tunneling of the ureters into the taenia of the cecum. Detubularization is usually accomplished by folding the opened superior portion of the reservoir over on itself (Heineke–Mikulicz reconstruction) (Fig. 26-12). Capacity of the pouch averages about 500 ml, and reflux has not been a prob-

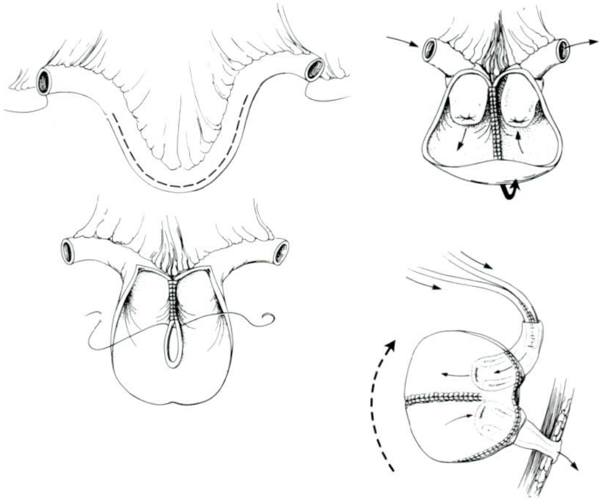

A

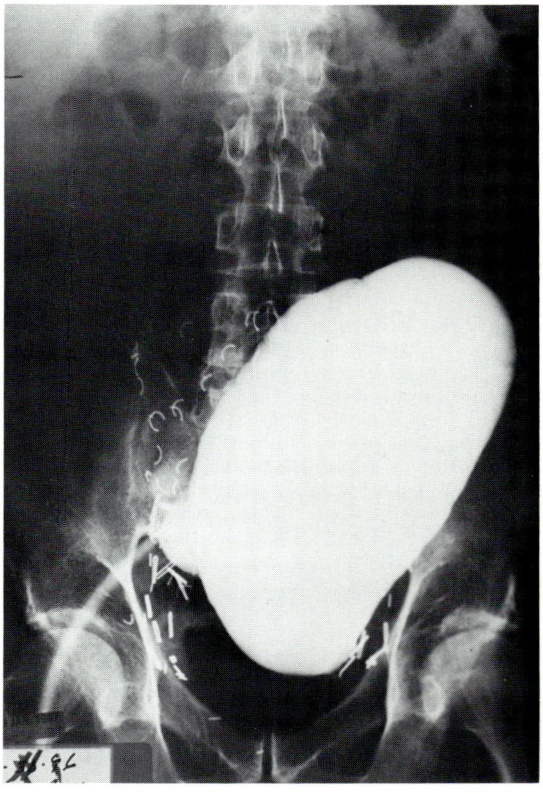

B

Figure 26-11. Kock continent urinary diversion. A. Diagram of surgical technique. B. Pouch study 1 year postoperatively reveals loss of ileal mucosal pattern, large capacity, and absence of reflux. (From E.S. Amis, Jr., J.H. Newhouse, and C.A. Olsson. Continent urinary diversion: Review of current surgical procedures and radiologic imaging. *Radiology* 168:395–401, 1988.)

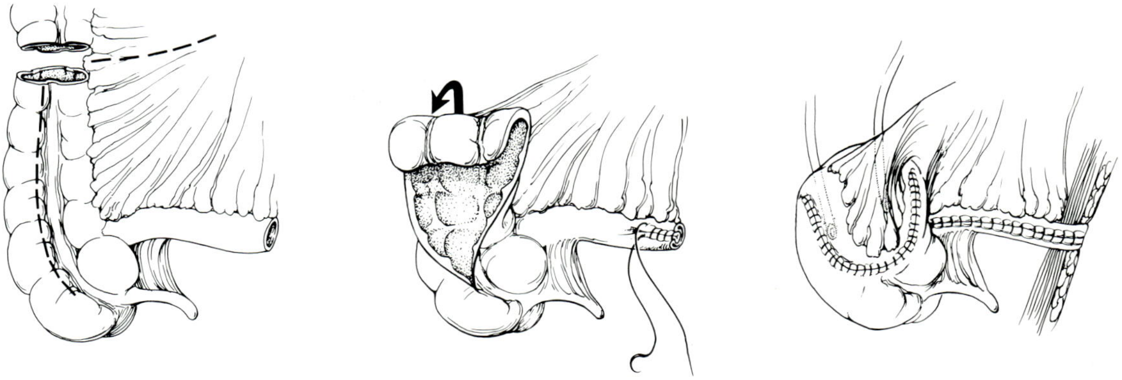

A

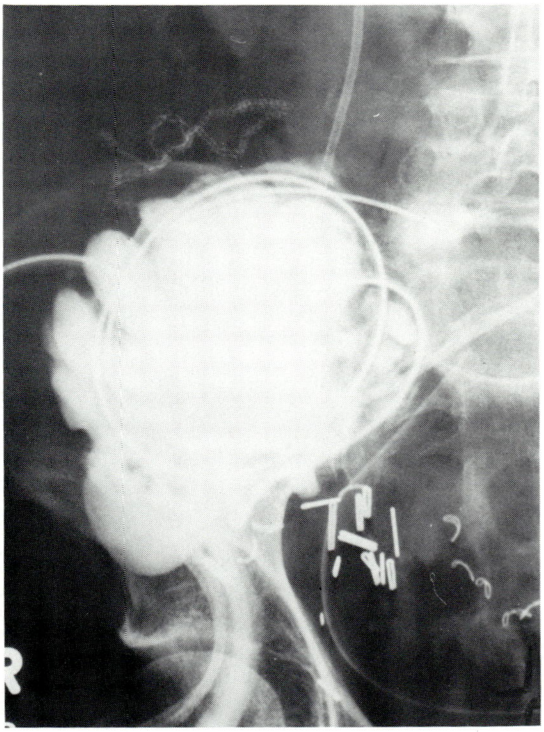

B

Figure 26-12. Indiana continent urinary diversion. A. Diagram of surgical technique. (From E.S. Amis, Jr., J.H. Newhouse, and C.A. Olsson. Continent urinary diversions: Review of current surgical procedures and radiologic imaging. *Radiology* 168:395-401, 1988.) B. Pouch study 10 days postoperatively demonstrates the expected large-bowel pattern. Ureteral stents are still in place.

lem. Satisfactory continence has been reported in 93 percent of patients.

Penn Pouch

Described at the Children's Hospital of Pennsylvania, the Penn pouch is constructed by folding the opened, attached terminal ileum into the opened cecum. Continence is provided by use of the Mitrofanoff technique, whereby a narrow tube, usually the appendix, is brought to the skin and used as the catheterizing port. As in other pouches, reflux is prevented by tunneling of the ureters in the posterior taenia of the cecal portion of the pouch. Early results indicate a continent, large-volume reservoir [7].

Postoperative Complications

Postoperative complications are similar for all the above pouches. Early problems include urine leaks, pelvic abscess, small-bowel obstruction, and pyelonephritis. Later complications are incontinence, calculus formation (especially on exposed staples), and difficulty in catheterizing the pouch. Pyelonephritis secondary to reflux or obstruction has been uncommon. Hyperchloremic acidosis also appears to be a minor problem, and it responds to a short course of medical management.

Postoperative Evaluation

The postoperative radiographic evaluation of continent diversions should be standardized. Furthermore, the radiologist should become familiar with the procedure performed, as well as with any tubes, stents, and drains placed at the time of surgery. It is common to find ureteral stents extending from the renal pelves through the anastomoses of the ureters to the pouch and exiting via the pouch stoma; a large-caliber catheter usually drains the pouch itself. A typical postoperative evaluation includes bilateral stent studies at about 1 week after surgery. Contrast medium is dripped into each stent, allowing documentation of stent position, status of the collecting systems, presence or absence of extravasation, and patency of the ureteral anastomoses. If all is satisfactory, the stents are removed shortly thereafter. At 10 days postoperatively, the pouch can be studied via its indwelling catheter. Again, drip technique and fluoroscopic control are used, and a maximum of 250 ml of contrast material is instilled to prevent stressing the fresh suture lines. Oblique views are obtained as necessary to examine all sides of the pouch for extravasation of contrast material. Studies performed after complete healing should document the capacity of the pouch, the presence or absence of reflux, and the postcatheterization residual urine. Urography is useful to document nonobstructed, functioning upper tracts.

When postoperative abscess is suspected, CT or sonography is often indicated. In such cases, it is imperative that the radiologist be aware of the location of the pouch and its appearance on these scanning methods, as the partially or completely filled pouch, often containing air introduced during catheterization, may resemble an infected fluid collection. Furthermore, pseudomasses in the pouch are usually due to bowel folds, clumps of mucus, or intussuscepted bowel segments.

REVERSAL OF URINARY DIVERSION AND BLADDER AUGMENTATION

Many patients, usually children having undergone urinary diversion in the past, are now being considered for reversal of the procedure, which has come to be called *undiversion.* This has been made possible by the development of innovative surgical techniques. Postoperatively, these patients may exhibit rather bizarre uroradiologic appearances, which can tax the radiologist attempting to render a useful evaluation [3, 8]. It is imperative for the radiologist to be aware of the exact procedure performed when he or she is studying these patients and attempting interpretation of the films. In many of these patients, there will be inadequate ureteral length to restore the urinary tract to its original state. In such cases, one or a combination of the ureteral lengthening techniques already discussed may be employed. Furthermore, the bladder may be found to be significantly reduced in capacity or nonfunctional because of chronic inflammation, contraction, or neurogenic dysfunction. If such is the case, the bladder must be augmented as an integral part of the undiversion procedure. This can be accomplished in various ways by the use of bowel segments. A common procedure is the ileocecal cystoplasty, in which the ileocecal region is isolated and rotated 180 degrees clockwise and the cecum anastomosed to the opened bladder dome or to the bladder base if the majority of the diseased bladder has been excised. The ileocecal valve is intussuscepted to prevent reflux, and the ure-

Figure 26-13. Ileocecal cystoplasty. Cystography shows the cecal appearance of the bladder, which has been almost entirely replaced in this augmentation procedure.

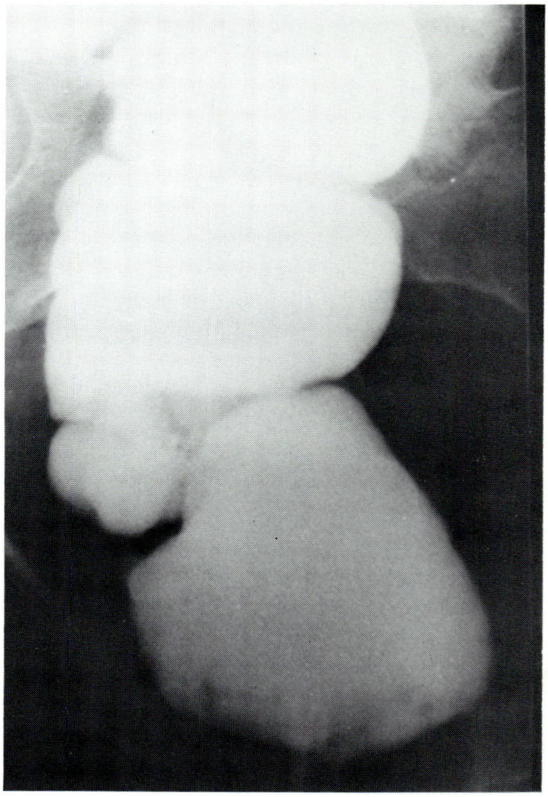

ters are anastomosed to the ileal segment. Cystography is such cases shows the cecal appearance of the augmented bladder (Fig. 26-13). As with the Camey orthotopic diversion, these patients void by relaxing their urethral sphincter and increasing intraabdominal pressure.

REFERENCES

1. Amis, E.S., Jr., Cronan, J.J., and Pfister, R.C. Filling defects in small bowel urinary conduits. *A.J.R.* 137:787, 1981.
2. Amis, E.S., Jr., Newhouse, J.H., and Olsson, C.A. Continent urinary diversions: Review of current surgical procedures and radiologic imaging. *Radiology* 168:395, 1988.
3. Amis, E.S., Jr., Pfister, R.C., and Hendren, W.H. Radiology of urinary undiversion. *Urol. Radiol.* 3:161, 1981.
4. Bricker, E.M. Bladder substitution after pelvic evisceration. *Surg. Clin. North Am.* 30:1511, 1950.
5. Camey, M. Bladder replacement by ileocystoplasty following radical cystectomy. *Semin. Urol.* 5:8, 1987.
6. Cronan, J.J., et al. Renal obstruction in patients with ileal loops: US evaluation. *Radiology* 158:647, 1986.
7. Duckett, J.W., and Snyder, H.Mc. The Mitrofanoff principle in continent urinary reservoirs. *Semin. Urol.* 5:55, 1987.
8. Fernbach, S.K., and Holland, E.A. Undiversion of the urinary tract: The pre- and postoperative evaluation. *RadioGraphics* 8:213, 1988.
9. Kock, N.G., et al. Urinary diversion via a continent ileal reservoir: Clinical results in 12 patients *J. Urol.* 128:469, 1982.
10. Lebowitz, R.L. *Postoperative Pediatric Uroradiology.* New York: Appleton-Century-Crofts, 1950. P. 15.
11. Middleton, A.W., and Hendren, W.H. Ileal conduits in children at Massachusetts General Hospital from 1955 to 1970. *J. Urol.* 115:591, 1976.
12. Papanicolaou, N., Harbury, O.L., and Pfister, R.C. Fat-filled postoperative renal cortical defects: Sonographic and CT appearance. *A.J.R.* 151:503, 1988.
13. Rowland, R.G., et al. Indiana continent urinary reservoir. *J. Urol.* 137:1136, 1987.
14. Shaver, W.A., Richter, P.H., and Orandi, A. Changes in the males urethra produced by instrumentation for transurethral resection of the prostate. *Radiology* 116:623, 1975.
15. Skinner, D.G., Lieskovsky, G., and Boyd, S.D. Continuing experience with the continent ileal reservoir (Kock Pouch) as an alternative to cutaneous urinary diversion: An update after 250 cases. *J. Urol.* 137:1140, 1987.
16. Thuroff, J.W., et al. The Mainz pouch (mixed augmentation ileum 'n zecum) for bladder augmentation and continent diversion. *World J. Urol.* 3:179, 1985.
17. White, P., and Lebowitz, R.L. Exstrophy of the bladder. *Radiol. Clin. North Am.* 15:93, 1977.

27

Impotence

The report on Human Sexual Inadequacy published by Masters and Johnson in 1970 [11] stated that physiologic causes of impotence were of "minor consideration." However, there has been significant research into the physiology of male erections since then, leading to the current estimate that an organic basis can be established in more than half of impotent patients. In fact, in one study of impotent men who complained of consistent erectile impairment for periods of longer than 1 year, a physical abnormality was found in 90 percent of cases [7]. Impotence is a major clinical problem; it has been estimated that up to 20 million American men suffer erectile insufficiency.

The term *impotence* denotes the inability to achieve or maintain an erection that allows mutually satisfactory intercourse. There are multiple causes of this condition, including emotional disease, diabetes mellitus and other endocrine disorders, neurologic disease or injury, vascular disease, and various drugs. In the past, diabetes mellitus was thought to be the most frequent cause of this dysfunction; however, current work indicates that there is a vascular cause for most cases of impotence [13], although diabetes can, of course, be associated with vascular disease. These patients frequently have no other symptoms, such as claudication or angina, to suggest vascular disease [8]. In one study, a vascular cause was found in 65 percent of unselected impotent patients [2]. It is in the area of vasculogenic impotence that radiology has a significant role both in diagnosis and treatment.

PHYSIOLOGY OF ERECTIONS

Given the proper hormonal and emotional environment, physical or mental stimulation results in generation of nerve impulses that travel from the spinal cord to the penile nerves. These impulses, by release of as yet poorly understood factors, cause smooth-muscle relaxation in the walls of sinusoids that fill each corpus cavernosum as well as in the walls of the cavernosal arteries.

As the muscular walls of the cavernosal sinusoids relax, there is a resultant decreased resistance to arterial flow into the cavernosa. This arterial flow, aided by the dilating walls of the cavernosal arteries, continues to increase until the pressure in the cavernosa is approximately the same as systolic pressure. As this is occurring, distention of the sinusoids with blood results in compression and blockage of flow in small perforating emissary veins between the peripheral sinusoids and the relatively rigid tunica albuginea surrounding the cavernosa (Fig. 27-1). Thus, increased inflow of blood in conjunction with decreased outflow results in an erection. After orgasm, muscle tone in the sinusoids begins to increase, resulting in emptying of the sinusoids, reinstitution of normal venous drainage, and an increased resistance to inflow of arterial blood. Venogenic impotence implies a loss in the ability to occlude venous outflow by filling of the sinusoids, whereas arteriogenic impotence indicates an inability to provide an increased inflow of cavernosal arterial blood. Combined venogenic and arteriogenic impotence account for about a third of cases of vasculogenic impotence.

The arterial supply to the penis is derived from the paired internal pudendal arteries, each arising as an anterior branch of the ipsilateral internal iliac (hypogastric) artery. Distally, each internal pudendal artery becomes the common penile artery, which gives rise to three branches: an artery to the bulb of the corpus spongiosum, the cavernosal artery, which passes through the middle of the ipsilateral corpus cavernosum, and one of the paired dorsal arteries of the penis (see Fig. 27-1). The blood flow necessary for achieving and maintaining an erection seems to be derived primarily from the cavernosal arteries. There is a significant degree of normal variability in the penile arterial system.

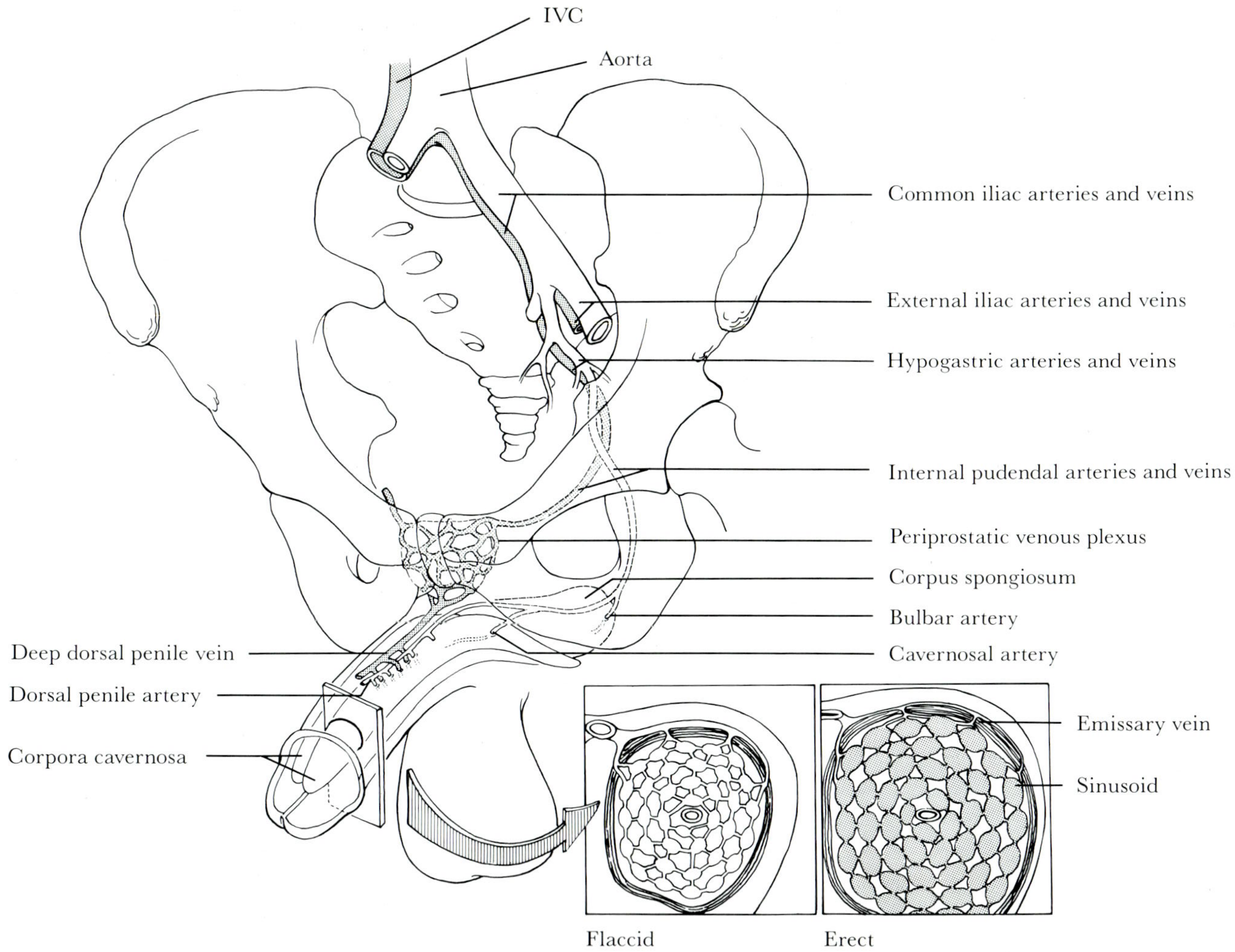

Figure 27-1. Simplified diagram of erectile function. Note that during erection the sinusoids in the corpora cavernosa distend and compress the emissary veins against the rigid tunica albuginea, thus occluding venous outflow. Leakage via these veins is the cause of venogenic impotence. Obstructive lesions (e.g., atherosclerotic plaques) at any level of the arterial supply to the penis can result in arteriogenic impotence. (IVC = inferior vena cava.)

The primary route of venous drainage from the erectile tissue is through emissary veins that drain lacunar spaces between the cavernosal sinusoids and the surrounding tunica albuginea. These veins pierce the tunica albuginea and drain into the deep dorsal vein of the penis, which is a single vein lying in the groove between the upper margins of the corpora cavernosa. Blood from the deep dorsal vein of the penis subsequently passes through the periprostatic plexus of Santorini before eventually reaching the systemic venous circulation via the internal iliac (hypogastric) vein. It is the emissary veins perforating the tunica albuginea that are compressed, and thus occluded, when the cavernosal sinusoids are filled during a normal erection.

EVALUATION OF IMPOTENCE

The first goal in the evaluation of impotence is to derive a preliminary diagnosis of the underlying cause. Evaluation should include a thorough medical history, physical examination, laboratory tests, and a series of specific tests designed to aid in the diagnosis of impotency.

If erections on awakening are absent by history, this suggests an organic cause for impotence. Evaluation for nocturnal erections can be performed with a penile tumescence monitor (a pressure gauge applied around the penis), which measures rigidity and expansion by continuously recording during sleep. Absent or abnormal nocturnal erections as determined by this study usually indicate organic impotence.

Several tests have been advocated for establishing a vasculogenic cause of impotence. Doppler scanning using a 10-MHz, high-resolution ultrasound probe can be used to measure the blood flow in the cavernosal artery. This is usually performed in conjunction with an injection of papaverine (a vasodilator) into the corpus cavernosum to permit evaluation of changes in luminal diameter of the vessels and peak flow velocity. After papaverine injection, normal arteries will exhibit at 75 percent increase in luminal diameter and a peak flow velocity of more than 30 mm per second. A lesser response indicates arteriogenic impotence.

The ratio of penile blood pressure to that in the arm is termed the penile–brachial index (PBI). This can be determined by the application of a pediatric blood pressure cuff around the base of the penis and then determining systolic penile pressure using a Doppler ultrasound probe applied to lateral surface of the corpora cavernosum. The normal PBI is greater than 0.75. A value of less than 0.60 indicates arterial obstruction [18]. This study has proven to be only moderately accurate.

Perhaps the simplest test for vasculogenic impotence is the injection into one corpus cavernosum of 30 mg of papaverine mixed with 0.5 mg of phentolamine mesylate (Regitine, Ciba, Edison, N.J.). After brief massage of the penis to ensure that these vasodilating drugs fill both corpora cavernosa, an erection will occur within 30 minutes in patients with no venogenic impotence. If erection does not occur, venogenic impotence is present in 75 percent of patients [2]. Although a normal response to this injection excludes venogenic impotence, it does not completely rule out arterial causes. Unfortunately, this test has some drawbacks. It has been shown that the response in the same patient may vary significantly depending on the dose, test environment, and degree of anxiety. If the response to this test is the development of a satisfactory erection in men with organic impotence of other than vasculogenic causes, this combination of drugs can be used for intracavernous pharmacotherapy. This requires self-injection of the drugs into one corpus by the patient at the time an erection is desired. However, there is a risk of developing priapism and subsequent cavernosal fibrosis with the use of this drug combination; other possible long-term adverse effects are not known at this time.

At this point in the evaluation of the impotent man, therapy apart from intracavernous injection of vasoactive drugs might include the insertion of a penile prosthesis. However, if surgical or transluminal alteration of the arterial or venous systems of the penis is being considered in the man with vasculogenic impotence, internal pudendal arteriography is indicated for the demonstration of arterial occlusive lesions and cavernosography with cavernosometry is useful in quantifying the extent of venous leakage.

INTERNAL PUDENDAL ANGIOGRAPHY

This study should be performed only on patients who are potential candidates for surgical arterial reconstructive procedures or for percutaneous transluminal angioplasty as treatment for arterial obstructive lesions. After catheterization of one femoral artery, a preliminary road map is obtained by filming in bilateral oblique views after injections of nonionic contrast media at the aortic bifurcation. This preliminary sequence also has the advantage of showing larger-vessel disease in the region of the aortic bifurcation or iliac arteries. Papaverine (60 mg) and phentolamine (1 mg) are then injected into one corpus cavernosum to facilitate maximal arterial flow into the penis [6]. Selective internal pudendal angiography is performed using nonionic contrast medium about 5 minutes after the intracavernosal injection [3].

It has been reported that the penile arterial system can be adequately visualized by means of nonselective angiography after intracorporal papaverine injection. In one series, adequate visualization of the penile arterial network was obtained in 97 percent of patients [17].

Although arterial obstruction may be observed at various levels, the most frequent sites of narrowing are in the distal internal pudendal or common penile arteries, as well as in the small arterial branches at the base of the penis. Because there is a tendency for bilateral symmetry in vascular disease in this region, selective arteriography may be limited to the initial side if there is visualization of normal ipsilateral cavernosal and dorsal penile arteries. Diffuse small-vessel disease is usually an indication that vascularization procedures will not be therapeutic. On the other hand, discrete posttraumatic or atheromatous narrowings may be amenable to angioplasty or surgical bypass procedures. Only a limited number of patients have been treated in this manner to date, with a variable rate of success.

CAVERNOSOGRAPHY/ CAVERNOSOMETRY

Cavernosography, in addition to its use in the evaluation of venogenic impotence, is useful in evaluating the extent of Peyronie's disease, which can be a factor in impotence. Patients with this condition complain of painful, deformed erections. The fibrous plaques involving the tunica albuginea of the cavernosa in Peyronie's disease can result in indentations on one or both sides of one or both corpora cavernosa, with a resultant deformity and narrowing. A widened intercorporal septum can also be found [14]. Standard cavernosography has been described in Chap. 25.

Cavernosography with cavernosometry should be reserved for patients in whom venous reconstruction or transluminal venous occlusion is being considered. There has been some variability in this technique as reported in the literature [1, 5, 10, 12, 15]. However, there is general agreement that the study should be performed after the intracavernosal injection of 60 mg of papaverine mixed with 1 mg of phentolamine. This injection can be performed through one of the 19-gauge butterfly needles that are inserted into each corpus cavernosum in the 2 and 10 o'clock positions, angling their tips toward the root of the penis. One needle is connected to a continuous-pressure-recording device. Heparinized saline (2500 units of heparin per liter) is then infused through the other needle at a rate sufficient to raise the intracorporal pressure to approximately 100 mm Hg or whatever specific pressure level is required to achieve an erection (80 to 150 mm Hg). This infusion rate is about 80 to 120 ml per minute in normal patients and 160 to 300 ml per minute in patients with venogenic impotence. Dilute contrast medium is then infused for visualization of the corpora as well as any venous leaks (Fig. 27-2). The rate of this infusion is that necessary to maintain the erection (15 to 50 ml per minute in normal males and 60 to 160 ml per minute in men with venogenic impotence). Significant venous leakage seen with the high flow rates necessary to maintain intracavernosal pressure in the 90 to 100 mm Hg range is considered evidence of venogenic impotence [16]. Abnormal venous leakage occurs most frequently via the deep dorsal penile vein into the periprostatic plexus. The rate of leakage can exceed 150 ml per minute. Leakage of less than 20 ml per minute is probably of little clinical significance. The total amount of contrast agent used should not exceed 300 ml. After the

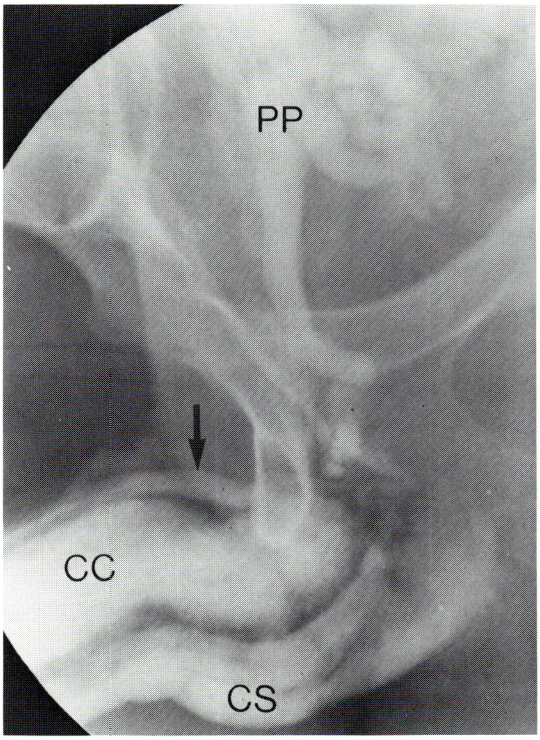

Figure 27-2. Venogenic impotence. Cavernosography shows significant venous leakage via the deep dorsal penile vein (arrow) into the periprostatic plexus. (CC = corpus cavernosum; CS = corpus spongiosum; PP = periprostatic plexus.) In this patient a flow rate approaching 100 ml per minute was required to maintain the penis in an erect state, with an intracavernosal pressure of about 100 mm Hg.

examination, residual contrast material should be washed from the corpora with heparinized saline.

Venous leakage has been treated surgically by ligation of the deep dorsal vein of the penis as well as arterialization of this vein with mixed results. The use of detachable balloons and coils for occluding the deep dorsal vein of the penis has also been reported [4].

PENILE PROSTHESES

There are many varieties of penile prostheses in current use [9]. The majority of men with organic impotence are treated by the implantation of one of these prostheses. The earliest prostheses used were autologous bone or cartilage grafts to mimic erectile tissue of the penis. These were eventually abandoned, as the grafts tended to become deformed or were resorbed. The development of successful penile prostheses since then has depended on the use of inert and durable synthetic materials. The first synthetic prostheses employed acrylic or silicone and were relatively rigid. There are still semirigid implants in use, some of them employing stainless steel or silver wires in the core to provide malleability (Fig. 27-3). Some of the newer prostheses have positionable cores composed of a series of articulating plastic segments and a central tensioning cable (Fig. 27-4).

In an attempt to imitate a physiologic erection, inflatable prostheses have been developed. These can be of the self-contained variety or may have a reservoir implanted in the lower abdomen (Fig. 27-5). The essential mechanism of operation is the same: Fluid is pumped into distensible cylinders implanted in the corpora cavernosa. A valve controlled by the patient regulates the flow in and out of the implants.

Figure 27-3. Jonas Malleable Penile Prosthesis (C.R. Bard, Covington, Ga.). Plain radiography of soft tissues below pubis clearly shows the braided wire cores in the cavernosal implants. Note the blastic metastatic involvement of the right pelvis in this patient who is impotent because of previous radical prostatectomy for prostate cancer. (From D.M. Hovsepian and E.S. Amis, Jr. Penile prosthetic implants: A radiographic atlas. *RadioGraphics* 9:707–716, 1989.)

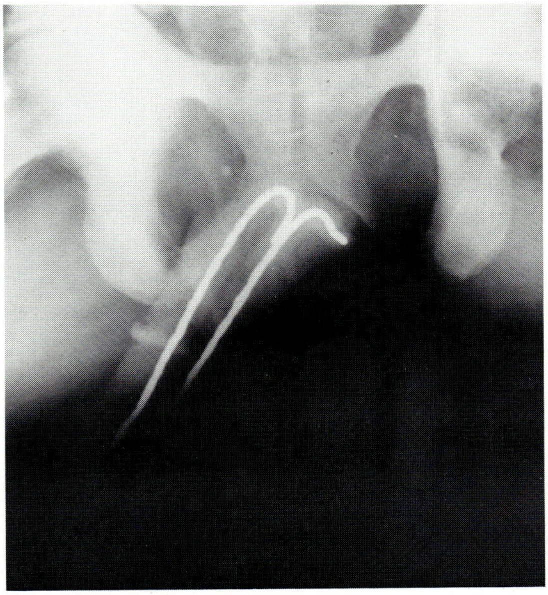

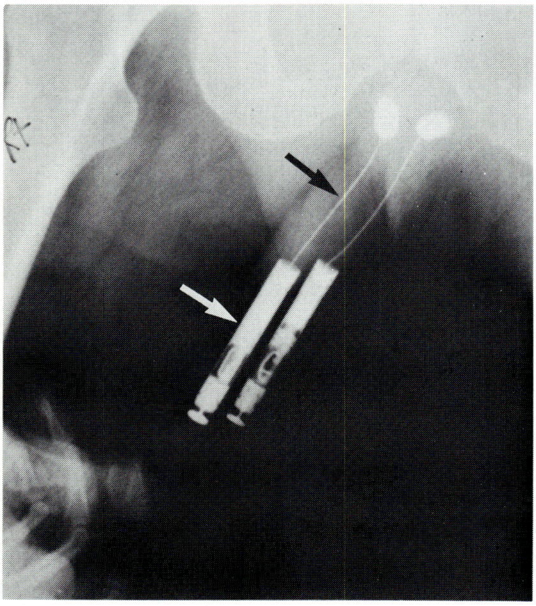

Figure 27-4. Omniphase Positionable Prosthesis (Dacomed, Minneapolis, Minn.). The distal activator switch (white arrow) shortens the tensioning cable (black arrow) to render the previously flaccid prosthesis positionable. Articulating plastic segments surrounding the cable are not visible. (From D.M. Hovsepian and E.S. Amis, Jr. Penile prosthetic implants: A radiographic atlas. *RadioGraphics* 9:707–716, 1989.)

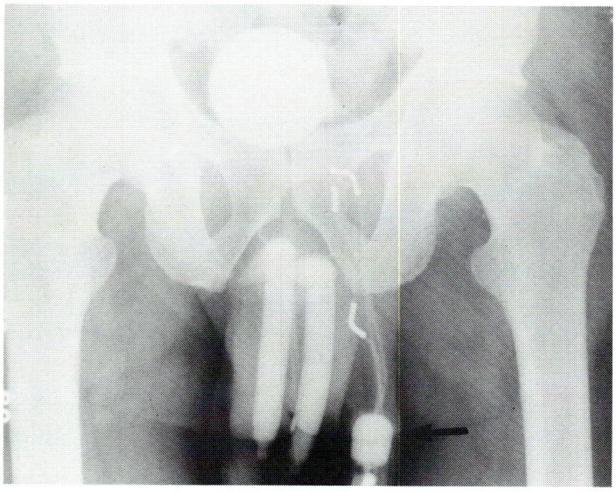

Figure 27-5. Scott Inflatable Penile Prosthesis (American Medical Systems, Minnetonka, Minn.). The system is filled with dilute contrast material, making the abdominal reservoir, corporal implants, and scrotal pump (arrow) easy to see, allowing evaluation of function. (From D.M. Hovsepian and E.S. Amis, Jr. Penile prosthetic implants: A radiographic atlas. *RadioGraphics* 9:707–716, 1989.)

Because these are more complex than the semirigid prosthesis, they are more expensive, often more difficult to implant, and generally more prone to failure.

Radiographic evaluation of prosthetic implants should begin with an anteroposterior and both oblique projections to include the entirety of the device [9]. In evaluating the inflatable prostheses, only those that contain contrast medium as the inflating fluid can be assessed for leakage. If the reservoir is remote, the connecting tubing should be evaluated for kinks or discontinuity. With the semirigid implants, the prosthesis should be scrutinized for fracture of the silicone shaft, the central wire core, or the central tensioning cable. Asymmetric position of the corporal implants may indicate migration and possible erosion through the tunica albuginea. Any prosthetic device may become infected, necessitating removal.

REFERENCES

1. Bookstein, J.J. Cavernosal venocclusive insufficiency in male impotence: Evaluation of degree and location. *Radiology* 164:175, 1987.
2. Bookstein, J.J. Penile angiography: The last angiographic frontier. *A.J.R.* 150:47, 1988.
3. Bookstein, J.J. Penile vascular catheterization in the diagnosis and treatment of impotence. In H.M. Pollack and G.W. Hartman (Eds.), *Uroradiology* (American Roentgen Ray Society Categorical Course Syllabus). Reston, Va.: American Roentgen Ray Society, 1989. Pp. 161–166.
4. Courtheoux, P., et al. Erectile dysfunction caused by venous leakage: Treatment with detachable balloons and coils. *Radiology* 161:807, 1986.
5. Delcour, C., et al. Impotence: Evaluation with cavernosography. *Radiology* 161:803, 1986.
6. Delcour, C., et al. Technical advances in penile arteriography. *A.J.R.* 150:803, 1988.
7. Goldstein, I., and Greenfield, A. Pathophysiology and Physiology of impotence. In H.M. Pollack and G.W. Hartman (Eds.), *Uroradiology* (American Roentgen Ray Society Categorical Course Syllabus). Reston, Va.: American Roentgen Ray Society, 1989. Pp. 155–159.
8. Gray, R.R., et al. Investigation of impotence by internal pudendal angiography: Experience with 73 cases. *Radiology* 144:773, 1982.
9. Hovsepian, D.M., and Amis, E.S., Jr. Penile prosthetic implants: A radiographic atlas. *RadioGraphics* 9:707, 1989.

10. Malhotra, C.W., et al. Cavernosography in conjunction with artificial erection for evaluation of venous leakage in impotent men. *Radiology* 161:799, 1986.
11. Masters, W.H., and Johnson, V.E. *Human Sexual Inadequacy* (1st ed.). Boston: Little, Brown, 1970. P. 185.
12. Melman, A. The evaluation of erectile dysfunction. *Urol. Radiol.* 10:119, 1988.
13. Miller, K., et al. The radiology of male impotence. *RadioGraphics* 2:131, 1982.
14. Ney, C., Miller, H.L., and Friedenberg, R.M. Various applications of corpus cavernosography. *Radiology* 119:69, 1976.
15. Puyau, F.A., et al. Dynamic corpus cavernosography: Effect of papaverine injection. *Radiology* 164:179, 1987.
16. Rosen, M.P., Walker, T.G., and Greenfield, A.J. Arteriography and radiology of impotence. *Urol. Radiol.* 10:136, 1988.
17. Schwartz, A.N., Freidenberg, D., and Harley, J.D. Nonselective angiography after intracorporal papaverine injection: An alternative technique for evaluating penile arterial integrity. *Radiology* 167:249, 1988.
18. Sidi, A.A., Koleilat, N., and Fraley, E.E. Evaluation and treatment of organic impotence. *Invest. Radiol.* 23:778, 1988.

Male Infertility

Infertility is defined as the failure of a couple to conceive after at least 12 months of unprotected sexual intercourse. Primary infertility is estimated to affect 15 percent of the married couples in the United States. Additionally, up to 10 percent of married couples may already have one or more children and be unable to conceive another [14]. In infertile couples, male infertility is the predominant factor in 30 percent, female infertility in another 30 percent, and in the remainder both partners may have problems or there may be no demonstrable cause [18]. Therefore, a male factor is present in, or contributes to, as many as 50 percent or more of infertility problems.

Once a couple has been classified as infertile, proper assessment of the male partner involves a comprehensive history and physical examination, followed by a semen analysis as the first laboratory test. The requirement for classifying a man as fertile is demonstration of sperm in the semen capable of fertilizing a human oocyte. There are multiple causes of failed production of normal sperm, which can usually be assigned to three general categories: testicular failure, hypothalamic–pituitary dysfunction, and posttesticular dysfunction [6]. Testicular failure, as typified by conditions such as Klinefelter's syndrome, bilateral cryptorchidism, or gonadal dysgenesis, accounts for 14 percent of male infertility. Endocrine dysfunction causes a further 9 percent of infertility, and posttesticular dysfunction is the cause of male infertility in the remaining 77 percent. The typical causes of posttesticular dysfunction are varicocele and obstruction or absence of the tubular structures that carry semen (epididymides, vasa deferentia, and ejaculatory ducts). A discussion of primary testicular failure or endocrine dysfunction is beyond the scope of this textbook. It is infertility secondary to obstructive phenomena or varicocele that necessitate involvement of the radiologist in both diagnosis and treatment. The remainder of this chapter will be devoted to these topics.

SEMEN ANALYSIS

The initial evaluation of the male partner should include a semen analysis. At least three specimens are recommended. These are obtained by masturbation after retraining from sexual activities for a period of 2 to 5 days. A normal semen specimen has a volume of 1 to 5 ml, the sperm count should be 20 million to 200 million per milliliter, and more than 50 percent of the sperm should have normal motility and morphology. A semen specimen is considered abnormal if any one or a combination of these parameters is found to be consistently abnormal. Probably the most important parameters in infertility are decreased motility of the sperm and an increased percentage of abnormal morphologic forms. The term *azoospermia* denotes the total absence of sperm in the semen sample.

Azoospermia is found in up to 20 percent of men undergoing evaluation for infertility. The main causes of this finding are testicular failure (about two-thirds of cases) and bilateral ductal obstruction (about one-third of cases) [10]. Of the patients with ductal obstruction, up to one-third may have bilateral vasal agenesis as the cause. Because the vasa are easily palpable at the neck of the scrotum, this condition can be diagnosed on physical examination. Azoospermic patients should also be tested for the presence of fructose in the semen; because it is secreted by the seminal vesicles, the absence of fructose suggests obstruction of the ejaculatory ducts or congenital absence of the seminal vesicles. Vasal agenesis can often be inferred when the seminal vesicles are congenitally absent. On the other hand, CT and ultrasonographic studies of the seminal vesicles in men with bilaterally absent vasa indicate that the seminal vesicles are normal in from 19 percent to 46 percent of cases; in the remaining cases the seminal vesicles may be unilaterally or bilaterally absent or hypoplastic [4, 10].

OBSTRUCTIVE AZOOSPERMIA

As previously noted, congenital absence of the vasa deferentia is one cause of obstructive azoospermia. When the vasa are present in the setting of normal hormonal function and normal testes, a search must be initiated for an obstruction in the ductal system between the testes and the posterior urethra. The proximal portion of this paired ductal system—the epididymis—is a 20-ft-long tubule that is pleated like an accordion into a 2-in. length; it is located posterolaterally to the testis. Spermatozoa are transmitted into the head of the epididymis via the efferent ductules of the testis. Inferiorly, near the lower pole of the testis, the epididymis connects with the vas deferens, which travels in the spermatic cord through the inguinal ring, after which it forms a sweeping loop in the pelvis before joining the duct of the ipsilateral seminal vesicle to form one of the paired ejaculatory ducts (Fig. 28-1). Each ejaculatory duct empties into the posterior urethra via a small ostium on the distal portion of the verumontanum. Obstruction at any point in this system can be congenital or may be a result of previous infection or trauma. Epididymitis is a frequent cause of obstruction at the epididymal level. If there is no history of epididymitis or scrotal trauma, bilateral obstruction at the epididymal level may due to Young's syndrome. Young's syndrome, in which bilateral epididymal obstruction is found in association with chronic sinus and pulmonary infections, has been reported to be the cause of obstructive azoospermia in some cases [9].

Previous vasectomy is by far the most common cause of obstruction of the vasa, although this diagnosis is obvious. Childhood surgery for repair of bilateral inguinal hernia is an unfortunate cause of vasal obstruction at the level of the groin. In azoospermic patients whose semen is fructose negative and whose vasa and seminal vesicles are present, the point of obstruction will

Figure 28-1. Diagram of male genital system.

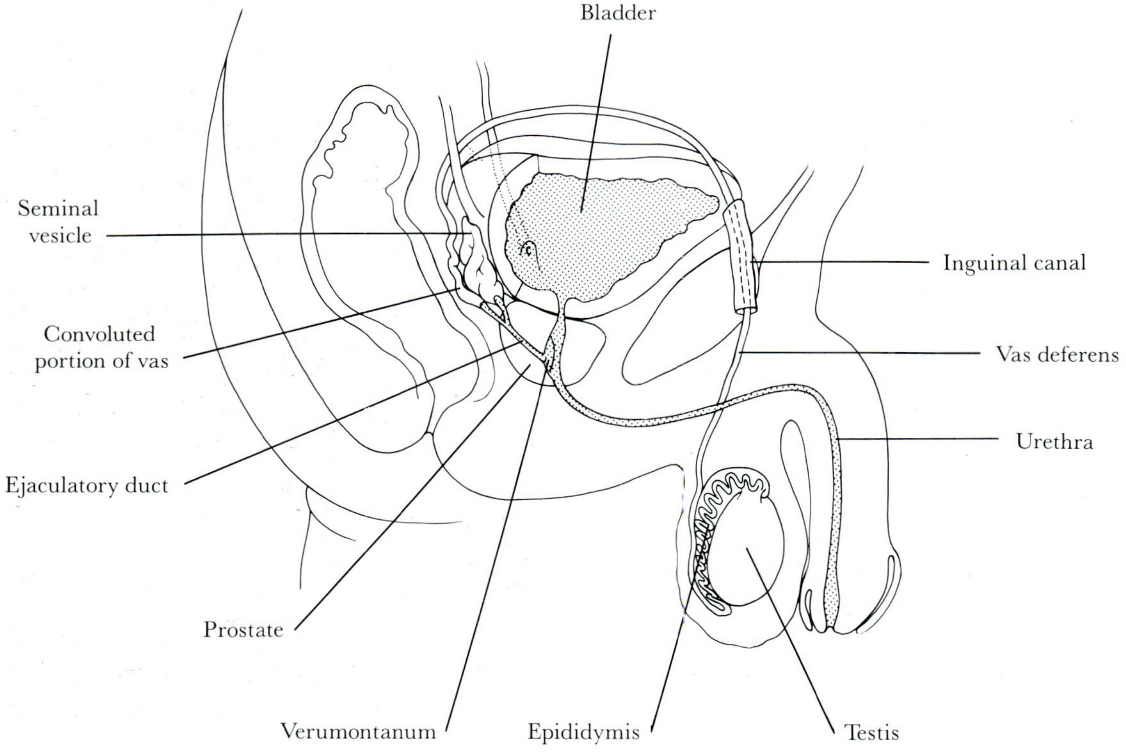

be in the ejaculatory duct, since fructose is elaborated only by the seminal vesicle. When the point of obstruction or its cause is unknown, the obstruction, whether developmental or acquired, is found most frequently at the junction of the epididymis with the vas [17].

Vasography is a technique for radiographically demonstrating the ductal system from epididymis to posterior urethra. This study is routinely performed by some urologists to determine a point of obstruction; however, other clinicians recommend microsurgical exploration of the epididymovasal junction in an effort to demonstrate and correct the blockage. This latter group feels that vasography may damage the vas deferens or the epididymal tubule and result in scarring and further obstruction.

Vasography is a surgical procedure conducted by the urologist. The vas deferens is surgically isolated at the neck of the scrotum and its lumen cannulated; it is then injected with contrast medium, and a radiograph is obtained. Vasography can demonstrate patency of the entire ductal system from epididymis to posterior urethra by injecting contrast material both cephalad and caudad into the lumen of the vas (Fig. 28-2), although sometimes only the portion above the injection site, including the seminal vesicle, is opacified (Fig. 28-3). Because these studies are usually referred to the radiologist for formal interpretation, familiarity with the appearance of this ductal system is essential. The lumen of the vas is small (0.5 to 1.0 mm) and smooth-walled; as the vas passes under the trigone of the bladder (ampulla of the vas), its

Figure 28-2. Bilateral complete vasograms. Contrast medium has been injected into the lumen of both vasa both cephalad and caudad from a point near the neck of the scrotum. The entire ductal system is patent bilaterally.

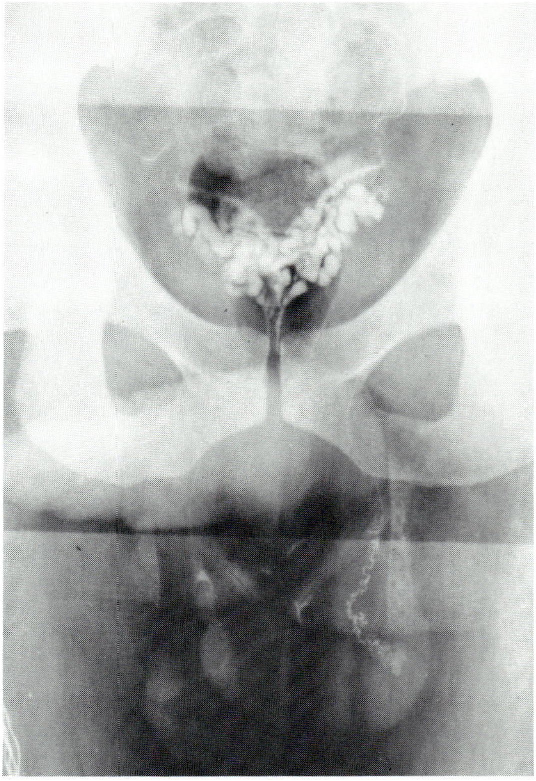

Figure 28-3. Partial left vasogram. The inguinal and pelvic portions of the left vas can be seen, as can the convoluted portion (ampulla) and the seminal vesicle. Contrast material is seen in the bladder, indicating normal communication with the urethra.

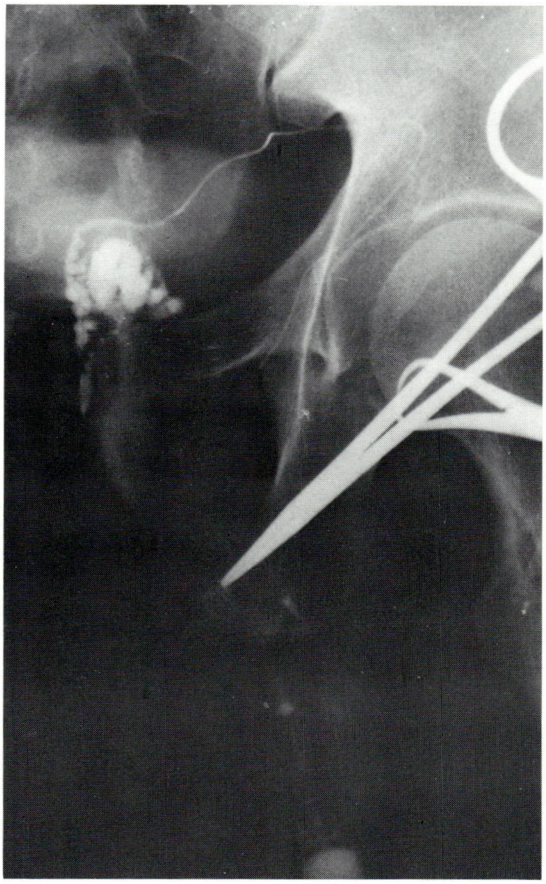

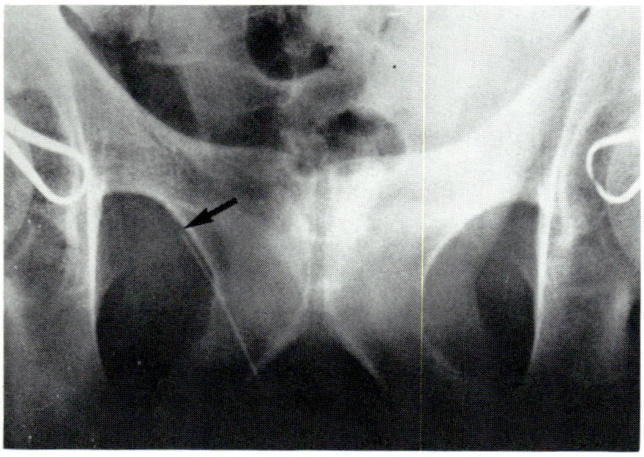

Figure 28-4. Obstruction of vasa secondary to bilateral hernia repair as a child. Right vasography shows obstruction of the right vas in inguinal area (arrow). The left vas was also obstructed in this azoospermic man.

lumen becomes larger and is irregular and tortuous. The ampulla then joins the duct of the seminal vesicle to form the 1.5- to 2.0-cm-long, smooth ejaculatory duct, which enters the posterior urethra. When contrast medium fails to pass beyond a given point, obstruction can be diagnosed (Fig. 28-4). With obstruction of an ejaculatory duct, the ipsilateral seminal vesicle and adjacent vas are usually dilated.

The development of microsurgical techniques in correcting obstructive azoospermia has resulted in significantly increased restoration of fertility in these patients.

VARICOCELE

A varicocele is an abnormal dilation of the pampiniform plexus of veins in the spermatic cord that results from absence or incompetence of the valves of the internal spermatic vein. This condition is the most common correctable cause of male infertility. Varicoceles occur in 10 to 20 percent of the general male population and, in some reports, in over half the men being evaluated for infertility.

Varicocele has classically been described as occurring predominantly on the left side. The prevalence of left-sided varicocele is probably due to the fact that the left internal spermatic vein drains into the left renal vein at a right angle. It has also been postulated that another cause of left varicocele is the compression of the left renal vein between the aorta and the superior mesenteric artery before it enters the inferior vena cava. On the other hand, the right internal spermatic vein drains directly into the inferior vena cava immediately adjacent to the origin of the right renal vein. However, studies have indicated that the incidence of bilateral varicoceles in infertile men may be as high as 50 to 60 percent [1, 11].

The mechanism by which varicoceles cause infertility is not known. Although several hypotheses have been suggested, none has been conclusively proven. These include increased scrotal temperature, circulation of toxic renal or adrenal metabolites to the testes, stasis of blood within the testes with subsequent hypoxemia and tissue degeneration, alteration in the size of intratesticular blood vessels resulting in modification in the transfer of nutrients, and deficient testicular hormone production. Of these, there is some evidence that elevated testicular temperature and altered testicular hormone production have a role in the abnormal spermatogenesis found in some men with varicoceles [8].

Varicoceles typically result in alterations in semen quality rather than azoospermia. A "stress pattern" of semen, consisting of altered morphology (tapered sperm heads) is typically found in association with varicoceles. However, this pattern is now considered nonspecific and is no longer considered diagnostic of varicoceles. A review of multiple series of infertile men treated by varicocelectomy indicates that semen improvement can be expected in 51 to 85 percent of patients [1]. Generally speaking, about 70 percent of infertile men who undergo this procedure will show an increase in sperm count and an improvement in sperm motility, with or without an improvement in the morphology of the sperm. Furthermore, up to 55 percent of infertile men treated by varicocelectomy have subsequently been reported to father children.

A large varicocele can be visualized on physical examination as an irregular scrotal mass in the upright patient; on palpation it is often described as a "bag of worms." The patient may need to perform the Valsalva maneuver while standing before a smaller varicocele can be palpated. The large majority of varicoceles will empty, and therefore become less easily palpable, when patients assume the supine position.

It has been reported that the improvement in semen quality after varicocelectomy is not related to the size of the varicocele on palpation. Therefore some studies have centered on detection of nonpalpable, subclinical varicoceles as a possible cause of infertility. In this regard, multiple techniques have been described for evaluating the upper scrotum. At the time of this writing, Doppler sonography has yielded only equivocal results. Thermography of the scrotum has been advocated as a screening method for diagnosing varicoceles because it can detect temperature differentials of 0.5 to 3°C between the involved hemiscrotum and the healthy contralateral side [7]. However, in patients with bilateral varicoceles this test will be unreliable and should be considered equivocal at best in its accuracy. Radionuclide blood-pool scanning has also been advocated for the detection of varicoceles [3]. However, this too has been found to be an equivocal method in patients with subclinical or bilateral varicoceles since no blood pooling is found in the former and no differential is found in the latter.

There are two techniques available to the radiologist that have been reported to be accurate in the detection of subclinical varicoceles: spermatic venography and scrotal ultrasonography. Although venography is probably the more specific method, it is invasive and associated with some morbidity, and it may require the expertise of an angiographer for adequate performance. High-resolution scrotal sonography has been reported as a noninvasive, relatively inexpensive technique that appears to be very sensitive in the diagnosis of subclinical varicoceles [5, 11].

In patients with subsequently proved varicocele, three or more veins can usually be detected sonographically in the spermatic cord adjacent to the testis. These abnormal veins measure more than 3 mm in diameter. The diagnosis is confirmed if these veins exhibit some increase in caliber during the Valsalva maneuver. The sonographic findings in clinically apparent varicocele have been described previously; they include a significant increase in size and tortuosity of the veins of the pampiniform plexus, seen as confluent, branching, echo-free tubular structures (Fig. 28-5). On occasion, varicoceles may appear as multicystic lesions that, because of their location just proximal to the upper pole of the testis, may be mistaken for other multicystic extratesticular masses, especially spermatocele [20].

The aim of internal spermatic venography is to confirm the extent of a palpable varicocele or to establish the presence of a subclinical one and to demonstrate the course of the spermatic vein before therapy is undertaken. Because of the previously mentioned work indicating a high percentage of bilaterality of varicoceles, both internal spermatic veins should be studied in infertile patients in whom subclinical varicoceles are suspected. Either the transfemoral or transjugular approach can be used for catheterizing the internal spermatic veins. Venograms are then obtained by injecting by hand 5 to 15 ml of low-osmolality contrast medium to define spermatic vein anatomy (Fig. 28-6). Filming is performed as necessary during fluoroscopic monitoring. After injection of contrast medium, its retrograde flow down the spermatic vein is seen only in patients with varicoceles.

Anomalies in the course of the internal spermatic veins are the rule rather than the exception in patients with varicoceles. The more common anomalies are double spermatic veins, variations in their terminations in the inferior

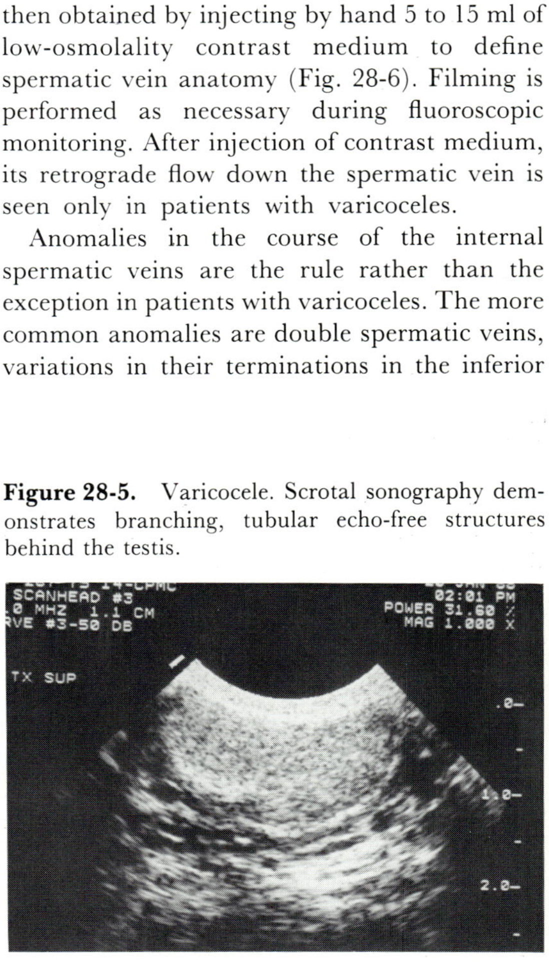

Figure 28-5. Varicocele. Scrotal sonography demonstrates branching, tubular echo-free structures behind the testis.

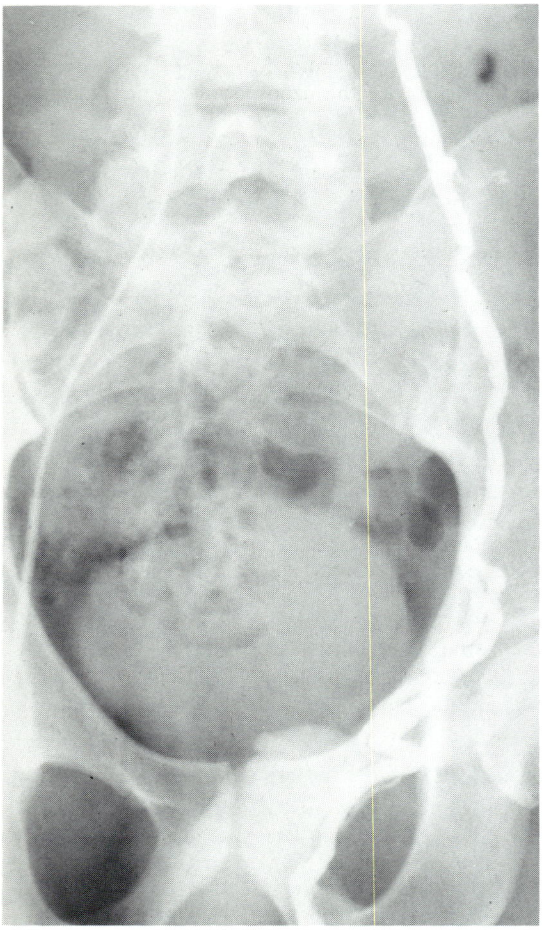

Figure 28-6. Varicocele. Left spermatic venography shows retrograde flow of contrast material in dilated left internal spermatic vein, which branches and becomes more tortuous in inguinal area.

vena cava or left renal vein, and cross connections to paravertebral, pelvic, and cremasteric veins [15]. Uncommonly, reflux down the internal spermatic vein may stop within the pampiniform plexus. More frequently, retrograde flow of contrast material in the caudad portion of the internal spermatic vein in patients with large varicoceles is seen passing into the cremasteric vein, the vein of the vas deferens, or both and finally emptying into one common iliac vein and the inferior vena cava [16].

After demonstration of a varicocele in the infertile patient, treatment is usually surgical ligation of the internal spermatic vein through an inguinal incision. The high rate of success with this treatment has been noted above. Complications of varicocelectomy have included hydrocele and recurrence. If the arterial supply to the testis is compromised during the procedure, testicular atrophy may occur. Microsurgical techniques have been advocated to allow identification and preservation of the testicular artery (thus avoiding testicular atrophy) and cord lymphatics (preventing hydrocele formation).

Interventional radiographic techniques have been reported for occluding the internal spermatic vein as a treatment for infertility [2, 12, 13, 19]. Agents used to date for occluding the internal spermatic vein include sclerosing solutions, stainless steel coils (Fig. 28-7), compressed

Figure 28-7. Occlusion of left internal spermatic vein by transluminal placement of stainless steel coils. Note that there is now no flow distal to the most caudad coil.

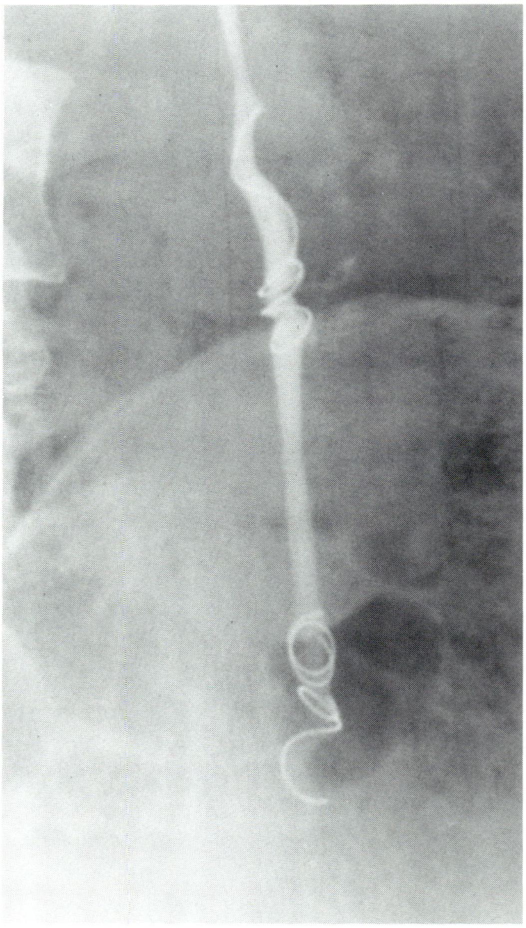

Ivalon plugs, and detachable balloons. The reported success rates with these interventional techniques rival those of surgical ligation of the internal spermatic vein. These procedures can be performed on outpatients with less expense and discomfort than with surgery, and there is no need for general anesthesia. Complications appear to be few.

REFERENCES

1. Dubin, L., and Amelar, R.D. Varicocelectomy: Twenty-five years experience. *Int. J. Fertil.* 33: 226, 1988.
2. Formanek, A., et al. Embolization of the spermatic vein for treatment of infertility: A new approach. *Radiology* 139:315, 1981.
3. Freund, J., et al. Detection of varicocele by radionuclide bloodpool scanning. *Radiology* 137: 227, 1980.
4. Goldstein, M., and Schlossberg, S. Men with congenital absence of the vas deferens often have seminal vesicles. *J. Urol.* 140:85, 1988.
5. Gonda, R.L., Jr., et al. Diagnosis of subclinical varicocele in infertility. *A.J.R.* 148:71, 1987.
6. Grunfeld, L. Work-up of male infertility. *J. Reprod. Med.* 34:143, 1989.
7. Hamm, B., et al. Varicoceles: Combined sonography and thermography in diagnosis and posttherapeutic evaluation. *Radiology* 160:419, 1986.
8. Hudson, R.W. The endocrinology of varicoceles. *Fertil. Steril.* 49:199, 1988.
9. Hughes, T.M., III, Skolnick, J.L., and Belker, A.M. Young's syndrome: An often unrecognized correctable cause of obstructive azoospermia. *J. Urol.* 137:1238, 1987.
10. Jarow, J.P., Espeland, M.A., and Lipshultz, L.I. Evaluation of the azoospermic patient. *J. Urol.* 142:62, 1989.
11. McClure, R.D., and Hricak, H. Scrotal ultrasound in the infertile man: detection of subclinical unilateral and bilateral varicoceles. *J. Urol.* 135:711, 1986.
12. Pochaczevsky, R., Lee, W.J., and Mallett, E. Management of male infertility: Roles of contact thermography, spermatic venography, and embolization. *A.J.R.* 147:97, 1986.
13. Riedl, P., Lungmayr, G., and Stackl, W. A new method of transfemoral testicular vein obliteration for varicocele using a balloon catheter. *Radiology* 139:323, 1981.
14. Ross, L.S. Diagnosis and treatment of infertile men: A clinical perspective. *J. Urol.* 130:847, 1983.
15. Seyferth, W., Jecht, E., and Zeitler, E. Percutaneous sclerotheraphy of varicocele. *Radiology* 139:335, 1981.
16. Sigmund, G., Gall, H., and Bahren, W. Stop-type and shunt-type varicoceles: Venographic findings. *Radiology* 163:105, 1987.
17. Silber, S.J. Microsurgery for male infertility. *Microsurgery* 9:251, 1988.
18. Swerdloff, R.S., Wang. C., and Kandeel, F.R. Evaluation of the infertile couple. *Endocrinol. Metab. Clin. North Am.* 17:301, 1988.
19. White, R.I., et al. Occlusion of varicoceles with detachable balloons. *Radiology* 139:327, 1981.
20. Wolverson, M.K., et al. High-resolution realtime sonography of scrotal varicocele. *A.J.R.* 141: 775, 1983.

Index

The abbreviations f and t stand for figure and table, respectively.